# Methods in Molecular Biology™



*Series Editor*
**John M. Walker**
**School of Life Sciences**
**University of Hertfordshire**
**Hatfield, Hertfordshire, AL10 9AB, UK**

For further volumes:
http://www.springer.com/series/7651

# Immunogenetics

## Methods and Applications in Clinical Practice

Edited by

**Frank T. Christiansen**

*Department of Clinical Immunology, PathWest Laboratory Medicine, Royal Perth Hospital; School of Pathology and Laboratory Medicine, University of Western Australia, Perth, WA, Australia*

**Brian D. Tait**

*National Transplant Services, Australian Red Cross Blood Service, The Royal Melbourne Hospital, Melbourne, VIC, Australia*

Humana Press

*Editors*
Frank T. Christiansen
Department of Clinical Immunology
PathWest Laboratory Medicine
Royal Perth Hospital
Perth, WA, Australia

School of Pathology and Laboratory
Medicine, University of Western Australia
Perth, WA, Australia

Brian D. Tait
National Transplant Services
Australian Red Cross Blood Service
The Royal Melbourne Hospital
Melbourne, VIC, Australia

ISSN 1064-3745 ISSN 1940-6029 (electronic)
ISBN 978-1-4939-5917-4 ISBN 978-1-61779-842-9 (eBook)
DOI 10.1007/978-1-61779-842-9
Springer New York Heidelberg Dordrecht London



Printed on acid-free paper

Humana Press is a brand of Springer
Springer is part of Springer Science+Business Media (www.springer.com)

# Preface

The ability of mice to distinguish "self" from "nonself" and recognize foreign organisms or tissues (an immune response) was found to be under genetic control by the seminal experiments of Peter Gorer in 1936 and his description of the H-2 system. This was later extended to the human with the discovery of the HLA system by Jean Dausset in 1958. Since that time the study and knowledge of the genes controlling such immune responses in the human has undergone a rapid expansion. These studies have been facilitated by the development of a range of molecular DNA techniques and a remarkable degree of international collaboration.

The HLA molecules, encoded by a highly polymorphic set of genes located with the major histocompatibility complex (MHC) on Chromosome 6, are important regulators of the immune response through mediating antigen presentation and interaction between key immune mediating cells. They are also the major histocompatibility barriers to transplantation, which is the clinical paradigm of the self vs. nonself concept. Within the MHC, one of the best characterized regions of the human genome, are a number of other gene clusters involved in controlling aspects of the immune response. These encode various accessory molecules such as TNF, components of the classical complement pathway, and heat shock proteins. In addition outside the MHC, many other genes encode components which can act as histocompatibility antigens or are involved in the function of the immune system. These include genes encoding polymorphic tissue-specific peptides presented within the context of HLA molecules which have been shown to give rise to a series of minor histocompatibility antigens which are barriers to allogeneic transplantation but which can also be exploited as targets for immunotherapy. Those polymorphic genes encoding the immunoglobulin and the T cell receptor molecules, important mediators of humoral and cell-mediated adaptive immune responses, also play a role in regulation of immune responses. The immune response is also mediated by a complex of cytokines and cell receptors and polymorphism in the structural and regulatory elements of the genes have been demonstrated and shown to have functional correlates. More recently a cluster of genes encoding receptors on NK cells, including the killer immunoglobulin-like receptors (KIR), which regulate NK cell activation largely through interaction with ligands encoded within the MHC, have been described and been shown to be important determinants in transplantation outcome and in conferring disease susceptibility.

It is now recognized that this diverse range of gene systems involved in the control of the immune response has been shown to be important in many aspects of clinical practice. As a result many new molecular and cellular methods have been developed for identifying these genes and their polymorphisms, and immunogenetic laboratories specializing in these methods have developed to support transplantation and other clinical programs. This volume focuses on such methods. The scope is exclusively for human clinical practice and the emphasis is on those assays which are of established or potential clinical utility and are likely to be included in the repertoire of tests provided by a routine diagnostic and service laboratory. In the tradition of *Methods in Molecular Biology* series, the methods provide details of the materials and equipment required and a step-by-step description of the laboratory method. Details of the critical factors in the performance and interpretation of these assays and other practical tips are provided through as series of Notes which we trust the reader will find particularly helpful.

The characterization of the HLA and other genes within the MHC is important to the routine diagnostic immunogenetics laboratory, particularly in supporting solid organ and hemopoietic stem cell transplant programs. We have included chapters describing HLA typing by molecular techniques including sequence-specific oligonucleotide hybridization (SSO) and sequence-specific priming (SSP) methods, solid phase bead-based assays and by direct DNA sequencing, and the use of specialist software for HLA allele assignment. An additional chapter focuses on a number of molecular methods adapted for the typing of specific HLA alleles which are of diagnostic utility in disease diagnosis and in drug hypersensitivity reactions. In addition to typing of the classical HLA molecules, we have included chapters describing typing of other MHC genes including the nonclassical HLA molecules HLA-E and HLA-G, the complement component C4, the MICA genes, and a panel of single nucleotide polymorphisms (SNPs) throughout the MHC. Methods for detecting the many non-MHC minor histocompatibility antigens which have been described and for detecting the functionally important polymorphisms in a range of cytokine genes are also included.

The detection and characterization of HLA antibodies directed at epitopes found on donor HLA molecules and the more recently described antibodies directed at MICA epitopes is known to be important in organ transplantation, and the recent development of solid phase bead-based assays to detect these antibodies has led to a new understanding of the role of HLA and MICA antibodies in organ transplant rejection. Chapters describing the methods for the detection of donor-specific antibodies using the traditional, but still gold standard, complement dependent cytotoxicity and the more sensitive flow cytometry-based crossmatches and bead-based antibody detection assays are included. Assays for the detection of T cell-mediated reactivity against alloantigens either directly or indirectly through the cross-reactivity of viral-specific T cells—so-called heterologous immunity—are also described.

The highly polymorphic KIR gene cluster, which encodes a family of NK cell receptors which are important in controlling NK cell function, has generated considerable interest recently. Methods detecting and characterizing the polymorphism of this complex gene system including PCR-SSP and direct sequencing and for detecting NK cell alloreactivity including a flow cytometry-based assay are described. Alloreactive NK cells have the potential to be effective therapeutic agents, and a detailed method for the clinical production of such cells is provided.

In addition to the method chapters we have included a series of overview chapters highlighting aspects of gene function or various methods available for their study. These include reviews of the MHC complex, the KIR complex, the human immunoglobulin allotypes, as well as reviews of the methods for the detection of alloreactive NK cells and the detection of HLA antibodies by solid phase assays. Because of their expertise and understanding of the complexity of the HLA system, many immunogenetics laboratories provide specialist advice to clinicians in their search for suitable unrelated hemopoietic stem cell donors. We have therefore included a chapter which provides a detailed and practical guide to cost-effective strategies for undertaking such searches.

Immunogenetic data is complex and the genes are highly polymorphic and have been extensively studied. These features have meant that extensive databases of such genes and the polymorphisms are now available. Included are chapters on methods for the establishment and management of immunogenetic databases and which describe the use of specialist HLA, immunoglobulin, and T cell receptor polymorphism databases. In addition two chapters are included which review the analytical methods available for the study and measurement of human population diversity and the identification, quantitation, and mapping of disease susceptibility genes respectively. These chapters also provide a number of worked examples and we trust the readers will find them particularly helpful.

We would like to thank all the contributors to what we believe is an outstanding collection of manuscripts which we are sure will be widely read and used by the immunogenetics community. These contributions represent many hours of work and the sharing of detailed methods and helpful tips gained by many years of experience in the field. We are delighted that they have been prepared to share this information with the wider scientific community.

We would also like to thank John Walker and Humana Press for inviting us to edit this volume of the very successful *Methods in Molecular Biology* series and for his excellent editorial guidance. We trust the final product has rewarded his trust in us.

Finally, we would like to express our special thanks to Natalie Caldwell for her outstanding clerical and editorial assistance. Her enthusiasm and skill has been invaluable as we have worked through the numerous editorial tasks.

***Perth, WA, Australia*** ***Frank T. Christiansen***
***Melbourne, VIC, Australia*** ***Brian D. Tait***

# Contents

## Contributors

ELTAF ALAMYAR • *IMGT®, the International ImMunoGeneTics Information System®, Université Montpellier 2, Laboratoire d'ImmunoGénétique Moléculaire (LIGM), Institut de Génétique Humaine (IGH), UPR CNRS 1142, Montpellier, France*

RICHARD J.N. ALLCOCK • *Lotterywest State Biomedical Facility Genomics, School of Pathology and Laboratory Medicine, University of Western Australia, Nedlands; Department of Clinical Immunology, PathWest Laboratory Medicine, Royal Perth Hospital, Perth, WA, Australia*

THOMAS BARNETCHE • *Rheumatology Service, Bordeaux University Hospital, Bordeaux, France*

MANDVI BHARADWAJ • *Department of Microbiology and Immunology, University of Melbourne, Parkville, VIC, Australia*

ERICK C. CASTELLI • *Molecular Genetics and Cytogenetics Laboratory, and Department of General Biology, Institute of Biological Sciences, Federal University of Goiás, Goiás, Brazil*

ALISON S.L. CASTLEY • *Department of Clinical Immunology, PathWest Laboratory Medicine, Royal Perth Hospital, Perth, WA, Australia*

MINGHUA CHEN • *Department of Pediatrics, CW Bill Young Marrow Donor Recruitment and Research Program, Georgetown University Medical Centre, Washington, DC, USA*

FRANK T. CHRISTIANSEN • *Department of Clinical Immunology, PathWest Laboratory Medicine, Royal Perth and Fremantle Hospitals, Perth, WA, Australia; School of Pathology and Laboratory Medicine (PaLM), University of Western Australia, Perth, WA, Australia*

ELISA CISNEROS • *Inmunogenética—HLA, Hospital Universitario Puerta de Hierro, Majadahonda, Spain*

FRANS H.J. CLAAS • *Department of Immunohematology and Blood Transfusion, Leiden University Medical Centre, Leiden, The Netherlands*

SARAH COOLEY • *Department of Medicine, University of Minnesota Cancer Centre, Minneapolis, MN, USA*

DIANNE DE SANTIS • *Department of Clinical Immunology, PathWest Laboratory Medicine, Royal Perth Hospital, Perth, WA, Australia*

LLOYD J. D'ORSOGNA • *Department of Immunohematology and Blood Transfusion, Leiden University Medical Centre, Leiden, The Netherlands; PathWest Laboratory Medicine, Perth, WA, Australia*

JONATHAN DOWNING • *Tissue Typing Laboratory, New Zealand Blood Service, Auckland, New Zealand*

ILIAS I.N. DOXIADIS • *Department of Immunohematology and Blood Transfusion, Leiden University Medical Centre, Leiden, The Netherlands*

HEATHER DUNCKLEY • *Australian Red Cross Blood Service, Sydney, NSW, Australia*

PATRICE DUROUX • *IMGT®, The International ImMunoGeneTics Information System®, Université Montpellier 2, Laboratoire d'ImmunoGénétique Moléculaire (LIGM), Institut de Génétique Humaine (IGH), UPR CNRS 1142, Montpellier, France*

FRANÇOIS EHRENMANN • *IMGT®, The International ImMunoGeneTics Information System®, Université Montpellier 2, Laboratoire d'ImmunoGénétique Moléculaire (LIGM), Institut de Génétique Humaine (IGH), UPR CNRS 1142, Montpellier, France*
SAMANTHA J. FIDLER • *Department of Clinical Immunology, PathWest Laboratory Medicine, Royal Perth Hospital, Perth, WA, Australia; School of Pathology and Laboratory Medicine (PaLM), University of Western Australia, Nedlands, WA, Australia*
BREE FOLEY • *Division of Hematology, Oncology and Transplantation, University of Minnesota Cancer Centre, Minneapolis, MN, USA*
VÉRONIQUE GIUDICELLI • *IMGT®, The International ImMunoGeneTics Information System®, Université Montpellier 2, Laboratoire d'ImmunoGénétique Moléculaire (LIGM), Institut de Génétique Humaine (IGH), UPR CNRS 1142, Montpellier, France*
NATALIA GÓMEZ-LOZANO • *Inmunogenética—HLA, Hospital Universitario Puerta de Hierro, Majadahonda, Spain*
ELS GOULMY • *Department of Immunohematology and Blood Transfusion, Leiden University Medical Center, Leiden, The Netherlands*
PIERRE-ANTOINE GOURRAUD • *Department of Neurology, University of California, San Francisco, CA, USA*
KATRI HAIMILA • *Clinical Laboratory, Finnish Red Cross Blood Service, Helsinki, Finland*
JILL A. HOLLENBACH • *Center for Genetics, Children's Hospital and Research Center Oakland, Oakland, CA, USA*
PETER A. HORN • *Institute for Transfusion Medicine, University Hospital Essen, Essen, Germany*
LIHUA HOU • *Department of Pediatrics, CW Bill Young Marrow Donor Recruitment and Research Program, Georgetown University Medical Centre, Washington, DC, USA*
CAROLYN K. HURLEY • *Department of Oncology, CW Bill Young Marrow Donor Recruitment and Research Program, Georgetown University Medical Centre, Washington, DC, USA*
DIANE M. KADIDLO • *Molecular and Cellular Therapeutics, University of Minnesota, St. Paul, MN, USA*
KANTHI KARIYAWASAM • *Department of Oncology, CW Bill Young Marrow Donor Recruitment and Research Program, Georgetown University Medical Centre, Washington, DC, USA*
GURVINDER KAUR • *Department of Transplant Immunology and Immunogenetics, All India Institute of Medical Sciences, New Delhi, India*
NINA LAUTERBACH • *Transplantation Immunology, Tissue Typing Laboratory, Maastricht University Medical Center, Maastricht, The Netherlands*
MARY S. LEFFELL • *Immunogenetics Laboratory, Department of Medicine, Johns Hopkins University School of Medicine, Baltimore, MD, USA*
GÉRARD LEFRANC • *IMGT®, The International ImMunoGeneTics Information System®, Université Montpellier 2, Laboratoire d'ImmunoGénétique Moléculaire (LIGM), Institut de Génétique Humaine (IGH), UPR CNRS 1142, Montpellier, France*
MARIE-PAULE LEFRANC • *IMGT®, The International ImMunoGeneTics Information System®, Université Montpellier 2, Laboratoire d'ImmunoGénétique Moléculaire (LIGM), Institut de Génétique Humaine (IGH), UPR CNRS1142, Montpellier, France*
DONNA P. LUCAS • *Immunogenetics Laboratory, Department of Medicine, Johns Hopkins University School of Medicine, Baltimore, MD, USA*

STEVEN J. MACK • *Center for Genetics, Children's Hospital and Research Center Oakland, Oakland, CA, USA*
MARI MALKKI • *Fred Hutchinson Cancer Research Centre, Seattle, WA, USA*
O. PATRICIA MARTINEZ • *Department of Clinical Immunology, PathWest Laboratory Medicine, Royal Perth and Fremantle Hospitals, Perth, WA, Australia; School of Pathology and Laboratory Medicine (PaLM), University of Western Australia, Nedlands, WA, Australia*
JAMES MCCLUSKEY • *Department of Microbiology and Immunology, University of Melbourne, Parkville, VIC, Australia*
DAVID H. MCKENNA • *Department of Laboratory Medicine and Pathology, Cancer Centre and Molecular and Cellular Therapeutics, University of Minnesota, Minneapolis, MN, USA*
NARINDER MEHRA • *Department of Transplant Immunology and Immunogenetics, All India Institute of Medical Sciences, New Delhi, India*
NICOLE A. MIFSUD • *Department of Medicine, Monash University, Alfred Hospital, Melbourne, VIC, Australia*
JEFFREY S. MILLER • *Department of Medicine, University of Minnesota Cancer Centre, Minneapolis, MN, USA*
MANUELA MORARU • *Inmunogenética—HLA, Hospital Universitario Puerta de Hierro, Majadahonda, Spain*
PHILIPPE MOREAU • *Commissariat à l'Energie Atomique, Service de Recherches en Hémato-Immunologie, I2BM, Institut Universitaire d'Hématologie, Hôpital Saint-Louis, Paris, France*
JENNIFER NG • *Department of Pediatrics, CW Bill Young Marrow Donor Recruitment and Research Program, Georgetown University Medical Centre, Washington, DC, USA*
HOLGER NÜCKEL • *Department of Haematology and Institute of Pharmacogenetics, University Hospital Essen, Essen, Germany*
CRISTA OCHSENFARTH • *Institute of Pharmacogenetics, University Hospital Essen, Essen, Germany*
GERHARD OPELZ • *Department of Transplantation Immunology, Institute of Immunology, University of Heidelberg, Heidelberg, Germany*
DAVID ORDÓÑEZ • *Inmunogenética—HLA, Hospital Universitario Puerta de Hierro, Majadahonda, Spain*
MACHTELD OUDSHOORN • *Department of Immunohematology and Blood Transfusion, Leiden University Medical Centre, Leiden, The Netherlands; Europdonor Foundation, Leiden, The Netherlands*
EFFIE W. PETERSDORF • *Fred Hutchinson Cancer Research Centre, Seattle, WA, USA*
RAJA RAJALINGAM • *UCLA Immunogenetics Center, Department of Pathology and Laboratory Medicine, David Geffen School of Medicine at UCLA, University of California, Los Angeles, CA, USA*
VERA REBMANN • *Institute for Transfusion Medicine, University Hospital Essen, Essen, Germany*
DAVE L. ROELEN • *Department of Immunohematology and Blood Transfusion, Leiden University Medical Centre, Leiden, The Netherlands*
PÄIVI SAAVALAINEN • *Research Program for Molecular Medicine, Department of Medical Genetics, Haartman Institute, Biomedicum Helsinki, University of Helsinki, Helsinki, Finland*
DAVID SAYER • *Conexio Pty Ltd, Fremantle, WA, Australia*

MICHELLE SETTERHOLM • *National Marrow Donor Program, Minneapolis, MN, USA*
RICHARD M. SINGLE • *Department of Mathematics and Statistics, University of Vermont, Burlington, VT, USA*
LINDA K. SMITH • *Department of Clinical Immunology, PathWest Laboratory Medicine, Royal Perth Hospital, Perth, WA, Australia*
ERIC SPIERINGS • *Department of Immunology, University Medical Centre Utrecht, Utrecht, The Netherlands*
PETER STASTNY • *Division of Transplant Immunology, Department of Internal Medicine, UT Southwestern Medical Centre, Dallas, TX, USA*
NORIKO STEINER • *Department of Oncology, CW Bill Young Marrow Donor Recruitment and Research Program, Georgetown University Medical Centre, Washington, DC, USA*
CANER SÜSAL • *Department of Transplantation Immunology, Institute of Immunology, University of Heidelberg, Heidelberg, Germany*
BRIAN D. TAIT • *National Transplant Services, Australian Red Cross Blood Service, The Royal Melbourne Hospital, Melbourne, VIC, Australia*
GABRIELLA TASSONE • *Department of Clinical Immunology, PathWest Laboratory Medicine, Royal Perth Hospital, Perth, WA, Australia*
GLENYS THOMSON • *Department of Integrative Biology, University of California, Berkeley, CA, USA*
MARCEL G.J. TILANUS • *Transplantation Immunology, Tissue Typing Laboratory, Maastricht University Medical Center, Maastricht, The Netherlands*
DANIEL TRAJANOSKI • *Department of Clinical Immunology, PathWest Laboratory Medicine, Royal Perth Hospital, Perth, WA, Australia*
ELLEN M.W. VAN DER MEER-PRINS • *Department of Immunohematology and Blood Transfusion, Leiden University Medical Centre, Leiden, The Netherlands*
MICHAEL D. VARNEY • *Victorian Transplantation and Immunogenetics Service, Australian Red Cross Blood Service, Melbourne, VIC, Australia*
RENATO M. VEGA • *Immunogenetics Laboratory, Department of Medicine, Johns Hopkins University School of Medicine, Baltimore, MD, USA*
ANDREA VELARDI • *Division of Haematology and Clinical Immunology, Department of Clinical and Experimental Medicine, University of Perugia, Ospedale Santa Maria della Misericordia, Perugia, Italy*
CARLOS VILCHES • *Inmunogenética—HLA, Hospital Universitario Puerta de Hierro, Majadahonda, Spain*
CHRISTINA E.M. VOORTER • *Transplantation Immunology, Tissue Typing Laboratory, Maastricht University Medical Center, Maastricht, The Netherlands*
CARLA WIRTZ • *Technical Support and Training, Conexio Genomics, Longmont, CO, USA*
CAMPBELL S. WITT • *Department of Clinical Immunology, PathWest Laboratory Medicine, Royal Perth Hospital, Perth, WA, Australia; School of Pathology and Laboratory Medicine (PaLM), University of Western Australia, Nedlands, WA, Australia*
ANDREA A. ZACHARY • *Immunogenetics Laboratory, Department of Medicine, Johns Hopkins University School of Medicine, Baltimore, MD, USA*
YVONNE M. ZOET • *Department of Immunohematology and Blood Transfusion, Leiden University Medical Centre, Leiden, The Netherlands*
YIZHOU ZOU • *Division of Transplant Immunology, Department of Internal Medicine, UT Southwestern Medical Centre, Dallas, TX, USA*

# Chapter 1

# The Major Histocompatibility Complex: A Paradigm for Studies of the Human Genome

**Richard J.N. Allcock**

## Abstract

The major histocompatibility complex (MHC) on chromosome 6 is one of the most intensively studied regions of the human genome and has many features which make it unique. It is the source of much research interest because of its role in autoimmune and infectious disease susceptibility, and of diagnostic interest because of its role in transplantation and rejection. It is the most gene-dense and SNP-rich region of the genome, with large number of complex haplotypes and other features which must be taken into account when analysing the MHC in the laboratory. This article provides a brief overview of the MHC highlighting some of the issues that must be considered when developing new methods and assays.

**Key words:** Major histocompatibility complex, Genetic polymorphism, HLA, Immune genes

## 1. Introduction

The major histocompatibility complex (MHC) is a 4 Mb region of chromosome 6 which is one of the most intensively studied regions of the human genome. It has been the subject of countless reviews over more than 20 years and was most recently reviewed in 2011 (1, 2).

The MHC has attracted the interest of researchers in many different fields, both medical and scientific, and was one of the first large regions of the human genome to be sequenced in its entirety in the 1990s (3). Study of this gene complex has led to a number of observations on genome structure and biology which have proven to be applicable to much of the rest of genome. The intense level of study of this region has meant that many genomic laboratory techniques have been pioneered or refined examining the MHC.

Frank T. Christiansen and Brian D. Tait (eds.), *Immunogenetics: Methods and Applications in Clinical Practice*, Methods in Molecular Biology, vol. 882, DOI 10.1007/978-1-61779-842-9_1, 

Given their important roles in disease and transplantation, the HLA genes (HLA-A, -B, -C, -DRA, -DRB1, -DRB3, -DRB4, DRB5, -DQA1, -DQB1, and -DPB1) have been the focus of many clinical and diagnostic studies. Many hundreds of thousands of individuals have been genotyped at high resolution at the six major HLA loci. The genotyping data from these loci are presented as numbered alleles, but it is important to note that an individual HLA allele can be made up of more than 50–60 individual single nucleotide polymorphisms (SNPs). Hence, individual alleles are in fact complex multi-SNP haplotypes, collectively named through a detailed and extensive nomenclature system (4). There are few comparably complex variable gene loci elsewhere in the genome and the methods for dealing with such a level of allelic variation have been to be developed by researchers in the field. Some of these issues are addressed elsewhere in this volume. As knowledge has advanced and new important genes within the MHC region have been identified, the methodological approaches and nomenclature system have been refined and revised to accommodate this new information. Investigators studying HLA and other genes in the MHC have had to become expert geneticists, genomicists, bioinformaticians, and statisticians in order to synthesise and integrate this knowledge. Because of complexity of the MHC and the need to develop specialised methods and nomenclature, the biology and genetics of the MHC has been perceived as an arcane niche. However, it is now increasingly apparent that many features once thought unique to the MHC apply more broadly to many other regions of the genome and that the MHC is rich and unique area for the study of general features of the human genome.

The MHC is known for a number of features including, but not limited to:

1. A very high gene density (1 locus every ~15 kb over its entire length), with a high proportion (20–30%) of the genes having a direct or indirect role in innate or adaptive immunity (for an exhaustive gene list and map, see ref. (2) and also see http://vega.sanger.ac.uk/Homo_sapiens/Location/Chromosome?r=6:1-171055067 for the current annotation of the region).
2. Very short intergenic lengths (<1 kb).
3. High numbers of SNPs including point variations and indels (1 every 200–300 base pairs (bp)), with many found in coding regions affecting amino acids (see refs. (5, 6) for descriptions and maps).
4. Whole-MHC haplotypes and smaller haplotype "blocks" of approximately 40–80 kb.
5. Variations in gene-content between haplotypes (e.g. the complement genes and the HLA-DRB region pseudogenes).

6. Low levels of recombination and, as a result, en bloc inheritance of highly conserved MHC haplotypes.

Between them this set of features combine to form a region whose properties are unique and therefore methods for their study must be adapted to take account of these features. Many diagnostic laboratory methods or genotyping techniques, which have been developed over time, have required revision due to, for example, unrecognised sequence variations which have led to allelic dropout during the polymerase chain reaction (PCR) and an inability to detect particular allele combinations. The modern sequence-based diagnostic tests for the HLA genes are able to identify the presence of new unrecognised alleles as well as being able to detect more than 1,500 alleles and 800 alleles of the class I loci and class II loci, respectively (7). Such progress reflects a long history of research and diagnostics effectively "crossing over" in MHC.

## 2. Physical Structure and Gene Content

The MHC lies on the short arm of chromosome 6, with the class I region at the telomeric end and the class II region at the centromeric end (reviewed in ref. (2)). Between them lies the class III, or central MHC, region of approximately 1 Mb. The class II region is relatively homogeneous, containing genes predominantly encoding HLA class II proteins (alpha and beta subunits), as well as a small number of genes involved in processing antigens for class I proteins (the TAP and PSMB genes). In contrast, the class I region encodes the classical (HLA-A, -B, -C) and non-classical (HLA-E, -F, -G) proteins, but is littered with the remnants of many evolutionary relics in the form of pseudogenes. In addition, the class I region encodes a significant number of Tripartite-motif (TRIM) family and butyrophilin (BTN) family genes, which may well have immune-related roles, and a large number of genes with functions outside the immune system.

The gene families found in the MHC are likely the result of multiple duplication events and individual pairs of genes can be almost identical (e.g. HLA-B and HLA-C), or highly similar to one another (e.g. the MIC family for MHC-class I-like genes—see ref. (8)) or much more divergent, sharing little more than broad intron–exon structures and having 20–25% sequence identity (e.g. TNF, LTA, and LTB—see ref. (9)).

The class I and II regions of the MHC are so named primarily because of the HLA genes encoded within them. Between them lies the class III region which has no such defining feature and contains a large number of genes of variable function, both within and outside the immune system. Some areas have been extensively studied (e.g. the complement genes, the TNF cluster and MICA genes), whilst others have been less well studied. The 1 Mb class III region has the highest gene density of the three major MHC regions.

## 3. Genetic Variation and Haplotypes

The MHC has long been known to harbour large numbers of SNPs, particularly in the MHC class I and II genes. However, it is now recognised that almost all MHC genes are more polymorphic than most genes elsewhere in the genome (2). These variations take the form of point mutations, small indels, large indels, and microsatellites. Within the HLA genes, particularly in the exons encoding the hypervariable regions, there may be 50–100 SNPs located within regions of 100–200 bp, many of which cause amino acid changes (5). Primer-design for PCR is fraught with problems in these regions and therefore many investigators site primers in introns or further afield where there are lower levels of variation. This problem is not limited to the HLA genes however, as variants are found throughout the MHC, sometimes in very close proximity to one another.

Initially, only a single MHC sequence, assembled from a variety of sources and individuals, was available (3) and the identification of sequence variations was based around "sample" sequencing of small regions of interest to particular investigators (e.g. see ref. (10)). Subsequently, the "MHC haplotype project" used standard mapping and sequencing techniques to resequence the entire MHC from eight hemi- or homozygous cells lines carrying well-defined and important haplotypes (11). The vast number of catalogued MHC variants generated by this project has allowed a greater insight into the existence of haplotypes blocks, both within the MHC, but also elsewhere (see refs. (5, 6)). The level of knowledge of block boundaries and number of the haplotypes within a given block is far greater in the MHC than elsewhere in the genome, largely as a consequence of the major interest in the region and the large number of variants identified. Whilst particular whole MHC haplotypes based on HLA class I and II combinations have been recognised for more than 20 years (12), it is now recognised that much smaller haplotype blocks of some 20–60 kb in length are present. The well-studied TNF block contains more than 100 SNPs but it can be defined by 20–30 SNPs (13), and the SNPs present in each haplotype appear to be found in many populations worldwide, and in similar combinations. Whilst populations differ in the frequency of individual haplotypes, the fundamental observation of a common set of haplotypes remains (14).

Overall genetic variation in the MHC, as elsewhere in the genome, is most frequent in intergenic and intronic regions. There are approximately 500–3,000 intronic variants, and a further 500–4,000 intergenic variants in any given haploptype (5). Coding region variants are less frequent, approximately 300–500 in a given haplotype, distributed in HLA and non-HLA genes alike. However, the HLA-genes contain approximately two thirds of the non-synonymous coding region variants, consistent with their functional importance (5). When the sequenced MHC haplotypes are considered as a whole, there are more than 70,000 identified and catalogued SNPs in the human MHC.

## 4. Assay Design and Approaches

To date, diagnostic assays have focussed on the amplification of small fragments and either hybridisation to labelled probes or sequencing using standard methods, such as fluorescent dideoxy chain terminators (Sanger sequencing). Diagnostic assays for other parts of the MHC have not been developed to the same extent. Assays for the detection of MICA polymorphisms have been developed and are described in this volume. Studies of the complement region, of interest to some groups, are complicated by a duplicated gene system in which there can be 0–4 genes present on each haplotype, all of which may be polymorphic (15). The recent significant interest in copy number variation has led to the development of methods to examine them effectively, and methods incorporating both CNV and SNP analysis are emerging. A similar situation exists at the telomeric end of the HLA class II region, where there is a variable gene content in the HLA-DRB pseudogenes, which once again can contain multiple alleles (16).

Arguably, the most complex bioinformatic analysis currently in use in the diagnostic world is the assignment of a pair of HLA alleles to a given individual. Currently, based on Sanger sequencing of the peptide binding-encoding exons, bulk heterozygous sequence is compared to a database of all combinations of known HLA alleles. Sophisticated analysis programmes have been developed for allele assignment and resolution of ambiguities. More recently, next-generation sequencing technologies have been applied to the study of MHC genes. One advantage of next-generation sequencing is the ability to sequence individual DNA strands, thus unambiguously defining the phase of identified SNPs (17). How these high-throughput methods will be applied in diagnostic laboratories is not yet clear, as cost and turn-around times remain significant. However, it is already evident approaches to enrich (capture) the MHC and sequence it in its entirety in a matter of days are technically feasible. Such approaches will result in a significant additional increase in our knowledge of sequences originating from the MHC and in turn pose new challenges for analysis and data handling.

## 5. The Future

Many autoimmune diseases have been associated with MHC alleles and haplotypes and the vast variety of functions encoded by MHC genes has led to a great deal of speculation as to the pathways that are implicated and whether immune system or non-immune system genes are responsible (recently reviewed in ref. (1)). To date no definitive answers have emerged and it remains possible than almost any gene within the MHC could be involved in autoimmune disease susceptibility. Greater understanding of MHC gene functions, genetic variability and haplotype structure, together with other information, such as methylation patterns (18) and how these epigenetic modifications affect expression, will be required to elucidate the mechanisms involved. In addition, a greater examination of variation in the HLA genes may lead to an improved understanding of the effects of the MHC on acceptance and rejection of allografts and ultimately further improvement in transplantation outcome.

## Acknowledgements

I am grateful to Winthrop Professor Frank Christiansen for his critical comments and suggestions during the preparation of this manuscript.

### References

1. Trowsdale J (2011) The MHC, disease and selection. Immunol Lett. doi:10.1016/j.imlet.2011.01.002
2. Shiina T, Hosomichi K, Inoko H et al (2009) The HLA genomic loci map: expression, interaction, diversity and disease. J Hum Genet 54: 15–39
3. The MHC Sequencing Consortium (1999) Complete structure and gene map of a major histocompatibility complex (MHC). Nature 401:921–923
4. Marsh SG, Albert ED, Bodmer WF et al (2010) Nomenclature for factors of the HLA system. Tissue Antigens 75:291–455
5. Horton R, Gibson R, Coggill P et al (2008) Variation analysis and gene annotation of eight MHC haplotypes: the MHC Haplotype Project. Immunogenetics 60:1–18
6. de Bakker PI, McVean G, Sabeti PC et al (2006) A high-resolution HLA and SNP haplotype map for disease association studies in the extended human MHC. Nat Genet 38:1166–1172
7. Smith LK, Sayer DC, Whidborne RS et al (2007) Sequencing-based typing identifies novel alleles due to single nucleotide polymorphisms in 'conserved' regions. Tissue Antigens 69(suppl 1):56–57

8. Choy MK, Phipps ME (2010) MICA polymorphism: biology and importance in immunity and disease. Trends Mol Med 16:97–106
9. Posch PE, Cruz I, Bradshaw D et al (2003) Novel polymorphisms and the definition of promoter 'alleles' of the tumour necrosis factor and lymphotoxin alpha loci: inclusion in HLA haplotypes. Genes Immun 4:547–558
10. Smith WP, Vu Q, Li SS et al (2006) Toward understanding MHC disease associations: partial resequencing of 46 distinct HLA haplotypes. Genomics 87:561–571
11. Stewart CA, Horton R, Allcock RJ et al (2004) Complete MHC haplotype sequencing for common disease gene mapping. Genome Res 14:1176–1187
12. Degli-Esposti MA, Leaver AL, Christiansen FT et al (1992) Ancestral haplotypes: conserved population MHC haplotypes. Hum Immunol 34:242–252
13. Allcock RJN, Windsor L, Gut IG et al (2004) High-density SNP genotyping defines 17 distinct haplotypes of the TNF block in the Caucasian population: implications for haplotype tagging. Hum Mutat 24:517–525
14. Valente FP, Tan CR, Temple SE et al (2009) The evolution and diversity of TNF block haplotypes in European, Asian and Australian Aboriginal populations. Genes Immun 10:607–615
15. Yang Z, Yu CY (2000) Organisations and gene duplications of the human and mouse MHC complement gene clusters. J Exp Med 191: 2183–2196
16. Traherne JA, Horton R, Roberts AN et al (2006) Genetic analysis of completely sequenced disease-associated MHC haplotypes identifies shuffling of segments in recent human history. PLoS Genet 2:e9
17. Erlich RL, Jia X, Anderson S et al (2011) Next-generation sequencing for HLA-typing of class I loci. BMC Genomics 12:42–55
18. Tomazou EM, Rakyan VK, Lefebvre G et al (2008) Generation of a genomic tiling array of the human major histocompatibility complex (MHC) and its application for DNA methylation analysis. BMC Med Genomics 1:19

# Chapter 2

## HLA Typing by SSO and SSP Methods

### Heather Dunckley

### Abstract

Human leukocyte antigen (HLA) typing, utilising the sequence-specific oligonucleotide (SSO) and sequence-specific primer (SSP) technologies, has been in routine use in many tissue typing laboratories worldwide for more than 20 years since the development of the polymerase chain reaction. Both methods are very useful for clinical and research purposes and can provide generic (low resolution) to allelic (high resolution) typing results. This chapter provides an overview of the SSO and SSP methods in relation to HLA typing.

**Key words:** HLA typing, PCR-SSP, PCR-SSO, Oligotyping, Reverse-SSO typing

## 1. Introduction

### *1.1. Sequence-Specific Primer Assay*

HLA-SSP typing of the HLA-DR genes was initially developed by Olerup and Zetterquist (1). Further developments of the method quickly followed which enabled sequence-specific primer (SSP) typing of other human leukocyte antigen (HLA) class I and II genes (2–5). In 1995 Bunce et al. developed a comprehensive SSP typing system for the HLA-A, -B, -C, -DRB1, -DRB3, -DRB4, -DRB5, and -DQB1 alleles where all the polymerase chain reactions (PCRs) were designed to work with identical thermocycler conditions (6). SSP typing involves the use of primers complementary to particular HLA allele sequences (e.g. HLA*02:03) or a group of similar alleles (e.g. all the A*02 alleles). Primers are designed so that the polymorphism to be detected is at the 3′ end of the primer. If there is a mismatch with the HLA allele at the 3′ end, the primer will not be extended by Taq DNA polymerase. In the case of HLA-A, -B, and -C typing, most primer sets detect polymorphisms in exons 2 and 3 of the class I genes as these regions cover most of the known

Frank T. Christiansen and Brian D. Tait (eds.), *Immunogenetics: Methods and Applications in Clinical Practice*, Methods in Molecular Biology, vol. 882, DOI 10.1007/978-1-61779-842-9_2, © Springer Science+Business Media New York 2012

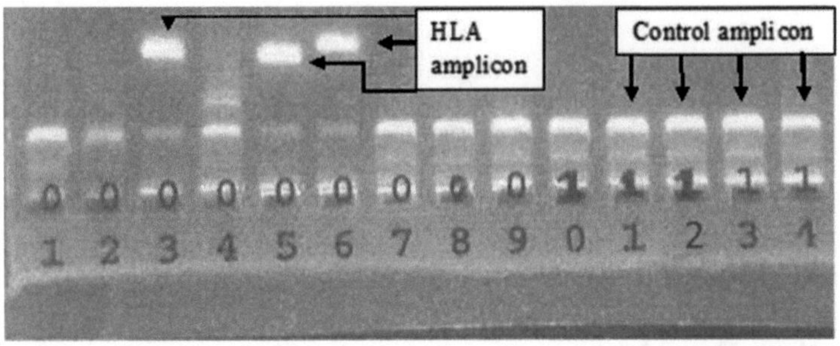


Fig. 1. Photo of a sequence-specific primer (SSP) gel. The photo shows amplification of the control gene and human leukocyte antigen (HLA) genes. The control amplicon is present in *all lanes* and the HLA amplicon is present in *lanes 3, 5,* and *6.* The control amplicon is weaker in *lanes 3, 5,* and *6.*

polymorphisms. For the HLA-DR, -DQ, and -DP genes, most primer sets cover exon 2 polymorphisms where the majority of the known sequence variation occurs. The SSP method can be used for either low resolution (generic) typing which resolves alleles to at least the antigenic level (the level detected by serological typing methods), or for high resolution (allele level) typing.

For HLA-SSP typing, primer sets are made up in advance and dispensed into microtitre trays or PCR tubes and stored frozen. If freeze dried, the primer sets can be stored at 2–8°C. When an individual requires HLA genotyping, DNA is extracted, usually from a blood sample, and added to a pre-made buffer containing dNTPs and Taq DNA polymerase and the mixture is then aliquotted into microtitre trays with the primer sets which are then subjected to the PCR process, (the same PCR conditions are used for all the primer sets). Amplification is detected by electrophoresing the PCR products through an agarose gel containing a dye, such as ethidium bromide, which binds to DNA. A photo taken while the gel is exposed to ultra violet light reveals the presence (or absence) of amplified HLA alleles. Positive amplification is recorded, and depending on which primer mixes have amplified, the HLA type of the sample can be assigned (see Fig. 1; Table 1).

In the initial years of SSP method development, there was a requirement by laboratories to purchase primers and prepare their own SSP typing trays and to maintain an up to date method as new HLA alleles were discovered. But the technology was quickly developed commercially and as a result it has been possible for some time to purchase SSP typing kits to type the HLA class I and II loci at either low or high resolution. This requires the laboratory only to extract DNA from clinical samples, add DNA and Taq DNA polymerase to the commercially pre-made buffer and primer sets, perform the PCR and run gels to observe amplification. With the ever increasing number of HLA alleles, result assignment requires the use of customised software and commercial HLA-SSP kit suppliers also have software to assist the result interpretation

**Table 1**
**SSP result interpretation and HLA typing from the gel in Fig. 1**

| | Well number | | | | | | | | | | | | | |
|---|---|---|---|---|---|---|---|---|---|---|---|---|---|---|
| | **1** | **2** | **3** | **4** | **5** | **6** | **7** | **8** | **9** | **10** | **11** | **12** | **13** | **14** |
| Control amplicon | + | + | + | + | + | + | + | + | + | + | + | + | + | + |
| HLA amplicon | – | – | + | – | + | + | – | – | – | – | – | – | – | – |
| DRB1* allele of HLA amplicon | 01 | 03 | 04 | 07 | 08 | 04, 07 or 09 | 09 | 10 | 11 | 12 | 13 | 14 | 15 | 16 |

"+" Means the amplicon is present; "–" means the amplicon is absent. Based on the positive reactions, the HLA type of the sample is DRB1*04, 08

and HLA genotyping assignment. The SSP method has the major advantage of being a very fast method of HLA genotyping, the process (including DNA extraction) being completed within 2–3 h. The technique therefore is well suited to the typing of urgent cases, such as patients requiring HLA-matched platelet transfusions, or genotyping of donors for organ transplantation. However, because of the number of PCRs required for each sample, the SSP method is not suited to the typing of large sample numbers, even with the use of multi-dispensing pipettes or robotics as there is also the consideration of the number of PCR machines required. Commercial kits are available which can perform low resolution HLA-A, -B, -DRB1 typing with 96 PCRs/sample. With the continually increasing large number of HLA alleles, it is becoming more difficult to resolve the major allele groups with a one-step SSP process. Additional primer mixes can be added to include newly found alleles, but there is a limit to the practicality of adding more and more primer mixes to resolve ambiguities.

### *1.2. Sequence-Specific Oligonucleotide Assay*

HLA-SSO typing was one of the first PCR-based HLA typing methods to be developed, initially for the HLA class II loci and then for the HLA class I genes (7–12). The technique involves extraction of DNA followed by amplification of a particular HLA gene locus, for example HLA-A or HLA-B or HLA-DRB1. Primers are selected to amplify in one PCR tube all known alleles of the particular HLA locus which requires genotyping. Generally, for HLA class I typing exons 2 and 3 are co-amplified as one PCR product while for HLA class II typing only exon 2 is amplified as these are the gene regions with the majority of the known sequence variation. The amplified DNA is blotted onto a nylon membrane which is positively charged permitting the negatively charged DNA to bind strongly. Many samples can be blotted onto the same membrane and the membrane size can be increased as sample numbers increase. Multiple membranes with the amplified DNA samples are prepared, one for each oligonucleotide probe used in the genotyping method.

The membrane with the bound DNA is placed in a container and mixed with a hybridisation solution containing an oligonucleotide labelled with a marker such as biotin and which has a DNA sequence that is specific for a particular HLA allele or group of alleles. When the amplified DNA sequence is complementary to the sequence of the oligonucleotide, hybridisation occurs. Non-hybridised oligonucleotides remain unbound in the solution and are easily removed in a series of stringency washing steps as are any oligonucleotides which are non-specifically bound to the amplified DNA on the nylon membrane. Oligonucleotides are designed so the polymorphism to be detected is in the middle of the oligonucleotide sequence which facilitates the strongest possible binding between the amplified DNA and the oligonucleotide. If there is sequence variation between the amplicon and the end of the oligonucleotide, then only one part of the oligonucleotide binds to the amplified DNA which increases the likelihood of washing off during the stringency washing step. A chemiluminescent or colourmetric reaction can be used to reveal the presence of bound oligonucleotide. The reaction of each sample with each oligonucleotide is recorded and the HLA type of the sample can be assigned based on the pattern of positive reactions.

The sequence-specific oligonucleotide (SSO) method is very well suited to the typing of large sample numbers, e.g. a routine typing lab using one to two 96-well microtitre trays can easily test 88–184 samples in one assay (with seven positive control samples of known HLA type and a negative control). New oligonucleotides to cover new alleles or resolve ambiguities can be added which only requires an additional membrane with the bound amplified DNA to be prepared. However, with the very high number of possible heterozygous HLA allele combinations, the SSO method struggles to resolve all ambiguities as the method does not distinguish between *cis* and *trans* polymorphisms. SSP typing on the other hand only detects alleles which have both the forward and reverse primer sequences on the same HLA allele thus linking two polymorphic regions to the same allele which assists in resolving some ambiguities. SSO typing takes approximately 2 days from the PCR stage to result assignment, so is not a rapid typing method, but as 88–184 samples can easily be typed in this time for one gene locus by one staff member it is a cost-effective method.

Because the primers used in SSO typing are designed to amplify all alleles for a particular locus they are selected from a non-variable part of the gene. Provided a new allele does not have a polymorphism in this region it will be amplified so the SSO method is generally able to detect new HLA alleles better than the SSP method. If a new allele has a polymorphism in one of the regions covered by an SSO, it should be detected and appear as a new pattern which does not match the expected patterns of known alleles.

But as the SSOs do not cover all regions of the gene, it is still possible for new alleles to be missed by this method and they would only be found if the sample was genotyped by another method such as DNA sequencing.

While the PCR-SSO method is not a suitable technique for low sample numbers, there is a method variation known as reverse-SSO (13, 14) which is well suited to the testing of individual samples or multiple samples concurrently. In the reverse-SSO technique, oligonucleotides are individually bound to membranes, each membrane having all the SSOs bound that are required for a particular HLA locus or allele group. These membranes are premade so they are available for testing at any time. Sample DNA is amplified using primers specific for the HLA locus to be typed, incorporating a label such as biotin. The amplified DNA is then hybridised to the membrane with the pre-bound oligonucleotides. Non-specifically bound amplicons are removed by washing and the hybridisation between the amplicon and membrane bound oligonucleotide is detected with a chemiluminescent or colour-based detection system.

A recently developed variation of the reverse-SSO system employs Luminex xMAP® technology. The Luminex xMAP® technique utilises polystyrene microspheres which are dyed internally with red and infrared fluorophores. The two dyes are incorporated in differing proportions on different beads allowing 100 unique sets of microspheres to be developed. Each of the 100 bead sets can be individually identified with a Luminex® analyser even when in the same reaction tube. For HLA genotyping, each of the microsphere sets is coated with a different oligonucleotide. Test DNA is amplified by PCR and hybridised to the bead sets in solution, the process is carried out in a 96-well PCR plate with one sample tested/well (each well contains all the different bead sets), allowing 96 samples to be tested simultaneously. Non-hybridised DNA is removed by washing and amplified DNA which has bound to the SSOs on the microspheres is detected by a fluorescent dye with a Luminex® analyser using flow cytometric technology. The analyser automates the data acquisition and provides quantitative results as well as HLA assignments. Because 100 different bead sets can be included in each reaction tube or tray well, it is easier to include a larger number of SSOs with Luminex xMAP® technology than other SSO or reverse-SSO methods, enabling a better level of HLA typing resolution.

While reverse-SSO typing still has the drawbacks of ambiguity resolution that the original SSO method has, it is well suited to genotyping of small sample numbers and there are several commercial kits available utilising this technology. Some commercial kits incorporate robotics for the hybridisation, washing and detection steps making the method also suitable for the typing of larger sample numbers.

### 1.3. Interpretation of Results

Because of the large and ever increasing number of HLA alleles, data analysis and HLA genotyping assignment now requires the use of software, commercial HLA typing kits generally provide software programs for this purpose. For the SSP, SSO and reverse-SSO methods, most analysis software follows the same principle. The reaction patterns of known alleles are established for the primer sets used in the SSP kit or the oligonucleotides in the SSO or reverse-SSO methods based on known HLA sequence data from the IMGT/HLA database (15, 16). When a sample is tested, the reaction pattern obtained is compared to the reaction patterns of known alleles. The software then provides a list of possible HLA types based on the patterns of known alleles which match the sample being tested. With the SSP and SSO methods, multiple results will sometimes be obtained as it is difficult for these methods to completely resolve all possible heterozygous allele combinations. However, provided the alternative results are within the same allele group and do not cross antigen specificities, this is not usually an issue particularly if a low resolution typing result is satisfactory. The SSO and SSP methods can also be used in conjunction with sequencing-based typing (SBT) by providing a generic result which determines the primers to be used in allele level SBT. In some cases, ambiguities can arise with SBT (with heterozygous sequences) in which case the SSP method can be used to help resolve an allele level typing. Because of the continual increase in the identification of new alleles, laboratories must keep all typing methods up to date which requires the databases used for SSO and SSP result interpretation to be updated at least every 6 months. The IMGT/HLA database of officially named HLA alleles is updated every month (15, 16).

While molecular HLA typing is more accurate and provides a higher level of resolution than serological tissue typing (17–20), molecular methods will not detect new alleles if a new polymorphism is not in the region where an amplification primer or SSO matches the gene. In addition, null or non-expressed alleles are usually detected when molecular typing is used in conjunction with serological methods. When only one method is used both serology and molecular techniques sometimes fail to detect null alleles. While null alleles are not common, tissue typing protocols for transplantation should be developed to avoid missing these non-expressed alleles, especially in matching for haematopoietic stem cell transplantation.

### 1.4. Clinical Applications

The SSP, SSO and reverse-SSO methods are all suitable for use in routine tissue typing laboratories as well as for research purposes. With a variety of commercial kits now available, laboratories can choose which method is most suitable for their work, and a combination of kits can be used for different requirements. In laboratories testing for clinical purposes like transplantation it is useful to have more than one method available so that any unusual results can be verified. If dealing with low sample numbers or urgent testing, then SSP is very practical. With low to large sample numbers reverse-SSO can be used, this method also gives a reasonable turnaround time for testing. For large sample batches and when the test time is less urgent, then SSO typing is a very cost-effective method.

As it is now easier to buy commercial HLA-SSP and reverse-SSO kits rather than developing in-house methods, the protocols described below summarise the steps that would be followed when using a commercial kit, some specific details being provided by the kit manufacturer supplier. When using commercial kits, each shipment and batch of kits needs to be checked before routine use. This can be accomplished using samples of known HLA type to verify the typing results obtained with the kit.

## 2. Materials

### 2.1. HLA-SSP Typing

1. Commercial kits will usually supply the primer sets (both HLA and control primers) already pre-dispensed into microtitre trays or tubes ready for use in a thermocycler. Some trays will also include the dNTPs and PCR buffer with the primers. Sometimes these mixes will be lyophilised, other times they will be in solution but covered with a layer of paraffin oil to avoid evaporation.
2. PCR buffer and dNTPs, if not included with the pre-dispensed primer sets, are usually included with the commercial kits as is the gel loading buffer.
3. Taq DNA Polymerase—may or may not be included with the commercial kit.
4. Tube caps or tray sealers for the PCR trays are usually included with the commercial kits.
5. Sterile molecular grade water (d$H_2O$).
6. Pipettes and sterile tips to dispense 1–10 μL, 10–200 μL, and 200–1,000 μL volume ranges. Electronic multi-dispensing pipettes are better if the sample numbers are high because of the large amount of pipetting involved.
7. Thermocycler with a heated lid.
8. Agarose horizontal gel tank equipment, gel casting trays, gel combs, and power supply.
9. Agarose (DNA grade).
10. Electrophoresis buffer as specified by the kit supplier.
11. Microwave or heating apparatus to dissolve the agarose.

12. DNA molecular weight marker to cover a range of 50–2,000 bp.
13. Ethidium bromide 10 mg/mL (see Note 1).
14. UV transilluminator and photographic equipment—a digital photo allows the photo to be stored electronically.
15. Gel documentation forms and worksheets if not included with the commercial kit.
16. Data analysis and HLA assignment software (from the kit supplier) and a computer.

### *2.2. HLA Reverse-SSO Typing*

1. A master mix containing biotinylated primers, dNTPs and buffer is usually supplied with commercial kits. $MgCl_2$ may be provided in a separate tube. These are normally supplied frozen.
2. Taq DNA polymerase may be included in the master mix, or may be provided in a separate tube, or may not be included with a commercial kit.
3. Strips with pre-bound oligonucleotides are provided with commercial kits.
4. Control DNA is usually supplied with a commercial kit.
5. Sterile molecular grade water ($dH_2O$).
6. Pipettes and sterile tips to dispense 1–10 μL, 10–200 μL, and 200–1,000 μL volume ranges. Electronic multi-dispensing pipettes are better if the sample numbers are high because of the large amount of pipetting involved.
7. PCR plastic ware—tubes or microtitre trays, caps or tray sealers.
8. Thermocycler with a heated lid.
9. Agarose horizontal gel tank equipment, gel casting trays, gel combs, and power supply.
10. Agarose (DNA grade).
11. Electrophoresis buffer as specified by the kit supplier.
12. Microwave or heating apparatus to dissolve the agarose.
13. Ethidium bromide 10 mg/mL (see Note 1).
14. UV transilluminator and photographic equipment—a digital photo allows the photo to be stored electronically.
15. Solutions required for denaturation, hybridisation, washing, and probe detection are included with commercial kits (see Note 2).
16. Some reverse-SSO kit suppliers provide automated assay equipment. Otherwise, the process can be carried out manually and requires a rocking platform, shaking water bath and containers for hybridisation, washing and probe detection steps as well as sterile pipettes (2–50 mL), and adjustable volume dispensers.

17. Water bath and filter forceps.
18. Ethanol.
19. Gel documentation forms and worksheets for recording oligonucleotide results if not included with the commercial kit.
20. Data analysis and HLA assignment software (from the kit supplier) and a computer.

## 3. Methods

### 3.1. HLA-SSP Method

1. Remove the PCR tray containing the primer sets and the kit components from the freezer or fridge in the pre-PCR area (see Note 3).
2. Following the manufacturer's instructions, add the required amount of $dH_2O$ to the PCR buffer provided in the kit, mix well and then add Taq DNA polymerase. Add the amount specified by the manufacturer to the negative control well of the PCR tray (see Notes 4 and 5).
3. Add the required amount of DNA to the remaining buffer/enzyme solution, mix well, and add the amount specified by the manufacturer to each of the test wells of the PCR tray. Seal or cap each tube tightly (see Notes 6–8).
4. Ensure the liquid of all the reaction mixes is at the base of the tray—hand flick the tray, or tap the tray gently on the bench, or pulse centrifuge the tray at a low speed (see Note 9).
5. In the PCR or post-PCR area, place the tray in the thermocycler and perform the PCR according to the kit supplier's specifications (see Notes 10–13).
6. When the PCR program is complete, remove the tray from the thermocycler.
7. In the post-PCR area, electrophorese the amplified samples and DNA molecular weight marker on an agarose gel containing ethidium bromide in the buffer recommended by the kit supplier. The supplier will provide details on the agarose concentration, gel size, well size, and voltage required (see Notes 14–17).
8. Take a photo of the gel under a UV light (see Note 18).
9. Check that the negative control is negative (no amplification product present). Score the positive PCRs (checking that the PCR product is the correct size) and note any wells where both the control PCR and HLA PCR failed as these cannot be scored as negative but as an unknown result (see Notes 19–22; Table 2).
10. Input the results of the PCRs (positive, negative, or unknown/no result) into the data analysis software program and obtain the HLA typing from the software (see Notes 23–28).

**Table 2**
**Interpretation of SSP gel results**

| HLA amplicon | Control amplicon | Result |
|---|---|---|
| Present | Present | Positive for the HLA amplicon |
| Present | Absent | Positive for the HLA amplicon |
| Absent | Present | Negative for the HLA amplicon |
| Absent | Absent | No result |

### *3.2. HLA Reverse-SSO Method*

1. In the pre-PCR area, make up the reaction mix as per the manufacturer's recommendations (buffer, water, dNTPs, primers, and Taq DNA polymerase). The amount of reaction mix made will depend on the number of samples to be amplified. Aliquot the reaction mix into the PCR tubes or tray (see Notes 3, 5, 7, and 29).
2. Add one DNA sample (amount as per the kit supplier specifications) to each reaction mix on the tray checking that the correct sample is added to each well or tube (see Note 30).
3. Seal or cap each tube tightly, ensure the liquid of all the reaction mixes is at the base of the tray—hand flick the tray, or tap the tray gently on the bench, or pulse centrifuge the tray at a low speed (see Notes 8 and 9).
4. In the PCR or post-PCR area, immediately place the tray in the thermocycler and perform the PCR according to the kit supplier's specifications (see Note 31).
5. When the PCR program is complete, remove the tray from the thermocycler.
6. In the post-PCR area, electrophorese the amplified samples on an agarose gel containing ethidium bromide in the buffer recommended by the kit supplier. The supplier will provide details on the agarose concentration, gel size, well size, and voltage required. Note: the agarose gel step is optional, some commercial kits do not include this step or steps 7 and 8 below.
7. Photograph the gel under a UV light (see Note 18).
8. Check that the negative control is negative (no amplification band present) and the PCR has worked for the test samples (amplification band evident on the gel).
9. Denature the amplified DNA sample as per the instructions in the kit and add the denatured DNA to the container with the

membrane strip which has the pre-bound oligonucleotides (see Note 32).

10. Incubate the amplicon DNA with the membrane for the hybridisation step and then remove unbound or non-specifically bound DNA by washing following the instructions in the kit (see Notes 33–35).
11. Add the conjugate to the membrane which binds to the labelled amplicons captured by the oligonucleotides. Remove unbound conjugate by washing following the kit instructions (see Note 36).
12. Incubate the membranes with the substrate solution from the kit for the colourimetric reaction. When the colour reaction has developed sufficiently, remove excess substrate by washing as per the kit instructions (see Note 37).
13. Add the short-term storage buffer from the kit to the membranes. A photo or scan (with a normal flat bed scanner) can be taken of the membrane strips for long-term digital record storage.
14. Use the strip template overlay provided with the kit to identify the probes correctly.
15. Check that the positive and negative controls give the correct results. Some kits also include an intensity reference probe. The reaction strength of the intensity reference probe is designed to be less than the reaction with all the HLA oligonucleotides on the strip. If the intensity reference probe signal is absent, there is a possibility that hybridisation with the HLA oligonucleotides has not been detected so the whole test will need to be repeated. Any HLA oligonucleotide signals that are equal to or greater than the intensity of the control probe should be scored as positive (see Note 38).
16. Score the hybridisation reactions with each oligonucleotide and input the results into the data analysis software program and obtain the HLA typing from the software (see Notes 24 and 27).

## 4. Notes

1. Ethidium bromide is a mutagen. Handle with appropriate personal protective equipment including gloves and eye protection.
2. The denaturation solution normally contains sodium hydroxide. The hybridisation and washing solutions usually contain a buffer

with sodium chloride, sodium phosphate and EDTA (SSPE), and sodium dodecyl sulphate (SDS). When using biotinylated primers, the conjugate is generally streptavidin-horseradish peroxide (HRP). The substrate for streptavidin-HRP which is used for probe detection depends on the kit supplier.

3. All work involving PCR requires the laboratory to have separate areas for pre- and post-PCR work so there is no risk of contaminating pre-PCR samples with PCR amplified product.

4. If an error is made during the PCR setup, this can lead to weak or no amplification of the internal control or test sample (one or multiple PCRs which may be incorrectly scored as negative reactions). The PCR must be set up exactly as specified in the kit instructions in relation to reagent volumes and concentrations. Ensure that pipettes are calibrated.

5. If the Taq DNA polymerase is not performing correctly, there will be weak or no amplification. Check the Taq DNA polymerase has been validated before use, re-verify if required with a known DNA sample.

6. If insufficient test DNA, poor quality or degraded DNA is used or PCR inhibitors are present in the DNA (e.g. too much EDTA), there may be no amplification of the internal control or the HLA alleles, or only weak amplification (one or multiple PCRs which may be incorrectly scored as negative reactions). If this occurs, the volume, concentration, and purity of the test DNA should be checked. If required re-precipitate the DNA (ethanol and salt step) and resuspend the DNA in a smaller volume of $dH_2O$ or repeat the whole DNA extraction with new reagents. DNA can be extracted from nucleated cells by any preferred method (in-house or commercial kit, manual or robotic system). If blood samples are used, the anticoagulant should be EDTA or ACD, not heparin which can inhibit the PCR. DNA should be kept in TE buffer for long-term storage but the aliquots for SSP work should be diluted in $dH_2O$, the final concentration of the DNA prior to amplification should be according to the recommendations of the kit supplier as this varies depending on the kit used. The $OD_{260/280}$ of the DNA should be between 1.6 and 1.9.

7. If the test DNA is not resuspended uniformly or the Taq DNA polymerase or PCR reagents are not mixed properly before use, there may be random PCR failures. Pipette the test DNA up and down several times to aid re-suspension; incubate test DNA on a heat block or in an incubator for 10 min at 70°C. Mix individual reagents briefly by vortexing (pulse only) before use. Reagents should also be centrifuged briefly (pulse only) so the reagent solutions are all at the base of the tube before use.

Ensure the Taq DNA polymerase/buffer/DNA mixture is also mixed well before dispensing into the PCR tray.

8. If the PCR tubes or tray are not capped or sealed tightly, there may be evaporation during the PCR leading to random amplification failure across the PCR plate. Make sure the caps or tray sealer are fixed properly (use a capping tool). Check the heated lid of the thermocycler is firmly in place.
9. If the PCR mix is not at the base of the tube in the PCR tray (some of the mix is on the side or lid of the tube), there may be random amplification failure leading to false negative results. Ensure all the PCR mix is under the paraffin oil if it is used.
10. A delay between the PCR setup and start of the PCR program can lead to false positive SSP reactions. Do not allow more than a 5 min delay between the PCR setup and commencing the PCR program.
11. Incorrect PCR conditions, for example an annealing temperature which is too high, can result in a low level of amplification or no amplification of the test DNA. One or multiple PCRs may be affected and incorrectly identified as negative. If this occurs the PCR program should be checked.
12. Temperature variation across the heat block in the thermocycler can cause random amplification failure across the PCR plate which may be falsely interpreted as negative reactions. Make sure the thermocycler is calibrated and re-calibrate if necessary to ensure the temperatures of the wells in the heat block are correct during thermocycling. Calibration verification is carried out by running a thermocycler program and measuring the temperature of the wells with a temperature probe to check the observed temperatures are within specification. If the observed temperatures are not within specification, the thermocycler will need to be re-calibrated following the equipment manufacturer's instructions.
13. Random amplification failure can be caused by inadequate contact between the thermocycler heat block and PCR tray or tubes. Ensure that the correct trays or PCR tubes are used for the thermocycler.
14. A DNA molecular weight marker should be run on the gel as the SSP method amplifies DNA of many different sizes so results need to checked against the size marker to ensure that a positive amplification result is of the correct size and not a false positive or primer dimer.
15. The presence of blurry amplification bands on the gel may be caused by the electrophoresis buffer becoming too hot due to excess voltage when running the gel; the wrong electrophoresis buffer composition; old electrophoresis buffer being used; or the agarose not being dissolved properly before pouring the gel. To avoid these problems lower the voltage during gel elec-

trophoresis, use fresh electrophoresis buffer and ensure the agarose is dissolved properly before pouring the gel.

16. Heavy streaking in random wells can be caused by uneven suspensions of DNA. Mix the PCR product up and down several times before loading the gel.
17. Occasional faint amplification bands may be due to a gel loading problem. Use slow, steady pipetting when loading the gel so the sample does not float away.
18. A photo can be taken of the gel on a UV transilluminator using a digital camera with an orange filter.
19. The negative control well contains the control primer set but no DNA. Any amplification seen when the negative control is run on the gel is evidence of DNA contamination at some stage of the test process and results of the test are invalid.
20. To avoid the risk of false negative reactions in the SSP method, internal controls must be used for every SSP PCR mix to verify the PCR conditions. Typically these controls are primers for a non-variable or conserved gene present in all samples and the control primer set is selected to amplify a DNA fragment of a different size to that expected from the HLA primer sets. In order to score a reaction with an HLA primer set as negative, the control amplification must be positive (amplified DNA detected) and the HLA amplicon absent. If the control amplicon is absent and the HLA amplicon is also absent, it cannot be assumed that this is a true negative result as there may be inhibition of the PCR in that tray well or tube. However, the presence of a specific HLA amplicon with no control amplification can be scored as a positive result. This conclusion is based on the fact that the PCR of the HLA gene usually amplifies better than the control PCR as the control primers are present in a lower concentration in order to favour the HLA specific reaction (see Fig. 1). Table 2 summarises the interpretation of SSP results.
21. Care must be taken when assigning homozygous results by the SSP method, particularly if any of the control amplicons are absent. The rates of homozygosity should be monitored, especially if there is a high rate of control amplification failure.
22. Interpretation of primer dimer as specific amplification bands can lead to false positive results. Always check the amplification band is the correct size.
23. Non-specific amplification (ladders or smears) may be seen if there are impurities in the test DNA or excess test DNA is used. Check the DNA quality and concentration. If required re-precipitate the DNA (ethanol and salt step) and resuspend the DNA in $dH_2O$ or repeat the whole DNA extraction with new reagents.

24. The presence of more than two specific HLA alleles indicates contamination between PCR products or between DNA samples during the DNA extraction or PCR preparation stages. Make sure the pre- and post-PCR work is kept separate (different rooms, lab coats, gloves, equipment and reagents); clean the working area with 10% bleach and ensure there is no mixing of PCR amplicons. Check there has been no mix up at the DNA extraction stage—check other test samples for a possible mix up.
25. False positive SSP reactions can be caused by contamination when dispensing reagents to set up the PCR or when loading the gel with the amplified product. Take more care when pipetting during the PCR setup or when loading the gel.
26. A false positive or false negative reaction may be due to an error in loading the gel so that the PCRs have been loaded in the wrong order. Check the alignment of the PCR mixes and gel lanes.
27. An unexpected positive or negative reaction may sometimes be due to the presence of a new allele. Repeat the typing and if the same reaction is seen verify the typing by SBT.
28. Persistent false negative or positive reactions with the same PCR mix may be due to a kit problem. Double check the kit with a control sample and advise the supplier if the control sample also gives the same false negative or positive result.
29. If an error is made during the PCR setup, this can lead to inefficient amplification and weak probe signals. The PCR must be set up exactly as specified in the kit instructions in relation to reagent volumes and concentrations. Ensure that pipettes are calibrated.
30. If insufficient test DNA, poor quality or degraded DNA is used, there may be inefficient amplification and weak probe signals. If this occurs, the volume, concentration, and purity of the test DNA should be checked. If required re-precipitate the DNA (ethanol and salt step) and resuspend the DNA in $dH_2O$ or repeat the whole DNA extraction with new reagents. DNA can be extracted from nucleated cells by any preferred method (in-house or commercial kit, manual or robotic system). If blood samples are used the anticoagulant should be EDTA or ACD, not heparin which can inhibit the PCR. DNA should be kept in TE buffer for long-term storage, the final concentration of the DNA prior to amplification should be according to the recommendations of the kit supplier as this varies depending on the kit used. The $OD_{260/280}$ of the DNA should be between 1.6 and 1.9.
31. Incorrect PCR conditions can result in a low level of amplification or no amplification of the test DNA (and consequently weak or no hybridisation signals). If this occurs, the PCR program should be checked.

32. Always handle the membranes at the end of the strips using forceps.
33. If the water bath, incubator, or wash solution temperature is too high when removing non-specifically bound probe (stringency wash step), it can result in weak hybridisation signals. If the wash temperature is too low, there can be false positive probe signals or high background on the probe support membrane. It is important to set the temperature with a calibrated thermometer and to monitor the temperature during the stringency wash step.
34. If the wash buffer solution is made up incorrectly, this can cause either weak hybridisation signals, high background on the probe support membrane or false positive probe signals. It is critical that wash buffer solutions are prepared carefully and that salt concentrations are correct.
35. High background on the probe support membrane can be caused by detergent residue in the hybridisation or wash containers. Do not use detergent when washing the containers or beakers used for making solutions but rinse the containers very well with water.
36. High background on the probe support membrane can be due to the conjugate step being performed at an incorrect temperature. Monitor this step with a calibrated thermometer.
37. Ensure the substrate incubation time is correct. If the time is too short, this can lead to weak hybridisation signals and if it is too long it can result in high background on the probe support membrane. Also check that the substrate is at room temperature before it is used.
38. If the positive control result is strong but the probe intensity of the test samples is weak, this is most likely due to a weak PCR because of insufficient test DNA or poor quality DNA. If this occurs, the volume, concentration, and purity of the test DNA should be checked. If required re-precipitate the DNA (ethanol and salt step) and resuspend the DNA in $dH_2O$ or repeat the whole DNA extraction with new solutions. Use non-heparinised blood to extract DNA.

## References

1. Olerup O, Zetterquist H (1992) HLA-DR typing by PCR amplification with sequence-specific primers (PCR-SSP) in 2 hours: an alternative to serological DR typing in clinical practice including donor-recipient matching in cadaveric transplantation. Tissue Antigens 39:225–235
2. Olerup O, Aldener A, Fogdell A (1993) HLA-DQB1 and -DQA1 typing by PCR amplification with sequence-specific primers (PCR-SSP) in 2 hours. Tissue Antigens 41:119–134
3. Bunce M, Taylor CJ, Welsh KI (1993) Rapid HLA-DQB typing by eight polymerase chain

reaction amplifications with sequence-specific primers (PCR-SSP). Hum Immunol 37: 201–206

4. Browning MJ, Krausa P, Rowan A et al (1993) Tissue typing the HLA-A locus from genomic DNA by sequence-specific PCR: comparison of HLA genotype and surface expression on colorectal tumor cell lines. Proc Natl Acad Sci USA 90:2842–2845
5. Sadler AM, Petronzelli F, Krausa P et al (1994) Low-resolution DNA typing for HLA-B using sequence-specific primers in allele- or group-specific ARMS/PCR. Tissue Antigens 44:148–154
6. Bunce M, O'Neill CM, Barnardo MCNM et al (1995) Phototyping: comprehensive DNA typing for HLA-A, B, C, DRB1, DRB3, DRB4, DRB5 & DQB1 by PCR with 144 primer mixes utilising sequence-specific primers (PCR-SSP). Tissue Antigens 46:355–367
7. Wordsworth BP, Allsopp CE, Young RP et al (1990) HLA-DR typing using DNA amplification by the polymerase chain reaction and sequential hybridization to sequence-specific oligonucleotide probes. Immunogenetics 32:413–418
8. Morel C, Zwahlen F, Jeannet M et al (1990) Complete analysis of HLA-DQB1 polymorphism and DR-DQ linkage disequilibrium by oligonucleotide typing. Hum Immunol 29:64–77
9. Scharf SJ, Griffith RL, Erlich HA (1991) Rapid typing of DNA sequence polymorphism at the HLA-DRB1 locus using the polymerase chain reaction and nonradioactive oligonucleotide probes. Hum Immunol 30:190–201
10. Kimura A, Sasazuki T (1992) Eleventh international histocompatibility workshop reference protocol for the HLA-DNA typing technique. In: Tsuji K, Aizawa M, Sasazuki T (eds) HLA 1991. Oxford University Press, Oxford, p 397
11. Gao X, Jakobsen IB, Serjeantson SW (1994) Characterization of the HLA-A polymorphism by locus-specific polymerase chain reaction amplification and oligonucleotide hybridization. Hum Immunol 41:267–279
12. Cereb N, Yang SY (1997) Dimorphic primers derived from intron 1 for use in the molecular typing of HLA-B alleles. Tissue Antigens 50:74–76
13. Erlich H, Bugawan T, Begovich AB et al (1991) HLA-DR, DQ and DP typing using PCR amplification and immobilized probes. Eur J Immunogenet 18:33–55
14. Bugawan TL, Apple R, Erlich HA (1994) A method for typing polymorphism at the HLA-A locus using PCR amplification and immobilized oligonucleotide probes. Tissue Antigens 44:137–147
15. Robinson J, Malik A, Parham P et al (2000) IMGT/HLA—a sequence database for the human major histocompatibility complex. Tissue Antigens 55:280–287. http://www.ebi.ac.uk/imgt/hla/
16. Robinson J, Mistry K, McWilliam H et al (2011) The IMGT/HLA database. Nucleic Acids Res 39(suppl 1):D1171–D1176
17. Mytilineos J, Scherer S, Dunckley H et al (1993) DNA HLA-DR typing results of 4000 kidney transplants. Transplantation 55:778–781
18. Mytilineos J, Lempert M, Middleton D et al (1997) HLA class I DNA typing of 215 "HLA-A, -B, -DR zero mismatched" kidney transplants. Tissue Antigens 50:355–358
19. Lorentzen DF, Iwanaga KK, Meuer KJ et al (1997) 25% Error rate in serologic typing of HLA-B homozygotes. Tissue Antigens 50:359–365
20. Mytilineos J, Christ U, Lempert M et al (1997) Comparison of typing results by serology and polymerase chain reaction with sequence-specific primers for HLA-Cw in 650 individuals. Tissue Antigens 50:395–400

# Chapter 3

# Methods for Diagnostic HLA Typing in Disease Association and Drug Hypersensitivity

**Michael D. Varney, Alison S.L. Castley, Katri Haimila, and Päivi Saavalainen**

## Abstract

This chapter describes the application of diagnostic HLA typing for disease association and five methods used for specific HLA genotypes. The methods utilise a combination of polymerase chain reaction (PCR) amplification to detect sequence polymorphism by the presence or absence of amplification, nucleotide sequencing of the PCR product, and hybridisation of the PCR product with labelled probes. The probes are specific for sequence polymorphism associated with the genotype and are attached to either a Micro Bead or a Solid Phase. In addition, the detection of single nucleotide polymorphism(s) which "tag" for the genotype using a real-time PCR is described.

**Key words:** HLA, Disease, Association, Hypersensitivity, Methods, B*27, B*57, Coeliac, B*1502, Narcolepsy, DQ

## 1. Introduction

Many diseases have been shown to be associated with antigens, alleles, epitopes, or haplotypes at different loci within the HLA region and yet the diagnostic value of these associations, with a number of exceptions, remains unclear. This chapter briefly outlines the challenges of disease association studies and their role in a diagnostic HLA typing laboratory and describes a combination of locally designed and commercially available HLA typing methods utilised for diagnostic HLA typing requests.

Typically in disease association studies, the frequency of a particular HLA polymorphism in a patient population is compared to a control population by constructing a 2 × 2 contingency table and

Frank T. Christiansen and Brian D. Tait (eds.), *Immunogenetics: Methods and Applications in Clinical Practice*, Methods in Molecular Biology, vol. 882, DOI 10.1007/978-1-61779-842-9_3, © Springer Science+Business Media New York 2012

testing the null hypothesis that no difference exists using the chi-squared test with Yates' correction or Fishers exact test. The strength of the association is measured by calculating the relative risk or odds ratio in the presence of a statistically significant difference (typically $p < 0.05$). To avoid a type 1 error (false positive finding) when many HLA polymorphisms are compared, the $p$ value may be conservatively corrected by multiplying it by the number of comparisons made (Bonferroni correction). Association studies in the HLA region are further complicated by the presence of linkage disequilibrium in that alleles at different loci are not always randomly associated. In association studies this makes the delineation of the causative loci problematic. Whilst appropriate statistical consideration is important in association studies, the selection of a clearly defined patient group and matched controls remains pivotal.

The use of HLA genotyping as a diagnostic test is dependent on the test sensitivity (proportion of disease positive patients correctly identified by the genotype i.e. true positive (TP) vs. false positive (FP)) and the test specificity (proportion of disease negative patients correctly identified by the genotype i.e. true negative (TN) vs. FP). However, the diagnostic relevance of the genotype result is the probability that it will positively predict disease (the probability that a genotype positive person will have the disease i.e. TP/TP+FP) or the absence of disease (the probability that a genotype negative person will not have the disease i.e. TN/TN+FN) (reviewed at (1, 2)). Whilst a positive predictive value may be requested of HLA genotyping, its value often lies in the negative predictive value. For example, the HLA genotypes associated with coeliac disease (Table 1) have a negative predictive value greater than 99%.

A large number of methods for HLA typing utilising the polymerase chain reaction (PCR) amplification of DNA have been published and described in collaborative workshops and this volume. This chapter has selected five methods and described their use in determining the genotypes associated with disease and drug hypersensitivity described in Table 1. However, it is recognised that each method has the potential to determine other genotypes and that the methods may be used in conjunction with one another.

Sequence Specific Priming (SSP) utilises the inefficient PCR amplification of a primer that contains a 3′ nucleotide mismatch. This inefficiency permits the design of PCR primers that, while specific for their target sequence, will not amplify closely related sequences (4). By standardising the PCR cycling conditions for a range of primers, multiple nucleotide differences in HLA genes can be detected using a pattern of amplification that corresponds to HLA alleles (5). The methods described below for HLA-DR and DQ are used locally to determine the genotypes associated with coeliac disease, narcolepsy, Type 1 diabetes, and carbamazepine hypersensitivity in conjunction with sequence-based typing (SBT) to resolve the DQB1*0302, 0602, and B*15 alleles.

**Table 1**
**Diagnostic HLA disease and hypersensitivity associations**

| Disease/hypersensitivity | HLA association | Notes |
|---|---|---|
| Ankylosing spondylitis | B-27 | High negative predictor B27 allele type may provide further discrimination; B*2702-08,10/14/15/19 positively associated, whereas B*2709 appears protective (3) |
| Narcolepsy | DQB1*0602 | DRB1*15 is in strong linkage disequilibrium with DQB1*0602 |
| Coeliac disease | DQA1*05, DQB1*02, DQB1*0302 | High negative predictor |
| Rheumatoid arthritis | DRB1*0401/04/05/13, 0101/02, 1402, 1001 | Positive DRB1 allele association reflects a "shared epitope" (QKRAA) at amino acids 70–75 |
| Type 1 diabetes | DRB1*03-DQB102, DRB1* 04-DQB1*0302 (DRB1* 15-DQB1*0602 protective) | May be used to assess familial risk |
| Abacavir hypersensitivity | B*5701 | High negative predictor |
| Carbamazepine hypersensitivity (Stevens–Johnson syndrome) | B*1502 | Restricted to Asian genetic background |

In addition, methods for the detection of HLA-B27 and B-57 using whole blood rather than DNA as a template are described.

SBT typically uses the Sanger approach with fluorescently labelled dideoxynucleotides in a cycle sequencing reaction using a purified PCR product. The subsequent reaction is "cleaned" of unincorporated dyes, dNTPs, and primers by precipitation or magnetic bead separation and the resulting fragments detected in an automated analyser. Nucleotide sequence is interpreted from the fragment analysis using an automated analysis program and compared to the known sequence of HLA alleles. The methods described below use PCR primer pairs specific for groups of alleles to allow sequencing of a single allele e.g. DQB1*02, *0302,*0602, DRB1*01,* 04, *14, *10, B*57, and B*15 allele combinations. Other approaches include sequencing of a single PCR product at each loci (6) using Sanger sequencing or the application of next generation sequencing (7). The reagents for both SSP and SBT at most HLA loci and analysis software packages are available commercially.

Micro Bead hybridisation assays utilise a series microsphere beads containing immobilised biotinylated oligonucleotide probes that are hybridised to PCR amplified DNA in a single well of a 96-well microtitre plate. Individual beads are recognised by a

**Table 2**
**Coeliac disease associated DQ2 and DQ8 haplotypes and their prediction by the six tagging single nucleotide polymorphisms (SNPs)**

| DQ haplotype | DRB1 | DQA1 | DQB1 | SNP rs number | Positive predicting allele (other allele) | Negative predicting allele (other allele) | Applied biosystems assay number |
|---|---|---|---|---|---|---|---|
| DQ2.5 | 03 | **0501** | **0201** | rs2187668 | T(C) | | C_58662585_10 |
| DQ8 | 04 | 0301 | 0302 | rs7454108 | C(T) | | C_29817179_10 |
| DQ7 | 11/12/13 | **0505** | 0301 | rs4639334 (rs79616158[a]) | A(G) | | C_42975350_10 |
| DQ2.2 | 07 | 0201 | **0202** | rs2395182 | T(G) | | C_11409965_10 |
| | | | | rs4713586 | | G(A) | C_27950246_10 |
| | | | | rs7775228 | C(T) | | C_29315313_10 |

The CD associated DQA1*05 and DQB1*02 alleles (marked bold) are located either *in cis* in the same DQ2.5 (DR-DQ2) haplotype or *in trans* in patients carrying both DQ7 and DQ2.2 haplotypes
[a]The TaqMan assay number C_42975350_10 for DQ7 refers currently to a changed SNP rs number (rs79616158) which is different to that in the referenced tables (8, 9)

combination of two internal fluorescent dyes and positive hybridisation by fluorescently labelled (Streptavidin-PE) captured PCR products in a flow cytometric analysis system. A number of commercial companies e.g. One Lambda (http://www.onelambda.com) and Lifecodes (http://www.gen-probe.com) provide complete HLA typing kits. The method described below is a summary of the commercial Luminex/Labtype (http://www.OneLambda.com) protocol with minor modifications.

A large number of solid phase hybridisation assays have been described which include the binding of either PCR product or oligonucleotide probe to a nylon membrane support and the colour or chemiluminescent detection of probes. The method described below utilises a biotinylated PCR product which is immobilised to streptavidin-coated microtitre plate and hybridised with a series of fluorescent probes in a single well of a microtitre plate. The probes are labelled with chelates of lanthanide metals which have distinct fluorescent profiles allowing the detection of several probes in the same assay. The method is a summary of the commercial DELFIA (http://www.las.perkinelmer.com) Coeliac Disease assay.

An alternative approach to HLA genotyping is the typing of single nucleotide polymorphisms (SNPs) which tag for HLA haplotypes. For coeliac disease, six tagging SNPs have been identified and validated in Caucasian populations only for the associated HLA-DQ2 and DQ8 haplotypes (Table 2). Whilst the specificities and sensitivities are high (8, 9) (97–100%), they are not complete due to the presence of rare haplotypes and so the method is not recommended for diagnostic testing but is cost effective and suitable for high-throughput screening assays. The method uses TaqMan® chemistry (http://www.AppliedBiosystems.com) and two allele-specific dual labelled probes with alternative 5′ dyes and a 3′ Quencher dye which bind to the SNP complementary target sequence in a real-time PCR. Positive hybridisation results in the release of a unique reporter dye detected by a fluorimeter allowing allelic discrimination.

## 2. Materials

### *2.1. Sequence Specific Priming and Sequence-Based Typing*

1. HLA-B 10× PCR Buffer: To prepare dissolve 8.11 g Trisma-Base in 80 mL $H_2O$ on a magnetic stirrer and adjust to pH = 8.8 using concentrated HCl. Add 2.19 g $(NH_4)_2$ $SO_4$ and dissolve. Make up to 95 mL, filter through a 0.22-μm filter, and add 1 mL Tween 20. Aliquot and store frozen.
2. SSP Buffer: To prepare 1,500 μL add 500 μL 10× 1.5 mM $MgCl_2$ PCR Buffer (as supplied with Taq DNA Polymerase), 500 μL 10× dNTPS, 250 μL Glycerol, 200 μL $H_2O$, 50 μL Cresol Red Solution (10 mg/mL diluted in $H_2O$).
3. 10× dNTPS: A stock solution is prepared containing a final concentration of 2 mM of dCTP, dGTP, dATP, and dTTP diluted in $H_2O$.
4. B*1502 Master Mix: For each sample a 39-μL Master Mix is prepared containing 5 μL HLA-B 10× PCR buffer, 2 μL dNTPs (40 mM), 2 μL 50 mM $MgCl_2$, 3.25 μL B*1502 primer mix, 35.35 μL $H_2O$.
5. B*27 Master Mix: For each sample a 39-μL Master Mix is prepared containing 5 μL HLA-B 10× PCR buffer, 0.3 μL dNTPs (40 mM), 6 μL B*27 primer mix, 27.7 μL $H_2O$.
6. B*57 Master Mix: For each sample a 39-μL Master Mix is prepared containing 5 μL HLA-B 10× PCR buffer, 2 μL dNTPs (40 mM), 3 μL 50 mM $MgCl_2$, 15.75 μL B*57 primer mix, 13.25 μL $H_2O$.
7. Formamide Master Mix: For each sample prepare a formamide mix containing 5 μL Deionised Formamide and 4 μL deionised $H_2O$.
8. 2.5 mM $MgCL_2$ DQB PCR Buffer: To prepare sufficient for 200 reactions (4,310 μL) add 500 μL 10× PCR Buffer (as supplied with Taq DNA Polymerase, no $MgCl_2$), 250 μL 50 mM $MgCl_2$, 500 μL 10× dNTPS, 250 μL DiMethyl Sulphoxide, 3,010 μL $H_2O$; 2.0 and 1.2 mM $MgCL_2$ DQB PCR Buffers are prepared by adjusting the proportion of 50 mM $MgCl_2$ and $H_2O$ appropriately.

9. 1.5 mM $MgCL_2$ DRB PCR Buffer: To prepare sufficient for 200 reactions (4,560 μL) add 500 μL 10× PCR Buffer (as supplied with AmpliTaq DNA Polymerase, no $MgCl_2$), 150 μL 50 mM $MgCl_2$, 500 μL 10× dNTPS, 3,410 μL $H_2O$; 2.0 mM $MgCl_2$ DRB PCR Buffer is prepared by adjusting the proportion of 50 mM $MgCl_2$ and $H_2O$ appropriately.
10. SBT HLA-B Master Mix: To prepare sufficient for 200 reactions (4,960 μL) add 500 μL HLA-B 10× PCR Buffer, 180 μL 50 mM $MgCl_2$, 500 μL 10× dNTPS, 150 μL Dimethyl Suphoxide, and HLA-B gen Primer Mix 600 μL, 2,670 μL $H_2O$ or HLA-B TA Primer Mix 600 μL, 500 μL 0.1 M β-Mercaptoethanol, 2,170 μL $H_2O$ or HLA-B CG Primer Mix 400 μL, 500 μL 0.1 M β-Mercaptoethanol, 2,370 μL $H_2O$.
11. Specialist equipment: Applied Biosytems 3730 DNA Analyser or equivalent.

### 2.2. Micro Bead Hybridisation Typing Assay

1. Denaturing Buffer, Neutralising Buffer, Hybridisation Buffer, Bead Mixtures, Wash Buffer, 100× SAPE, SAPE buffer as supplied by the manufacturer (OneLambda).
2. Specialist equipment: Luminex® LABScan™ Analyser or equivalent.

### 2.3. DELFIA Hybridisation

1. Wash Concentrate, Bio-Hybridization Control, Hybridization Buffer, labelled probes, Enhancer Solution, Enhancement Solution, streptavidin coated microtitration strips as supplied by the manufacturer.
2. dNTP mix (10 mM).
3. Sodium Hydroxide solution (20 mmol/L): Prepare the solution: 2.0 mL NaOH Titrisol 1 mol/L, add ultrapure water to a volume of 100 mL, store maximum 2 months, the solution is corrosive.
4. Tris buffer 10 mM, pH 8.0, Tris, p.a. 0.61 g, ultrapure water add 500 mL, store maximum 1 year, the solution is irritating.
5. Specialist equipment: automatic microplate washer, e.g. DELFIA Platewasher, plateshaker, a time-resolved fluorometer e.g. VICTOR.

### 2.4. TaqMan® Typing of HLA-Tagging SNPs in Coeliac Disease

1. TaqMan® (2×) Genotyping Master Mix (Applied Biosystems).
2. TaqMan® (20×) SNP Genotyping Assay Mix (Applied Biosystems).
3. PCR-quality $H_2O$.
4. Specialist equipment: ABI 7900HT real-time PCR system (Applied Biosystems) or equivalent with 84- or 96-well optical PCR plates and lids.

## 3. Methods

### 3.1. Sequence Specific Priming

1. The identification of an individual or group of alleles is determined by the presence or absence of the correctly sized test PCR product (Table 3) using standard agarose or polyacrylamide gel electrophoresis. In addition, a control PCR product indicates the success of the assay which may or may not be present when the test PCR is positive.
2. DRB/DQ. For each primer mix (see Note 1) being tested, prepare an SSP Master Mix containing 5 μL of the primer mix, 3 μL SSP Buffer, and 0.1 μL Taq DNA Polymerase (5 U/μL).
3. Aliquot 8 μL of SSP Master Mix into a 200-μL PCR strip tube or plate and add 2 μL DNA (50 ng/μL) (see Note 2).
4. Seal the tubes/plates and cycle in a PCR machine for 96°C-120 s, 96°C-10 s, 65°C-60 s ×10 cycles, 96°C-10 s, 61°C-50 s, 72°C-30 s ×20 cycles, 20°C hold.
5. HLA-B*1502. For each sample add 0.4 μL of AmpliTAQ DNA polymerase to 47.6 μL of B*1502 Master Mix (see Note 1), mix by gently flicking and add 2 μL DNA (30 ng/μL).
6. Seal the tubes and cycle in a PCR machine for 96°C-60 s ×1 cycle, 96°C-25 s, 70°C-45 s, 72°C-45 s ×4 cycles, 96°C-625 s, 65°C-50 s, 72°C-45 s ×24 cycles, 96°C-25 s, 55°C-60 s, 72°C-80 s ×10 cycles, 15°C hold.
7. HLA-B*27 and B*57 (whole blood, see Note 2). Add 9.0 μL of formamide mix to a PCR microtube and 1 μL of whole blood, cap the tube, and mix by gently flicking.
8. Incubate at 95°C in a thermal cycler for 5–10 min, remove the tubes and immediately place them on ice for at least 2 min.
9. For each sample add 1.0 μL of AmpliTAQ DNA polymerase to 39 μL of B*27 or B*57 Master Mix (see Note 1) and add to the denatured blood sample. Mix by gently flicking.
10. Seal the tubes and for B*27 cycle in a PCR machine for 85°C-120 s, 55°C-45 s, 60°C-60 s ×7 cycles, 85°C-60 s, 50°C-45 s, 60°C-90 s ×15 cycles, 85°C-60 s, 45°C-45 s, 60°C-120 s ×10 cycles, 15°C hold. For B*57 cycle for 85°C-120 s, 86°C-25 s, 60°C-45 s, 62°C-45 s ×4 cycles, 86°C-25 s, 55°C-50 s, 62°C-45 s ×24 cycles, 86°C-25 s, 45°C-45 s, 62°C-45 s ×10 cycles, 15°C hold.

### 3.2. Sequence-Based Typing

1. Select the PCR reaction(s) for the association to be tested using the primer pair specificities listed in Table 4. Additional primer pairs e.g. DQB1*0201/02/03, B CG are described to assist in the resolution of ambiguous results.

**Table 3**
**SSP primer pair sequences and specificity used in diagnostic HLA disease and hypersensitivity association testing**

| Primer pair specificity[a] (PCR product size) | Primer sequences (direction) | Primer mix final concentration (μM) |
|---|---|---|
| DQA1*05 (186 bp) | GGTCCCTCTGGCCAGTTC (f) | 1.5 |
| | GTTGGAGCGTTTAATCAGAC (r) | 1.5 |
| DQB1*0201-05 (200 bp) | TGCGTCTTGTGAGCAGAAG (f) | 1.5 |
| | CGTGCGGAGCTCCAACTG (r) | 1.5 |
| DQB1*0302/03/07/11/12/15/18/20/23/26,*0604/05/07/09/25/27/32/34-39 (170 bp) | GACGGAGCGCGTGCGTCT (f) | 1.5 |
| | AACTCCGCCCGGGTCCT (r) | 1.5 |
| DQB1*0501-05, 0601-39 (285 bp) | TTCCCCGCAGAGGATTTCGT (f) | 1.5 |
| | CTCTCCTCTGCARGATCCC (r) | 1.5 |
| DRB1*1501-43 except 150107,1521/27/34 (215 bp) | TTCCTGTGGCAGCCTAAGAGG (f) | 1.0 |
| | TCCACCGTGGCCCGCGC (r) | 1.0 |
| DQB1*0601-39 except 0623 (220 bp) | GACGGAGCGCGTGCGTCT (f) | 0.5 |
| | GACGGAGCGCGTGCGTTA (f) | 0.5 |
| | GCAAGATCCCGCGGAACG (r) | 0.5 |
| | GCAGGATCCCGCGGTACC (r) | 0.5 |
| PCR amplification control used in all DQ primer pairs (693 bp) | TGCCAAGTGGAGCCCCAA (f) | 0.2–0.4 |
| | GCATCTTGCTCTGTGCAGAT (r) | 0.2–0.4 |
| B*1502[b] (357 bp) | CGGAACACACAGATCTCCAAGACC (f) | 3.57 |
| | GCCATACATCCTCTGGATGAT (r) | 3.57 |

| | | |
|---|---|---|
| B*1502 amplification control (439 bp) | CAGTGCCTTCCCAACCATTCCCTTA (f) | 0.71 |
| | ATCCACTCACGGATTTCTGTTGTGTTTC (r) | 0.71 |
| B*27 (141 bp) | AGT CTG TGC CTT GGC CTT GC (f) | 6.67 |
| | GCT ACG TGG ACG ACA CGC (r) | 6.67 |
| B*27 amplification control (439 bp) | CAGTGCCTTCCCAACCATTCCCTTA (f) | 0.42 |
| | ATCCACTCACGGATTTCTGTTGTGTTTC (r) | 0.42 |
| B*57 (130 bp) | TGTAAAACGACGGCCAGTGTCTCACATCATCCAGGT (f) | 1.82 |
| B*57 amplification control (439 bp) | CAGGAAACAGCTATGACCATCCTTGCCGTCGTAGGCGG (r) | 1.82 |
| | CAGGAAACAGCTATGACCATCCTTGCCGTCGTAGGCAG (r) | 1.82 |
| | CAGTGCCTTCCCAACCATTCCCTTA (f) | 1.09 |
| | ATCCACTCACGGATTTCTGTTGTGTTTC (r) | 1.09 |

[a]IMGT database 2.28

[b]The HLA-B*1502 primers also amplify some rarer HLA-B alleles, all positive results must be confirmed by an alternative HLA-B PCR/SBT assay

**Table 4**
**SBT primer pair sequences and specificity used in diagnostic HLA disease and hypersensitivity association testing**

| Primer pair Id and specificity[a] (sequencing primer, PCR product size) | Primer sequence (direction) | Primer mix concentration |
|---|---|---|
| DQB2,3,4 | TGTAAAACGACGGCCAGTTATTCCCCGCAGAGGATTTCG (f) | 6.25 μM |
| DQB1*0201-05,*0301-26,*0401-04 (M13, 285 bp) | TGTAAAACGACGGCCAGTTATTCCTCGCAGAGGATTTCG (f) | 6.25 μM |
| | TGTAAAACGACGGCCAGTCTCGCCGCTGCAAGGTCGT (r) | 12.5 μM |
| DQB5,6 | TGTAAAACGACGGCCAGTTATTCCCCGCAGAGGATTTCG (f) | 12.5 μM |
| DQB1*0501-05, 0601-39 (M13, 285 bp) | CAGGAAACAGCTATGACCCTCTCCTCTGCAAGATCCC (r) | 6.25 μM |
| | CAGGAAACAGCTATGACCCTCTCCTCTGCAGGATCCC (r) | 6.25 μM |
| PCR amplification control (693 bp) | TGCCAAGTGGAGCCCCAA (r) | 2.5 μM |
| | GCATCTTGCTCTGTGCAGAT (r) | 2.5 μM |
| DQB2 | TGTAAAACGACGGCCAGTAGGAAGGCGGATTCCCGAAGA (f) | 12.5 μM |
| DQB1*0201-03 (M13, 584 bp) | CAGGAAACAGCTATGACCCTGTCCTCTGGGGTGGAACA (r) | 12.5 μM |
| DQB7 | TGTAAAACGACGGCCAGTAGGAAGGCGGATTCCCGAAGA (f) | 12.5 μM |
| DQB1*0301/04 (M13, 591 bp) | CAGGAAACAGCTATGACCTGTCCCCTGGGGTGGAACG (r) | 12.5 μM |
| DR1 (M13, 463 bp) | TGTAAAACGACGGCCAGTTCCCAGTGCCCGCTCCCT (f) | 12.5 μM |
| | CAGGAAACAGCTATGACCACACACTCAGATTCTCCGCTT (r) | 12.5 μM |
| DR3/11/13/14 (M13, 501 bp) | TGTAAAACGACGGCCAGTTGGTGGGCGTTGGGGCG (f) | 12.5 μM |
| | CAGGAAACAGCTATGACCACACACACACTCAGATTCCCA (r) | 12.5 μM |
| DR4 (M13, 528 bp) | TGTAAAACGACGGCCAGTAGCCACTGGGTGCGTGTT (f) | 12.5 μM |
| | CAGGAAACAGCTATGACCACACACACACTCAGATTCTCC (r) | 12.5 μM |

| | | |
|---|---|---|
| DR10 (M13, 495 bp) | TGTAAAACGACGGCCAGTGGCGTTGCGGGTCGGCG (f) | 12.5 μM |
| | CAGGAAACAGCTATGACCACACACAGAGTCAGATTCCCA (r) | 12.5 μM |
| DR15/16 (M13, 756 bp) | TGTAAAACGACGGCCAGTGGTGGGTGCTGTTGAAGGT (f) | 12.5 μM |
| | CAGGAAACAGCTATGACCACACACACACTCAGATTCCCA (r) | 12.5 μM |
| B CG | TGTAAAACGACGGCCAGTCGGGGGCGCAGGACCCGG (f) | 10 μM |
| B*13,15,18,27,37,38,39,40,41,44, 45,46,47,49,50,54,55,56, 57,59,82 (M13, ~1 kb) | CAGGAAACAGCTATGACCCCATCCCSGGCGAYCTAT (r) | 10 μM |
| B TA | TGTAAAACGACGGCCAGTGGCGGGGGCGCAGGACCTGA (f) | 5 μM |
| B*07,08,14,1502,35,42,48,51,52, 53,58,67,78,81 (M13, ~1 kb) | CAGGAAACAGCTATGACCCCATCCCSGGCGAYCTAT (r) | 5 μM |
| M13 sequencing primers | TGTAAAACGACGGCCAGT (f) | 3.2pM |
| | CAGGAAACAGCTATGACC (r) | 3.2pM |
| B gen (B gen, ~1 kb size) | GGGTCCCAGTTCTAAAGTCCCCACG (f) | 3.33 μM |
| | CCATCCCCGGCGACCTATAGGAGATG (r) | 3.33 μM |
| | AGGCCATCCCGGGCGATCTAT (r) | 3.33 μM |
| B gen sequencing primers | GGGCGCAGGACCYGRGGA (f) | 3.2 pM |
| | GGAGGCCATCCCCGGCGACCTAT (r) | 3.2 pM |

[a]IMGT database 2.28

2. DQB1 PCR: A 25-μL PCR is prepared for each sample containing 21.5 μL DQB PCR Buffer (DQB234 = 2.5 mM $MgCl_2$, DQB56 and DQB7 = 1.5 mM $MgCl_2$, DQB2 = 1.2 mM $MgCl_2$), 1 μL DQB Primer Mix (see Note 3), 1.25 μL Glycerol, 0.2 μL Taq DNA Polymerase (5 U/μL), 1 μL DNA (100 ng/μL) in a 200-μL PCR strip tube or plate.
3. Seal the tubes/plates and cycle in a PCR machine for 96°C-120 s ×1 cycle, 96°C-10 s, 65°C-60 s ×10 cycles, 96°C-10 s,61°C-50 s, 72°C-30 s ×20 cycles, 20°C hold. Proceed to step 7.
4. DRB1 PCR: A 25-μL PCR is prepared for each sample containing 22.5 μL DRB PCR Buffer (DR4 = 1.5 mM $MgCl_2$, DR1, DR3/11/13/14, DR10 = 2.0 mM $MgCl_2$), 1 μL DRB Primer Mix (see Note 3), 0.2 μL AmpliTaq DNA Polymerase (5 U/μL), 1 μL DNA (100 ng/μL) in a 200-μL PCR strip tube or plate.
5. Seal the tubes/plates and cycle in a PCR machine for (DR1, DR15/16, DR4, DR3/11/13/14) 96°C-120 s ×1 cycle, 96°C-10 s, 71°C-60 s ×15 cycles, 96°C-30 s, 61°C-40 s, 72°C-30 s ×20 cycles, 72°C-10 min, 20°C hold or (DR10) 96°C-120 s ×1 cycle, 96°C-10 s, 65°C-60 s ×10 cycles, 96°C-10 s, 59°C-50 s, 72°C-30 s ×20 cycles, 20°C hold. Proceed to step 8.
6. HLA-B PCR: A 25-μL PCR is prepared for each sample containing 23.9 μL HLA-B PCR Master Mix (see Note 3), 0.1 μL AmpliTaq DNA Polymerase (5 U/μL), 1 μL DNA (100 ng/μL) in a 200-μL PCR strip tube or plate.
7. Seal the tubes/plates and cycle in a PCR machine for 96°C-6 min ×1 cycle, 96°C-30 s, 70°C-60 s, 72°C-30 s ×10 cycles, 96°C-30 s, 68°C-60 s, 72°C-30 s ×15 cycles, 96°C-30 s, 66°C-60 s, 72°C-30 s ×6 cycles, 96°C-25 s, 55°C-60 s, 72°C-120 s ×4 cycles, 72°C-10 min, 1 cycle, 20°C hold.
8. The PCR products may be visualised and approximate size determined using standard agarose or polyacrylamide gel electrophoresis.
9. For each PCR product, remove excess dNTPS and primers by adding 5 μL of PCR product to 5 μL of Exo SAP-IT and incubating at 37°C-15 min, 80°C-15 min, 4°C hold using a PCR machine. Dilute the cleaned PCR product by adding 30 μL of sterile water.
10. Cycle sequencing: Use a 96-well PCR plate to aliquot per sample; 4 μL cleaned PCR product, 10 μL $H_2O$, 4 μL 5× Sequencing Buffer (Applied Biosystems), 1 μL M13 or B gen Sequencing Primer, 1 μL Big Dye Terminator (version 3.1, Applied Biosystems) and cycle for 96°C-10 s ×1 cycle, 96°C-10 s, 50°C-5 s, 60°C-4 min ×25 cycles, 4°C hold. Pulse centrifuge the PCR plates prior to amplification and store the product at 2–8°C in the dark.

11. Dye Terminator Removal: Prepare a Master Mix containing 50 μL 95% Ethanol and 2 μL 3 M Sodium Acetate per sample and aliquot 52 μL into each sequencing reaction. Replace the PCR caps in their original order and invert the plate at least ten times to mix.
12. Centrifuge the plate for 1 min at approximately 800 × *g* and leave at room temperature in the dark for 15 min.
13. Spin the plate at approximately 2,060 × *g* for 45 min, carefully remove from the centrifuge, remove the lids, and immediately discard the supernatant by inverting and flicking the plate onto an absorbent towel (see Note 4).
14. Place the inverted plate on new absorbent towel in the centrifuge centrifuging at approximately 800 × *g* for 1 min.
15. Remove the plate from the centrifuge and add 200 μL of 70% ethanol to each pellet. Discard the absorbent towel from the centrifuge.
16. Recap the plate, invert two to three times to mix and centrifuge at approximately 2,060 × *g* for 10 min.
17. Discard the supernatant by removing the caps, inverting and flicking the plate, and blotting onto an absorbent towel and centrifuging at approximately 800 × *g* for 1 min (see Note 4).
18. Repeat steps 14–16.
19. Dry the upright plate in the 70°C oven for at least 30 min and discard the absorbent towel from the centrifuge.
20. Resuspend in 12 μL Hi-Di formamide, denature at 95°C, cool on an ice bath prior to loading on the Applied Biosytems 3730 DNA Analyser according to the manufacturers' instructions. The analyser separates the dye labelled DNA fragments in a polymer-filled capillary array by electrophoresis. The fragments are detected by excitation of the fluorescent dye which is displayed as an electropherogram by the data collection software. Base calling software is then used to assign a sequence.
21. HLA alleles are assigned by comparing the sequence obtained to a library of reference sequences (http://www.ebi.ac.uk/imgt/hla/). A number of analysis programs have been described (10–12) and detailed elsewhere in this volume to accommodate the HLA reference library and the analysis of both multiple and heterozygote templates.

### 3.3. Micro Bead Hybridisation Typing Assay (Luminex/Labtype)

1. A 10-μL PCR is prepared for each sample containing 6.9 μL D-mix, 2.0 μL Primer Set, 0.1 μL Taq DNA Polymerase (not supplied) and 1 μL DNA (20 ng/μL). Cycle in a Perkin Elmer PCR machine with ramp setting at 9600 for 96°C-180 s ×1 cycle, 96°C-20 s, 60°C-20 s, 72°C-20 s ×5 cycles, 96°C-10 s, 60°C-15 s, 72°C-20 s ×30 cycles, 72°C-10 min, 4°C hold.

2. The PCR products may be visualised and approximate size determined using standard agarose or polyacrylamide gel electrophoresis.
3. Start the Luminex® LABScan™ Analyser according to the manufacturers' instructions and set a PCR machine to a 60°C hold at least 30 min before use.
4. For each sample aliquot 2.5 μL of PCR product and 1.3 μL of Denaturing Buffer into a 96-well PCR microtitre plate, seal the plate, pulse centrifuge, vortex gently, and incubate for 10 min at room temperature.
5. Carefully remove the tray seal and add 2.5 μL of Neutralising Buffer, seal the plate, pulse centrifuge, vortex gently, and place the tray on crushed ice or a tray cooler. Note the colour change from pink to yellow (see Note 5).
6. Prepare the hybridisation mixtures by vortexing the required bead mixtures for 1 min and adding 2 μL of bead mixture to 17 μL of Hybridisation Buffer for each sample being tested.
7. Carefully remove the tray seal, add 19 μL of hybridisation mixture per sample, remove from the ice/cooler, place in a tray holder, seal, and vortex thoroughly.
8. Remove the tray from the holder and place in a thermocycler held at 60°C for exactly 15 min.
9. Immediately place in tray holder, remove the seal and add 50 μL Wash Buffer, seal and centrifuge for 5 min at approximately 1,200 × *g*.
10. Retaining the plate in the holder, remove the seal and remove the Wash Buffer by firmly flicking the tray over a sink or wet waste bin. Maintaining the tray in an inverted position, firmly blot the tray on an absorbent towel immediately followed by five gentle taps of the tray on the towel. Return the tray to an upright position and gently vortex.
11. Repeat steps 9–10 twice for a total of three washes.
12. Prepare sufficient SAPE solution (0.25 μL 100× SAPE stock and 24.75 μL SAPE buffer per sample). Keep refrigerated and protected from light until ready to use.
13. Add 25 μL of SAPE solution to each well, seal the tray, vortex, remove from the holder and place in the thermocycler maintained at 60°C for exactly 5 min.
14. Immediately place in tray holder, remove the seal and add 50 μL Wash Buffer, seal and centrifuge for 5 min at approximately 1,200 × *g*.
15. Retaining the plate in the holder, remove the seal and remove the Wash Buffer by firmly flicking the tray and whilst inverted firmly blot the tray on an absorbent towel followed by five

gentle taps on a clean towel. Return the tray to an upright position and gently vortex.

16. Add 70 μL of Wash Buffer to each well, gently mix using a pipette and transfer entire well contents to a 96-well round bottom reading plate. Store at 2–8°C in the dark until ready to read.
17. Refer to the manufacturers' instructions for the calibration, operation, and data acquisition by the Luminex® LABScan™ Analyser and analysis by the HLA Fusion software.

***3.4. Solid Phase Hybridisation Typing (DELFIA Coeliac Disease)***

1. Prepare a 45-μL PCR Master Mix for each sample and a negative control containing 19 μL ultrapure $H_2O$, 5 μL AmpliTaq Gold 10× PCR Buffer, 5 μL dNTP (2 mM), 5 μL DQA1fo (10 pml/μL), 5 μL DQA1re (10 pml/μL), 2.5 μL DQB1fo (10 pml/μL), 2.5 μL DQB1re (10 pml/μL), 1 μL AmpliTaq Gold per sample (see Note 6).
2. Pipette 45 μL of the Master Mix to each PCR well/tube and add 5 μL of DNA (optimally 20 ng/μL) and cycle at 95°C-15 min ×1 cycle, 95°C-50 s, 54°C-60 s, 72°C-60 s ×40 cycles, 72°C-5 min, 4°C hold. The PCR products may be stored at 2–8°C for 2 days or at approximately −20°C for 2–3 weeks prior to assay.
3. The PCR products may be visualised and approximate size determined using standard agarose or polyacrylamide gel electrophoresis.
4. Binding the PCR products: Dilute the Wash Concentrate (50 + 1,200 mL) and warm half of it in an incubator at 43°C (see Note 7). Dilute the Bio-Hybridization Control to DELFIA Hybridization Buffer (0.5 + 49.5 μL).
5. Pipette 10 μL of water to the wells 1–4 (background control for hybridization), 10 μL of diluted Bio-Hybridization Control to the wells 5–8, 10 μL of negative control to the wells 9–12, 10 μL of each PCR product to 4 wells, 50 μL Hybridization Buffer to each well mentioned above.
6. Incubate 30 min at room temperature on a plateshaker.
7. Dilute the probes with the Hybridization Buffer, 100 μL is required per well. Prepare two solutions: A including Europium (Eu)-DQB1*0302 (1 ng/well) and Terbium(Tb)-DQB1*02 (1 ng/well), and B including Samarium (Sm)-DQA1*05 (3 ng/well), Tb-DQB1 Control (3 ng/well), and Eu-DQA1 Control (0.5 ng/well). The dilutions must be kept on ice and used within 30 min. The probes must be on ice and returned to a freezer as quick as possible (see Note 8).
8. Denaturation and hybridization: Wash the plate four times with 400 μL of prewarmed washing dilution using the automatic washer.

9. Add 150 μL of NaOH solution to each well and incubate for 5 min at room temperature on a plateshaker.
10. Wash the plate four times with 400 μL of prewarmed washing dilution using the automatic washer.
11. Pipette 100 μL of solution A to the wells 1–2, 5–6, 9–10 and 100 μL of solution B to wells 3–4, 7–8, 11–12, etc. There are four replicates for each sample on a plate.
12. Seal the plate and incubate for 2 h (±10 min) at 37°C.
13. Wash the plate six times with 400 μL of prewarmed washing dilution using the automatic washer.
14. Quantitation: Add 200 μL of Enhancement Solution at room temperature (see Note 9) and incubate for 30 min at room temperature on a plateshaker (see Note 10).
15. Measure the Eu and Sm labels by a time-resolved fluorometer.
16. Add 50 μL of Enhancement Solution to each well (see Note 9) and incubate for 5 min at room temperature on a plateshaker.
17. Measure the Tb label using a Time-resolved fluorometer (see Note 11).
18. The probes detect alleles DQB1*0302 (also *0304-5 and *0307-8), DQB1*02 (specific for *0201-03), and DQA1*05 (specific for *0501-05). Homozygotes and heterozygotes cannot be separated.

### 3.5. TaqMan® Typing of HLA-Tagging SNPs in Coeliac Disease

1. For a 384-well microplate, a 4-μL PCR is prepared for each sample containing 2.0 μL TaqMan® (2×) Genotyping Master Mix (Applied Biosystems), 0.2 μL TaqMan® (20×) SNP Genotyping Assay mix and 1.8 μL DNA (10 ng/reaction) suspended in PCR-quality $H_2O$. Prepare a pre-mix of the Genotyping Master Mix and SNP Genotyping Assay mix for the required number of samples and aliquot 2.2 μL to each well of an empty plate followed by 1.8 μL of DNA using a multichannel pipette. Alternatively, first transfer the DNA using a pipette robot into the wells of six identical 384 plates and let the DNA dry into the bottom of the wells at room temperature or 37°C. After drying, the plates can be stored covered with lid at room temperature. To the plates add the pre-mix, described above but including 1.8 μL PCR-quality $H_2O$ instead of DNA, using a multichannel or stepper pipette. To reduce reagent use, the pre-mix may be modified to 1.5 μL Genotyping Master Mix, 0.12 μL SNP Genotyping Assay mix, and 0.58 μL $H_2O$ (or 2.38 μL $H_2O$ if plate dried DNA is used). This may also improve the amplification of some of the SNPs (see Note 12).

2. Leave at least two wells as negative controls with pre-mix but no DNA. The computer program is designed to use these two values to exclude background. They also act as a quality control for the Master Mix, SNP Assay mix and water for contamination. Seal the plate and pulse centrifuge to bring the fluid down. Start ABI 7900HT real-time PCR cycler and complete the assay and well information data according to the instructions of the system.
3. Perform a PCR run of 10 min at 95°C (on the first cycle only), followed by at least 50 cycles of 15 s at 92°C and 1 min at 60°C (see Note 13). Perform these amplification steps with program SDS Standard Curve (Absolute Quantification, AQ). After the plate is ready, run an end-point analysis using program SDS Allelic Discrimination (AD) to obtain allele assignment. The results for each sample are listed as "allele 1" (homozygous FAM), "allele 2" (homozygous VIC), or "both" (heterozygote). Check from the SNP assay data sheet which allele of the SNP is labelled with FAM, and which one with VIC.
4. Check also the *X*-*Y*-plot of the signal intensities from all 384 samples together to double check that three well separated genotype clusters and the negative control cluster are seen. Samples with unclear clustering are removed from the analysis and may require re-examination of the real-time amplification curve and/or classical HLA typing. For the DQ7 tagging, SNP rs4639334 four genotype clusters instead of three are sometimes seen. This is likely to be caused by additional SNPs within the probe or primer target sequence carried by some donors. Attention should be paid to allele calling in addition to checking Hardy-Weinberg equilibrium of the observed genotypes.
5. Export the results from Allelic Discrimination (AD) file into text file. Once all six SNP results are complete, order the detected genotypes of each SNP into Excel for interpretation of the predicted HLA-haplotypes (Table 2).
6. For DQ2.5, DQ8, and DQ7, there is only one SNP for each, and hetero/homozygosity of the predicted SNP alleles usually predicts hetero/homozygosity of these HLA haplotypes. For DQ2.2, one needs the predictive alleles of all three tagging SNP alleles for best prediction value. Report the interpreted HLA types e.g. DQ2.5/DQ8, DQ2.2/DQ7, DQ2.5/DQ2.5, DQ2.5/DQX, DQX/DQX, etc. where DQX means any other allele than the detected DQ2.5, DQ8, DQ7, or DQ2.2.
7. For some rare haplotypes, there might be more than two DQ alleles suggested by the tagging SNPs, and in such cases classical DQ (and possibly also DR typing) is recommended. Exclusion of false negative results by traditional HLA typing is also recommended for confirmed celiac disease patients for which

the tagging SNP method does not predict any DQ2/DQ8 risk haplotypes. Discrepancies between the tagging SNP method and classical HLA-DQ typing may be resolved with reference to the published reference tables (8, 9).

## 4. Notes

1. SSP primer mixes (Table 3) have been designed locally or are drawn from existing literature (13–17).
2. DNA. With the exception of the whole blood SSP method, genomic DNA is used in each method described. A number of published and commercial DNA extractions methods have been described. Heparin is typically avoided as an anti-coagulant as it may inhibit the PCR and must not be used in the HLA-B*27 and B*57 whole blood protocols. The purity and concentration of the DNA can be critical in PCR-based assays.
3. Primer sequences (Table 4) have been selected from previous publications with minor modifications or derived locally based on published sequences (18–23). The DQB*02/03/04 and *05/06 primer mixes contain a PCR amplification control.
4. Be careful not to discard the pellets, if the supernatant cannot be discarded immediately re-spin the plate for 2 min before discarding.
5. The colour must be yellow to proceed; if it remains pink add an additional 1 μL of Neutralising Buffer until yellow.
6. The PCR primer sequences for the celiac disease assay are: DQA1fo Bio TATGGTGTAAACTTGTACCAGT, DQA1re GGTAGCAGCGGTAGAGTTG, DQB1fo GCATGTGCTA CTTCACCAACG, DQB1re Bio-CCTTCTGGCTGTTCCA GTACT. The Biotin labelled primers must be HPLC purified, the unlabelled primers may be desalt purified. Dilute the primers to 100 pmol/μL in Tris buffer to store at −20°C or to 10 pmol/μL in Tris buffer for use (maximum storage is 3 months at −20°C).
7. Diluted Wash Concentrate can be stored for a maximum of 2 weeks.
8. Empty tubes for the dilutions should be cooled down on ice beforehand.
9. It is recommended to use a separate pipette because of high contamination risk.
10. It is recommended not to seal the plate because a plastic seal easily spreads liquids from well to well cross-contaminating samples.

11. The hybridization control must be over 100 cps, the DQA1 control over 700 cps, and the DQB1 control over 60 cps. Washes must be done very carefully as background signal can easily interfere with quantification.
12. In many populations, over 90% of patients with coeliac disease are positive for the DQA1*05-DQB1*02 haplotype. Whenever possible, it is therefore advisable to have both patients and controls within each genotyped 384-well plate to provide a good cluster definition of the three genotypes in the analysis step.
13. A long number of cycles may be required to see a clear plateau phase when the SNPs are not working optimally due to the difficult template sequence.

## Acknowledgements

The DR/DQ SSP, SBT, and micro bead hybridisation methods are a culmination of input by the molecular typing staff of the Transplantation and Immunogenetics Service of the Australian Red Cross Blood Service.

### References

1. Warrens AN (2000) Statistical considerations in analyzing HLA and disease associations. In: Lechler R, Warrens A (eds) HLA in health and disease, 2nd edn. Academic, London
2. http://www.dorak.info/hla/stat.html
3. Brown MA (2009) Genetics and the pathogenesis of ankylosing spondylitis. Curr Opin Rheumatol 21:318–323
4. Wu DY, Ugozzoli L, Pal BK, Wallace RB (1989) Allele-specific enzymatic amplification of beta-globin genomic DNA for diagnosis of sickle cell anemia. Proc Natl Acad Sci USA 86:2757–2760
5. Olerup O, Zetterquist H (1992) HLA-DR typing by PCR amplification with sequence-specific primers (PCR-SSP) in 2 hours: an alternative to serological DR typing in clinical practice including donor-recipient matching in cadaveric transplantation. Tissue Antigens 39:225–235
6. Sayer DC, Whidborne R, De Santis D, Rozemuller EH, Christiansen FT, Tilanus MG (2004) A multicenter international evaluation of single-tube amplification protocols for sequencing-based typing of HLA-DRB1 and HLA-DRB3,4,5. Tissue Antigens 63:412–423
7. Lind C, Ferriola D, Mackiewicz K, Heron S, Rogers M, Slavich L, Walker R, Hsiao T, McLaughlin L, D'Arcy M, Gai X, Goodridge D, Sayer D, Monos D (2010) Next-generation sequencing: the solution for high-resolution, unambiguous human leukocyte antigen typing. Hum Immunol 71:1033–1042
8. Monsuur AJ, de Bakker PI, Zhernakova A, Pinto D, Verduijn W, Romanos J, Auricchio R, Lopez A, van Heel DA, Crusius JB, Wijmenga C (2008) Effective detection of human leukocyte antigen risk alleles in celiac disease using tag single nucleotide polymorphisms. PLoS One 3:e2270
9. Koskinen L, Romanos J, Kaukinen K, Mustalahti K, Korponay-Szabo I, Barisani D, Bardella MT, Ziberna F, Vatta S, Széles G, Pocsai Z, Karell K, Haimila K, Adány R, Not T, Ventura A, Mäki M, Partanen J, Wijmenga C, Saavalainen P (2009) Cost-effective HLA typing with tagging SNPs predicts celiac disease risk haplotypes in the Finnish, Hungarian, and Italian populations. Immunogenetics 61:247–256
10. Helmberg W, Lanzer G, Zahn R, Weinmayr B, Wagner T, Albert E (1998) Virtual DNA analysis—a new tool for combination and

standardised evaluation of SSO, SSP and sequencing-based typing results. Tissue Antigens 51:587–592

11. Sayer DC, Goodridge DM, Christiansen FT (2004) Assign 2.0: software for the analysis of Phred quality values for quality control of HLA sequencing-based typing. Tissue Antigens 64:556–565
12. Rozemuller EH, Ploeger LS, Mulder W (2008) SBTengine; the ultimate solution for high resolution HLA typing. Hum Immunol 69:131
13. Olerup O, Aldener A, Fogdell A (1993) HLA-DQB1 and -DQA1 typing by PCR amplification with sequence-specific primers (PCR-SSP) in 2 hours. Tissue Antigens 41:119–134
14. Olerup O (1994) HLA-B*27 typing by group specific PCR amplification. Tissue Antigens 43:253–256
15. Sayer DC, Cassell HS, Christiansen FT (1999) HLA-B*27 typing by sequence specific amplification without DNA extraction. Mol Pathol 52(5):300–301
16. Martin AM, Nolan D, Mallal S (2005) HLA-B*5701 typing by sequence-specific amplification: validation and comparison with sequence-based typing. Tissue Antigens 65:571–574
17. Man CB, Kwan P, Baum L, Yu E, Lau KM, Cheng AS, Ng MH (2007) Association between HLA-B*1502 allele and antiepileptic drug-induced cutaneous reactions in Han Chinese [Erratum in: epilepsia 2008]. Epilepsia 48:1015–1018
18. Kotsch K, Wehling J, Blasczyk R (1999) Sequencing of HLA class II genes based on the conserved diversity of the non-coding regions: sequencing based typing of HLA-DRB genes. Tissue Antigens 53:486–497
19. Voorter CE, Kik MC, van den Berg-Loonen EM (1998) High-resolution HLA typing for the DQB1 gene by sequence-based typing. Tissue Antigens 51:80–87
20. Van Dijk A, Melchers R, Tilanus M, Rozemuller E (2007) HLA-DQB1 sequencing-based typing updated. Tissue Antigens 69(Suppl 1): 64–65
21. Dunn PP, Day S, Williams S, Bendukidze N (2005) HLA-DQB1 sequencing-based typing using newly identified conserved nucleotide sequences in introns 1 and 2. Tissue Antigens 66:99–106
22. Tilanus MGJ (ed) (2000) IHWG technical manual. Genomic analysis of the human MHC. DNA based typing for HLA Alleles & linked polymorphisms. Fred Hutchinson Cancer Research Centre, Seattle, USA
23. Cereb N, Yang SY (1997) Dimorphic primers derived from intron 1 for use in the molecular typing of HLA-B alleles. Tissue Antigens 50:74–76

Chapter 4

# HLA Typing Using Bead-Based Methods

Daniel Trajanoski and Samantha J. Fidler

## Abstract

The LABType® SSO (One Lambda, Inc) and Gen-Probe LIFECODES HLA-SSO HLA Typing tests are rapid and efficient assays for determining human leukocyte antigens (HLAs). The principle of these assays involves the hybridization of reverse sequence-specific oligonucleotide probes each attached to a unique colour coded microsphere to identify HLA class I and class II alleles. Target DNA is polymerase chain reaction (PCR) amplified using group-specific primers and then biotinylated which allows it to be detected using R-Phycoerythrin-conjugated Streptavidin. The PCR product is then denatured and allowed to hybridise to complementary DNA probes conjugated to fluorescently code microsperes. The Luminex® Flow Analyser achieves detection by determining the fluorescent intensity of PE on each microsphere. The assignment of HLA alleles is based on the reaction pattern of the various beads compared to patterns with known HLA alleles.

**Key words:** LABType® SSO, Luminex®, Denaturation, Gen-Probe LIFECODES HLA-SSO, Hybridisation, R-Phycoerythrin-conjugated streptavidin, Polymerase chain reaction, Human leukocyte antigen, Microsphere

## 1. Introduction

Over the past few decades, human leukocyte antigen (HLA) typing methods have utilized advances in technology to provide assays with higher resolution whilst reducing cost and time. Historically, HLA typing was first performed by serological typing of HLA antigens using antisera with defined specificities (1, 2), but this procedure has largely been replaced by DNA typing methods. The polymerase chain reaction (PCR) assay developed by Saiki et al. in 1985 (3) was a major breakthrough technology for HLA genotyping, and methods using PCR-amplified DNA are now widely used by HLA laboratories throughout the world. Currently there are numerous DNA-based methods available that can detect HLA alleles from PCR-amplified DNA, such as restriction fragment

Frank T. Christiansen and Brian D. Tait (eds.), *Immunogenetics: Methods and Applications in Clinical Practice*, Methods in Molecular Biology, vol. 882, DOI 10.1007/978-1-61779-842-9_4, © Springer Science+Business Media New York 2012

length polymorphism (RFLPs) (4), direct sequencing (5), sequence-specific primers (SSPs) (6), and many others. Several of these are described elsewhere in this volume. However, all these methods have their limitations in one way or another in terms of speed, lack of resolution, low throughput of sample number, and high cost.

A novel method has been developed by combining PCR-amplified DNA and sequence-specific oligonucleotide probe (SSO) protocols with the Luminex® xMAP® technology.

The LABType® SSO (One Lambda, Inc) and Gen-Probe LIFECODES SSO HLA Typing Assays use SSOs bound to fluorescently coded microspheres to identify alleles encoded by the sample DNA. The principle involves adapting Luminex® xMAP® technology to the reverse SSO DNA typing method. Initially target genomic DNA is PCR amplified using a group-specific primer. The PCR product is biotinylated, which allows it to be detected using R-Phycoerythrin-conjugated Streptavidin (SAPE). The PCR product is denatured and allowed to rehybridise to complementary DNA probes conjugated to fluorescently coded microspheres. After washing the beads, bound amplified DNA from the test sample is tagged with SAPE. Using the Luminex® Flow Analyser, the amount of PE on each specifically identified microsphere is detected. The assignment of the HLA typing is based on the pattern of reactivity of each bead compared to patterns associated with published gene sequences.

## 2. Materials

### 2.1. LABType SSO (One Lambda)

#### 2.1.1. Instrument Requirements

1. Luminex®100 or 200 Flow Analyser.
2. Luminex® XY Platform.
3. Centrifuge
   - Mikro 22 Hettich Zentrifugen or equivalent for 1.5-mL microtube.
   - Sigma Laboratory Centrifuge 4–15 or equivalent for 96-well microplate.
4. Vortex mixer with adjustable speed.
5. Thermal cycler—ABI 9700 or Equivalent (see Note 1).
6. Electrophoresis apparatus.
7. UV transiluminator with photographic image software.
8. Freezer (−20 to −80°C).
9. Refrigerator (4–8°C).

#### 2.1.2. Materials and Reagent Requirements

1. Genomic DNA—patient samples and controls (see Note 2).
2. Deionised water.
3. 70% Ethanol.

4. 20% Chlorine Bleach solution or equivalent.
5. Luminex Sheath Fluid.
6. Luminex Calibrator beads.
7. Luminex Control beads.
8. AmpliTaq polymerase 1,000 U, 5 U/μL (ABI Part# N808-0101) (see Note 3).
9. Isorack (Eppendorf).
10. Crushed Ice bath.
11. 1.5-mL Microtube (Eppendorf or equivalent).
12. 5-, 20-, and 50-mL Disposable tubes (for making dilutions).
13. Disposable pipette tips (10, 20, 100, 200, 1,000 μL).
14. PCR pad.
15. Timers.
16. 10-, 20-, 100-, 200-, and 1,000-μL pipette–Gilson or equivalent.
17. PCR 96-well microplates.
18. 96-well, 250-μL V-bottom, white polystryene microplates.
19. Aluminium foil.
20. Adhesive Tray seal (OLI Cat# SSPSEA300) or equivalent.
21. PCR plate cap strips.
22. Wash Troughs/Trays.
23. 1% Seakem ME agarose.
24. Electrophoresis loading Dye—6× DNA loading dye (Fermentas) or equivalent.
25. DNA lambda ladder—Generuler 100 bp DNA Ladder (Fermentas) or equivalent (see Note 4).
26. 1× TBE buffer.
27. 5 mg/mL Ethidium Bromide.
28. SAPE (One Lambda, Inc).
29. One Lambda SSO Genotyping Kit (see Note 5) containing
    - LABType® SSO Bead Mixture (Pre-optimised and tested mixture of microspheres with covalently attached probes).
    - LABType® SSO Hybridisation Buffer.
    - LABType® SSO Wash buffer.
    - LABType® SSO Denaturation Buffer.
    - LABType® SSO Neutralisation Buffer.
    - LABType® SSO Primer Set (Pre-optimised HLA loci-specific primer mix).
    - LABType® SSO D-Mix.
    - LABType® SAPE Buffer.

### 2.2. Gen-Probe LIFECODES SSO

Refer to Subheading 2.1.1.

#### 2.2.1. Instrument Requirements

#### 2.2.2. Materials and Reagent Requirements

The same as Subheading 2.1.2 except replace One Lambda SSO Genotyping kit with:

- Gen-Probe LIFECODES HLA-SSO Typing Kit (see Note 6) containing
  - LifeCodes HLA master mix.
  - LifeCodes Probe Mix.
  - Dilution Solution.
  - SAPE.

## 3. Methods

The methods in this chapter have been written according to current manufacturer's protocols. Any changes to these methods such as volumes of reagents and thermal cycler conditions can be found in the kit insert and the appropriate websites (http://www.onelambda.com and http://www.gen-probe.com). These should also be checked following any lot change.

### 3.1. LABType® SSO HLA Typing Method

#### 3.1.1. DNA Amplification

1. Create a LABType® PCR program on your thermal cycler as shown in Table 1.

**Table 1**
**LABType® SSO polymerase chain reaction (PCR) program**

| Step | Temperature and incubation time | Number of cycles |
|---|---|---|
| Step 1 | 96°C for 03:00 min | 1 |
| Step 2 | 96°C for 00:20 min<br>60°C for 00:20 min<br>72°C for 00:20 min | 5 |
| Step 3 | 96°C for 00:10 min<br>60°C for 00:15 min<br>72°C for 00:20 min | 30 |
| Step 4 | 72°C for 10:00 min | 1 |
| Step 5 | 4°C forever | 1 |

**Table 2**
**LABType® amplification mixture**

| Number of reactions | D-mix (μL)[a] | Amplification primer (μL)[a] | AmpliTaq polymerase (μL) |
|---|---|---|---|
| 1 | 13.8 | 4 | 0.2 |
| 10 | 138.0 | 40 | 2.0 |
| 50 | 690.0 | 200 | 10.0 |
| 96 | 1,491.0 | 432 | 21.6 |

[a]As provided in the One Lambda SSO genotyping kit

2. Turn on thermal cycler to keep heated lid warm.
3. Select the appropriate HLA typing kit (locus and resolution) and thaw out amplification primers and D-mix (see Note 7). Make sure to keep on ice until ready to use (see Note 8).
4. Vortex D-mix and amplification primer for at least 15 s and perform a quick centrifuge (5 s) to spin down any liquid trapped under lid.
5. Create the amplification mixture by adding correct volumes of D-mix and amplification primers in a 1.5-mL Eppendorf tube according to Table 2 (see Note 9).
6. Pipette 2 μL of each DNA template (see Note 10) into a 96-well PCR microplate.
7. Add the correct amount of AmpliTaq Polymerase (see Table 2) to the amplification mixture and vortex for 5s (see Note 11).
8. Aliquot 18 μL of amplification mixture into each well containing DNA (see Note 12).
9. Cap or seal the plate and give a quick vortex to mix contents in plate.
10. Place PCR plate in thermal cycler and start the "LABType® PCR program" shown in Table 1.
11. After the "LABType® PCR program" is finished, remove PCR plate and store in a 4°C fridge.
12. Pour agarose in a gel tray with the correct numbers of combs needed to electrophorese all the PCR products. (It is recom-

mended you electrophorese all samples to confirm an amplification product band is present.)

13. Once the agarose gel is set, place gel tray in electrophoresis tank and pour 1× TBE buffer until agarose is fully immersed in the 1× TBE buffer.
14. Mix 5 μL of DNA lambda ladder and 5 μL of loading dye and pipette into first well of each row of the agarose gel (see Note 13).
15. In a separate clean PCR plate, mix 5 μL of PCR product and 5 μL of loading dye and pipette into remaining empty wells. Repeat this for all the samples.
16. Place the cover on the electrophoresis tank and run at 150 V for 20 min.
17. Take out gel and place on UV transilluminator to inspect PCR products. Save photo and check all samples have correctly amplified (see Note 14).

*3.1.2. Denaturation/ Neutralisation*

1. Turn on thermal cycler and run program to 60°C hold. Make sure lid is heated to optimum temperature before use.
2. Remove reagents listed in Tables 3 and 4 and supplied in the SSO genotyping kit from −80°C freezer to room temperature to thaw and then prepare all reagent volumes in an appropri-

**Table 3**
**LABType® reagent volumes**

| Number of tests[a] | Denaturation buffer (μL)[b] | Neutralisation buffer (μL)[b] | Hybridisation buffer (μL)[b] | Wash buffer (μL)[b] | Bead mixture (μL)[b] |
|---|---|---|---|---|---|
| 1 | 2.5 | 5 | 34 | 480 | 4 |
| 10 | 25 | 50 | 340 | 4,800 | 40 |
| 20 | 50 | 100 | 680 | 9,600 | 80 |
| 50 | 125 | 250 | 1,700 | 24,000 | 200 |
| 96 | 240 | 480 | 3,264 | 46,080 | 384 |

[a]Number of tests includes all samples to be tested including appropriate controls and extra volume (see Notes 2 and 9 for comments)
[b]As provided in the One Lambda SSO genotyping kit

**Table 4**
**LABType® R-Phycoerythrin-conjugated Streptavidin (SAPE) and SAPE buffer volumes**

| Number of tests | SAPE stock volume (μL) | SAPE buffer volume (μL)[a] |
|---|---|---|
| 1 | 0.5 | 49.5 |
| 10 | 5.0 | 495.0 |
| 20 | 10.0 | 990.0 |
| 50 | 25.0 | 2,475.0 |
| 96 | 48.0 | 4,752.0 |

[a]As provided in the One Lambda SSO genotyping kit

ately sized disposable tube as necessary according to Tables 3 and 4 (see Notes 8 and 15).

3. Return any unused reagents to 2–8°C (do not re-freeze bead mixture after thawing).
4. Prepare a crushed ice bath.
5. Transfer 5 μL of each amplified DNA sample into the corresponding well of a clean 96-well PCR plate (see Note 16).
6. Add 2.5 μL Denaturation Buffer to each well of the PCR plate and mix thoroughly by pipetting up and down. Incubate at room temperature (20–24°C) for 10 min.
7. Add 5 μL Neutralisation Buffer with pipette to each well of the PCR plate and mix thoroughly (see Note 17).
8. Place PCR plate on ice bath or 96-well ice rack.

*3.1.3. Hybridisation*

1. Prepare Hybridisation Mixture by combining appropriate volumes of Bead Mixture and Hybridisation buffer according to Table 3 (see Note 18).
2. Add 38 μL hybridisation mixture to each well.
3. Cover with tray seal and give the PCR plate a quick mix using the vortex (see Note 19).
4. Place PCR plate into the pre-heated (60°C) thermal cycler, cover with PCR pad, and close and tighten lid. Incubate for 15 min.
5. Remove the PCR plate seal and quickly add 100 μL wash buffer to each well (see Note 20).
6. Cover PCR plate with plate seal and centrifuge plate for 5 min at 1,000–1,300 × *g*.

7. Remove the tray seal, then remove the wash buffer by dumping/flicking plate upside down (see Note 21). Gently pat on absorbant paper three times to remove any residual liquid.
8. Repeat steps 4–6 two more times for a total of three wash steps.
9. Prepare the 1× SAPE solution at the third centrifugation stage according to Table 4.

*3.1.4. Labelling*

1. Add 50 μL of 1× SAPE solution to each well of the PCR plate.
2. Cover plate with seal and vortex thoroughly at low speed.
3. Place PCR plate into the pre-heated (60°C) thermal cycler, cover with PCR pad, and close lid. Incubate for 5 min.
4. Remove the PCR plate seal and quickly add 100 μL wash buffer to each well (see Note 20).
5. Cover PCR plate with plate seal and centrifuge plate for 5 min at 1,000–1,300 × *g*.
6. Remove wash buffer by dumping/flicking plate upside down (see Note 12).
7. Add 70 μL wash buffer to each well and gently mix by pipetting.
8. Transfer contents of each well to a 96-well V-bottom microplate (reading plate) using an 8-channel pipette. To avoid contamination use fresh pipette tips each time.
9. Cover reading plate with seal and aluminium foil. Keep in dark and at 4°C until ready to read using LABScan™ Flow Analyser (see Note 22).

*3.1.5. Sample Acquisition on Luminex® Flow Analyser*

1. Turn on the system and set up the Luminex® Flow Analyser for sample acquisition and calibration. *(Further details of how to use the* Luminex® *Flow Analyser can be found in the Luminex® user's manual.)*
2. Verify the levels of sheath fluid and waste fluid (see Note 23).
3. Perform Warm up by selecting "Warm Up" button in the Luminex opening system. The warm up requires no plate or solution.
4. Prime the instrument by selecting "Prime". Again this step requires no plate or solution.
5. Perform a 70% alcohol flush, followed by four washes with sheath fluid.
6. A calibration should be performed every time the instrument is turned on or if the temperature of the instrument has increased or decreased by more than 3°C from the time of calibration.

7. To calibrate instrument, vortex calibration (CAL1 and 2) and control (CON1 and 2) beads thoroughly (see Note 24).
8. Place four drops of the bead solutions in each of four wells (e.g. A1, B1, C1, and D1) in the following order: CAL1, CAL2, CON1, and CON2.
9. In the acquisition software, select "CAL1" indicating the location of the bead solution. The instrument will then perform the calibration for CAL1. If the calibration is successful, this will be indicated in the "diagnostic" tab.
10. Repeat steps 8 and 9 for CAL2, CON1, and CON2 (see Note 25).
11. Once calibration has been performed, perform four washes.
12. Select the correct template according to the product catalogue and lot number being used (see Note 26).
13. Create a filename for the samples to be run, for example DATE_LOCUS_USERINITIALS.
14. Check all template settings are correct (see Note 27).
15. Load the 96-well reading plate from Subheading 3.1.4 step 9 into instrument and select "Start".
16. Once run is finished, wash three times with sheath fluid, sanitise once with 20% bleach, wash three times with distilled water and soak with distilled water twice.
17. Shut down Luminex® instrument.

#### 3.1.6. Data Analysis: One Lambda HLA Fusion™

1. Data analysis for the HLA Class I and II assays are performed with the software package HLA Fusion™. The LABType® analysis feature of the program analyses Luminex .csv output files and is based on catalogue specifications provided with the software. Import the data files as specified by the manufacturer (see Note 28).
2. The analysis software establishes the HLA type by firstly categorising each of the beads via its internal fluorescence, then determining whether a probe is bound or not by the strength of external fluorescence on that bead produced by the SAPE. For a particular sample, the bead/probe fluorescence for each of the beads bearing a particular probe is visualised in the lower left-hand quadrant of the software (Fig. 1) as a bar chart. Any probe can be selected from this bar chart for further scrutiny. The upper left quadrant shows the manufacturer's QC panel reactivity with the selected probe. In this example, the QC for probe A107 (Bead 512) is shown (see Note 29). The upper right quadrant shows the probe reactivity for all samples in the run being analysed (see Note 30). The lower right quadrant shows the software analysis derived HLA type of the sample based on the positive and negative probe reactions (see Note 31).

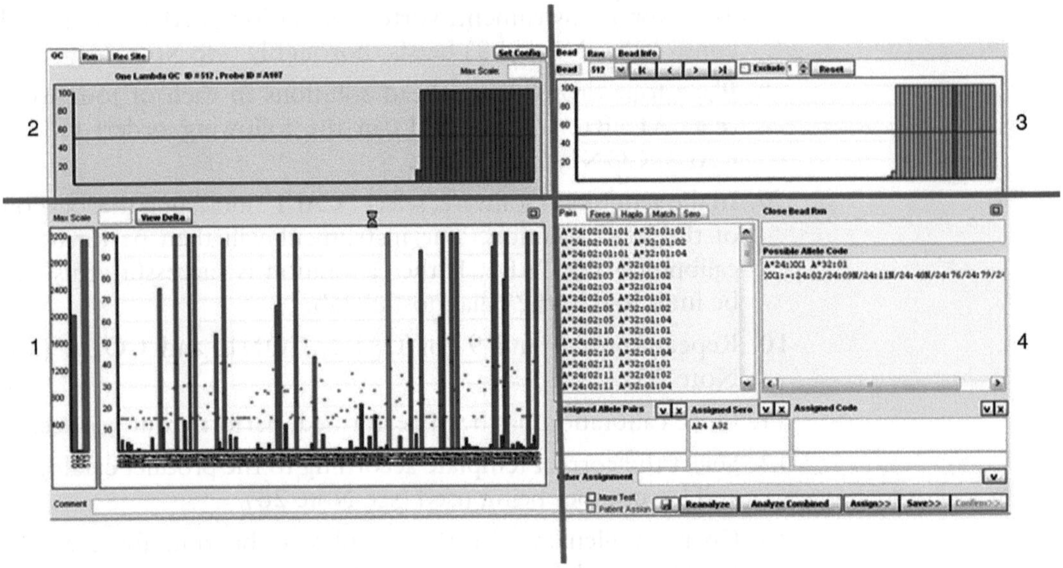


Fig. 1. HLA-Fusion® analysis software. Quadrant 1 shows the bead/probe fluorescence for each of the beads bearing a particular probe. Any probe can be selected from this bar chart for further scrutiny. Quadrant 2 shows the manufacturer's QC panel reactivity with the selected probe (see Note 29). Quadrant 3 shows the probe reactivity for all samples in the run being analysed (see Note 30). Quadrant 4 shows the software analysis derived HLA type of the sample based on the positive and negative probe reactions (see Note 31). Courtesy of One Lambda, Inc. Used with permission.

**Table 5**
**Gen-Probe LIFECODES components for amplification mix**

| Component | Volume per PCR sample reaction |
|---|---|
| LIFECODES master mix[a] | 15 μL |
| Genomic DNA | 4 μL (see Note 34) |
| Taq polymerase | 0.5 μL (2.5 U) |
| Water | 30.5 μL |

[a]As provided in the Gen-Probe SSO genotyping kit

3. The reporting function in the Fusion™ software allows resulting via a printed hard-copy report, or export of results via a . csv file (see Note 32).

### 3.2. Gen-Probe LIFECODES HLA-SSO Typing Method

#### 3.2.1. DNA Amplification

1. Select the appropriate SSO kit for the HLA locus to be typed.
2. Allow the master mix (containing amplification primers) to thaw to room temperature (see Note 8).
3. Using Table 5, prepare the components for amplification for $n+2$ reactions using the indicated amount of each component per reaction (except for DNA) (see Note 33).

**Table 6**
**Gen-Probe LIFECODES thermal cycler conditions for amplification**

| Step | Temperature and incubation time | Number of cycles |
|---|---|---|
| Step 1 | 95°C for 05:00 min | 1 |
| Step 2 | 95°C for 00:30 min<br>60°C for 00:45 min<br>72°C for 00:45 min | 8 |
| Step 3 | 95°C for 00:30 min<br>63°C for 00:45 min<br>72°C for 00:45 min | 32 |
| Step 4 | 72°C for 15:00 min | 1 |
| Step 5 | 4°C forever | 1 |

4. Bring to a final volume of 50 μL (minus the volume of DNA template) per reaction with nuclease free water. Gently vortex, spin down, and place on ice (see Note 9).
5. Pipette the appropriate amount of DNA template into the PCR tubes (see Note 34).
6. Aliquot the amplification mix into the PCR tubes containing the DNA. (The total volume of amplification mix and DNA template should equal 50 μL for each sample reaction.)
7. Cap or seal wells tightly to prevent evaporation during PCR.
8. Place samples in the thermal cycler and run program (see Table 6).
9. After the program is finished, remove PCR plate and store in a 4-C fridge.
10. Pour agarose in a gel tray with the correct number of combs needed to electrophorese all the PCR products. (It is recommended you electrophorese all samples to confirm amplification product band is present).
11. Once the agarose gel is set, place gel tray in electrophoresis tank and pour 1× TBE buffer until agarose is fully immersed in the 1× TBE buffer.
12. Mix 5 μL of DNA lambda ladder and 5 μL of loading dye and pipette into first well of each row of the agarose gel (see Note 12).
13. In a clean PCR plate, mix 5 μL of PCR product and 5 μL of loading dye and pipette into the remaining empty wells of the agarose gel. Repeat this for all the samples.

14. Place the cover on the electrophoresis tank and run at 150 V for 20 min. Take out gel and place on UV transilluminator to inspect PCR products. Save photo and check all samples have correctly amplified (see Note 35).

*3.2.2. Hybridisation*

1. Warm probe mix in a 55–60°C heat block for at least 5–10 min to thoroughly solubilise components in probe mixture.
2. Vortex briefly for about 15 s to thoroughly suspend the beads (see Note 18).
3. Aliquot 5 μL of locus-specific PCR product from Subheading 3.2.1 step 7 into a 96-well PCR plate (see Note 12).
4. Aliquot 15 μL of corresponding probe mix for the locus-specific product into each well. When aliquoting probe mix to more than 10 wells, gently vortex probe mix after each set of ten. Seal plate with film.
5. Hybridize samples under the incubation conditions indicated in Table 7.
6. While the samples are hybridizing, prepare a 1:200 Dilution Solution/SAPE mixture. Combine 170 μL Dilution Solution (DS) and 0.85 μL 1 mg/mL SAPE per sample (follow Table 8 and see Notes 15, 36, and 37).

**Table 7**
**Gen-Probe LIFECODES thermal cycler conditions lfor hybridization**

| Step | Temperature and incubation time | Number of cycles |
|---|---|---|
| Step 1 | 95°C for 05:00 min | 1 |
| Step 2 | 47°C for 30:00 min | 1 |
| Step 3 | 56°C for 10:00 min | 1 |
| Step 4 | 56°C | HOLD |

**Table 8**
**Gen-Probe LIFECODES SAPE and dilution solution volumes**

| Number of samples | Dilution solution (DS) μL[a] | SAPE stock volume (μL)[b] |
|---|---|---|
| 1 | 170 | 0.85 |
| 5 | 850 | 4.25 |
| 10 | 1,700 | 8.5 |
| 20 | 3,400 | 17 |
| 50 | 8,500 | 42.5 |

[a]As provided in the Gen-Probe SSO genotyping kit

7. At the 56°C hold step (i.e. step 4, Table 7), while the tray is on the thermal cycler, dilute each sample with 170 μL of the prepared DS/SAPE mixture. It is critical to dilute all samples within 5 min (following the 10 min 56°C step i.e. step 3, Table 7) (see Note 15).
8. Transfer contents of each well to a 96-well V-bottom microplate (reading plate) using an 8-channel pipette. To avoid contamination use fresh pipette tips each time.

   *NOTE: The Gen-Probe LIFECODES HLA-SSO assay requires no centrifugation or wash steps.*
9. Cover reading plate with seal and aluminium foil. Keep in dark and at 4°C until ready to read using LABScan™ 100 Flow Analyser (see Note 22).

*3.2.3. Sample Acquisition on Luminex® Flow Analyser*

The procedure for sample acquisition for the Gen-Probe LIFECODES SSO method is the same as that for the ONE LAMBDA method. Follow Subheading 3.1.5 steps 1–17.

*3.2.4. Data Analysis-Gen-Probe LifeMatch Quick-Type™*

1. Data analysis for the HLA Class I and II assay is performed with the software package LifeMatch™. The Quick-Type™ analysis feature of the program analyses Luminex .csv output files and is based on catalogue specifications provided with the software. Import the data files as specified by the manufacturer (see Note 38).
2. The analysis software establishes the HLA type by firstly categorising each of the beads via its internal fluorescence, then determining whether a probe is bound or not by the strength of external fluorescence on that bead produced by the SAPE. The probe reactivity thresholds and probe assignments for an individual sample are shown in the table in section A (Fig. 2). In the example shown in Fig. 2, for probe 331 the positive and negative thresholds are 0.624 and 0.511, respectively. For the sample tested, for probe 331 the fluorescence observed is 0.992 which is greater than the positive threshold. This is scored positive. An assignment can be changed from positive to negative or vice versa in this table (see Notes 30 and 39). The drop-down in section B allows selection of an individual probe. In this section, the probe reactivity for all samples in the run under analysis can be viewed. In the example in Fig. 2, probe 202 gave a fluorescence above the positive threshold for three of the samples displayed. Section C shows the selected probe reactivity for all historical samples. These local data can be used to allow the user to modify the cut-offs as required. The final HLA type is displayed in section D, including any results from other analyses of the same sample. In this example, the final HLA type is A*01, A*02. The suggested allelic combination for an individual sample is shown in section E. In this example, possible combinations

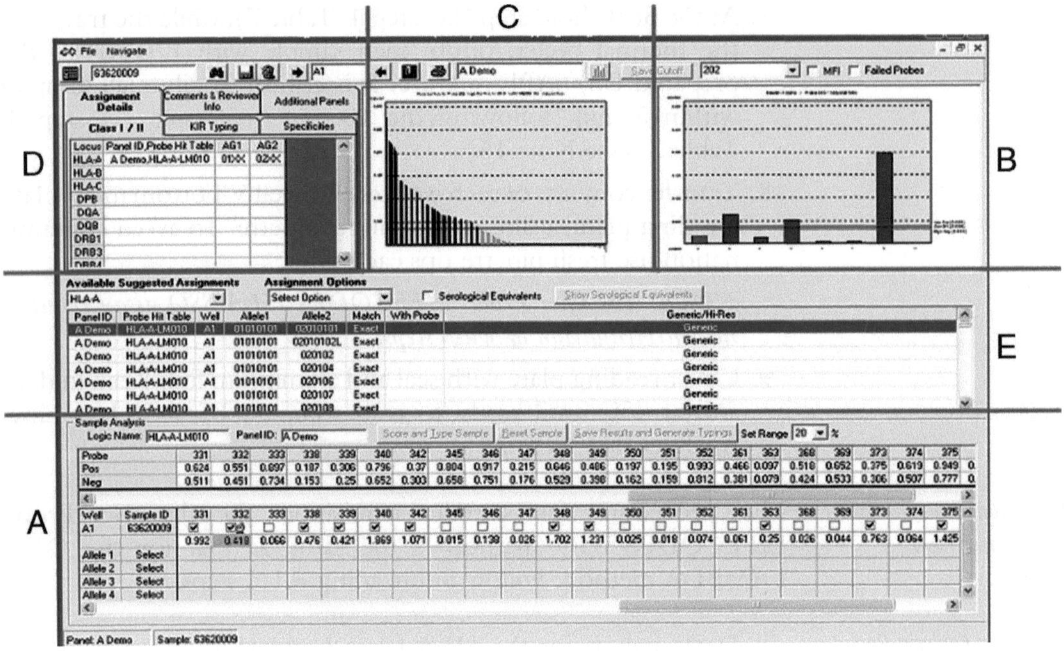


Fig. 2. LIFECODES® Quick-Type™ analysis software. Section A shows the probe reactivity thresholds and probe assignments for an individual sample. An assignment can be changed from positive to negative or vice versa in this table (see Notes 30 and 39). The drop-down in section B allows selection of an individual probe. In this section, the probe reactivity for all samples in the run under analysis can be viewed. Section C shows the selected probe reactivity for all historical samples. The final HLA type is displayed in section D, including any results from other analyses of the same sample. The suggested allelic combination for an individual sample is shown in section E. Courtesy of Gen-Probe, Inc. Used with permission.

are A*01:01:01:01, A*02:01:01:01 or A*01:01:01:01, A*02:01:01:02L or A*01:01:01:01, A*02:01:02, etc.

3. The reporting function in the LIFECODES™ software allows resulting via a printed hard-copy report or export of results via a .csv file (see Note 23).

## 4. Notes

1. Ramping speed is critical for this PCR reaction. If an ABI 9700 thermal cycler is not available, a detailed work-up of the assay may be required adjusting ramping speed as appropriate.
2. At least one control DNA of well-established HLA type should be included in each typing run. This control can be used as an amplification control, hybridisation control, and as a run control (sample order control). The concentration of DNA required is defined by the manufacturer in the kit insert.

3. AmpliTaq is recommended by the manufacturer. If an alternative is used, it will need careful QC to ensure appropriate amplification of DNA occurs.
4. A DNA ladder from 100 to 1,000 bp is sufficient to size any product from the LABType SSO range.
5. The LABType SSO range includes HLA typing kits specific for HLA-A, -B, -C, -DRB1, -DRB3,4,5, -DQB1, -DQA1, -DPB1. Intermediate resolution kits are available for all loci and high resolution kits are available for some. For the full range refer to http://www.onelambda.com.
6. The LifeCodes SSO range includes HLA typing kits specific for HLA-A, -B, -C, -DRB1,-DRB3,4,5, -DQB1, -DQA1, -DPB1. Intermediate resolution kits are available for all loci. For the full range refer to http://www.gen-probe.com.
7. D-mix is generic and may be used with any HLA typing kit. However, the amplification primers are specific for each kit and lot specific and therefore must not be interchanged.
8. Once the reagents are thawed at room temperature, vortex the vials at medium speed for 20 s followed by a quick centrifuge spin. This is done to spin down any liquid present in the lid. After centrifuging, place them in a cold isorack or crushed ice to keep cool.
9. When making up the amplification mixture always make extra volume for the required number of tests needed. The extra volume may be needed depending on pipetting techniques and calibration status of equipment.
10. ONE LAMBDA recommend DNA at 20 ng/μL concentration with A260/A280 ratio 1.65:1.8. DNA should not be resuspended in EDTA. Where DNA concentration is less than 20 ng/μL, the assay may be modified by adding a greater volume of DNA, and reducing the volume of D-mix as appropriate.
11. When adding Taq polymerase, gently mix using vortex on low speed or by flicking tube with fingers. Excessive fast mixing may denature the Taq polymerase resulting in poor PCR amplification of the template DNA.
12. Take care not to crosscontaminate samples with one another. Either use a fresh tip each time or if you are multidispensing, place the tip on the top left side of each well and dispense. This should not cause contamination as the tip touches a clean part of the well each time.
13. Make sure to use an 8-channel pipette as this will reduce pipetting time, and always use fresh clean tips for each dispense. Never re-use tips, as this will cause contamination.
14. The size of the PCR amplification product differs according to the HLA typing kit used. The expected product size can be found

in the manufacturer's kit insert or at http://www.onelambda.com. If no band is present, the DNA concentration and quality should be rechecked and the PCR repeated. If the band is of the wrong size, it is possible the amplification primers used for that particular loci were incorrect. The PCR should be repeated carefully checking the amplification primers before use.

15. Once thawed, the 100× SAPE solution should be kept refrigerated. Do not remove the 100× SAPE solution from the fridge until needed. The SAPE is light sensitive and must always be kept in the dark. Prepare the SAPE solution during the third wash step and immediately use after.
16. Make sure sample location and sample identification are correctly noted by following a proforma or spreadsheet. It is easy to mix up sample locations, especially if you are testing 96 samples.
17. Note a colour change from clear to pale yellow. If there is no colour change, add a further 1 μL of neutralisation buffer, which should trigger a colour change. If there is still no colour change, then there is a possibility that the sample did not denature properly. It is good practice to note down which wells did not change colour just in case they fail during the reading of the samples. This way you can identify where a problem has occurred.
18. Make sure to vortex Bead Mixture vigorously to give a homogenous bead mixture. This is best done by vortexing the vial three times for 10 s each time.
19. Hold the PCR plate firmly and flat on the vortex to avoid splashing of liquid onto the tray seal.
20. Use an 8-channel pipette and a wash trough. Or alternatively you can use an electronic pipette set to multidispense. This will enable you to quickly add wash buffer to all wells. To eliminate contamination, make sure not to dispense the wash buffer to the bottom of the well, but the top side of the well. If, however, you do dispense to the bottom of the well, make sure to use fresh tips each time.
21. Make sure to do this in one very quick flick in order to avoid loosing beads. If done slowly, the wash buffer can wash away the beads that are in the bottom of the well as it runs on the side of the well walls. Speed and correct techniques are vital at this step. A good flick will get rid of any excess wash buffer and/or reagents and produce a good strong signal. Once the tray has been flicked and returned to the upright position, do not invert the tray for a second time before blotting, as this will cause the beads to be flushed out onto the paper towel. If

this has occurred, repeat steps 4 and 5 in Subheading 3.1.4 before blotting.

22. For best results, read the plate as soon as possible. Prolonged storage of samples (more than 4 h) may result in signal loss. If samples cannot be read immediately, cover in aluminium foil and store at 4°C. Mix the samples thoroughly with gentle vortexing before reading as the beads may have set over time.
23. Waste container levels must always be monitored. The run 0.2 and 0.3 batch tab displays a warning when the sheath fluid container needs to be refilled. Check all tubes are running freely and there is no line blockage or breakage.
24. The calibration beads are in larger 10 mL vials and vigorous mixing is needed. Vortex for at least 1 min at high speed to get a homogenous bead mixture.
25. The calibrator microspheres are used to normalise the settings for the reporter, classification, and the doublet discriminator channels. If calibration of any of the calibration or control beads fails, then the calibration must be performed again. Failure could be due to either air in the lines of the instrument or bead mix was insufficiently vortexed. Performing a couple of wash steps will eliminate air in the lines of the instrument.
26. Templates can be found and downloaded from ONE LAMBDA via its website http://www.download.onelambda.com or from Gen-Probe via its website http://www.gen-probe.com.
27. It is extremely important that the correct lot number is selected. Incorrectly assigning the lot will result in invalid data.
28. The HLA Fusion™ software has many import features and can be adapted to suit the laboratories' reporting systems. Full training on the software is commonly provided by ONE LAMBDA or its distributors, but basic functionality can be easily followed in the user manual.
29. The manufacturer's QC shows the probe reactivity under ideal conditions. The default probe cut-off is set in the software by the manufacturer using the QC panel.
30. Different DNA extraction methods (quality of DNA) and differences in thermal cyclers may contribute to differences in probe reactivity from the manufacturer's QC. The probe cut-off can therefore be adjusted according to the individual laboratory QC.
31. The "Force" tab shows the antigen assignment possible if an individual probe has false positive or false negative reactivity. The "Close Bead Reaction" section shows any probes which are close to the set cut-off for positivity. Adjusting any of the

cut-offs may change the antigen assignment and should be checked carefully.

32. The .csv file export format allows import directly into the laboratory reporting system, thereby minimising transcription errors.
33. The master mix contains locus-specific amplification primers and therefore cannot be interchanged for amplification of other loci.
34. Gen-Probe recommends DNA at 10–200 ng/μL concentration with A260/A280 ratio 1.65:1.8. Two hundred nanogram of DNA template is required per reaction. Based on an average yield of 50 ng/μL (for robotic DNA extraction systems), 4 μL of template is required per test. This volume will be altered according to the DNA concentration of an individual sample, alternatively all samples could be standardised to the same concentration by dilution.
35. The size of the PCR amplification product differs according to the HLA typing kit used. The expected product size can be found in the manufacturer's kit insert or at http://www.gen-probe.com.
36. It is recommended to make enough Dilution Solution Mixture for $n+2$ samples to account for pipetting loss.
37. The Dilution Solution may, if required, be warmed at 45°C for 5 min and vortexed to ensure all components are in solution. Dilution Solution must be at room temperature (18–30°C) before making the SAPE/DS mixture.
38. The LIFECODES™ software has many import features and can be adapted to suit the laboratories' reporting systems. Full training on the software is commonly provided by Gen-Probe or its distributors, but basic functionality can be easily followed in the user manual.
39. Adjusting any of the cut-offs may change the antigen assignment and should be checked carefully.

## Acknowledgments

HLA Fusion screenshots reproduced with kind permission from One Lambda, Inc; LIFECODES Quick-Type™ screenshots reproduced with kind permission from Gen-Probe.

We wish to acknowledge the following for assistance with writing this manuscript: Peter Brescia (One Lambda, Inc) and Rob Vorhaban (Gen-Probe, Inc).

## References


1. Claas FH, van der Poel JJ, Castelli-Visser R, Pool J, Chen RB, Xu KY, van Rood JJ (1985) Interaction between des-Tyr1-gamma-endorphin and HLA class I molecules: serological detection of HLA-A2 subtype. Immunogenetics 22:309–314
2. Kojima S, Inaba J, Yoshimi A et al (2001) Unrelated donor marrow transplantation in children with severe aplastic anaemia using cyclophosohamide, anti-thymocyte globulin and total body irradiation. Br J Haematol 114:706–711
3. Saiki RK, Scharf S, Faloona F et al (1985) Enzymatic amplification of beta-globulin genomic sequences and restriction site analysis for diagnosis of sickle cell anaemia. Science 230:1350–1354
4. Olerup O (1990) HLA class I typing by digestion of PCR-amplified DNA with allele specific restriction endonucleases. Tissue Antigens 36:83–87
5. Sayer D, Whidborne R, Brestovac B et al (2001) HLA-DRB1 DNA sequencing based typing: an approach suitable for high throughput typing including unrelated bone marrow registry donors. Tissue Antigens 57:46–54
6. Olerup O, Zetterquist H (1992) HLA-DR typing by PCR amplification with sequence-specific primers (PCR-SSP) in 2 hours: an alternative to serological DR typing in clinical practice including donor-recipient matching in cadaveric transplantation. Tissue Antigens 39:225–235

# Chapter 5

# HLA Typing by Direct DNA Sequencing


## Linda K. Smith



## Abstract

Sequencing-based typing is a high resolution method for the identification of HLA polymorphisms. The majority of HLA Class I alleles can be discriminated by their exon 2 and 3 sequence, and for Class II alleles, exon 2 is generally sufficient. There are polymorphic positions in other exons which may require additional sequencing to exclude certain alleles with differences outside exon 2 and 3, depending on the clinical requirement and relevant accredition guidelines. The process involves selective amplification of target alleles by PCR, agarose gel electrophoresis of the PCR products to assess the quantity and quality, followed by purification of PCR amplicons to remove excess primer and dNTPs. Cycle sequencing reactions using Applied Biosystems™ BigDye® Terminator Ready Reaction v1.1 or v3.1 Kit are performed, then purification of sequence reactions before electrophoresing using Applied Biosystems™ 3730 or 3730*XL* Genetic Analyser (or similar). Data is processed by specialised software packages, which compare the sample sequence to the sequences of all possible theoretical allele combinations to assign an accurate genotype. Examination of all nucleotides, both at conserved and polymorphic positions enables the direct identification of new alleles, which may not be possible with techniques such as SSP and SSO typing.



**Key words:** PCR, Sequencing, HLA, Sequencing-based typing


## 1. Introduction

### *1.1. Amplification of Target Region Using PCR*

Sequencing is carried out using a PCR product as the template. The PCR amplifies a specific region of the gene/locus of interest, which is then sequenced from both directions to generate a high-quality DNA sequence. Bi-directional sequencing is required to achieve the desired level of accuracy and confidence in the base calls at critical positions throughout the length of the sequence (see Fig. 1 for overview).

Two of the most common strategies for designing PCR methods for sequencing-based typing (SBT) include:

(a) Designing primers with a sequencing "tail" or "tag" (Fig. 2). The most common tail (or tag) sequence is M13, which was


Frank T. Christiansen and Brian D. Tait (eds.), *Immunogenetics: Methods and Applications in Clinical Practice*, Methods in Molecular Biology, vol. 882, DOI 10.1007/978-1-61779-842-9_5,

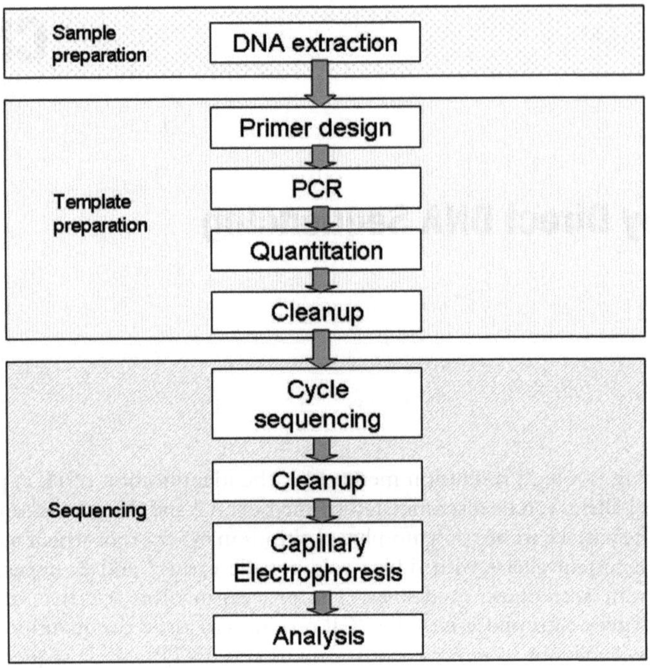


Fig. 1. Steps for sequencing of PCR templates.

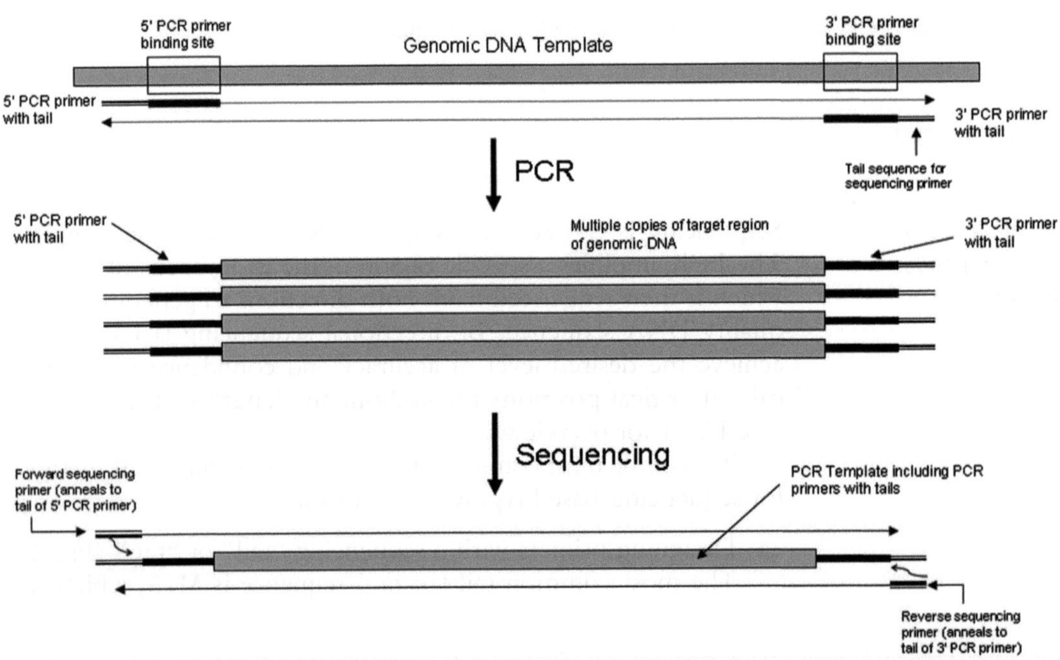


Fig. 2. Sequencing with tailed PCR primers.

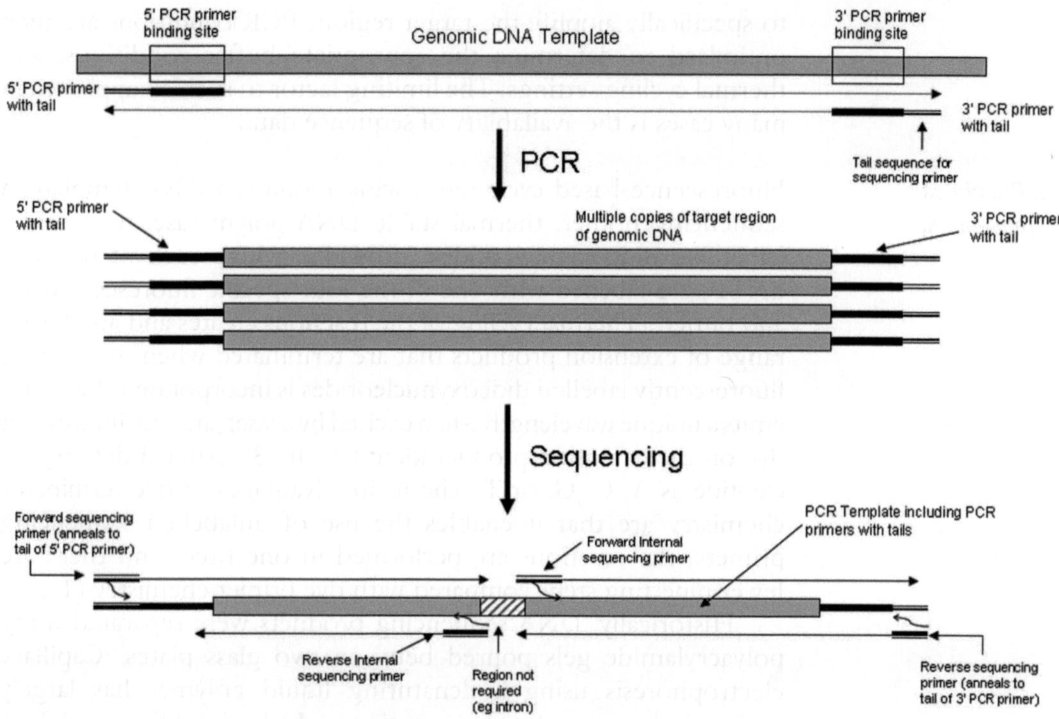


Fig. 3. Sequencing with internal sequencing primers and tailed PCR primers.

initially used for sequencing clones constructed in the M13 bacteriophage. The potential disadvantage of using tailed primers is the increase in primer length, which requires higher quality oligonucleotides, and to a lesser extent, challenges in designing primers with a tail.

(b) Using nested (internal) sequencing primers (Fig. 3). Internal primers may be required for sequencing of long PCR fragments, where the length of good quality sequence from each end of the PCR template is insufficient to cover the entire region required. This applies mainly to HLA Class I loci, where data from more than one exon is required. This approach may also be used if the entire gene is amplified in the PCR, but only certain exons are intended to be sequenced (1).

There are now commercial kits available from several sources which include both PCR and sequencing primers for the majority of HLA loci. Alternatively, there are a number of published protocols (2–15), which can be reproduced in a laboratory planning to implement HLA typing using direct sequencing. This latter approach is likely to require a degree of optimisation, as the instrumentation and other operating conditions may vary from the original reporting laboratory. If there are no suitable commercial kits, or published protocols suitable for the specific target of interest, then the available sequence data for the gene can be examined to determine whether primers can be designed in conserved regions to specifically amplify the target region. PCR conditions are then optimised to determine the appropriate buffer conditions, and thermal cycling settings. The limiting factor to such an approach in many cases is the availability of sequence data.

### 1.2. Principles of Sequencing

Fluorescence-based cycle sequencing requires a DNA template, a sequencing primer, thermal stable DNA polymerase, nucleotides (dNTPs), dideoxynucleotides (ddNTPs) where each of the four dNTPs are labelled with one of the four specific fluorescent dyes, and buffer . Thermal cycling of the reactions creates and amplifies a range of extension products that are terminated when one of four fluorescently labelled dideoxynucleotides is incorporated. Each dye emits a unique wavelength when excited by a laser, and the fluorescent dye on the extension product identifies the 3′ terminal dideoxynucleotide as A, C, G, or T. The main advantages of dye terminator chemistry are that it enables the use of unlabelled sequencing primers, the reactions are performed in one tube, and there are fewer pipetting steps compared with dye primer chemistry (1).

Historically, DNA sequencing products were separated using polyacrylamide gels poured between two glass plates. Capillary electrophoresis using a denaturing liquid polymer has largely replaced the use of gel separation, which simplifies workflow, increases throughput, and is easier to use. During capillary electrophoresis, the extension products of the sequencing reaction enter the capillary via electrokinetic injection. High voltage is applied to the buffered sequence reaction, which forces the negatively charges fragments into the capillaries. Products are separated by size based on their total charge. As the fragments reach the positive electrode, they pass through the path of a laser beam, which causes the dyes to fluoresce. An optical detection device captures the signal, and the software converts this to digital data (16).

The data is then examined using specialised software which will align the resulting sequences, allow the operators to edit the base calls if required, and compare the final consensus sequence to a reference library to determine the allele combination present (see Chapter 6).

The method included in this chapter is based on reagents and software developed by Conexio Genomics Pty Ltd (CG-HLA Sequence Based Typing Kits™) (17). Note that the kits are designed to amplify a larger region of many loci than what is required by many tissue typing accrediting bodies, but they allow resolution of certain Class I null alleles as required by the National Marrow Donor Program (NMDP). The regions amplified for each locus are as follows:

| | |
|---|---|
| HLA-A: exons 1–4 | DRB1: exons 2 + 3 |
| HLA-B: exons 1–4 | DQB1: exons 2 + 3 |
| HLA-C: exons 1–8 | |

In a medium to high throughput situation, it is advisable, where possible, to use robotic workstations (automated liquid handling platforms) to reduce the incidence of repetitive pipetting injury.

## 2. Materials

### *2.1. Specimen Requirements (See Note 1)*

1. Sterilised tissue culture grade water (negative/no template control).
2. High molecular weight human genomic DNA (concentration range 20–100 ng/μL and OD 260/280 ratio >1.8) extracted from ACD or EDTA anticoagulated whole blood specimens. Do not use samples containing Heparin (see Note 2).

### *2.2. PCR Amplification of Target DNA and Agarose Gel Electrophoresis*

1. CG-HLA Sequence Based Typing Kits™ (see Table 1 for components).
2. Sterile molecular grade or tissue culture grade deionised water.
3. Adjustable pipettes (manual or electronic, various volumes) and aerosol resistant pipette tips.
4. Thermal Cycler with heated lid.

   Conexio Genomics kits have been tested using the following thermal cyclers: Applied Biosystems™ (by Life Technologies™) GeneAmp PCR system 9700, Biorad DYAD™ (previously MJ Research DNA Engine DYAD), and Eppendorf Mastercycler Pro™. Use of other thermal cyclers will require validation by the user.
5. 0.2-mL thin walled reaction tubes either in 8-tube strips or 96-well plates. Use those to suit your thermal cycler as not all plates fit all thermal cyclers.
6. Strip lids to fit 96-well PCR plates.
7. Sterile 1.5-mL tubes.
8. Vortex mixer.
9. Sterile biological safety cabinet or hood.
10. Agarose gel electrophoresis apparatus.
11. 1% Agarose gel (molecular biology grade) in 0.5× TBE, containing 0.1 g/mL ethidium bromide.
12. 0.5× TBE electrophoresis buffer, diluted from 10× TBE which is prepared as follows:

**10× TBE (for 2 L)**

| | |
|---|---|
| Trizma base | 215.6 g |
| Boric acid | 110 g |
| EDTA (di-sodium salt) | 16.4 g |

**Table 1**
**Conexio genomics HLA sequencing-based typing kit details**

| | | | Pre-PCR contents | | Post PCR contents | |
|---|---|---|---|---|---|---|
| Kit | Catalogue number | No of tests | Reagent | Volume (μL) | Primer name | Volume (μL) |
| HLA-A | XH-PD1.1-2(50) | 50 | DNA Pol | 1 × 55 | AEX1F, AEX1R, AEX2F, AEX2R, AEX3F, AEX3R, AEX4F, AEX4R | 1 × 110 of each |
| | | | CG-HLA-A mix | 1 × 880 | | |
| | XH-PD1.1-2(100) | 100 | DNA Pol | 1 × 110 | AEX1F, AEX1R, AEX2F, AEX2R, AEX3F, AEX3R, AEX4F, AEX4R | 1 × 220 of each |
| | | | CG-HLA-A mix | 2 × 880 | | |
| HLA-B | BS-PD2.1-2(50) | 50 | DNA Pol | 1 × 55 | BEX1F, BEX2F, BEX2R, BEX3F, BEX3R, BEX4F, BEX4R | 1 × 110 of each |
| | | | CG-HLA-B mix | 1 × 880 | | |
| | BS-PD2.1-2(100) | 100 | DNA Pol | 1 × 110 | BEX1F, BEX2F, BEX2R, BEX3F, BEX3R, BEX4F, BEX4R | 1 × 220 of each |
| | | | CG-HLA-B mix | 2 × 880 | | |
| HLA-C | HH-PD 3.2-2(50) | 50 | DNA Pol | 1 × 55 | CEX1F, CEX1R, CEX2F, CEX2R, CEX3F, CEX3R, CEX4F, CEX4R, CEX5F, CEX5R, CEX6F, CEX6R, CEX7F, CEX7R, CEX8F | 1 × 110 of each |
| | | | CG-HLA-C mix | 1 × 880 | | |
| | HH-PD 3.2-2(100) | 100 | DNA Pol | 1 × 1101 | CEX1F, CEX1R, CEX2F, CEX2R, CEX3F, CEX3R, CEX4F, CEX4R, CEX5F, CEX5R, CEX6F, CEX6R, CEX7F, CEX7R, CEX8F | 1 × 220 of each |
| | | | CG-HLA-C mix | 2 × 880 | | |

| | | | | | | |
|---|---|---|---|---|---|---|
| DRB1 | HH-PD5.2-4(50) | 50 | DNA Pol | 1×18 | DRB1EX2F, DRB1EX3R, DRB1EX3R, RB-TG344-R | 1×110 of each |
| | | | CG-HLA-DRB1 mix | 1×920 | | |
| | HH-PD5.2-4(100) | 100 | DNA Pol | 1×36 | DRB1EX2F, DRB1EX3R, DRB1EX3R, RB-TG344-R | 1×220 each |
| | | | CG-HLA-DRB1 mix | 2×920 | | |
| DQB1 | PQ-PD6.2-1(50) | 50 | DNA Pol | 1×18 | DQB1EX2F, DQB1EX2R, DQB1EX3F. DQB1EX3R | 1×110 of each |
| | | | CG-HLA-DQB1 mix | 1×920 | | |
| | PQ-PD6.2-1(100) | 100 | DNA Pol | 1×36 | DQB1EX2F, DQB1EX2R, DQB1EX3F. DQB1EX3R | 1×220 of each |
| | | | CG-HLA-DQB1 mix | 2×920 | | |

The PRE-PCR component of each kit consists of a vial/s of a locus-specific PCR mix (e.g. CG-HLA-A mix) consisting of PCR buffer, dNTPs, $MgCl_2$, locus-specific PCR primers, and a single vial of DNA polymerase (DNA Pol). The POST-PCR kit contains sequencing primers (e.g. AEX1F)

Weigh each of the reagents and place into a clean sterile 2-L conical flask. Dissolve in 1.2 L of Milli-Q water with continuous mixing on a magnetic stirrer. When dissolved make up to 2 L with Milli-Q water. Place buffer into 2 × 2 L clean sterile autoclavable containers. The buffer is divided into two containers so as not to spill over during autoclaving. Autoclave to sterilise. Store in the dark.

13. Electrophoresis loading buffer. Prepare as follows:

    Place 20 mL of Milli-Q water into a clean sterilised glass beaker; add 8 g of sucrose and 0.05 g Bromophenol Blue. Mix using a magnetic stirrer. Once dissolved, make the solution up to 160 mL with Milli-Q water. Store at 4°C for immediate use, or for long term storage at −20°C.

14. PCR Marker ("Lambda ladder") suitable to cover range of 300–1,300 bp (e.g. TrackIt 100 bp DNA ladder or TrackIt 1 Kb Plus DNA ladder, from Invitrogen™).
15. BIO-RAD™ GEL DOC 2000 Transilluminator or similar.

#### 2.3. PCR Purification

1. ExoSAP-IT® (USB Products).
2. 2 mM $MgCl_2$.
3. Shaker.

#### 2.4. Sequencing, Purification, and Denaturation

1. BigDye® Terminator (BDT) Sequencing Kits v3.1 or v1.1 Ready Reaction mix (from Applied Biosystems™ by Life Technologies™).
2. BigDye® Terminator v1.1/3.1 5× Sequencing Buffer.
3. 96-Well half skirt PCR plates to fit Applied Biosystems™ sequencers (e.g. Axygen™: PCR-96-ABC).
4. CR cooler 200-μL starter kit (Eppendorf™) or ice bath to fit 96-well plate.
5. Table top centrifuge with plate adapters and ability to reach 2,500 × *g* (e.g. Heraeus™ Megafuge 2.0).
6. 125 mM EDTA, pH 8.0.
7. Absolute ethanol. Each run requires freshly prepared 80% ethanol consisting of Absolute ethanol and tissue culture grade water. DO NOT USE DENATURED ALCOHOL.
8. Hi-Di™ Formamide (Applied Biosystems™).
9. Vacuum pump and vacuum apparatus.
10. Automated DNA sequencer and accessories (e.g. Applied Biosystems™ ABI Prism® 3730 or 3730-XL Genetic Analyser) including Data Collection software.

    Conexio Genomics kits have been tested and validated on Applied Biosystems™ ABI Prism® 3100, 3730 or 3730-XL capillary sequencers and software. The use of other sequencing platforms requires validation by the user prior to use.

11. HLA Sequencing analysis software, e.g. Assign SBT™, version 3.5 or higher, or Assign ATF™ (Conexio Genomics Pty Ltd) as described in Chapter 6.

## 3. Methods

### *3.1. PCR Amplification of Target DNA (17)*

1. For each locus set up one reaction for each sample being amplified (see Note 3). Include appropriate positive controls of known genotype (see Note 4) and at least one negative control (see Note 5) for each group of samples being amplified.
2. CG-HLA Sequence Based Typing Kits™ are supplied as separate aliquots of primer mix and polymerase. The polymerase needs to be added to the primer mix just prior to setting up the PCR reactions. Thaw the required number of vials of the appropriate PCR Mix. For example, for a run of 15 samples including controls, make up enough primer/polymerase mix for 16 samples. This allows for slight pipetting inaccuracies which can be due to a small amount of the solution adhering to the outside of the tips. Once thawed, vortex briefly to mix components.
3. Calculate the number of samples to be tested and dispense the required amount of PCR mix and DNA polymerase into a sterile tube. Refer to Table 2 for volumes required per sample. Vortex the solution three to four times, for approximately 1 s each time.
4. Dispense 17 μL of the primer/polymerase mix prepared in step 3 above into each reaction well of either a 96-well plate or 8-tube strips.
5. Add 3 μL of sample DNA or appropriate positive control DNA to each reaction well. Add 3 μL of sterile water to the negative control reaction well.

**Table 2**
**PCR mastermix volumes—per sample**

| Locus | HLA-A (μL) | HLA-B (μL) | HLA-C (μL) | HLA-DRB1 (μL) | HLA-DQB1 (μL) |
|---|---|---|---|---|---|
| Locus-specific PCR mix (e.g. CG-HLA-A mix) | 16 | 16 | 16 | 16.7 | 16.7 |
| DNA-Pol | 1 | 1 | 1 | 0.3 | 0.3 |

6. Seal the reaction wells or tubes. Mix thoroughly but gently by vortexing, then centrifuge briefly to ensure all reaction components are at the bottom of the wells (i.e. turn centrifuge on, allow it to reach a speed of approximately 185 × *g*, and then turn off).
7. Place the 96-well plate or tube strips into a thermal cycler and amplify the target sequence according to the thermal cycling conditions below.

**Thermal cycling program**

| | | |
|---|---|---|
| 95°C | 10 min | |
| 96°C | 20 s | 33 cycles |
| 60°C | 30 s | 33 cycles |
| 72°C | 3 min | 33 cycles |
| 15°C | Hold | |

NB: Amplification takes approximately 2.5 h to complete.

8. When the PCR is completed, remove the plate from the thermal cycler and either proceed directly to gel electrophoresis or store at 4°C until required. Purification of amplicons by ExoSap-IT® treatment (see Subheading 3.3) should occur within 24 h of completion of PCR.

### 3.2. Agarose Gel Electrophoresis

1. Confirm successful amplification of the template DNA by agarose gel electrophoresis using 2 μL of each PCR product combined with 5 μL loading buffer (If different volumes of loading buffer are to be used, this should be validated prior to use). The use of 1% agarose gel is recommended (17). See Note 6 for voltage and running time recommendations.
2. Photograph the gel using a BIO-RAD GEL DOC 2000 Transilluminator or similar. The ethidium bromide-labelled DNA bands are illuminated by the UV light.

**Table 3**
**Expected number of PCR products and respective sizes for each locus**

| Locus | Expected band sizes |
|---|---|
| HLA-A | ≈2 kb |
| HLA-B | ≈2 kb |
| HLA-C | ≈1 and 1.4 kb |
| HLA-DRB1 | ≈450–650 bp (banding pattern will vary depending on which of the specific allele groups are present, maximum of two bands expected) |
| HLA-DQB1 | ≈300 and 350 bp |

3. The number and expected sizes of the resultant amplicons will vary according to the locus and sample genotype. Expected PCR amplicon sizes are indicated in Table 3. Band intensities should be reproducible within each assay if DNA quality is consistent. A sample with a slightly weaker band can still be processed for sequencing using a lower post-ExoSAP-IT® dilution volume. Very weak products should not be sequenced (17). See Note 7 for interpretation of positive and negative PCR controls.

### 3.3. Purification of PCR Products for Sequencing

PCR products contain excess primers and unconsumed dNTPs which require removal before sequencing reactions can be performed. They may interfere with the efficiency of the sequencing reaction, or can result in background "noise" in the sequence. There are a number of options for purifying PCR products: Spin columns, enzyme digestion, or magnetic bead-based technology. Purification systems other than ExoSAP-IT® (e.g. Agencourt® AMPure® XP or column-based systems) can be used to purify these PCR products. It is strongly recommended that users validate these procedures before proceeding. If ExoSAP-IT® is used; it is recommended that users follow the procedure described below (17).

1. Prepare a mastermix consisting of 4 μL of ExoSAP-IT® and 8 μL of 2 mM $MgCl_2$ per sample. Dispense 12 μL of the mastermix into each PCR sample to be sequenced. (This is determined by the band intensities seen following agarose gel electrophoresis as described in Subheading 3.2. Very weak products are not suitable for sequencing and therefore do not need to be treated with ExoSAP-IT®.) Seal the tubes or plates, vortex or place on shaker for 2 min, and centrifuge as described in Subheading 3.1, step 6 to ensure all reagents are at the bottom of the wells, before placing into the thermal cycler.
2. Run the thermal cycler according to the following protocol:

   37°C-30 min

   80°C-15 min

   4°C-hold
3. Upon completion, dilute the purified product 1:8 with sterile water. This dilution step will ensure that there is sufficient template to perform the sequencing reactions and ensure that the concentration of the template is sufficient to produce good quality sequence data. Note that weaker PCR products may require a lower dilution factor than 1:8.
4. ExoSAP-IT® treated samples may be stored at 4°C until ready for use.

### 3.4. Sequencing of PCR Amplified Template

All sequencing reactions must be set up in a designated ("post-PCR") area. This cannot be the same area as used to set up the PCR reactions.

In instances where heterozygous ambiguities are to be resolved with hemizygous sequencing primers, such as HARPs® (Heterozygous Ambiguity Resolving Primer), the procedure is the same as described in this method.

The RB-TG344-R included in the CD-HLA-DRB1 kit (Table 4) is a HARP® directed towards the codon 86 dimorphism. Its use is optional (17).

1. Allow the vial of BDT and other reagents to thaw at room temperature. Expose BDT to light as little as possible. Once thawed, transfer reagents to ice. Reagents should be kept on ice and the sequencing reactions should be prepared on a cooling block or on an ice bath (see Note 8 for Quality testing of BDT and buffer batches).
2. For each reaction, prepare a fresh sequencing primer reaction mix as follows (3).

| Reagent | Volume required (μL) |
|---|---|
| Sequencing primer | 2.0 |
| BDT v3.1 ready reaction mix | 1.0 |
| 5× Sequencing buffer | 3.5 |
| Water | 11.5 |

   For multiple samples requiring the same sequencing primer, make a large mix of the components above, allowing for pipetting error (e.g. for nine samples, make enough mix for ten reactions). See Note 9 regarding optimisation of these reagent ratios for different instruments.

3. Mix each sequencing primer reaction mix gently by pulse (2–3 s) vortexing.

**Table 4**
**Sequencing primers provided for use with each locus**

| Locus | Sequencing primers |
|---|---|
| HLA-A | AEX1F, AEX1R, AEX2F, AEX2R, AEX3F, AEX3R, AEX4F, AEX4R |
| HLA-B | BEX1F, BEX2F, BEX2R, BEX3F, BEX3R, BEX4F, BEX4R |
| HLA-C | CEX1F, CEX1R, CEX2F, CEX2R, CEX3F, CEX3R, CEX4F, CEX4R, CEX5F, CEX5R, CEX6F, CEX6R, CEX7F, CEX7R, CEX8F |
| HLA-DRB1 | DRB1EX2F, DRB1EX3R, DRB1EX3R, RB-TG344-R |
| HLA-DQB1 | DQB1EX2F, DQB1EX2R, DQB1EX3F, DQB1EX3R |

4. Dispense 18 μL of the sequencing reaction mix to each appropriate reaction tube or well of a 96-well plate. If 8-tube strips or individual tubes are used, they should be placed in a carrier so as to avoid mixing up the positions during the procedure.
5. Add 2 μL of purified PCR product (from Subheading 3.3, step 3 and 4) to each appropriate well (see Note 10).
6. Cap or seal wells or plate tightly, mix gently then centrifuge briefly as previously described in Subheading 3.1, step 6 to ensure all reagents are at the bottom of the tubes.
7. Place the reaction tubes or plate into a thermal cycler and run according to the following program (17) (see Note 11):

| | |
|---|---|
| 96°C for 10 s | 25 cycles |
| 50°C for 5 s | |
| 60°C for 2 min | |
| Then 4°C indefinitely | |

8. Once the program is complete, remove the reaction tubes or plate from the thermal cycler and either proceed directly to purification of the sequencing reaction products or store at 4°C until required. It is recommended that sequence reaction samples are purified and run on the DNA sequencer within 24 h (17).

### 3.5. Purification and Concentration of Big Dye Terminator Sequencing Products Using Ethanol Precipitation (17, 18)

See Note 12 for additional information.

1. Remove the reaction tubes or 96-well plate from the thermal cycler (or 4°C storage) and centrifuge briefly as previously described in Subheading 3.1, step 6. If reusable lids/caps have been used during thermal cycling, label the lids/caps to avoid cross-contamination.
2. Each reaction requires 5 μL of 125 mM EDTA and 60 μL ethanol (see Note 13). Make a mix of the following for a full 96-well plate:

   550 μL of 125 mM EDTA.

   6.6 mL of 100% ethanol.

   Add 65 μL of the above mix to each sample.

   The final ethanol concentration is 70%.
3. Replace caps and invert tubes or plate four times to ensure thorough mixing.
4. Centrifuge briefly as previously described in Subheading 3.1, step 6.

5. Leave at room temperature, protected from light, for 15 min to precipitate the extension products. Slightly longer precipitation times are acceptable, preferably no longer than 1 h (18) (see Note 14).
6. Place the tubes or plate in a centrifuge and spin according to the following guidelines:

   Centrifuge speed 1,400–2,000 × *g*: 45 min.

   Centrifuge speed 2,000–3,000 × *g*: 30 min.

   *Important*: Proceed to the next step immediately. If this is not possible, then spin the tray for an additional 10 min immediately before performing the next step.
7. Without disturbing the precipitates, remove the strip lids and discard the supernatant, by inverting the tubes or plate onto absorbent tissues (e.g. facial tissues).
8. Place the inverted tubes or plate with the tissues into the centrifuge and spin briefly as described previously in Subheading 3.1, step 6.
9. Remove the plate from the centrifuge, discard tissues, and then add 60 μL of freshly prepared 80% ethanol to each pellet. Cap the tubes and then invert the tubes or plate four times to mix.
10. Place the tubes or plate in centrifuge and spin at approximately 1,700 × *g* for 15 min.
11. Repeat steps 8–10, then remove from centrifuge, and discard tissues. Vacuum dry for 15 min, or air dry for 1 h, in the dark. Reseal plate if not proceeding immediately to denaturation step.
12. Resolubilise pellets by adding 12 μL of Hi-Di™ formamide. Thoroughly vortex tubes or plate for approximately 15 s.
13. Denature samples by placing in a thermal cycler which is already at 98°C, for 5 min.
14. At the end of 5 min, remove from thermal cycler and immediately place on ice for at least 5 min. Centrifuge briefly as described previously in Subheading 3.1, step 6 to bring down any condensation.

    *ENSURE THAT THERE ARE NO AIR BUBBLES IN THE WELLS. THESE CAN ENTER AND DAMAGE THE CAPILLARY.*
15. Load the reaction plate onto the automated sequencer and prepare the data collection file according to the sequencer manufacturer specifications. Samples should be run within 24–36 h; otherwise, the Hi-Di™ formamide will begin to break down to formic acid and there will be significant loss of resolution. If it is not possible to run the plate within this time frame, it should be stored at 4°C (17, 18).

**Table 5**
**Data collection settings for ABI 3730 or 3730xl**

| Parameter | Setting |
|---|---|
| Dye set | Z-BigDye V3 |
| Mobility file | KB_3730_POP7_BDTV3 |
| Basecaller | KB.bcp |
| Run module | Regular FastSeq50_POP7 |
| Injection time | 15 s |
| Run time | 2.5 h |

### 3.6. Electrophoresis of Sequencing Products on 3730 Sequencer

1. Run the sequencing product plates according to the instrument parameters in Table 5. These have been validated by the manufacturer using POP-7™. These parameters may require user validation for other polymers and instruments. Please refer to the appropriate instrument user's manual for detailed instructions and guidance (17).
2. Use the instrument's data collection software to process the raw collected data and create the sequence files. Please refer to the appropriate instrument user's manual for detailed instructions and guidance (19).
3. See Note 15 for brief sequence quality troubleshooting guide.

### 3.7. Allele Assignment

Sequence analysis may be performed using Assign SBT™ or Assign ATF™ software. For more details, please refer Chapter 6 or the Conexio Genomics Pty Ltd. Web site (http://www.conexio-genomics.com). See Notes 16–19 for some critical issues in allele assignment.

## 4. Notes

1. Care should be taken to ensure reagents are sterile and the water is of high quality for PCR and sequencing. DNases and RNases can degrade DNA and PCR products, resulting in poor quality sequence. The presence of salts or other contaminants can inhibit PCR and sequencing reactions and can compete with DNA product in electrochemical injection on capillary-based sequencers.
2. Genomic DNA from anticoagulated whole blood, buffy coat or buccal mucosa swabs is suitable for HLA typing by DNA sequencing. ACD or EDTA is the preferred anticoagulant,

whereas heparin inhibits PCR reactions and is therefore not recommended. There are many commercial kits for DNA extraction, both manual and automated. The concentration and purity of the isolated DNA should be determined using a spectrophotometer before proceeding to the PCR. Some commercial kits recommend a specific concentration to which the DNA is diluted. Others may use a particular volume of DNA within a range of concentrations. Very low DNA concentrations (<15 ng/μL) should be avoided as the failure rate will be increased, and there is some potential for uneven amplification of heterozygous samples.

3. PCR set-up is to be performed on ice or a cold-brick in a dedicated ("pre-PCR") area (e.g. biological safety cabinet). Mastermix preparation should be performed in a separate area to that used for addition of DNA.
4. DNA samples with known HLA types should be included in each PCR assay to ensure the primers are amplifying the target region as expected. For example, it should be possible to cover all of the broad DRB1 allele groups using four controls, such as DRB1*01 + 03, DRB1*04 + 07, DRB1*09 + 15, and DRB1*01 + 10. For DQB1, a combination of control samples to cover DQB1*02, 03, 04, and 05/06 is suggested. For Class I loci, it is sufficient to use a single heterozygous sample. These controls should be sequenced to confirm the identity of the sample.
5. A negative or blank control (water) should be included on each PCR run to detect contamination. This sample should have all reaction components except DNA. Any PCR run where there is amplification evident in the negative control should be repeated, as there is likely to be contamination of one or more reagents.
6. The maximum voltage for electrophoresis is dependent upon the size of the tank. For a large tank (42 cm), the maximum voltage is approximately 150 V for 20–30 min. The maximum voltage for a medium and small size tank is 130 V for 20–30 min. The smaller the gel, the lower the voltage required. Good resolution of PCR products are obtained if gels are run at a lower voltage and for a longer period of time.
7. If the positive control has failed (no band visible on gel, or a band of the incorrect size), or there is a band visible in the negative control, the PCR run must be repeated. If desired, all samples can be visualised in this manner. It is advisable to do this until you are satisfied with the reproducibility of the assay. It should also be considered when starting a new batch of primers or master mix.

8. The Big Dye Terminator and Sequencing Buffer must be tested together and the two test lots should be used together routinely. If ordering large-scale BDT kits, extra bottles of buffer may need to be ordered in order to keep the batches coordinated.
9. These volumes apply only to the Applied Biosystems™ 3730/3730xl sequencer referred to in this chapter. Other sequencers may require different combinations. Less sensitive instruments may require a higher concentration of BDT, or more template. It is advisable to carry out a titration of BDT and template to determine the optimum combination for your laboratory. When increasing the volume of BDT, the volume of 5× sequencing buffer should be decreased proportionately. If increasing primer or template volume, the volume of water should be adjusted accordingly so that total volume is still 20 μL.
10. Care must be taken to prevent cross-contamination of sequence reactions. Fresh tips must be used for each sequencing primer reaction mix and each PCR product. PCR plates should be briefly centrifuged, as previously described in Subheading 3.1, step 6, before lids or seals are removed so that any condensation that may have formed does not flick into another well during removal.
11. Note that the sequencing thermal cycling conditions are slightly different from Applied Biosystems™ recommended cycling conditions, which are as follows:

| | | |
|---|---|---|
| 96°C | for 10 s | 25 cycles |
| 50°C | for 5 s | |
| 60°C | for 4 min | |
| Then 4°C indefinitely | | |

The use of these standard conditions in place of Conexio Genomics' recommended protocol would require validation by the user. This may be necessary if using an outside sequencing service, as opposed to having access to your own instrument. In a sequencing service with multiple sample types from different "customers", it may not be possible to have specific sequence cycling conditions for a particular assay. An initial comparison between the two cycling conditions is suggested, for all loci being tested, as the extent to which they are affected may vary.

12. Purification of the sequencing reaction products may be carried out by procedures other than the ethanol precipitation method described here. It is strongly recommended that users validate these procedures before proceeding.

13. Absolute ethanol absorbs water from the atmosphere, gradually decreasing its concentration. This can lead to inaccurate final concentrations of ethanol, which can affect sequencing protocols. Ethanol should be stored in small aliquots so that there is limited opportunity for repeated use of each aliquot, which reduced exposure to the atmosphere.
14. Precipitation times <15 min will result in the loss of very short extension products. Precipitation times >24 h will increase the precipitation of unincorporated dye terminators (1).
15. Poor sizing precision or allele calling, poor sequence resolution and/or decreased signal intensity may be an indication that the capillary array on the sequencer requires renewal. Capillary arrays degrade over time. They should last at least 300 runs (will probably last 600 runs). However, these symptoms are similar to those seen when poor grade Hi-Di™ formamide is used, or has been exposed to air for too long (19).
16. It should be noted that mutations at amplification or sequencing primer sites are possible and may result in allele drop-out. Samples that suggest a homozygous typing result should be confirmed by alternative procedures. These may include serology, or other PCR-based assays, such as SSP or SSO typing.
17. The nature of HLA sequence-based typing is such that factors other than the PCR mix may result in preferential amplification or allele drop out. As a consequence, apparent homozygous typing results should be confirmed using alternative methods as mentioned above in Note 16, or family genotyping.
18. If sequence electropherograms have high background, there is potential for errors in base calling which may result in incorrect allele assignment. Laboratory personnel should be capable (through experience and training) of assessing the quality of sequence data and excluding those samples which are not of sufficient quality to interpret reliably. If using the Assign software package described in Chapter 6, there will be a visual indication of sequence quality (the degree or intensity of "redness") of each base. The user will be prompted by the software to confirm the base at each position with low quality, if that function is selected in the Editing Tool. See Chapter 6 for further details.
19. SBT generally results in high resolution typing, however not all allele combinations can be resolved. The location and specificity of the PCR and sequencing primers will determine which ambiguous allele combination can occur. Three different categories of ambiguity are recognised (20):
    - Single alleles that cannot be distinguished because the resolving positions are outside the region amplified. For example, where exons 2 and 3 are amplified for Class I loci, and the difference between the alleles is in exon 4.

- Several allele pairs that result in the same heterozygous sequence. This occurs when the alleles share sequence motifs, but in different combination, so it is impossible to determine whether the motifs are in *cis* or *trans* linkage.
- Combinations of alleles where one of the alleles has incomplete sequence for the region analysed.

The only way to resolve ambiguities of the first type is to employ an assay that amplifies the additional region required. Separation of alleles followed by additional sequencing can be employed to resolve the other kinds of heterozygous ambiguities. This may be by means of additional allele or group-specific PCR amplification or by the use of allele or group-specific sequence primers to separate the alleles in the primary heterozygous PCR product. If using the Assign software package, the user can produce a list of suggested resolving primers from the "Reports" menu.

## References


1. Applied Biosystems (2000) Automated DNA sequencing chemistry guide. © Copyright 2000, Applied Biosystems
2. Cereb N, Maye P, Lee S, Kong Y, Yang SY (1995) Locus-specific amplification of HLA class I genes from genomic DNA: locus-specific sequences in the first and third introns of HLA-A, -B and -C alleles. Tissue Antigens 45(1):1–11
3. Petersdorf EW, Hansen JA (1995) A comprehensive approach for typing the alleles of the HLA-B locus by automated sequencing. Tissue Antigens 46(2):73–85
4. Blasczyk R, Wehling J, Weber M, Salama A (1996) Sequence analysis of the 2nd intron revealed common sequence motifs providing the means for a unique sequencing based typing protocol of the HLA-A locus. Tissue Antigens 47(2):102–110
5. Cereb N, Yang SY (1997) Dimorphic primers derived from intron 1 for use in the molecular typing of HLA-B alleles. Tissue Antigens 50(1):74–76
6. Kotsch K, Wehling J, Kohler S, Blasczyk R (1997) Sequencing of HLA class I genes based on the conserved diversity of the noncoding regions: sequencing-based typing of the HLA-A gene. Tissue Antigens 50(2):178–191
7. Voorter CE, de Bruyn-Geraets D, van den Berg-Loonen EM (1997) High-resolution HLA typing for the DRB3/4/5 genes by sequence-based typing. Tissue Antigens 50(3): 283–290
8. Voorter CE, Kik MC, van den Berg-Loonen EM (1998) High-resolution HAL typing for the DQB1 gene by sequence-based typing. Tissue Antigens 51(1):80–87
9. Van der Vlies SA, Voorter CE, van den Ber-Loonen EM (1998) A reliable and efficient high resolution typing method for HLA-C using sequence-based typing. Tissue Antigens 52(6):558–568
10. Kurz B, Steiert I, Heuchert G, Muller CA (1999) New high resolution typing strategy for HLA-A locus alleles based on dye terminator sequencing of haplotypic group-specific PCR-amplicons of exon 2 and exon 3. Tissue Antigens 53(1):81–96
11. Kotsch K, Wehling J, Blasczyk R (1999) Sequencing of HLA class II genes based on the conserved diversity of the non-coding regions: sequencing based typing of HLA-DRB genes. Tissue Antigens 53(5):486–497
12. Sayer D, Whidborne R, Brestovac B, Trimboli F, Witt C, Christiansen F (2001) HLA-DRB1 DNA sequencing based typing: an approach suitable for high throughput typing including unrelated bone marrow registry donors. Tissue Antigens 57(1):46–54
13. Sayer DC, Whidborne R, De Santis D, Rozemuller EH, Christiansen FT, Tilanus MG (2004) A multicenter international evaluation of the single-tube amplification protocols for sequencing-based typing of HLA-DRB1 and HLA-DRB3,4,5. Tissue Antigens 63(5): 412–423

14. Dunn PP, Day S, Williams S, Bendukidze N (2005) HLA-DQB1 sequencing-based typing using newly identified conserved nucleotide sequences in introns 1 and 2. Tissue Antigens 66(2):99–106
15. Van Dijk A, Melchers R, Hilkes Y, Rozemuller E, Tilanus M (2007) HLA-DRB sequencing-based typing: an improved protocol which shows complete DRB exon 2 sequences and includes exon 3 of HLA-DRB4/5. Tissue Antigens 69(Suppl 1):61–63
16. Applied Biosystems (2002) 3730/3730*xl* DNA analyzers sequencing chemistry guide. © Copyright 2002, Applied Biosystems
17. Conexio Genomics Pty Ltd (2011) CG-HLA sequence based typing kits™ Instructions for Use, PCR amplification and sequencing of HLA Class I and II Loci, Version No: 6.0, Feb 2011
18. Applied Biosystems (2002) BigDye® Terminator v3.1 cycle sequencing kit protocol. © Copyright 2002, Applied Biosystems
19. Applied Biosystems (2002) 3730/3730*xl* DNA analyzers user guide. © Copyright 2002. Applied Biosystems
20. Rozemuller E (2000) SBT resolution and ambiguities (Chapter 6). In: Tilanus MGJ, Hansen JH, Hurley CK (eds) IHWG technical manual genomic analysis of the human MHC: DNA-based typing for HLA alleles and linked Polymorphisms. Publication of the 13th International Histocompatibility Working Group. Fred Hutchinson Cancer Research Centre, Seattle, USA

# Chapter 6

# Data Analysis of HLA Sequencing Using Assign-SBT v3.6+ from Conexio

**Carla Wirtz and David Sayer**

## Abstract

DNA Sequencing is now a standard frontline high-throughput HLA typing procedure with some unrelated bone marrow donor registry typing laboratories performing tens of thousands of tests per year. The advantage of DNA sequencing is that, by definition, sequencing *directly* identifies all bases in the DNA template. Alternative molecular-based assays such as the use of sequence-specific PCR primers (PCR-SSP) and oligonucleotide probes (PCR-SSO) provide information only for those regions to which the oligos are designed and no information is obtained for the regions between primers and probes.

The era of routine high-throughput sequencing-based typing (SBT) was made possible by the development of locus-specific PCR-based assays and the development of the HLA sequencing-based typing software, Assign-SBT v3.2.7 by Conexio Genomics. A single PCR per locus simplified the template preparation stage of the test and Assign-SBT simplified the sequence analysis and allele assignment stage. Together these developments dramatically simplified the SBT procedure, making SBT cost effective.

This chapter provides a comprehensive description of Assign-SBT sequence analysis software for use in a HLA typing laboratory.

**Key words:** High throughput DNA sequencing, Sequence analysis, Assign-SBT, HLA

## 1. Introduction

### *1.1. Background*

DNA Sequencing is now a standard frontline high-throughput HLA typing procedure with some unrelated bone marrow donor registry typing laboratories performing tens of thousands of tests per year. The advantage of DNA sequencing is that, by definition, sequencing *directly* identifies all bases in the DNA template. Alternative molecular-based assays such as the use of sequence-specific PCR primers (PCR-SSP) and oligonucleotide probes (PCR-SSO) provide information only for those regions to which the oligos are designed and no information is obtained for the regions between primers and probes. As a result of the increase of

Frank T. Christiansen and Brian D. Tait (eds.), *Immunogenetics: Methods and Applications in Clinical Practice*, Methods in Molecular Biology, vol. 882, DOI 10.1007/978-1-61779-842-9_6, 

HLA typings that are now performed by sequencing, there has been an explosion in the description of new HLA alleles (see IMGT/HLA Database, http://www.ebi.ac.uk/imgt/hla/).

The era of routine high-throughput sequencing-based typing (SBT) was made possible by the development of locus-specific PCR-based assays by Malcolm McGinnis, Pete Krausa, and Jason Stein at Applied Biosystems (Foster City, CA, USA) and then Forensic Analytical (South San Francisco, CA, USA) and the development of the HLA sequencing-based typing software, Assign-SBT v3.2.7 by David Sayer and Damian Goodridge at Conexio Genomics (Fremantle, WA, Australia). A single PCR per locus simplified the template preparation stage of the test and Assign-SBT simplified the sequence analysis and allele assignment stage. Together these developments dramatically simplified the SBT procedure, making SBT cost effective.

Assign-SBT v3.2.7 was specifically designed for HLA typing in a high-throughput routine laboratory. It contained a unique base caller designed for accurate base calling of heterozygous sequence and a unique quality scoring system that enabled poor quality sites within a sequence to be identified and base call errors, if present to be easily identified. Any editing resulted in an immediate change to the results. Furthermore, the software was the first of its kind to provide a quantitative quality control system, in the vein of Shewhart analysis, which enabled sample-to-sample, run-to-run, and assay-to-assay assessment of quality.

Assign-SBT has continued to evolve, not only to keep up with the complexities of HLA typing but also to provide researchers with the tool for continuing the research into HLA complexity and its role in transplantation biology and disease susceptibility.

Assign-SBT v3.6+ is the latest version of HLA sequence analysis software from Conexio; it represents a new breakthrough in HLA sequence analysis software.

Features of Assign-SBT v3.6+ include:

(a) The choice for the user to decide if they wish to genotype by comparing against cDNA and genomic DNA reference sequences from the IMGT/HLA database.

(b) The most significant improvement over Assign-SBT v3.6, providing multiple report formats, includes:
   - Indicators of which alleles are rare and which have been reported in a quantifiable frequency, the so-called CWD alleles.
   - Grouping alleles according to their nucleotide sequence identity in exons 2 and 3 of class I HLA genes and exon 2 of class II HLA genes (G groups).
   - Grouping alleles according to their amino acid sequence identity in exons 2 and 3 of class I HLA genes and exon 2 of class II HLA genes (P groups).

– Improved reporting of hemizygous sequencing primers for the resolution of heterozygous ambiguities.

Maximum benefits of Assign-SBT v3.6+ are obtained when using Conexio's *Resolver* SBT assays.

### 1.2. About Assign SBT 3.6+

#### 1.2.1. Compatibility

1. Computer operator system's
   Assign is a Windows-based program and will run on Windows XP, Windows Vista, and Windows 7 operating systems. Microsoft Excel 97 or above is required for the creation of reports.
2. Data files supported
   Assign requires .ab1, .abd, or .scf files from automated DNA sequencers. Sequence files from non-Applied Biosystems DNA Sequencers can be analysed. All files must be processed with Sequence Analysis software prior to importing into Assign.

#### 1.2.2. Overview

1. Functions and features
   (a) Sequences from multiple loci can be imported into the same layout.
   (b) The sample identifier, sequence electropherogram, and allele assignment results are all visible on one screen.
   (c) Sequence editing includes priority analysis of positions of low quality and positions that are mismatched with closely related alleles.
   (d) Simultaneous analysis of sequences for the resolution of heterozygous ambiguities is possible.
   (e) Analysis of non-coding sequence for Class I alleles is possible.
   (f) Assign 3.6+ can report CWD alleles, G groups, and P groups (see Note 1).
   (g) Assign 3.6+ includes sample-to-sample and run-to-run QC analysis.
2. Performance characteristics
   (a) Throughput: Assign 3.6+ has successfully imported over 5,000 sequence electropherograms into a single project.
   (b) Base Call Accuracy: Assign contains a unique base caller developed to improve the accuracy of heterozygous base calls. However, base call accuracy is influenced by sequence data quality. Generally, samples with a base call quality score (described in detail below) of >85 do not have incorrect base calls.
3. Limitations
   (a) Sequence with background noise and poorly separated peaks may result in incorrect base calls and the potential for incorrect typing results. This is true for all sequence analysis

software. However, this limitation is offset as poor quality data are easily identified within the software, so that it can be reviewed for incorrect base calls. Such data can be excluded from analysis, so that an incorrect genotype cannot be performed.

(b) Assign-SBT v3.6+ compares a sample sequence with a library of sequences from known alleles. The report lists those alleles/allele combinations in the library that are identical to the sample sequence. It is possible that the same sequence could be derived from alleles yet to be described and whose sequence is not yet part of the library. Therefore caution must be taken when interpreting the genotype report as an HLA type.

## 2. Getting Started and Using the Software

### *2.1. Installation*

Assign-SBT v3.6+ is a standalone computer software program and should be installed on the computer on which SBT analysis is performed. It is recommended that Assign is installed by a user with complete administrator access to the computer. The installer package can be acquired by contacting Conexio via their website, http://www.conexio-genomics.com. It is also helpful if the computer has access to the Internet to facilitate the system updates with new libraries and other files as needed.

1. To install: Double click on the installer file icon and follow the instructions for installation. During installation, a 16-digit computer-specific hardware identifier will be generated. Copy and paste this ID into an e-mail and send to key@conexio-genomics.com to obtain licence keys. The software will not be functional until the key files are successfully installed.
2. Reference libraries and NMDP codes, if required, need to be installed. Go to the Conexio Genomics website, http://www.conexio-genomics.com, and click on the **Downloads** tab on the left side of the screen. Click on the **Libraries** tab. Click on the library version that you require. A zip file will be downloaded to your computer. Unzip the file and save the **References** folder to the desktop or other convenient location. The References folder will contain the gene-specific reference files, P Group file, and G Group file.

   (a) Next, launch the software. Use the default operator (admin) and password (cg01) login. Click on **Help | Update System** on the top menu bar.

   (b) Click on the **References** button and navigate to the unzipped References folder. Highlight the .xml reference

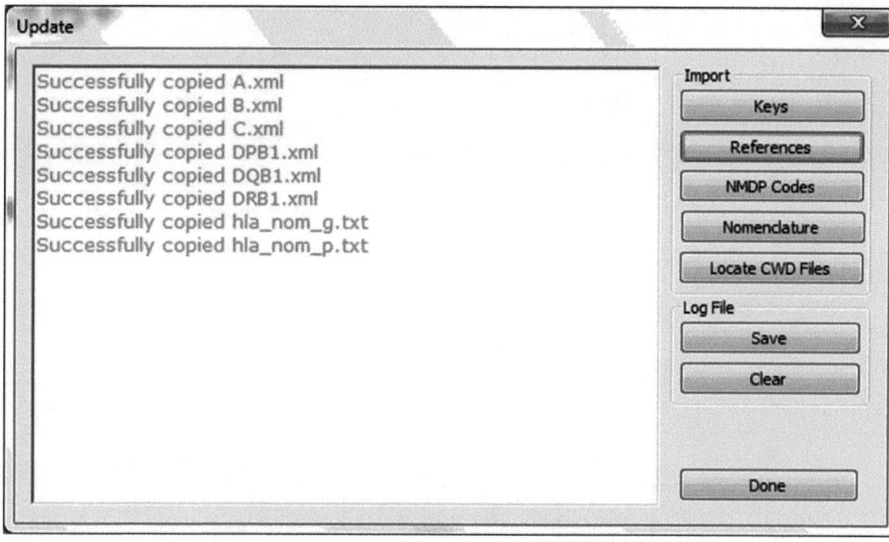


Fig. 1. The Update screen is used to update Keys, Reference files, and NMDP Codes.

files to update then click Open. The references will be imported to the correct location within the software. A message will appear indicating if the reference file update is successful or not. If the update is unsuccessful, the process should be repeated to verify that the correct file was chosen for the update (Fig. 1).

3. Repeat the process with the NMDP codes by clicking on the **NMDP Codes** tab on the Conexio website. The NMDP code file is named "numer.txt" and must not be renamed. Save the .txt file to your computer. Log into the software and click on **Help | Update System | NMDP codes**. Navigate to the numer.txt file and highlight it. Click Open. The code file will be imported to the proper location within the software.
4. When the licence key(s) are received, use the Keys update function within the software by clicking **on Help | Update System | Keys.**

### *2.2. Login and Adding Users*

1. Launch the software by double clicking on the Assign 3.6+ icon on the desktop. The default operator is "admin" and the default current password is "cg01". It is recommended that the admin password is never changed.
2. Additional users can be added. Enter the admin login and password then click "More". Below will be a section to add additional users. Type in the new operator's name in the Edit Operator section. Type in a password for that user. Re-type the password. Select the Operator Level. Click Add/Update directly next to the Retype Password box. Repeat for additional users (Fig. 2).

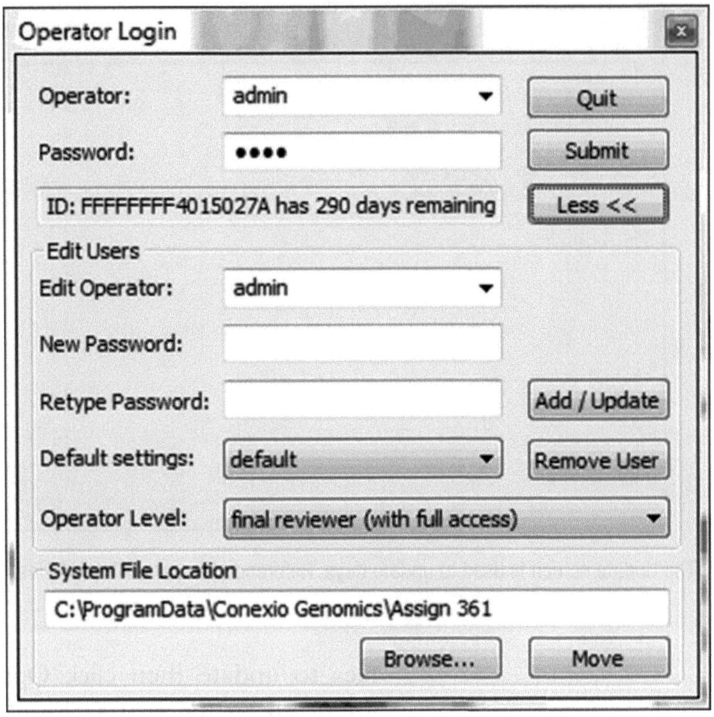


Fig. 2. The Operator Login screen is used to add/edit users and select Settings files.

3. To launch the software under a particular user, double click on the Assign icon. In the Operator drop down, select the user. Type in the password then click **Submit.**

### *2.3. Settings*

The settings menu enables the user to configure the software for their requirements. Settings can be saved as different settings files to enable the software to be individualized for different users.

#### *2.3.1. General*

General Settings allow modifications to the interface such as changes in font size, electropherogram's colours, and electropherogram's line thickness.

1. To open the default settings file, click on **Edit | Settings** on the top menu bar in the software. The 'General' tab displays the default settings and allows for creation of new settings files.
2. Customize the display
   (a) Click on **Display** in the General tab.
   (b) The Display options will appear.
   (c) Adjust the base colours, background colours, text size, and line width (EPG tracing width) then click Done (Fig. 3).
3. To create a new settings file if desired, type in a new settings file name and proceed to the Advanced tab to create the naming conventions and locus alias names.

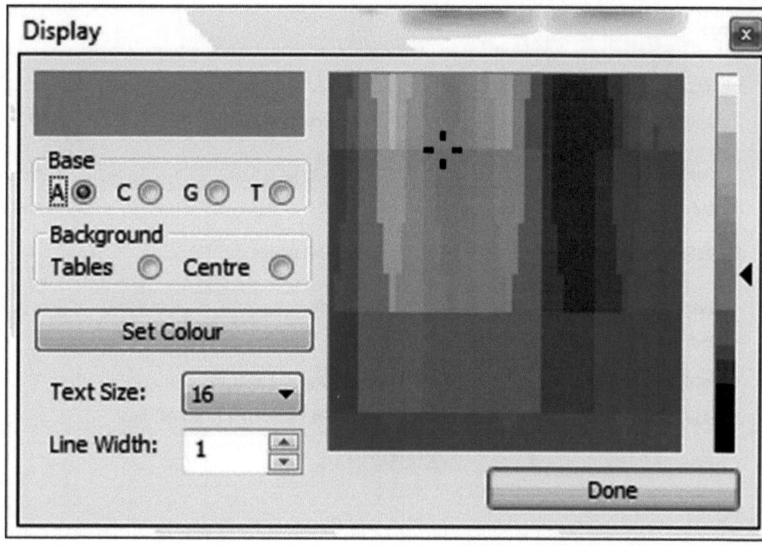


Fig. 3. The screen display is modified by selecting a colour scheme customized for the user.

### 2.4. Naming Conventions

In the **Advanced** tab, the user can enter the parameters that define the sample name and the locus identifier in sample sequence filename. The sequence filename must be unique for sequencing reaction for a sample and contain the sample name and an identifier that can be used as an alias for the locus being genotyped. If a standard system is used by the operator, analysis will occur automatically and different data from different loci can be entered into the same layout (Fig. 4).

#### 2.4.1. Sample Delimiters

**Sample Delimiters** have been used to separate the components of the sequence-file name.

Example:

Sequence-file name A01[12345_DQ2F_A01

**Delimiters** have been used to separate the components of the sequence-file name

[ has been used to separate the PCR number (A01) and the sample name (12345).

_ has been used to separate the sample name and the locus (HLA-DQB1) and primer (exon 2 Forward).

_ has also been used to separate the locus and well location (A01).

Set the Naming convention by defining the **Sample Delimiters**.

In the example above, the sample name begins with [ and the sample name ends with _Enter [ in the Start string box, and enter _ in the End string box.

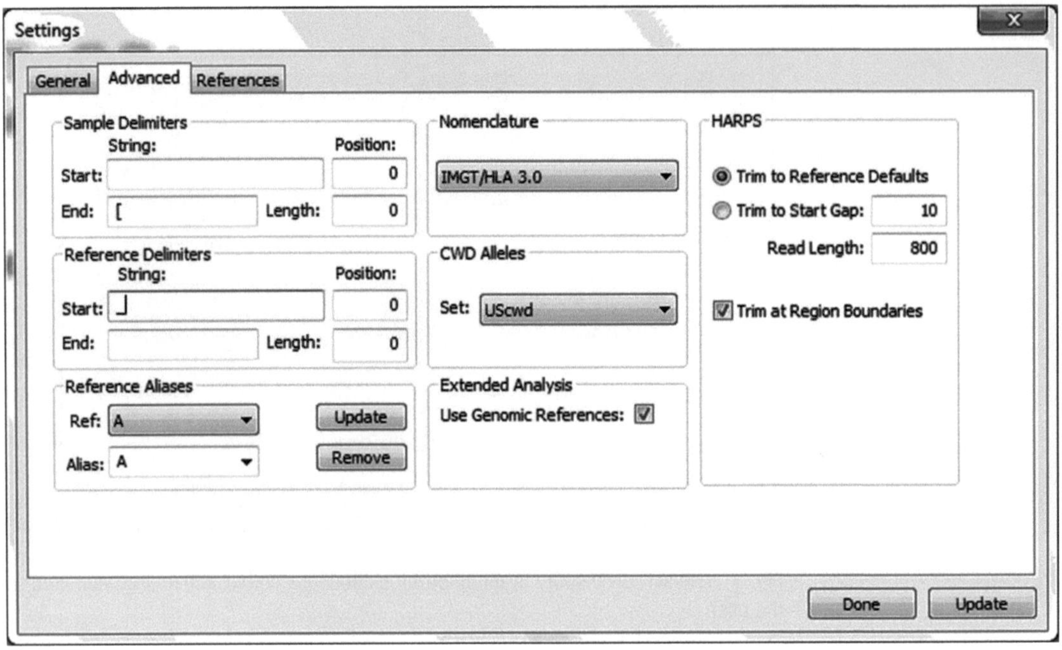


Fig. 4. Settings | Advanced tab is used to customize sample naming conventions and reference aliases, select Nomenclature output naming, CWD Allele set, and to indicate if genomic references are to be used.

*2.4.2. Alias Names*

1. In the example above, DQ is used as a symbol for HLA-DQB1. In Subheading 2.4.7, use the Ref: drop down menu to select the locus. Next, in the Alias drop down menu select the alias used (DQ). If the alias is not present, type it into the Alias box, and then click **Update** directly to the right of the Ref box.
2. Repeat this for each locus alias you will be using. After all aliases have been added, click on the Update button in the lower right-hand corner of the Settings box.

*2.4.3. Nomenclature*

The HLA nomenclature standards changed in April 2010 from v2 to v3.0. In **Select the Output Naming Standard**, either IMGT/HLA3.0 or 2.0 can be selected for the naming convention of the reported alleles.

*2.4.4. Heterozygous Ambiguity Resolving Primers*

Heterozygous Ambiguity Resolving Primers (HARPs) are sequencing primers designed to sequence only one of the alleles in a heterozygous sample. HARPs are used for the resolution of heterozygous ambiguities, by producing hemizygous sequence for one of the alleles. The sequence data from an HARP is combined with the existing sequence data from the sample to produce a high-resolution genotype report. Setting the **Start Gap** enables only good quality sequence to be analysed by eliminating the poor quality data at the start of a sequence. The Start Gap will vary between laboratories according to the sequence reaction clean-up method used, the DNA Sequencer make and model, and the polymer in the sequencer capillaries.

1. Enter the number of base pairs between the end of the primer and the first usable sequence generated in the **Start Gap**.

*2.4.5. CWD Alleles*

The CWD alleles are stored in a text file. A default set of CWD alleles based on those described by Cano et al. (1) are provided with the software. However, laboratories may want to create their own list.

1. Set the **CWD** allele set you will be utilizing, if any.

*2.4.6. Extended Analysis*

By selecting **Genomic References**, the sequence analysis will enable the comparison of the sample sequence with the Genomic References provided by the IMGT/HLA database. This analysis improves typing accuracy by enabling those alleles that are characterized by polymorphisms to be genotyped. By leaving the **Genomic References** box unchecked, analysis will be performed against the standard cDNA reference.

1. If the laboratory will utilize analysis of the non-coding regions, put a check in the Use **Genomic References** box.

*2.4.7. Reference Aliases*

Reference aliases are used in the sequence filenames to indicate the HARP being used for sequencing.

1. Click on the **References** tab of the **Setting** menu to establish alias names for primers used.
2. Click on the **Load Reference** box at the top right of the screen. Navigate to the References folder and click on the reference needed. Click OK.
3. The reference information will populate the screen.
4. To establish a reference alias for the Codon 86 resolution primer, highlight the DRB1.xml file and click OK.
5. In the References tab, in the lower left corner drop down menu, select the Codon 86 primer. To the right of the primer will be the alias drop down menu. Click the drop down menu to determine if your naming alias is present.
6. To add an alias, type the alias into this box. For example, DR86 as an alias for the Codon 86 GTG primer. Next, click on Add Alias directly below the alias drop down menu box. Then, click on Update in the lower right corner. After all aliases have been added, click on Done.

*2.4.8. Variant Positions*

**Variant Positions** is a tool to draw attention to sequence artefacts that may result in base call errors, or other positions within a sequence where automated base calls may be frequently incorrect.

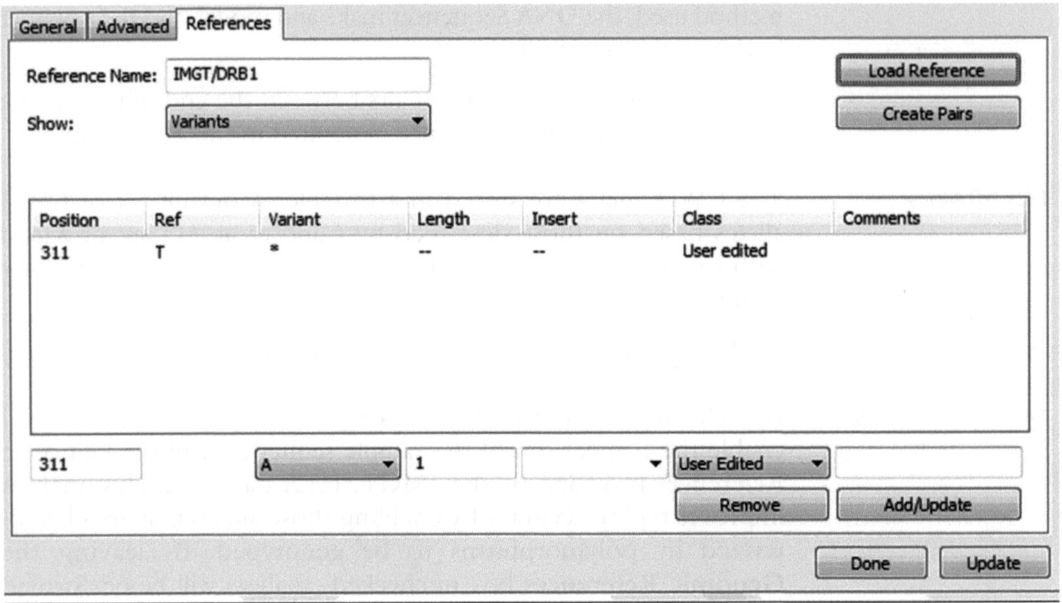


Fig. 5. User Defined Variant positions are established using the References tab in the Update Settings menu.

Such positions can be included as those positions within the sequence that must be validated by the user in order to generate a report (Fig. 5).

1. Load the reference for which you want to create a variant position following the instructions above.
2. Once the reference is loaded, click on **Show** then **Variants**. This will open the variant position box.
3. In the lower left corner, in the blank box under Position, type in the position for the variant.
4. In the Variant drop down, select the variant base type (usually * so any call at that position is flagged).
5. Enter the length of the variant in bases.
6. In the Insert box, enter bases if this variant includes an insertion. Leave blank if no insertion is expected.
7. Select the Class of variant (usually User Edited). Enter any comments desired.
8. Click on Add/Update to add the variant position.
9. Repeat for additional variants.
10. Click on Update then Done when complete. A purple box will be displayed at each variant position indicated.

### 2.5. Importing Sequences

If the sequence file-naming convention is defined in the software **Settings**, sequences can be imported by browsing to a directory and importing the contents or by importing the

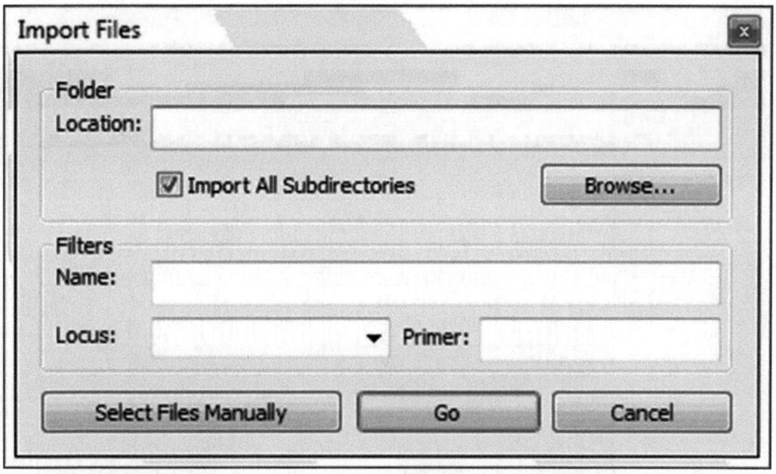


Fig. 6. The Import Files menu is accessed by selecting File | Import | Electropherograms from the top menu bar.

sequence files individually. Importing from a directory also allows filters to be applied, so that only specific samples are imported, or only sequences from a particular locus or from a sequencing primer can be imported.

*2.5.1. Importing Sequences by Directory*

1. To import sequences by directory (import all electropherograms in a given folder), Select **File | Import | Electropherograms** on the top menu bar.
2. In the pop up window, click on **Browse** and navigate to the folder that contains the sequences. Highlight the folder and click OK (Fig. 6).
3. The folder location will populate the Import Files menu. Check the Import All Subdirectories box if all subdirectories are to be imported. Click Go.

*2.5.2. Importing Sequences Individually*

1. To import only selected electropherograms from a folder, click on **Select Files Manually**. Navigate to the folder containing the necessary sequences. Highlight all the sequences to be imported using the Ctrl or Shift key. Then click Open.
2. Use the **Filters** dialogue to import to search for an import samples of a specific **Name**, or all samples for a **Locus** or specific sequence files for a sequencing **Primer**.

***2.6. The Screen Layout, Editing, and Analysis***

Once the sequence data has been imported, the software screen becomes populated with sample, sequence, and result information. There is a predominance of white to red shading used to demonstrate sequence data quality.

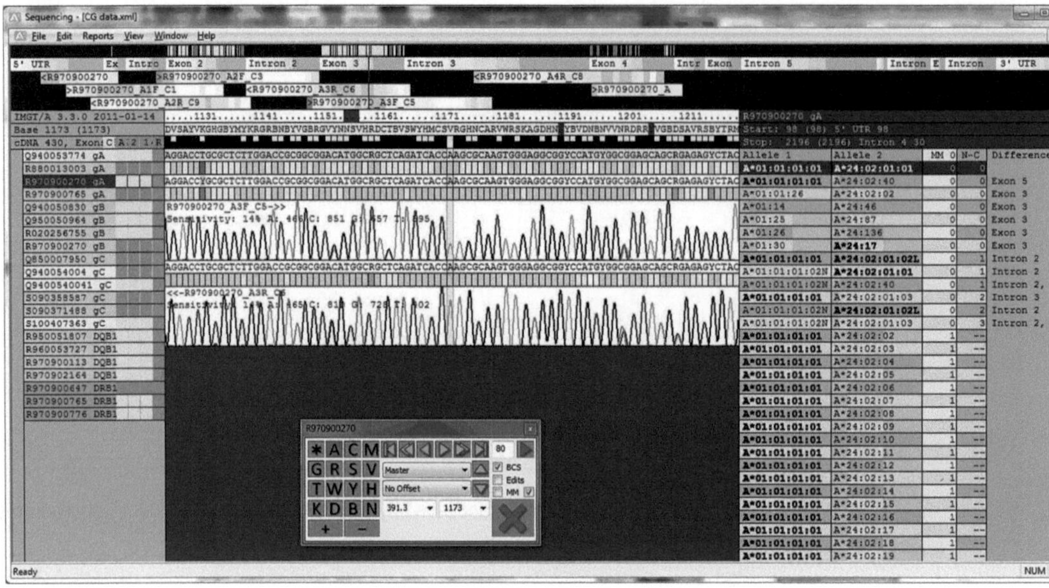


Fig. 7. Shading within the electropherogram coverage indicates quality of given sequences.

*The use of shading to indicate sequence data quality*

SBT errors may occur if a base call error is made, and the probability of a base call error is increased if the quality of the data is poor. Assign-SBT contains a quality scoring algorithm that assesses the quality of a sequence peak based on the peaks shape, whether or not it is well separated from neighbouring peaks and whether or not there is non-specific background.

A Base Call Score (BCS) from 0 to 50 is calculated from each peak and is represented in a box under the base call as a shade of red to white, where red is a BCS of 0 and white has a BCS of 50, shading in between 0 and 50 is shaded accordingly. The consensus sequence BCS is calculated from the BCS of sequences that contribute to a consensus.

The BCS for positions within a sequence can be used to calculate a quality score of a sample.

The use of colour coding enables a sample with poor quality data and poor quality positions within the sequence to be readily identified and checked for base call errors (Fig. 7).

*2.6.1. Sample ID Pane*

The screen layout shows information for a particular sample. It includes the sample ID, the electropherograms data, the aligned sequences for a sample, and the best-matched allele combinations (Fig. 8).

The samples imported are listed on the left side of the screen. Sample names are colour coded to indicate data quality.

1. The sample pane also includes five columns of boxes.

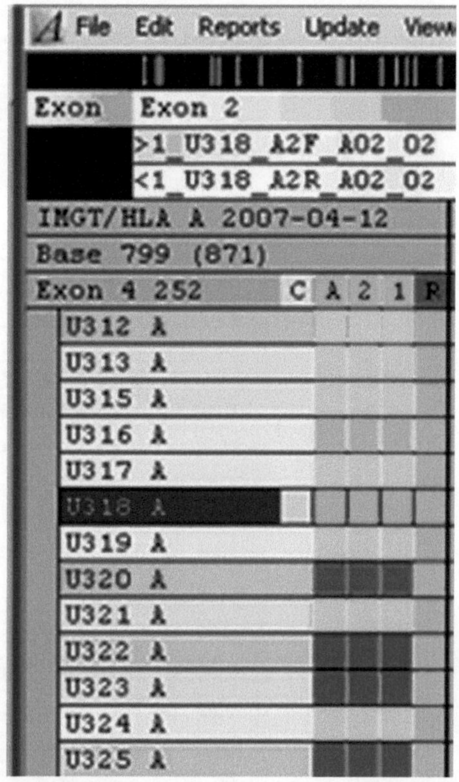


Fig. 8. The Sample ID Pane shows information about the samples in the project.

(a) A light blue box in the **C** column indicates if **comments** have been made about a sample. Right clicking on the sample allows the comments to be added and reviewed. The comments are also included in the genotype report.

(b) A green box in the **A** column indicates that the sample has been verified at all positions indicated in the Navigator. This box changes to green once all the positions requiring confirmation have been confirmed using the navigator (see below for Navigator bar use).

(c) A green box in the **1** column indicates that the sample has undergone **first review**. After the first reviewer has performed the analysis, the yellow box in the 1 column is clicked, changing it to green.

(d) A green box in the **2** column indicates the sample has undergone **secondary review**. Checking this box will lock the sample and prevent any further edits unless the box is manually unchecked.

(e) A green box in the **R** column indicates the sample can be reported using the **Report Generator**.

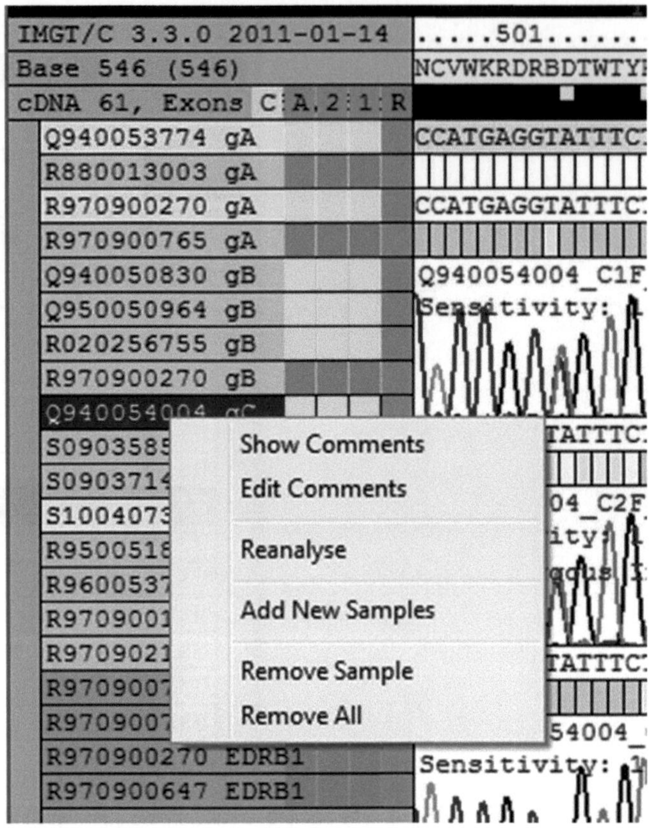


Fig. 9. Right click on Sample ID to access Sample Options section.

2. Right click on the sample name in the Sample Pane to access sample options (Fig. 9).
   (a) **Show Comments** will display any quality warnings about a sample.
   (b) **Edit Comments** gives a text box to record any comments about a sample. These comments will appear on the report. A light blue box in the C column will indicate that a comment is present.
   (c) **Reanalyze** will remove any edits and trims that have been made.
   (d) **Add New Samples** will launch the import files menu.
   (e) **Remove Sample** will remove the highlighted sample from the project.
   (f) **Remove All** will remove all samples from the project.

*2.6.2. Sequence Electropherograms*

Importing the sequence electropherograms results in a display of how the sequence files are orientated according to the gene

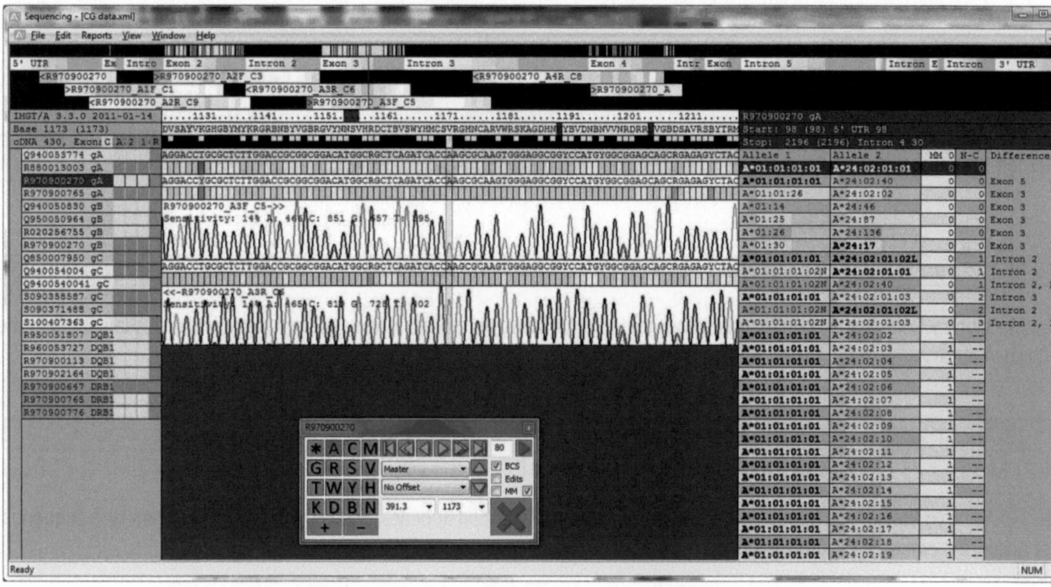

Fig. 10. Sequence Electropherogram information is contained in the Sample layout screen, including the structure of the gene being sequenced, sample sequence alignments, consensus sequences, and sample sequence data.

Fig. 11. The structure of the gene being sequenced is represented at the top of the screen.

structure, the sequence electropherograms themselves, and the Assign-SBT base calls and quality score information (Fig. 10).

The Assign layout contains important information to assist with the analysis of DNA sequence data.

1. The Structure of the Gene being sequenced
   The blue band shows the genetic structure of the reference sequence and the yellow bars above indicate those positions within the sequence that when the base call is changed will result in change to an alternative allele combination in the results pane (Fig. 11).
2. Sample Sequence Alignments
   The bands shaded white to red show the sequence data alignments. They are shaded white to red according to quality. This enables "at-a-glance" to be able to locate poor data quality positions for manual review. The sequence filename and direction of sequencing (< or >) is included (Fig. 12).
3. The Library Consensus sequence
   Beneath the sequence alignment map is consensus sequence of alleles within the library (Fig. 13). The sequence is shaded yellow to indicate exon sequence and white to indicate intron

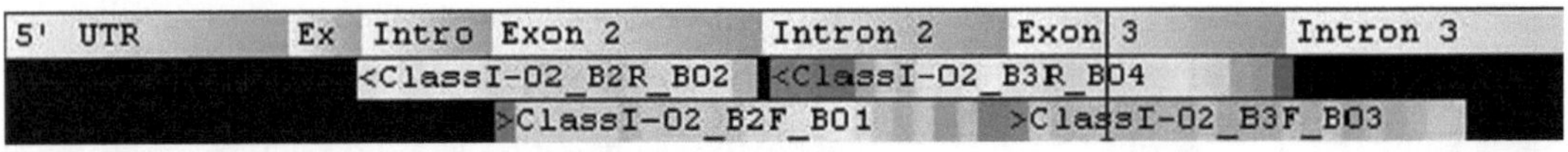


Fig. 12. The sample sequence alignment shows sequence quality shaded within each electropherogram. Lighter electropherograms represent better quality sequence.

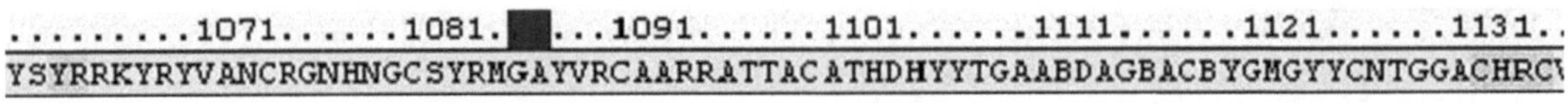


Fig. 13. Library Consensus sequence is colour coded depending on region. This sequence represents all alleles within the reference library.

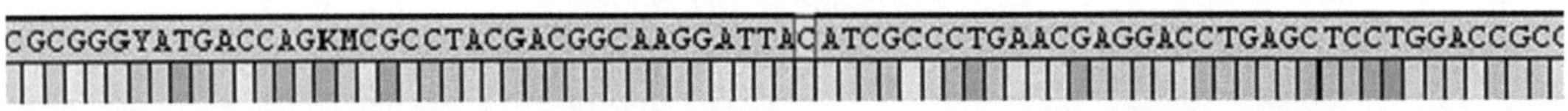


Fig. 14. Sample Consensus Sequence of the sample being sequenced appears just below the Library Consensus sequence, just above the electropherogram tracings.

sequence. In addition, positions shaded light blue indicate there are alleles in the library that contain deletions at this position and dark blue regions indicate the position of insertions in some alleles.

4. The Sample Consensus Sequence
   The sequence data below the consensus sequence of alleles within the library is the consensus sequence of the sample being sequenced. The boxes underneath the base calls are shaded white to red to indicate the quality of the consensus base call. It is the consensus sequence that is compared to the sequence library and it is only the consensus sequence where base call edits can be made (Fig. 14).

5. The Sample Sequence Data
   Beneath the sample consensus sequence is the sample sequence electropherograms data, the software base calls, and the quality indicator. The electropherogam panels contain the sequence filename, the "Sensitivity" of heterozygous base calls. That is, the percentage that one peak needs to be within another before a heterozygous base call is made on data with no background. The signal intensities of the four bases are also indicated (Fig. 15).

6. Right clicking on a given electropherogram gives access to options for each electropherogram (Fig. 16).
   (a) **Set Start Base** will trim off all data to the left of the cursor.
   (b) **Set End Base** will trim off all data to the right of the cursor.
   (c) **Less Sensitivity** will filter out background noise, raising the threshold 5%.
   (d) **More Sensitivity** will increase sensitivity, calling more heterozygous bases.

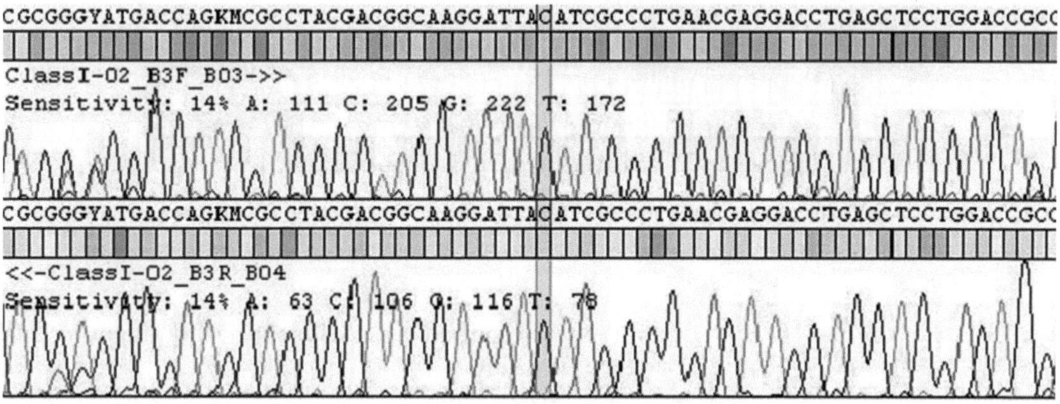


Fig. 15. Sample sequence data, software base calls, and quality indicators are represented within the electropherogram tracing.

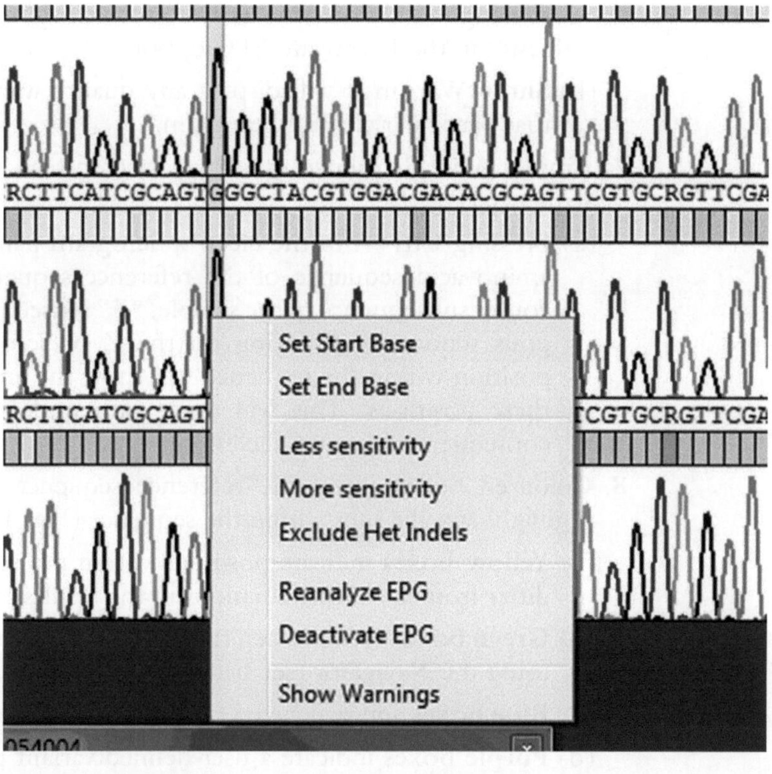


Fig. 16. Right click on the electropherogram to view Electropherogram options.

(e) **Exclude Het InDels** will filter out excess background in the sequence due to a co-amplified stretch of DNA. When the signal to noise is relatively low, the extra signal can be interpreted as a heterozygous InDel. Choosing "Exclude Het InDel" informs the software that the additional signal

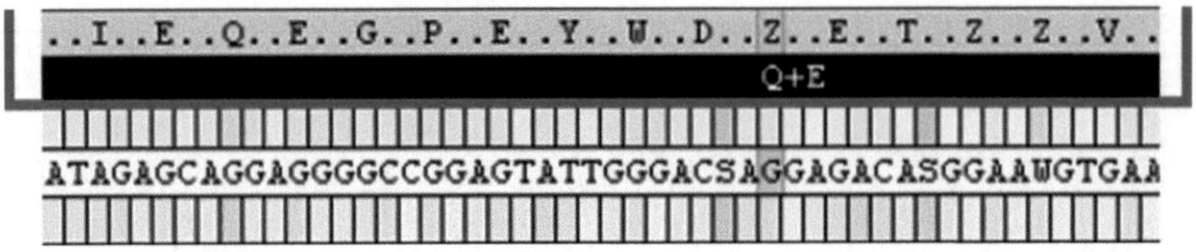


Fig. 17. Amino Acid sequence can be viewed instead of base pair sequence by pressing Ctrl+A in the electropherogram pane.

should be interpreted as background and not as a real sequence feature.

(f) **Reanalyse EPG** will remove any user edits and trims from the electropherogram.

(g) **Deactivate EPG** will remove the electropherogram from analysis, but does not remove it from the layout. Right clicking on the deactivated electropherogram again will result in the Reactivate EPG option.

(h) **Show Warnings** will display any quality warnings about that particular electropherogram.

7. **Amino Acid Sequence** can be viewed instead of base pair sequence (Fig. 17).

(a) Pressing Ctrl+A in the electropherogram pane shows the amino acid sequence of the reference sequence and the consensus sequence of the sample. "Z" is used for heterozygous sequences. Clicking on the Z or scrolling to the position within the sequence will show the amino acids at these positions. This will assist with understanding the consequence of novel alleles.

8. Coloured boxes above the reference sequence are used to highlight specific sites within the sequence (Fig. 18).

(a) **Yellow boxes** indicate positions within the sequence that differ from allele combinations in the results pane.

(b) **Green boxes** appear when the base call has been confirmed using the Navigator (see below).

(c) **Blue boxes** appear when a position has been edited.

(d) **Purple boxes** indicate a user-defined variant position (see Subheading 2.4.8).

*2.6.3. Results Pane*

The **Results pane** includes the sample name, the start and stop positions of the test sequence, and the allele combination with the best-matched sequence to the test sequence. Bolded alleles are CWD alleles whilst those unbolded are and rare alleles (Fig. 19).

1. **Allele 1** and **Allele 2** columns display the allele pairs best matched to the test sequence.

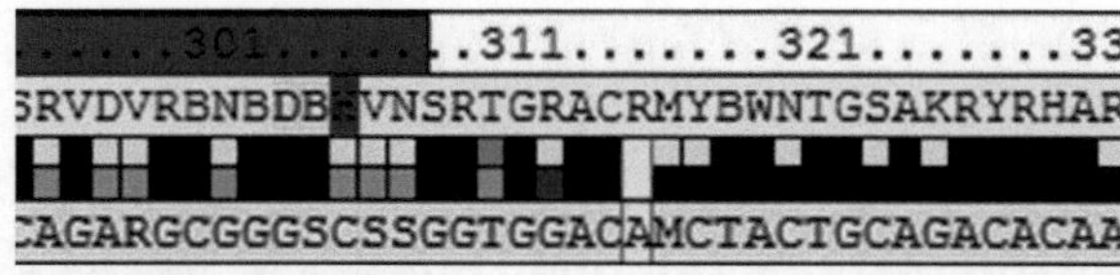


Fig. 18. Coloured boxes above the Sample Consensus sequence indicate points of interest in the sequence.

R970900776 DRB1
Start: 14 (101) Exon 2 1
Stop: 509 (596) Exon 3 226

| Allele 1 | Allele 2 | MM 0 | MM 1 | Differences |
|---|---|---|---|---|
| DRB1*01:01:01 | DRB1*03:01:01:01 | 0 | 0 | |
| DRB1*01:01:01 | DRB1*03:01:01:02 | 0 | 0 | |
| DRB1*01:18 | DRB1*03:06 | 0 | 1 | Exon 2 |
| DRB1*01:20 | DRB1*03:05:01 | 0 | 24 | Exon 2 |
| DRB1*01:01:01 | DRB1*03:01:02 | 1 | -- | |
| DRB1*01:01:01 | DRB1*03:01:03 | 1 | -- | |
| DRB1*01:01:01 | DRB1*03:01:04 | 1 | -- | |
| DRB1*01:01:01 | DRB1*03:01:05 | 1 | -- | |
| DRB1*01:01:01 | DRB1*03:01:06 | 1 | -- | |
| DRB1*01:01:01 | DRB1*03:01:07 | 1 | -- | |
| DRB1*01:01:01 | DRB1*03:01:08 | 1 | -- | |
| DRB1*01:01:01 | DRB1*03:01:09 | 1 | -- | |
| DRB1*01:01:01 | DRB1*03:01:10 | 1 | -- | |
| DRB1*01:01:01 | DRB1*03:01:11 | 1 | -- | |

Fig. 19. The Results pane includes sample name, start/stop positions, and best-matched allele combination.

2. The **MM0 column** is the number of mismatches between the test sequence and the sequence of the alleles.
3. Additional columns, labelled **MM1**, **MM2**, etc., will be present when heterozygous ambiguity resolving sequencing primers are used. These columns indicate the number of mismatches between the test sequence and sequence of the allele.
4. The **N-C column** indicates the number of mismatches in the non-coding region (Fig. 20).
5. The **IND column** contains mismatch information in the heterozygous insertion/deletion (indel) data. The software is sensitive to runs of mixed bases since many introns do have heterozygous indels.

   When there is background in the sequence due to a co-amplified stretch of DNA or when the signal to noise is relatively low, the extra signal can be interpreted as a heterozygous InDel. Choosing “Exclude Het InDel” informs the software that the

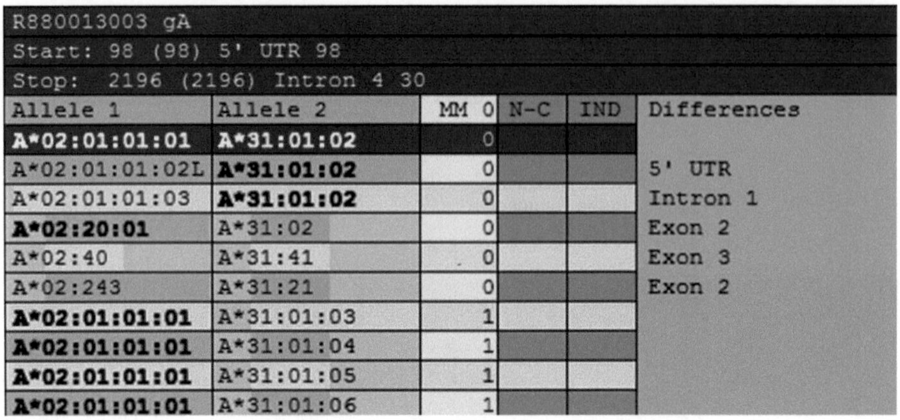


Fig. 20. Non-coding and Indel data are viewed in the N-C and IND columns, respectively.

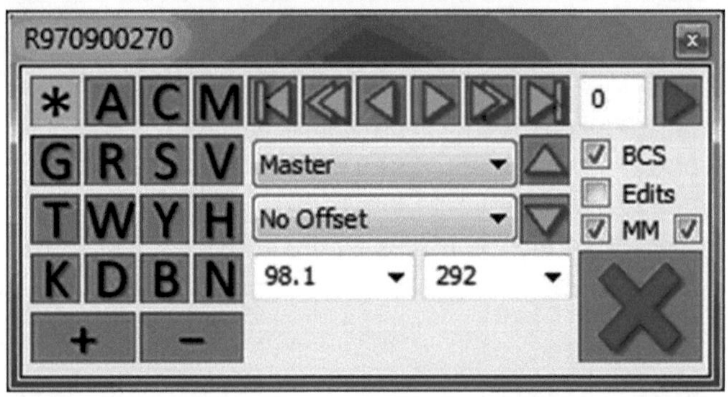


Fig. 21. The Navigator enables editing, review, and movement from sample to sample within the project.

additional signal should be interpreted as background and not as a real sequence feature.

If either the N-C or IND column is shaded pink, the data from these regions are NOT included in the analysis. To activate the N-C and IND layers to include the data in the analysis, click on the appropriate column. Clicking again will deactivate the layers. When the N-C and IND layers are activated, the data are included in the analysis and the data within these layers must be edited (see Notes 2 and 3).

6. The **Differences column** indicates the regions within the reference sequence that contain the sequence differences between the ambiguities.

### *2.7. Navigator*

The navigator enables sequence editing, moving between samples, and moving between positions within a sequence. Importantly, the Navigator is used to Validate automated base calls (Fig. 21).

1. Positions for **Validation** can include positions with a low **Base Call Score** (BCS), **Edited** positions, potential **MisMatch** positions, and user-defined **variant** positions (box to the right of the MM).
   (a) **Base Call Score** (BCS) is a quality measurement that is determined by peak spacing, presence of background noise, and signal strength. The BCS for each base appears above the BCS in the navigator.
   (b) Bases with a BCS of lower than 70 (or lower than 35 for single direction sequences) will be included in the priority review using the red X or the double arrows.
2. Moving to positions for Validation is performed by selecting the double arrow buttons or using the red X button. The presence of the red X means that the cursor is at a position that has not been validated by the operator. Clicking the red X validates the base call and changes the red X to a green tick.
3. Selecting either single arrow button moves the EPG one position left or right.
4. Selecting the up arrow moves to the sample above and selecting the down arrow moves to the sample below in the Sample Pane.
5. The Master drop down menu selects between master sequences, HARP sequences, Master-intron, or Master-indel sequences.
6. The No Offset drop down menu allows the user to chose the base numbering motif desired.
7. Underneath the No Offset drop down menu are the codon and base location.

   To navigate to a particular base, enter the base position in the right drop down and hit enter.
8. Clicking on the red X will confirm the base call and move to the next position that meets the "to be validated" criteria. As the red X is clicked, a green box will appear above the base indicating that it has been confirmed. Once ALL validation positions have been verified, the yellow box under the Audit column in the Sample Pane will turn green.
9. If a base call needs to be edited, the call can be changed manually using the base letters on the Navigator. The raw data are not changed with edits. The consensus sequence is changed, and these changes are recorded in the saved project. When the project is opened, the changes are applied again to the raw data.

#### 2.8. Other Sample and Sequence Editing Functions

1. Resizing the EPG

   The EPG can be resized by pressing the Shift key and the up/down or left/right arrows on the computer keyboard.

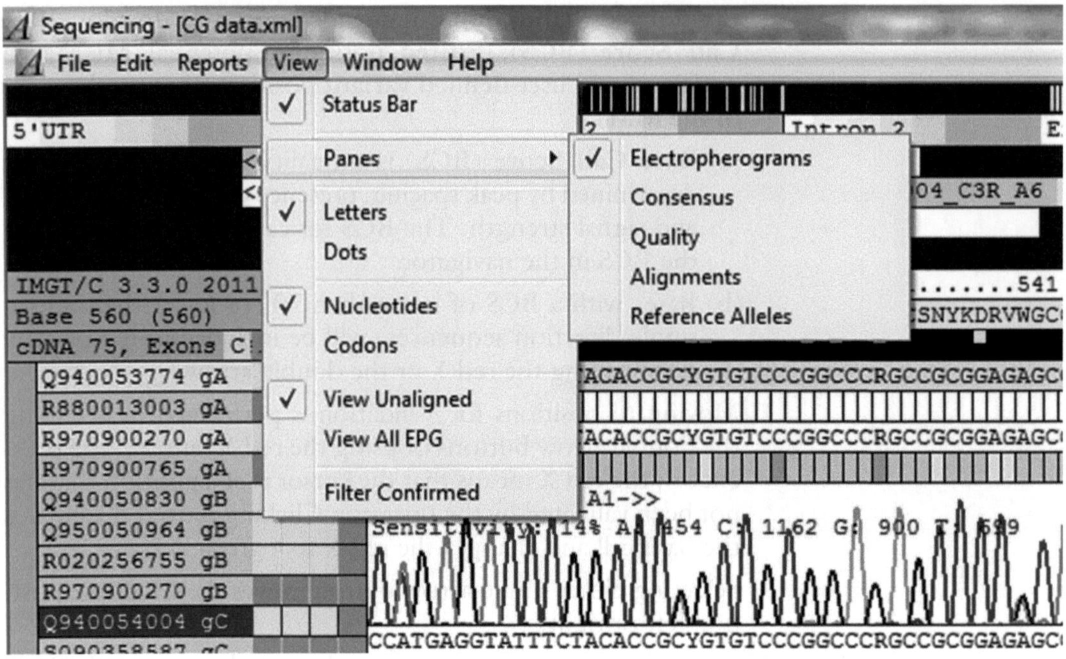


Fig. 22. View options allows the data and reference library data to be viewed in different ways.

2. Hiding EPG traces

   Pressing the computer keyboard Shift key and one of the letters representing the four bases simultaneously will remove the trace of this base from the EPG. Repeating the process will return the trace.

   This function is useful if heterozygyous peaks are perfectly overlaid and the base call requires confirmation.

### 2.9. View Options

The **View** options enable the samples sequence data and the sequence data from the alleles in the library to be viewed in different ways (Fig. 22).

1. **Status Bar** shows the status of the project at the bottom of the screen.
2. **Panes**
   (a) **Electropherogram** is the default and displays the electropherogram tracings of the sample.
   (b) **Consensus displays** the consensus sequence for all samples in a project.
   (c) **Quality** displays the consensus sequence shaded according to the consensus sequence BCS for each base for every sample in the project.
   (d) **Alignments** displays the consensus sequence for each of the possible allele combinations for a given sample. Mismatches with the sample consensus appear highlighted in yellow.

(e) **Reference Alleles** shows the sequence of alleles within the library compared to the sequence of the selected sample. Differences are highlighted in yellow. The alleles are shown in the results pane.
The user can select specific allele sequences to align together by typing the allele names in the Navigator.

3. **Letters or Dots**
   (a) Selecting letters will show the bases for alignments and reference as letters.
   (b) Selecting Dots will show dots at each base where the alignment or reference matches with the consensus sequence. Bases that differ will be shown as letters.
4. **Nucleotides or Codons**
   (a) Selecting Nucleotides will show the base numbering.
   (b) Selecting Codons will show the codon numbering.
5. When using the coding sequence reference, the **View Unaligned** option will include or exclude the intronic overlap of the sequences between exons.
6. **View All EPG** enables the HARP electropherograms to be seen with the EPG of the F and R sequences. Note that the highlighted sequence in the results pane (yellow column) is highlighted in the EPG pane. By selecting the HARPs layer, the HARPs EPGs become highlighted.
7. **Filter Confirmed**
   As positions are confirmed using the red X, alleles within the results pane are excluded and only those alleles with 0 mismatches with the test sequence remain. To restore the list of possible allele combinations, unclick on the Filter Confirmed option in the view pane.

### 2.10. Data Analysis and Editing EPGs

#### 2.10.1. Logging on

Log into the Assign 3.6+ software and select the settings file desired by clicking on **Edit** then **Settings**. Select the settings file and click **Done**.

#### 2.10.2. Importing Data

1. Import the desired dataset using either the **Browse** option to import an entire folder of data or the **Select Files Manually** to selectively import files.
2. Imported samples will be displayed as a list on the left side of the screen.
3. The Electropherogram data will be in the centre of the screen.
4. The Allele assignments for the active (highlighted in blue) sample will be displayed at the right side of the screen.

5. Each of these panes can be sized by dragging the frame to the desired width to optimize the amount of electropherogram data displayed.
6. Resize the electropherogram peaks if desired.

*2.10.3. Navigation*

1. The Navigator box is used to navigate through the data checking the critical bases.
2. Set the desired bases to be audited in the Navigator box: BCS, Edits, MM, and variant positions.
3. Highlight the sample to be reviewed by clicking on it in the left sample pane.
4. Navigate to the first base in the sample by clicking on the left arrow with the bar in the navigator.
5. Using the red X button, navigate through the sequence verifying all desired bases. As each base is confirmed, the red X will change to a green check and the cursor will move to the next base to be verified. A green box will appear above each base pair that has been verified using this method.
   (a) There should be at least one allele pair in the Results Pane on the right that indicates no mismatches in the MM0 column.
   (b) Once the Master Layer has been reviewed, the Navigator will take the user to any resolution primer layers that are present. These layers must also be reviewed before the sample analysis is complete.
   (c) Once all priority review bases have been verified, the red X will change to a green check mark indicating no additional bases need confirming. In the Sample Pane, the box under the A column (Audit) will turn green.
   (d) Clicking on the box under the 1 column will indicate the sample has been reviewed once.
   (e) At this point, the project should be saved to prevent any accidental loss of data review. Click on File then Save As. Select a file name and location to save the project. The saved project (.xml format) indicates which electropherograms were used including their saved location, any edits and confirmations that were done, and information about the user.
   (f) If Genomic References were selected, the N-C and IND column may be present. Refer to the differences column to determine if analysis of the non-coding region would be beneficial. Click on the N-C column to highlight it in yellow. Navigate to the mismatch positions and make any edits necessary. Once all review and edits have been made, click back on the MM0 column to view the allele pairs.

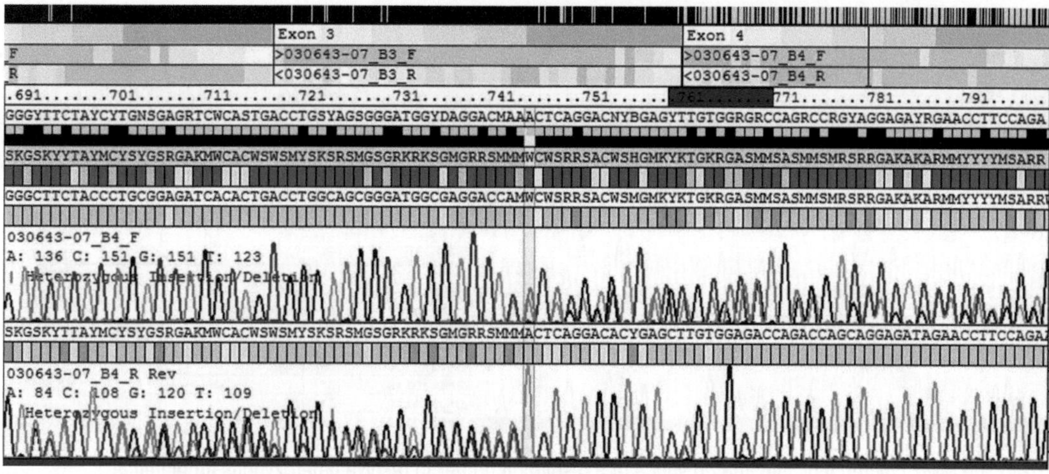

Fig. 23. Example of a sample with an Insertion or Deletion (InDel) in exon 4.

(g) Repeat on the IND column if desired. The IND column should be reviewed only when there is a clear insertion or deletion in the sample. Poor quality or mobility shifts can trigger the Heterozygous Insertion or Deletion warning. Use the Exclude Het InDel option to eliminate any warnings due to background noise and not true InDels. Below is an example of a clear InDel (Fig. 23).

6. Once all the review has been completed on the first sample, click on the second sample and repeat the process.

   (a) Save your work often to prevent any loss of review.

7. If a secondary review is desired, the project should be opened by the second reviewer to preserve the audit trail. The second reviewer logs onto the software and selects **Open** in the **File** menu. Navigate to the saved project (.xml file). The software will locate the raw data, import it, and apply all changes and verifications that have been performed by any previous reviewers.

   (a) Select the desired priority review positions in the Navigator box. Use the left double arrow button to navigate to the required positions. Using the big red X will cancel and reapply the audited positions.

   (b) Once all positions have been reviewed, the second reviewer can click on the box in the 2 column in the sample pane.

   (c) Once the second review box is checked, the sample is "locked" and no more edits can be made unless the box is manually unchecked.

   (d) Save often to prevent the accidental loss of data review.

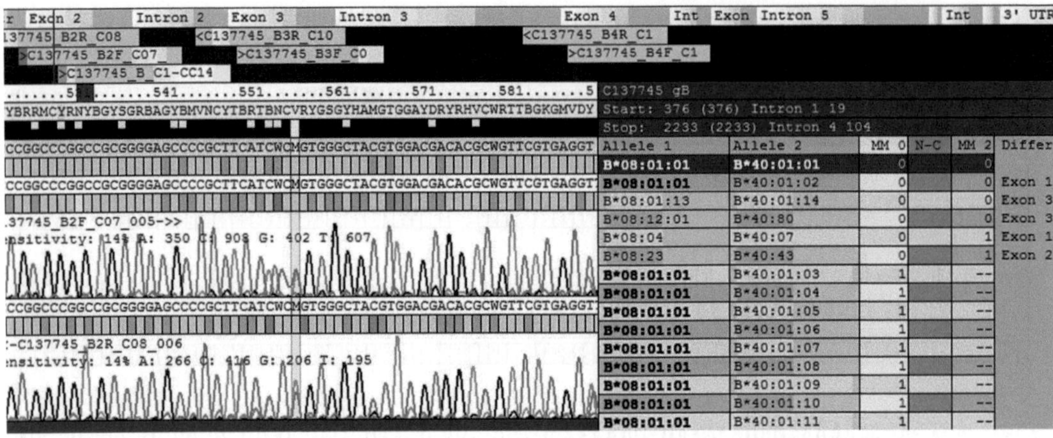


Fig. 24. The MM2 column indicates the presence of a resolution primer to resolve heterozygous ambiguities.

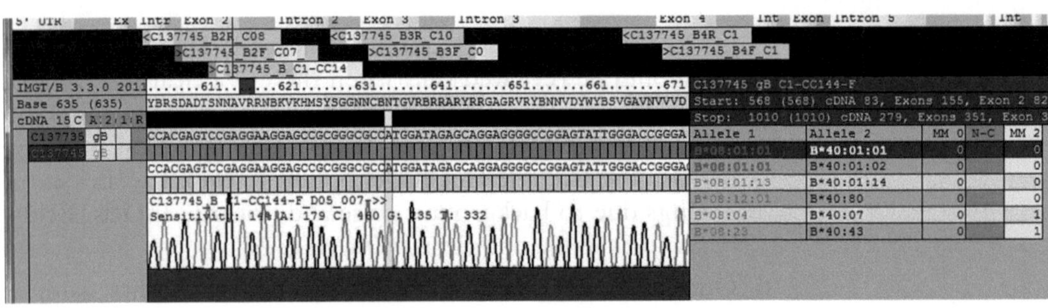


Fig. 25. The Resolving layer is activated to allow review of resolution primer data.

*2.10.4. Resolution Primer Layers*

1. HARPs are used to resolve heterozygous ambiguities within the regions sequenced. HARPs target one of the alleles present, creating a hemizygous sequence. In the example below, multiple ambiguities exist after analysing the master sequence as indicated in the MM0 column highlighted in yellow. Heterozygous sequence is present (Fig. 24).
2. Selection of an HARP that will detect only one of the alleles in the pair will result in a hemizygous sequence in the MM1 layer. This will eliminate some of the heterozygous ambiguities. Allele combinations with no mismatches in the MM0 and MM1 column will be included in the report. Alleles with mismatches in the MM1 column have been eliminated by the HARP sequence (Fig. 25).

*2.10.5. Auditing*

All user interaction is logged in the audit trail. The software logs time and date any edit was made, when the project was saved and the user performing the action. This information can be printed on the allele report along with the sample allele assignments.

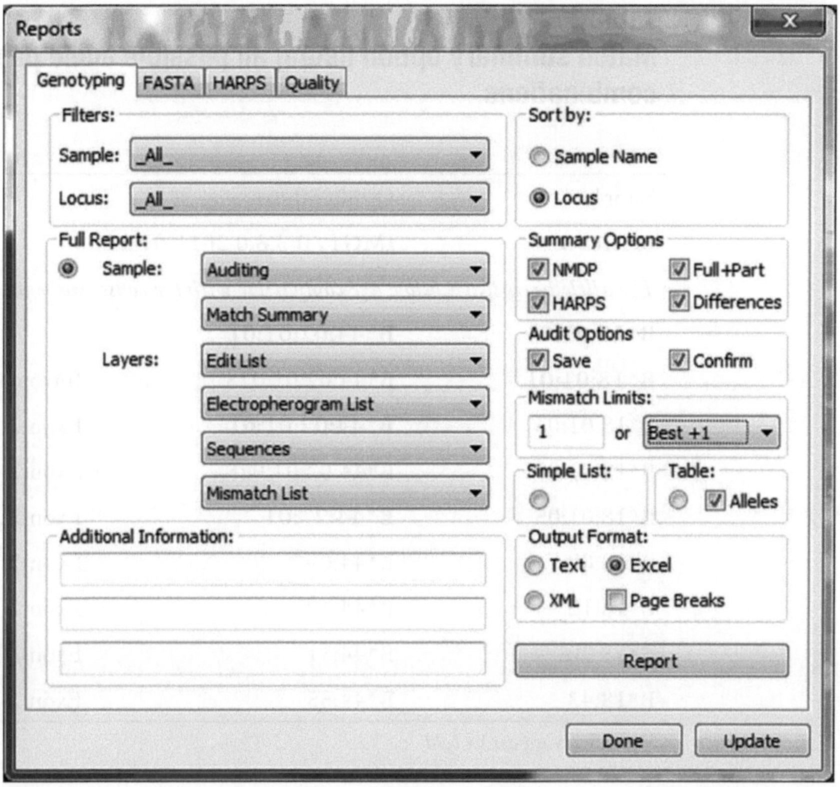


Fig. 26. Genotyping Report options allows for customized reports.

### 2.11. Reporting

The Assign-SBT reports enable a comprehensive assessment of the sequence data. A genotyping report lists the best-matched alleles to the sample sequence and also enables CWD alleles to be indicated. The genotype report also enables alleles to be reported as functional groups by reporting G groups and P groups and enables the user to structure the report specific for their requirements. The software can also report the HARPs required to resolve the heterozygous ambiguities.

To access the report functions, click on **Reports** then **Report Generator** on the top menu bar.

#### 2.11.1. Genotyping Report

The Genotyping report is used to report the allele combinations that have identical sequence to the sequence of the sample (Fig. 26).

1. The **Full Report Section** enables laboratories to create their report format. The Sample drop down menus enable the lab to include or exclude specific items from the report.
   (a) The **Sample** section contains the Auditing, Match Summary, G Groups, and P Groups reports.
   (b) **Match Summary** will list all the possible allele pair combinations. If the CWD option is selected, the CWD alleles will appear in bold type in the report (Table 1).

**Table 1**
**Match summary option listing all possible allele pair combinations**

| | | |
|---|---|---|
| Sample | Q950050964 | |
| Reference | IMGT/B 3.3.0 2011-01-14 | |
| *The allele pairs listed below are compatible with the consensus sequence* | | |
| **B*18:01:01** | **B*44:02:01:01** | |
| **B*18:01:01** | B*44:02:01:02S | Intron 4 |
| B*18:01:05 | **B*44:02:01:01** | Exon 2 |
| B*18:01:05 | B*44:02:01:02S | Exon 2, Intron 4 |
| B*18:01:05 | **B*44:27:01** | Exon 2 |
| B*18:09 | B*44:09 | Exon 2 |
| B*18:12 | B*44:12 | Exon 2 |
| B*18:20 | B*44:51 | Exon 3 |
| B*18:43 | B*44:55 | Exon 2 |

CWD alleles appear in *bold*

(c) The **G Group Report** enables those Class I alleles with identical nucleotide sequence in exons 2 and 3 to be reported under the same code and class II alleles that are identical in exon 2. If the CWD option is selected, those alleles that have been reported at a significant allele frequency groups will appear in bold type in the report. HLA alleles that have identical nucleotide sequences across the exons encoding the peptide binding domains (exons 2 and 3 for HLA class I and exon 2 only for HLA class II alleles) will be designated by an upper case "G" which follows the first three fields of the allele designation of the lowest numbered allele in the group (Table 2).

(d) The **P Group Report** will list the alleles grouped according protein sequences as encoded by exons 2 and 3 for HLA class I alleles, and for HLA class II alleles this is based on identical protein sequences as encoded by exon 2. P groups containing CWD alleles will be bolded on the report (Table 3).

(e) The Auditing option will include a comprehensive audit report including date, time, and identification of the operator validating the results.

2. The **Layers** section contains the Edit List, Electropherogram List, Sequences, Mismatch List, and Mismatch table. These can be included or excluded according to the needs of the laboratory.

**Table 2**
**G group report**

| | |
|---|---|
| Sample | Q950050964 |
| Reference | IMGT/B 3.3.0 2011-01-14 |
| *The allele pairs listed below are compatible with the consensus sequence* | |
| **B*18:01:01G** | **B*44:02:01G** |
| B*18:09 | B*44:09 |
| B*18:12 | B*44:12 |
| B*18:20 | B*44:51 |
| B*18:43 | B*44:55 |

**Table 3**
**P group report**

| | |
|---|---|
| Sample | Q950050964 |
| Reference | IMGT/B 3.3.0 2011-01-14 |
| *The allele pairs listed below are compatible with the consensus sequence* | |
| **B*18:01P** | **B*44:02P** |
| B*18:09 | B*44:09 |
| B*18:12 | B*44:12 |
| B*18:20 | B*44:51 |
| B*18:43 | B*44:55 |

3. The **Additional Information** section can be used to add comments specific for a typing run. These comments appear at the top of the report.
4. **Sort** by is used to sort the report by Sample Name or Locus.
5. **Summary Options** includes options to add to the report: NMDP Codes, HARPs used, Full + Part indicates which alleles are fully typed in the IMGT database, and Differences indicates where each allele pair differs from the others.
6. **Audit Options** allows the operator to choose to record all the Save events for the project by clicking the Save box. Confirm records change and priority base confirmation.

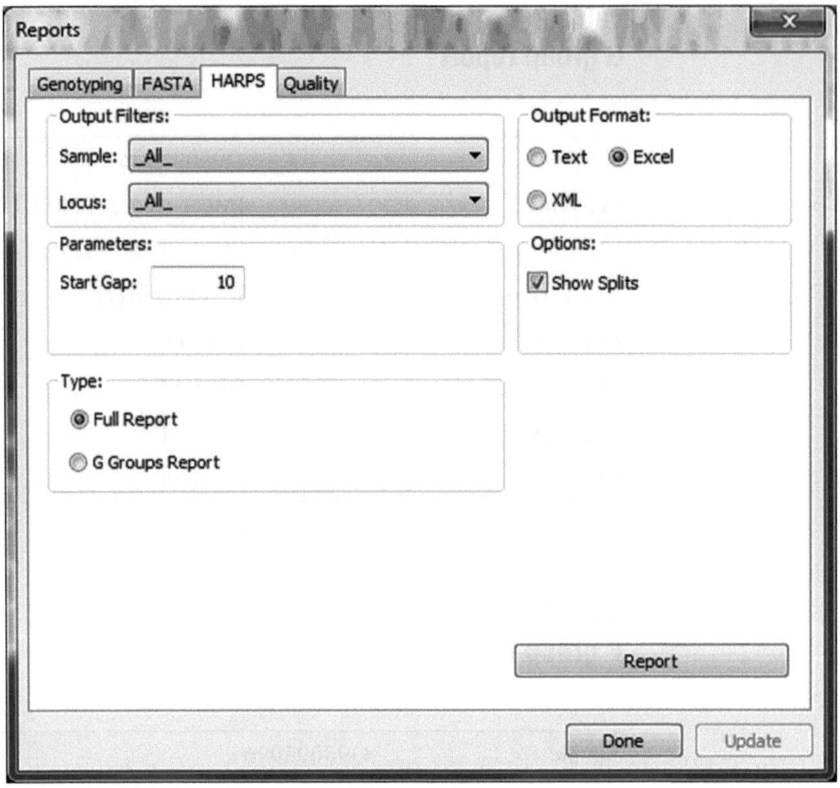


Fig. 27. The heterozygous ambiguity resolving primers (HARPs) report indicates which resolution primers are required to resolve ambiguities.

*2.11.2. HARPs Report*

1. The HARPs report indicates to the operator which HARPs are required to resolve heterozygous ambiguities and which exons are required to be sequenced to resolve allele ambiguities (Fig. 27).
   (a) The **Output Filters** can be used to filter for a single sample/locus or all samples/loci in a project.
   (b) The **Start Gap** under Parameters can be set depending on the gap between the end of the sequencing primer and usable data. This is generally around ten for POP6 users and longer for POP7 users.
   (c) The operator can choose between a **Full Report** and a **G Groups Report** under the Type section.
   (d) The **Full Report** will list the HARP resolution for each allele pair (Table 4).
   (e) The **G Group Report** will group the resolution based on the broader G Grouping of the allele pairs (Table 5).

**Table 4**
**Example of a full HARPs report listing resolution for each allele pair and HARPs required to resolve the ambiguities**

| | | | |
|---|---|---|---|
| Sample | Q950050964 | | |
| Reference | IMGT/B 3.3.0 2011-01-14 | | |
| Use ONE primer from group 1 | C1-AC559-R-520 | C1-TG539-R-507 | C1-CT559-R-494 |
| Use ONE primer from group 2 | C1-GAA309-R-953 | | |
| Splits | B*18:01:01 | B*44:02:01:01 | |
| | B*18:01:01 | B*44:02:01:02S | Intron 4 |
| | B*18:01:05 | B*44:02:01:01 | |
| | B*18:01:05 | B*44:02:01:02S | Intron 4 |
| | B*18:01:05 | B*44:27:01 | Exon 4 |
| | B*18:09 | B*44:09 | |
| | B*18:12 | B*44:12 | |
| | B*18:20 | B*44:51 | |
| | B*18:43 | B*44:55 | |

Unresolved ambiguities remain within exon 4, intron 4

**Table 5**
**Example of a G group HARPs report**

| | | | |
|---|---|---|---|
| Sample | Q950050964 | | |
| Reference | IMGT/B 3.3.0 2011-01-14 | | |
| Use ONE primer from group 1 | C1-AC559-R-520 | C1-TG539-R-507 | C1-CT559-R-494 |
| Use ONE primer from group 2 | C1-GAA309-R-953 | | |
| Splits | **B*18:01:01G** | **B*44:02:01G** | |
| | B*18:01:05 | B*44:02:01G | |
| | B*18:09 | B*44:09 | |
| | B*18:12 | B*44:12 | |
| | B*18:20 | B*44:51 | |
| | B*18:43 | B*44:55 | |

Unresolved ambiguities remain within exon 4, intron 4
Resolution is based on the broader G grouping of the allele pairs

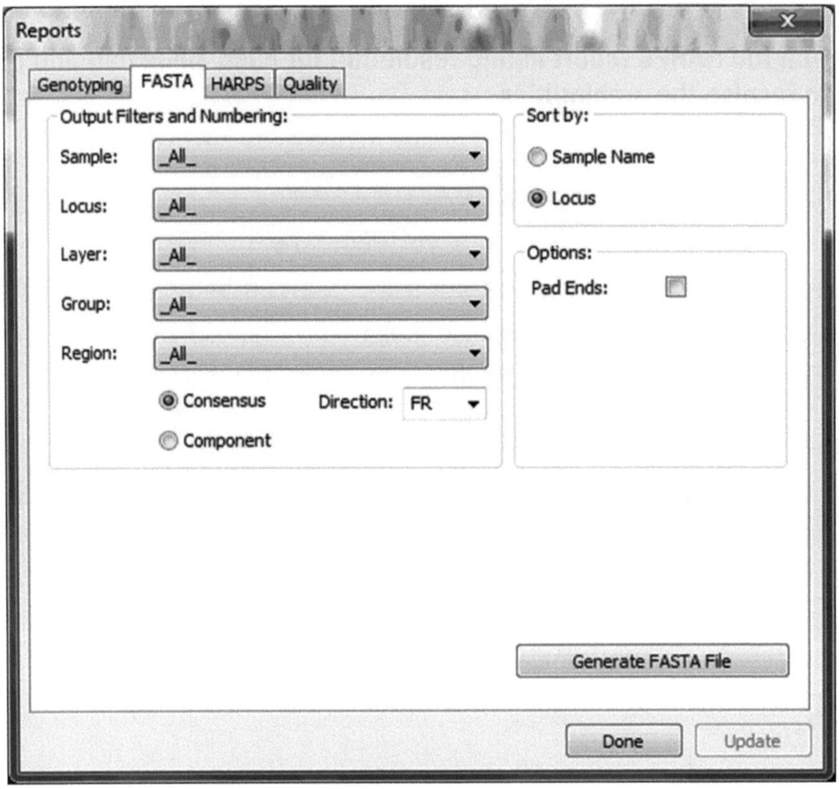


Fig. 28. The FASTA report enables sequences in FASTA text format to be produced.

(f) The **Output Format** can be in a Text file, Excel (default), or XML format.

(g) The **Options** section will determine if the report is generated using Splits or not. Clicking **Show Splits** will list all the allele combinations and the HARPs needed to resolve them. Leaving it unclicked will result in a list of required HARPs only.

*2.11.3. FASTA*

The FASTA report enables sequences in FASTA text format to be produced. Selecting the sample, locus, layer, group, and region provides a detailed description of the FASTA file in the FASTA file name (Fig. 28).

*2.11.4. Quality Reports*

The quality reports utilizes the BCS at each position to create quality control information for a sample, which can then be compared between different samples to create quality control information for the assay. The principle is that if the mean and standard deviation of BCS for a number of sequence positions can be calculated, this will provide a quality score for the region of sequence from which the mean and standard deviation were calculated. This information can

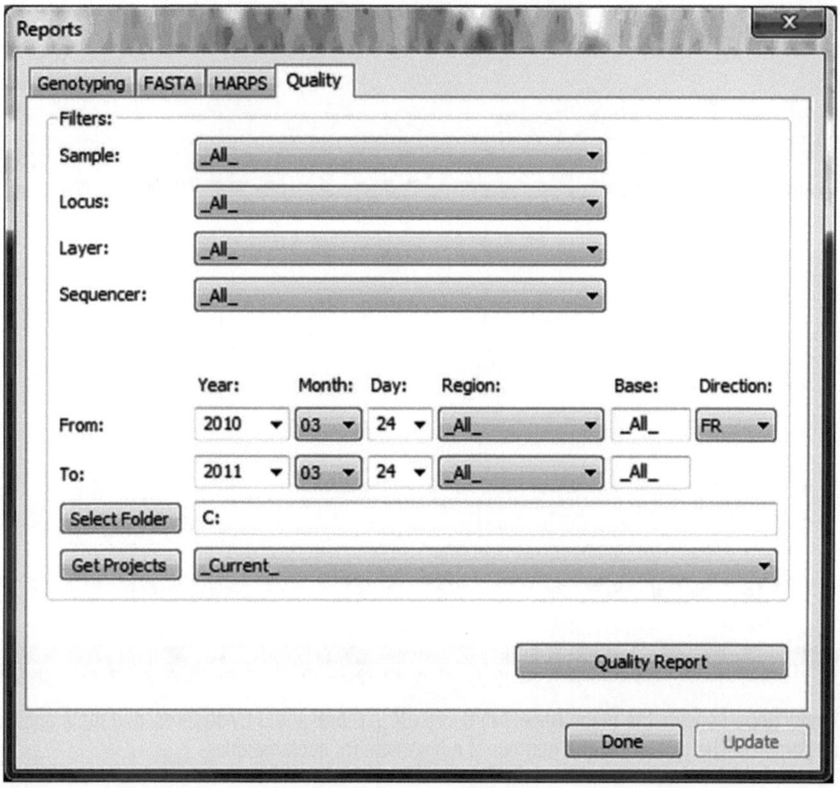


Fig. 29. The Quality Report utilizes the base caller score at each position to create a comparison between different samples, providing quality control information for the assay.

then be used to calculate quality information for specific sequencing primers, for different assays and different samples. The data can be used to monitor the performance of a test and set performance criteria that can be used when assessing changes, such as reagent batch changes, or DNA extraction procedures, for example (Fig. 29).

1. The **Quality** report dialogue enables the user to select parameters for quality analysis. In addition to the sample information, the user can select across regions (i.e., an exons) within the sequence to analyse, or a specific range of bases within a region.
2. Leaving the **Get Projects** default at **_Current_** will produce a quality report in the active Assign-SBT layout.
3. By Clicking **Get Projects** and then browsing to directories in the **_Current_** drop down menu, a quality report can be generated from saved layouts within the browsed directories (Fig. 30).

The Quality Report shows the mean BCS in blue and the standard deviation in pink for all samples HLA-B exon 2 for a SBT run. The red dots show the number of edits made for each sample.

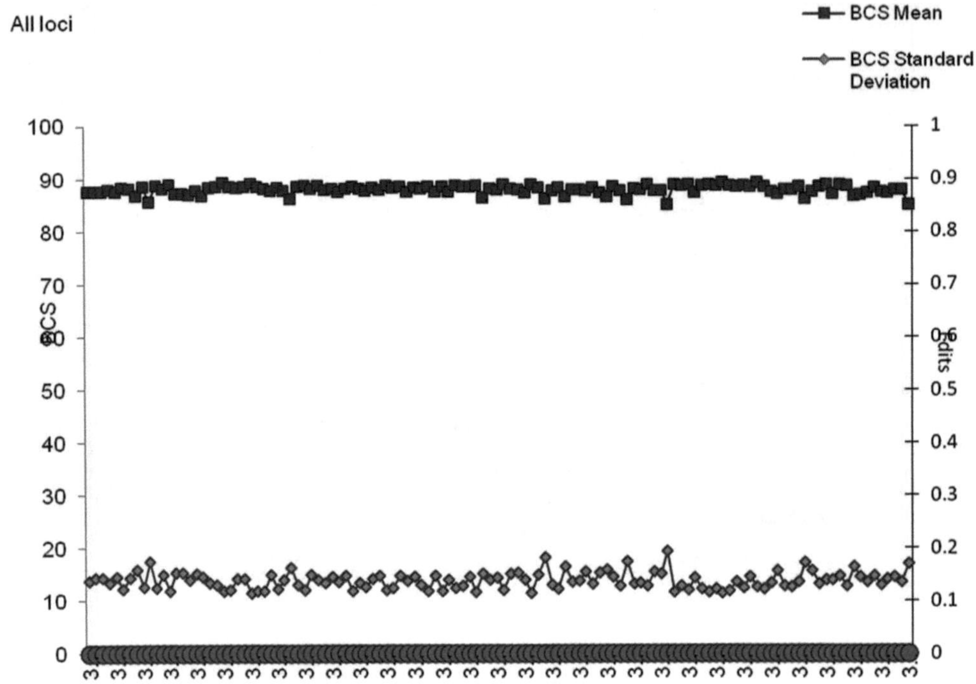


Fig. 30. The Quality Report shows the mean Base Call Score (BCS) represented by squares, and the standard deviation in diamonds for all samples. The dots show the number of edits made for each sample.

## 3. Notes

1. CWD alleles, or common and well-documented alleles, are those alleles with a calculated allele frequency in one or more populations, G groups are those groups of alleles that share the same nucleotide sequence in exons 2 + 3 of class I and exon 2 of class II, and P groups are those alleles that share the same amino acid sequence in exons 2 + 3 of class I and exon 2 of class II alleles. These options enable laboratories to determine the probability of a particular allele or allele combination within an ambiguous report, or if an ambiguous report contains functional differences between alleles).
2. Note: If the software does not detect heterozygous insertion/deletion data, the IND column is not created.
3. Note: If the **Use Genomic References** box is not checked in the Edit/Settings/Advanced tab, the N-C column is not created.

## 4. Conclusion

This chapter provides a comprehensive description of the use of Assign-SBT sequence analysis software for use in HLA sequencing-based typing.

The sequencing of HLA genes was one of the first applications for DNA re-sequencing. Currently the applications of DNA sequencing seem endless and sequencing is used for the identification of sequence differences in a countless number of genetic systems. In order to accommodate the increasing needs of DNA sequencing, Conexio has developed Assign-ATF. Assign-ATF includes all the quality control, auditing, and editing features of Assign-SBT but enables the user to create his own references and libraries and use the software for whatever application is required. Assign-ATF software operates in two modes: a genotyping mode, which compares a sequence against a library of allele/or variant sequences (similar to HLA typing) and is used for applications such as Hepatitis C genotyping, and a variant detection mode, which compares a sequence against a single reference sequence (usually a "wildtype" sequence). In the variant detection mode, all sequence differences between the sample and the reference sequence are reported; the software also enables nucleotide changes to be reported as predicted amino acid changes. Assign-ATF is ideal for the detection of variants associated with genetic disorders.

DNA sequencing technology has advanced significantly in recent years. Of the Next Generation (NG) technologies, the 454 Sequencing Technology is the first to be used for HLA typing (2–4). As was the case for Sanger Sequencing and the original development of SBT, it is software that is making HLA typing using NG sequencing technology possible. NG sequencing presents new challenges including, shorter sequencing read lengths, the generation of up to hundreds of thousand strings of sequence data and the presence of non-specific sequence data. At Conexio, we have developed a version of Assign for use with Next Generation sequencing technology, and, despite the challenges, we have created a user friendly, high-throughput sequence analysis software that enables high resolution HLA typing.

## References

1. Cano P, Klitz W, Mack SJ et al (2007) Common and well-documented HLA alleles: report of the Ad-Hoc committee of the American society for histocompatibility and immunogenetics. Hum Immunol 68(5):392–417
2. Bentley G, Higuchi R, Hoglund B et al (2009) High-resolution, high-throughput HLA genotyping by next-generation sequencing. Tissue Antigens 74(5):393–403
3. Lind C, Ferriola D, Mackiewicz K et al (2010) Next-generation sequencing: the solution for high resolution, unambiguous human leukocyte antigen typing. Hum Immunol 71(10):1033–1042
4. Holcomb CL, Höglund B, Anderson MW et al (2011) A multi-site study using high-resolution HLA genotyping by next generation sequencing. Tissue Antigens 77(3):206–217

# Chapter 7

# Simple Methods for the Detection of HLA-G Variants in Coding and Non-coding Regions

**Holger Nückel, Erick C. Castelli, Philippe Moreau, Crista Ochsenfarth, Peter A. Horn, and Vera Rebmann**

## Abstract

The non-classical human leukocyte antigen (HLA)-G plays a crucial role in the induction of tolerance at the feto–maternal interface as well as in transplantation, cancer, inflammation, and autoimmune diseases. To understand gene regulation and the impact of polymorphic sites on the function, simple and easy feasible approaches are needed for the detection of HLA-G variants in coding and non-coding regions. Here we summarize a set of methods for the identification of variants in the exon 2–4, in the 3′ untranslated region and in the gene promoter region of the HLA-G gene.

**Key words:** HLA-G, Polymorphism, 14 bp Fragment ins/del, 3′ Untranslated region, Human leukocyte antigen, Coding region, Non-coding region, Gene promoter region

## 1. Introduction

The non-classical human leukocyte antigen (HLA)-G is strongly expressed at the feto–maternal interface but only marginally on healthy tissues including thymus, cornea, and erythroid cells as well as blood cells. In a non-physiological situation HLA-G is found to be expressed in grafted tissue, in cancer, or in inflammation and autoimmune diseases. The expression of this molecule is always associated with the induction of tolerance by the inhibition of the adaptive and innate immune response (for review see ref. (1)).

The gene structure of HLA-G is homologous to the classical HLA class I genes: The HLA-G gene exhibits seven introns and eight exons. Exon 1 encodes the peptide signal, exons 2, 3, and 4, the extracellular α1, α2, and α3 domains, respectively, exon 5 the

Frank T. Christiansen and Brian D. Tait (eds.), *Immunogenetics: Methods and Applications in Clinical Practice*, Methods in Molecular Biology, vol. 882, DOI 10.1007/978-1-61779-842-9_7, © Springer Science+Business Media New York 2012

transmembrane region and exon 6 the cytoplasmic tail; exon 7 is always absent from the mature mRNA; and exon 8 is not translated because of a premature stop codon in exon 6 (2). HLA-G exhibits only a limited variability within the coding region. But an extended polymorphism has been reported in the 5′ upstream regulatory region (5′URR) and in the 3′-untranslated region (3′UTR) of the gene. According to the International Immunogenetics Database (IMGT database 2.28.0, January 2010) (3), 44 different HLA-G variants have been assigned; 33 single nucleotide polymorphisms (SNPs) are found within the encoding region of HLA-G; and only 13 variations result in an amino acid exchange. Nevertheless it has to be pointed out that at least 24 of the 44 alleles reveal a substitution detected only in one or in a few individuals worldwide (2).

The nucleotide variations that result in amino acid exchanges at the protein level may lead to conformational changes and thereby may affect the biological function. With regard to the consensus

**Table 1**
**HLA-G polymorphisms in exon 1–4 and in 3′UTR**

| Position | Exon 2 | | | | | | | | | | | Exon 3 | | | |
|---|---|---|---|---|---|---|---|---|---|---|---|---|---|---|---|
| Rel. to ATG = 0 | 234 | 239 | 280 | 292 | 297 | 306 | 324 | 361 | 366 | 372 | 408 | 706 | 726 | 738 | 741 |
| Codon | 11 | 13 | 27 | 31 | 32 | 35 | 41 | 54 | 55 | 57 | 69 | 93 | 100 | 104 | 105 |
| Amino acid | A | S/F | Y/H | T/S/M | Q | R | A | Q/R/- | E | P | A | H | G/D | G/V | S/C |
| G*01:01:01 | GCC | TCC | TAC | ACG | CAG | CGG | GCG | CAG | GAG | CCG | GCC | CAC | GGC | GGG | TCC |
| G*01:01:02 | --- | --- | --- | --- | --- | --- | --- | --- | --- | --A | --- | --T | --- | --- | --- |
| G*01:01:03 | --- | --- | --- | --- | --- | --- | --- | --- | --- | --A | --- | --- | --- | --- | --- |
| G*01:01:04 | --- | --- | --- | --- | --- | --- | --- | --- | --- | --A | --T | --- | --- | --- | --- |
| G*01:01:05 | --- | --- | --- | --- | --- | --- | --- | --- | --- | --- | --- | --- | --- | --- | --- |
| G*01:01:06 | --- | --- | --- | --- | --- | --- | --- | --- | --- | --- | --- | --- | --- | --- | --- |
| G*01:01:07 | --- | --- | --- | --- | --- | --- | --- | --- | --- | --A | --- | --T | --- | --- | --- |
| G*01:01:08 | --- | --- | --- | --- | --- | --- | --- | --- | --- | --A | --- | --- | --- | --- | --- |
| G*01:01:09 | --- | --- | --- | --- | --- | --- | --- | --- | --- | --- | --- | --- | --- | --- | --- |
| G*01:01:11 | --- | --- | --- | --- | --- | --- | --- | --- | --- | --- | --- | --- | --- | --- | --- |
| G*01:01:12 | --- | --- | --- | --- | --- | --- | --T | --- | --- | --A | --- | --T | --- | --- | --- |
| G*01:01:13 | --- | --- | --- | --- | --- | --- | --- | --- | --- | --A | --- | --T | --- | --- | --- |
| G*01:01:14 | --- | --- | --- | --- | --- | --A | --- | --- | --- | --A | --- | --T | --- | --- | --- |
| G*01:01:15 | --- | --- | --- | --- | --- | --- | --- | --- | --A | --- | --- | --- | --- | --- | --- |

allele HLA-G*01:01 only 4 out of the 33 SNPs within the coding region of HLA-G are related to an amino acid exchange, which do present frequencies above 1% in population studies (4–9). One of them is located at codon 31 in exon 2 exchanging a threonine for serine, being typical for the G*01:03 allele (Table 1). Two are found at codon 110 and codon 130 in exon 3. The first one results in the amino acid exchange of leucine to isoleucine typical for the G*01:04 group. A deletion of a cytosine at the first nucleotide of codon 130 in exon 3 (Table 1) changes the reading frame and leads to a stop signal (TGA) in codon 189 at exon 4. As this allele misses substantial information of the full length transcript, it is designated as G*01:05N allele (N = null allele) (10, 11). The fourth variation comprises a variation at codon 258, exchanging threonine for methionine, being typical for the G*01:06 allele. The other SNPs are synonymous substitutions.

| | | | | | | | Exon 4 | | | | | | 3′UTR (6) | |
|---|---|---|---|---|---|---|---|---|---|---|---|---|---|---|
| 748 | 755 | 778 | 814 | 871 | 902 | 394 | 1590 | 1659 | 1681 | 1734 | 1799 | 1827 | 3741 | |
| 107 | 110 | 117 | 130 | 148 | 159 | 169 | 188 | 211 | 219 | 236 | 258 | 267 | | |
| G | A | L/I | L/- | E | Y/H | H | H | A | R/W/Q | A | T/M | p | | Frequencies in Brazilians (2) |
| GGA | CTC | GCC | CTG | GAG | TAC | CAC | CAC | GCG | CGG | GCA | ACG | CCG | −14 bp | 39.8 |
| --- | --- | --- | --- | --- | --- | --- | --- | --- | --- | --- | --- | --- | +14 bp | 19.9 |
| --T | --- | --- | --- | --- | --- | --- | --- | --- | --- | --- | --- | --- | +14 bp | 5.34 |
| --- | --- | --- | --- | --- | --- | --- | *** | *** | *** | *** | *** | *** | *** | 0.49 |
| --T | --- | --- | --- | --- | --- | --- | --- | --- | --- | --- | --- | --- | −14 bp | 0 |
| --- | --- | --- | --- | --- | --- | --- | --T | --- | --- | --- | --- | --- | *** | 0.97 |
| --T | --- | --- | --- | --- | --- | --- | --- | --- | --- | --- | --- | --- | *** | 0 |
| --- | --- | --- | --- | --- | --- | --- | --- | --- | --- | --- | --- | --- | −14 bp | 4.37 |
| --- | --- | --- | --- | --A | --- | --- | --- | --- | --- | --- | --- | --- | *** | 0 |
| --- | --- | --G | --- | --- | --- | --- | --- | --- | --- | --- | --- | --- | *** | 0.49 |
| --- | --- | --- | --- | --- | --- | --- | --- | --- | --- | --- | --- | --- | *** | 0 |
| --- | --- | --- | --- | --- | --- | --T | *** | *** | *** | *** | *** | *** | *** | 0 |
| --- | --- | --- | --- | --- | --- | --- | --- | --- | --- | --- | --- | --- | *** | 0 |
| --- | --- | --- | --- | --- | --- | --- | --- | --- | --- | --- | --- | --- | *** | 0 |

(continued)

**Table 1 (continued)**

| Position | Exon 2 | | | | | | | | | | | Exon 3 | | | |
|---|---|---|---|---|---|---|---|---|---|---|---|---|---|---|---|
| Rel. to ATG = 0 | 234 | 239 | 280 | 292 | 297 | 306 | 324 | 361 | 366 | 372 | 408 | 706 | 726 | 738 | 741 |
| Codon | 11 | 13 | 27 | 31 | 32 | 35 | 41 | 54 | 55 | 57 | 69 | 93 | 100 | 104 | 105 |
| Amino acid | A | S/F | Y/H | T/S/M | Q | R | A | Q/R/- | E | P | A | H | G/D | G/V | S/C |
| G*01:01:16 | --G | --- | --- | --- | --- | --- | --- | --- | --- | --A | --- | --T | --- | --- | --- |
| G*01:01:17 | --- | --- | --- | --- | --- | --- | --- | --- | --- | --A | --- | --T | --T | --- | --- |
| G*01:01:18 | --- | --- | --- | --- | --- | --- | --- | --- | --- | --A | --- | --T | --- | --- | --- |
| G*01:01:19 | --- | --- | --- | --- | --- | --- | --- | --- | --- | --A | --- | --T | --- | --- | --- |
| G*01:01:20 | --- | --- | --- | --- | --- | --- | --- | --- | --- | --- | --- | --T | --- | --- | --- |
| G*01:02 | --- | --- | --- | --- | --- | --- | --- | -G- | --- | --- | --- | --- | --- | --- | --- |
| G*01:03 | --- | --- | --- | T-- | --- | --- | --- | --- | --- | --- | --- | --- | --- | --- | --- |
| G*01:04:01 | --- | --- | --- | --- | --- | --- | --- | --- | --- | --A | --- | --- | --- | --- | --- |
| G*01:04:02 | --- | --- | --- | --- | --- | --- | --- | --- | --- | --A | --- | --- | --- | --- | --- |
| G*01:04:03 | --- | --- | --- | --- | --- | --- | --- | --- | --- | --- | --- | --- | --- | --- | --- |
| G*01:04:04 | --- | --- | --- | --- | --- | --- | --- | --- | --- | --A | --- | --- | --- | --- | --- |
| G*01:04:05 | --- | --- | --- | --- | --A | --- | --- | --- | --- | --A | --- | --- | --- | --- | --- |
| G*01:05N | --- | --- | --- | --- | --- | --- | --- | --- | --- | --A | --- | --T | --- | --- | --- |
| G*01:06 | --- | --- | --- | --- | --- | --- | --- | --- | --- | --A | --- | --T | --- | --- | --- |
| G*01:07 | --- | -T- | --- | --- | --- | --- | --- | --- | --- | --A | --- | --- | --- | --- | --- |
| G*01:08 | --- | --- | --- | --- | --- | --- | --- | --- | --- | --A | --- | --T | --- | --- | --- |
| G*01:09 | --- | --- | --- | --- | --- | --- | --- | --- | --- | --A | --- | --T | --- | --- | --- |
| G*01:10 | --- | --- | --- | -T- | --- | --- | --- | --- | --- | --- | --- | --- | --- | --- | --- |
| G*01:11 | --- | --- | --- | -T- | --- | --- | --- | --- | --- | --A | --- | --- | --- | --- | --- |
| G*01:12 | --- | --- | C-- | --- | --- | --- | --- | --- | --- | --A | --- | --- | --- | --- | --- |
| G*01:13N | --- | --- | --- | --- | --- | --- | --- | T-- | --- | --A | --- | --T | --- | --- | --- |
| G*01:14 | --- | --- | --- | --- | --- | --- | --- | --- | --- | --A | --- | --- | -A- | --- | --- |
| G*01:15 | --- | --- | --- | --- | --- | --- | --- | --- | --- | --A | --- | --- | --- | -T- | --- |
| G*01:16 | --- | --- | --- | --- | --- | --- | --- | --- | --- | --A | --- | --T | --- | --- | -G- |
| G*01:17 | --- | --- | --- | --- | --- | --- | --- | --- | --- | --A | --- | --T | --- | --- | --- |

Nucleotide sequence variations observed in exon 1–4 of the coding region of HLA-G according to the IMGT (3) *A* alanine; *S* serin; *F* phenylalanine; *Y* tyrosine; *T* threonine; *M* methionine; *Q* glutamine; *R* arginine; *E* glutamine; Table 1 indicates SNP identified by the primer mentioned in Table 2

| | | | | | | | | | | | | | | |
|---|---|---|---|---|---|---|---|---|---|---|---|---|---|---|
| | | | | | | | **Exon 4** | | | | | | **3′UTR (6)** | |
| **748** | **755** | **778** | **814** | **871** | **902** | **394** | **1590** | **1659** | **1681** | **1734** | **1799** | **1827** | **3741** | |
| **107** | **110** | **117** | **130** | **148** | **159** | **169** | **188** | **211** | **219** | **236** | **258** | **267** | | |
| **G** | **A** | **L/I** | **L/-** | **E** | **Y/H** | **H** | **H** | **A** | **R/W/Q** | **A** | **T/M** | **p** | | **Frequencies in Brazilians (2)** |
| --- | --- | --- | --- | --- | --- | --- | --- | --- | --- | --- | --- | --- | *** | 0 |
| --- | --- | --- | --- | --- | --- | --- | --- | --- | --- | --- | --- | --- | *** | 0 |
| --- | --- | --- | --- | --- | --- | --- | --- | --A | --- | --- | --- | --- | *** | 0 |
| --- | --- | --- | --- | --- | --- | --- | --- | --- | --- | --- | --A | --- | *** | 0 |
| --- | --- | --- | --- | --- | --- | --- | --- | --- | --- | --- | --- | --- | *** | *** |
| --- | --- | --- | --- | --- | --- | --- | --- | --- | --- | --C | --- | --- | *** | 0 |
| --- | --- | --- | --- | --- | --- | --- | --T | --- | --- | --- | --- | --- | +14 bp | 8.74 |
| --- | A-- | --- | --- | --- | --- | --- | --- | --- | --- | --- | --- | --- | −14 bp | 8.25 |
| --- | A-- | --- | --- | --- | --- | --- | --T | --- | --- | --- | --- | --- | *** | 0 |
| --- | A-- | --- | --- | --- | --- | --- | --- | --- | --- | --- | --- | --- | *** | 0 |
| --- | A-- | --- | --- | --- | --- | --- | --- | --- | --- | --- | --- | --A | *** | 3.88 |
| --- | A-- | --- | --- | --- | --- | --- | --- | --- | --- | --- | --- | --- | *** | 0 |
| --- | --- | --- | ~TG | --- | --- | --- | --- | --- | --- | --- | --- | --- | +14 bp | 0.97 |
| --- | --- | --- | --- | --- | --- | --- | --- | --- | --- | --- | -T- | --- | +14 bp | 4.85 |
| --- | A-- | --- | --- | --- | --- | --- | --- | --- | --- | --- | --- | --- | *** | 0 |
| --- | --- | --- | --- | --- | --- | --- | --- | --- | T-- | --- | --- | --- | *** | 0 |
| --- | --- | --- | --- | --- | C-- | --- | *** | *** | *** | *** | *** | *** | *** | 0.49 |
| --- | --- | --- | --- | --- | --- | --- | *** | *** | *** | *** | *** | *** | *** | 0 |
| --- | A-- | --- | --- | --- | --- | --- | *** | *** | *** | *** | *** | *** | *** | 0 |
| --- | --- | --- | --- | --- | --- | --- | --- | --- | --- | --- | --- | --- | *** | 0 |
| --- | --- | --- | --- | --- | --- | --- | --- | --- | --- | --- | --- | --- | *** | 0 |
| --- | --- | --- | --- | --- | --- | --- | --- | --- | -A- | --- | -T- | --- | *** | 0 |
| --- | A-- | --- | --- | --- | --- | --- | --- | --- | --- | --- | --- | --- | *** | 0 |
| --- | --- | --- | --- | --- | --- | --- | --- | --- | --- | --- | -T- | --- | *** | 0 |
| --- | --- | --- | --- | --- | --- | -G- | *** | *** | *** | *** | *** | *** | *** | *** |

*+14 bp* insertion (presence) of 14 bp; *−14 bp* deletion (absence) of 14 bp; *** not evaluated; ~ deleted; amino acid codes: *H* histidine; *P* proline; *G* glycine; *D* asparagine acid; *V* valine; *C* cysteine; *L* leucine; *W* tryptophan; ***grey background*** in

As exon 7 is absent from the mature mRNA and exon 8 is not translated due to the stop codon in exon 6, this gene segment is considered to be the 3′UTR of the mature RNA (2). Here the HLA-G gene exhibits at 3′UTR, a 14 bp fragment insertion/deletion (ins/del) polymorphism. HLA-G alleles with a 14 bp insertion are associated with alternative splicing products missing 92 bases from 3′UTR. Although such truncated mRNAs are reported be more stable, the 14 bp insertion itself is related to low mRNA production (2).

Currently, there are more than 29 variation sites in the promoter region (27 SNPs and 2 insertions/deletions) (8, 12, 13) (Castelli et al. 2010, unpublished data). Many of the promoter region polymorphisms either coincide with or are close to known or putative regulatory elements, and thus may affect the binding of HLA-G regulatory factors.

The realization that HLA-G strongly suppress the immune system, and that certain HLA-G variations are associated with high and low expression levels which might be of functional relevance, has emphasized the need for simple, practical approaches for the typing of the coding and non-coding regions of the HLA-G gene. Here we describe a two-pronged approach to such typing. The first uses PCR to generate six amplicons which are then used in either (a) pyrosequencing (PSQ) to detect the most relevant SNPs (codon 31, 35, 57, 93, 100, 107, 100, 130, 188, or 258) or (b) a simple electrophoretical separation of the specific PCR product for the identification of the 14 bp fragment ins/del polymorphism in 3′UTR. Using this strategy all HLA-G* alleles with frequencies above 1% can be defined, whereas HLA-G* alleles with nucleotide substitutions within introns are not taken into consideration. Secondly, for the further evaluation of the HLA-G promoter region variation, a PCR-amplified fragment of approximately 1,852 bp encompassing the −1445 (5′URR) and +407 (exon 2) nucleotides is produced and sequenced.

## 2. Materials

### 2.1. Materials for HLA-G* Allele Typing and the Identification of the 14 bp Fragment ins/del Polymorphism in 3′ UTR

#### 2.1.1. Polymerase Chain Reactions

1. 2× Master Mix RED for PCR: 150 mM Tris–HCl, pH 8.5, 40 mM $(NH_4)_2SO_4$, 3 mM, $MgCl_2$, 0.2% Tween 20®, 0.4 mM DNTPs, 0.05 units/μL Ampliqon Taq DNA polymerase, inert red dye, and a stabilizer (Ampliqon, Skovlunde, Denmark).
2. Template DNA: A good quality DNA at a concentration of approximately 50 μg/μL.
3. Oligonucleotides primers for PCR (Table 2): All primers are diluted with sterile and nuclease-free water to a concentration

**Table 2**
**Primers to identify SNPs within the coding region and the 14 bp fragment insertion/deletion (ins/del) polymorphism at 3′UTR of HLA-G**

| Primer number | Name | 5′–3′ Sequence | Target | Use |
|---|---|---|---|---|
| 1 | HLA-Gex2-SEBT | TCATCGCCATGGGCTACG | Exon 2 | First amplification |
| 2 | HLA-Gex2-AS | CTGGCCTCGCTCTGGTTGTAG | | |
| 3 | HLA-Gex2_31_35-seq | CGAGTCGCTGTCGAA | Exon 2; codons 31, 35 | Pyrosequencing |
| 4 | HLA-Gex2_57-seq | TGTCTCCTCTTCCCAATA | Exon 2; codons 57 | Pyrosequencing |
| 5 | HLA-Gex3-SEBT | CCGGGTACTCCCGAGTCT | Exon 3 | First amplification |
| 6 | HLA-Gex3-AS | TCGTTCAGGGCGAGGTAATC | | |
| 7 | HLA-G_93_100seq | GGACCCCAGGTCGCA | Exon 3, codons 93, 100 | Pyrosequencing |
| 8 | HLA-G_107_110seq | ATACTGTTCATACCCGC | Exon 3; codons 107, 110 | Pyrosequencing |
| 9 | HLA-G130-SE | GGTGGGGCCAGGTTCTC | Exon 3 codon 130 | First amplification |
| 10 | HLA-G130-ASbt | GGAGATCTGAGCCGCAGTGTC | | |
| 11 | HLA-G130seq | GCCCTGAACGAGGAC | Exon 3 codon 130 | Pyrosequencing |
| 12 | codon188-SE | TCAGACCCCCCCAAGACA | Exon 4 | First amplification |
| 13 | codon188-AS.bt | GGGTGGCCTCATAGTCAAAGAC | | |
| 14 | codon188-seq | GACCCCCCCAAGACA | Exon 4, codon 188 | Pyrosequencing |
| 15 | codon258SEBT | TGCGGAGATCATACTGACCTG | Exon 4 | First amplification |
| 16 | codon258AS | CGACCCTGTTAAAGGTCTTCAGAG | | |
| 17 | codon258-seq | CATGCTGCACATGGCA | Exon 4, codon 258 | Pyrosequencing |
| 18 | HLAG3utr-SE | GTGATGGGCTGTTTAAAGTGTCACC | Exon 8 | First amplification |
| 19 | HLAG3utr-AS | GGAAGGAATGCAGTTCAGCATGA | | |

*SE* sense; *AS* anti-sense; *BT* 5′biotinylation of the primer at the time of synthesis; *seq* sequencing primer of 100 pmol for storage and diluted to a concentration of 10 pmol for usage.

4. PCR tubes or plates (depending on the amount of samples), with corresponding lids or covers.
5. Thermal cycler for PCR.

*2.1.2. Gel Electrophoresis*

1. Biozym LE agarose for gel electrophoresis (Biozym Scientific GmbH, Oldendorf, Germany).
2. 10× Tris buffered ethelene-diamine-tetra-acetic acid (EDTA): 108 g Tris base, 55 g boric acid, 7.44 g EDTA to 1 L with double distilled water.
3. Sybr Safe DNA gel stain or ethidium bromide (Invitrogen, Darmstadt, Germany).
4. Electrophoresis chambers and sufficient power supply.
5. UV-transilluminator of a Gel Documentation System with UV light.
6. DNA marker—pBR322DNA/AluI Marker (Fermentas GmBH, St. Leon-Rot, Germany).

*2.1.3. Pyrosequencing*

1. Pyrosequencing machine, for example, PSQ96MA (Biotage, Uppsala, Sweden) to be used in conjunction with the computer program PSQ96MA 2.1.1 which is a part of this system. Software however may differ according to which pyrosequencing machine is used.
2. Vacuum Prep Tool (Biotage, Uppsala, Sweden).
3. Vacuum source with a minimum vacuum of 300 mmHg.
4. Liquid waste container (must withstand absolute vacuum).
5. Mixer/shaker for microtiter plates, one at room temperature and one which can be heated to 80°C.
6. PSQ™ 96 Sample Prep Thermoplate (Biotage, Uppsala, Sweden).
7. PyroMark™ Q96 Plate Low (Qiagen, Hilden, Germany).
8. PyroMark™ Gold Q96 reagents (Qiagen, Hilden, Germany).
9. PyroMark™ binding buffer, annealing buffer, and wash buffer (Qiagen, Hilden, Germany).
10. 70% Ethanol to be prepared from 100% pure ethanol with double distilled water.
11. 0.5 M NaOH to be prepared with double distilled water.
12. Biotinylated PCR product.

13. Streptavidin sepharose high performance beads (GE Healthcare, Munich, Germany).
14. Sequencing primers (see Table 2).
15. High purity and nuclease free water.

### 2.2. Materials for the HLA-G Gene Promoter Region Variations

1. DNA polymerase: this protocol was optimized and tested using three different DNA polymerases (a) Platinum Taq DNA polymerase (Invitrogen, Carlsbad, CA), (b) PCR Long PCR enzyme mix (Fermentas, Maryland, USA), and (c) Platinum Taq DNA polymerase high-fidelity (Invitrogen, Carlsbad, CA).
2. 0.2-mL PCR tubes or plates.
3. Ultra-pure deionized and autoclaved water, DNAse and RNAse-free.
4. dNTPs: this method was optimized using a 100 mM dNTP set (Invitrogen) but any set of dNTP should do.
5. 5 mM dNTP solution: 5 μL of each dNTP from the 100 mM dNTP Set and 80 μL of ultra-pure deionized water, resulting in a solution of 5 mM of each dNTP.
6. 50 mM Magnesium chloride or 50 mM magnesium sulphate: typically this is provided with the polymerases described in step 1.
7. Primers: Primers used in this protocol are given in Table 3. Each primer was diluted to a final concentration of 10 pmol/μL.
8. DNA samples diluted to 50 ng/μL.
9. This protocol was standardized using the Veriti 96-well Thermal Cycler (Applied Biosystems), but any thermal cycler should do.
10. Agarose, horizontal electrophoresis cube apparatus, and ethidium bromide to assemble a 1% agarose gel.
11. Any non-denaturant load buffer.
12. DNA ladder that allows the identification of a 1,852-bp fragment. This protocol was standardized using the 1 Kb GeneRuler Express (Fermentas).
13. UV-transilluminator or Gel documentation system with UV light.
14. Exonuclease I enzyme (EXO) and Shrimp alkaline phosphatase (SAP).
15. Sequencer and reagents for sequencing according to the sequencer available.

**Table 3**
**Primers to amplify and sequence the HLA-G promoter region**

| Primer name | Type | 5′–3′ Sequence | Target[a] | Use | References |
|---|---|---|---|---|---|
| GPromo.S | Forward | ACATTCTAGAAGCTTCACAAGAATG | −1445 to −1421 | First amplification | (12, 22) |
| GPromo.R | Reverse | GCCTTGGTGTTCCGTGTCT | +389 to +407 | | Castelli et al. 2010, unpublished data |
| G-908R | Reverse | TTCACCTCACAGTTGTAAGTGTTC | −930 to −907 | Sequencing | (22) |
| G-830F | Forward | CACACGGAAACTTAGGGCTACG | −829 to −808 | Sequencing | (22) |
| G-304R | Reverse | GCCAAGCGTTCTGTCTCAGTGT | −302 to −282 | Sequencing | (22) |
| GPR-247 | Forward | CTCAAGCGTGGCTCTCAGGGTC | −245 to −225 | Sequencing | (22) |
| HG01F | Forward | TAAAGTCCTCGCTCACCCAC | −47 to −28 | Sequencing | (21) |
| GPROMO3R | Reverse | GTTGGTATATAAATGCATCTAAAAG | −713 to −689 | Sequencing | Castelli et al. 2010, unpublished data |
| GIN1-98 | Reverse | GTTTCCCTCCTGACCCCGCACT | +77 to +98 | Sequencing | (22) |

[a]According to the IMGT (3)

## 3. Methods

### 3.1. HLA-G* Allele Typing and the Identification of the 14 bp Fragment ins/del Polymorphism in 3′UTR

#### 3.1.1. Polymerase Chain Reaction

See Table 2 for a detailed outline of individual PCR products and their representative mutations with codon names. A total of six PCR products will be produced: Exon 2 (including codons 31, 35, and 57), exon 3 (including codons 93, 100, 107, 110), exon 3 codon 130, exon 4 codon 188, and exon 4 codon 258, and 3′UTR. It is recommended to make a master mix in order to simplify the pipetting and reduce the chance of any single error (see Note 1).

1. Exon 2 codons 31, 35, 57 PCR: Each individual PCR reaction has a total volume of 50 μL; this includes 25 μL Ampliqon Master Mix RED, 20 μL high purity water, 2 μL of each primer numbers 1 and 2 (Table 2), and 1 μL DNA. Thermal cycler was set as following: 5 min at 95°C (hot start), 30 s at 95°C (denaturation), 40 s at 65°C (annealing), 30 s at 72°C (extension), and finally, 10 min at 72°C. Steps 2–5 are repeated 38 times before the final extension time. The amplified product is 208 bp long (see Note 2). This product will be used for pyrosequencing—see Subheading 3.1.3, step 1.
2. Exon 3 codons 93, 100, 107, 110 PCR: Each individual reaction has a total volume of 30 μL; this includes 15 μL Amplicon Master Mix RED, 12 μL high purity water, 1 μL of each primer numbers 5 and 6 (Table 2), and 1 μL DNA. Thermal cycler conditions are exactly as for Exon 2 PCR. End product should be 278 bp long. All of the 30 μL of PCR product will be for pyrosequencing—see Subheading 3.1.3, step 2 (see Note 2).
3. Exon 3 codon 130 PCR: Use the same master mix recipe as for exon 3 (30 μL) (step 2), using primer numbers 9 and 10 (Table 2). Thermal cycler conditions are the same as for Exon 2 PCR with the following exception: The annealing temperature is changed to 65.5°C and the extension is changed from 30 to 15 s. PCR product is 167 bp long. 15 μL of this product will be used for pyrosequencing—see Subheading 3.1.3, step 3. The rest can be frozen at -20°C until all genotypes are confirmed.
4. Exon 4 codon 188 PCR: Use the same master mix recipe as for exon 3 (30 μL) (step 2), using primer numbers 12 and 13 (Table 2). Thermal cycler conditions are the same as for Exon 2 PCR with one exception: The annealing temperature is changed to 60°C. PCR product is 58 bp long. 15 μL of this PCR product will be used for pyrosequencing—see Subheading 3.1.3, step 4. The rest can be frozen at -20°C until all genotypes are confirmed.
5. Exon 4 codon 258 PCR: Use the same master mix recipe as for exon 3 (30 μL) (step 2), using primer numbers 15 and 16

(Table 2). Thermal cycler conditions are the same as for Exon 2 PCR with one exception: The annealing temperature is changed to 60°C. PCR product is 267 bp long. 15 μL of this PCR product will be used for pyrosequencing—see Subheading 3.1.3, step 5. The rest can be frozen at −20°C until all genotypes are confirmed.

6. 3′UTR PCR: Use the same master mix recipe as for exon 3 (30 μL), using primer numbers 18 and 19 (Table 2). Thermal cycler conditions are exactly as for Exon 2 PCR. PCR product should be 434 bp long. 10 μL of this PCR product will be used for Gel Electrophoresis—see Subheading 3.1.2, steps 3–5. The rest can be frozen at −20°C until all genotypes are confirmed.

*3.1.2. Electrophoretical Separation of the PCR Products of the Coding and the 3′ UTR Region*

1. To confirm that the PCR of the coding region worked properly, the PCR products (i.e. products from Subheading 3.1.1, steps 1–5) are applied to a 2% agarose gel. To prepare the gel add 2 g agarose to 100 mL of 0.5× TBE and cook in the microwave for approximately 3–5 min until all agarose is dissolved (see Note 3). Thereafter Sybr Safe DNA gel stain or ethidium bromide is added (0.5 μg/mL). Keep in mind that you need enough wells in the gel for all the samples, plus negative and positive PCR controls, as well as for the DNA Marker. A negative PCR control would consist of PCR master mix which was run in the thermal cycler exactly like the patient samples, only without template DNA. A positive PCR control would be PCR master mix which was run in the thermal cycler exactly like the test samples except that here a DNA sample with known HLA-G allele (14) would be used being already proven to function in PCR.
2. Place the agarose gel in the gel chamber and make sure it is sufficiently covered by 0.5× TBE.
3. Load the samples completely in the gel and attach the power supply. Run at 180 V until good separation is acquired.
4. Put the gel into a UV-Transilluminator of a Gel Documentation System with UV light. The presence of a fragment with the expected bp indicates that the amplification ran properly (see Note 4).
5. For the SNP in the 3′UTR, 10 μL of the product (i.e. from Subheading 3.1.1, step 6) is applied to a 3% agarose. This is prepared by mixing 3 g agarose with 100 mL 0.5× TBE and cooking for approximately 5 min. Microwaving times may vary. Thereafter Sybr Safe DNA gel stain or ethidium bromide is added (0.5 μg/mL).
6. After the gel has cooled off, place in the gel chamber, make sure that it is covered by 0.5× TBE, and load 10 μL of each

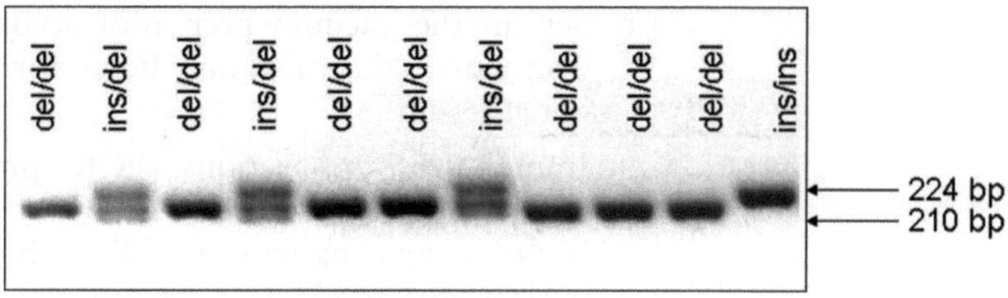


Fig. 1. Typing of 14 bp ins/del polymorphism in 3′UTR. PCR product is run on a 3% agarose gel until good separation is acquired.

PCR product onto the gel. Run at 180 V until good separation is acquired. Put the gel into a UV-Transilluminator of a Gel Documentation System with UV light. The two different PCR products of 210 and 224 bp should be present.

7. A sample with only one band at 210 (deletion 14 bp) or 224 (insertion 14 bp) indicates a homozygosity for the given genotype, for example del/del or ins/ins. A sample with two bands visible (one at 210 and the other at 224) indicates a heterozygote del/ins (Fig. 1).

#### 3.1.3. Pyrosequencing

All steps here are to be performed at room temperature unless otherwise stated. In addition, all buffers should be stored at 4°C, but allowed to warm up to room temperature before starting. Also before use, all sequences to be analysed should be entered into the computer as indicated by the software instructions.

1. The exon 2 codons 31, 35, 57 PCR product will be used for two individual sequencing reactions. The first, using primer number 3, sequences SNPs in codon 31 and 35. The second, using primer number 4, sequences one SNP in codon 57.
2. The exon 3 codons 93, 100, 107, 110 PCR product will also be used for two individual sequencing reactions. The first, using primer number 7, sequences SNPs in codons 93 and 100. The second, using primer number 8, sequences SNPs in codons 107 and 110.
3. The exon 3 codon 130 PCR product will be used for only one sequencing reaction using primer number 11 for the SNP in codon 188.
4. The exon 4 codon 188 PCR product will be used for only one sequencing reaction using primer number 14 for the SNP in codon 188.
5. The exon 4 codon 258 PCR product will be used for only one sequencing reaction using primer number 17 for the SNP in codon 258.

6. Set up the vacuum prep tool according to manufacturer's instruction (this must only be performed once, at the time of initial set-up).
7. Immobilize the various PCR products obtained from Subheading 3.1.1 to the Streptavidin Sepharose beads. Do this by preparing a master mix of 37 μL binding buffer, 15 μL high purity water, and 3 μL of *very well* mixed Streptavidin Sepharose beads per reaction. To each well in a Pyro Mark Low plate, pipette 55 μL of binding buffer-beads mixture. To this "binding" plate, add 15 μL of PCR product (biotinylated), see Note 5. Using a shaker, incubate at room temperature with constant agitation to keep the beads in motion.
8. While the binding plate is mixing, prepare the "annealing" plate. Do this by preparing a master mix of 40 μL annealing buffer and 2 μL of above mentioned (Subheading 3.1.3, steps 1–5) primer (10 pmol stock solution). To each well in a new Pyro Mark Low plate, pipette 40 μL of annealing buffer mixture. Each different SNP sequence must be separately analysed. This means one cannot combine primers; you have to use only *one* primer per reaction. Set this annealing plate aside.
9. Prepare the washing troughs for the vacuum prep tool. Fill with approximately 180 mL of the solutions; 70% ethanol, 0.5 M NaOH, washing buffer, and double distilled water. Turn the vacuum on.
10. After 5 min (see Note 6), remove binding plate from shaker and *quickly* but gently lower the vacuum prep tool into the binding plate. This will collect the beads, which are now bound to the DNA from the PCR and filter out all other solutions. Make sure that the liquid has been aspirated completely from the binding plate and that little to no beads are remaining at the bottom of the plate (see Note 7).
11. Place the vacuum prep tool in the 70% ethanol solution and let the solution flush through the filters for approximately 5 s. Move to the NaOH trough and once again, let the solution flow through the filters for approximately 5 s. Finally, move the prep tool to the washing buffer and flush through for 5 s. Allow all liquid to drain completely from the probes (filter tips) by turning the prep tool to a 90° angle, and then back to a horizontal position a few times. Make sure it is very dry.
12. Holding the vacuum prep tool over the sequencing plate (annealing), which has already been filled with annealing buffer and specific primer, turn the vacuum off. Release the vacuum prep tool into the buffer and shake to remove all beads from the filters into the annealing buffer.
13. Place the annealing plate, including primer and bead-DNA complex, at 80°C and shake for 2 min using the PSQ 96 Sample

Prep thermoplate. During this time, start to wash the vacuum prep tool in high purity water to prepare for the next run. Also prepare the enzyme and substrate cartridge including the necessary nucleotides.

14. Remove the annealing plate from the heat block and let cool to room temperature. Continue with the sequencing reaction according to the programme specifications for the PSQ96MA 2.1.1.
15. After the PSQ run has been completed, the results (genotypes) are ready for proofing and adding to the text document. With one simple click on "Analyze Results" the computer analyzes all of the pyrograms created (results) and reports to you whether or not the sample was successful (passed, check, or failed) as well as the genotype of the sample. The results should also be manually proofed in order to exclude mistakes possibly made by the computer. First all other genotyping methods must be completed. The quality of the PSQ results are checked by the control samples (see Subheading 3.1.2, step 1).

### 3.2. Methods for the HLA-G Gene Promoter Region Variations

#### 3.2.1. HLA-G Promoter Amplification by PCR

1. Separate the reagents for PCR amplification (DNA polymerase, dNTPs, ultra-pure deionized water, and the primers for the first amplification GPromo.S and GPromo.R—Table 3), thaw and keep them on ice.
2. On a separate bench, thaw the DNA samples and keep them on ice.
3. Prepare a mix of reagents for the amplification. The following protocol is for one reaction and the volumes are adjusted to the reagents in proposed final concentration. Amplification is performed in a final volume of 50 μL containing:
   (a) 33.7 μL of ultra-pure water (or a quantity enough to a final volume of 50 μL if any of the volumes given below changed);
   (b) 1× PCR buffer (typically 5 μL of the buffer provided with the polymerases described in Subheading 2);
   (c) 3 μL of magnesium chloride (for Platinum Taq Polymerase from Invitrogen and Long PCR enzyme Mix from Fermentas) or 3 μL of magnesium sulphate (Platinum Taq Polymerase High-Fidelity from Invitrogen), giving a final concentration of 1.5 mM;
   (d) 2 μL of the 5 mM dNTP, giving a final concentration of 0.2 mM of each dNTP;
   (e) 2 μL of each primer for the first amplification, giving a final amount of primer of 20 pmol each per reaction;
   (f) 0.3 μL of DNA polymerase (1.5 units);
   (g) Gently homogenize this solution by pipetting up and down. Cap the tube.

4. On the other bench, add 2 μL of the diluted DNA sample into the mix and gently homogenize the solution by pipetting up and down. Cap the tube.
5. Put the reaction mix at the thermal cycler using the following cycling protocol:
6. Initial denaturation cycle at 94°C for 2 min.
   (a) 32 cycles at 94°C for 30 s, 59°C for 30 s, and 72°C (for regular Platinum Polymerase) or 68°C (for High-Fidelity Platinum and Long PCR enzyme Mix) for 135 s.
   (b) Final extension step at 72°C (for regular Platinum Polymerase) or 68°C (for High-Fidelity Platinum and Long PCR enzyme Mix) for 5 min. Keep them on ice before going to the next step.
7. Assemble a common 1% agarose gel (using TBE or TAE buffer) stained with ethidium bromide and load 5 μL of the amplification reaction together with a non-denaturant load buffer of your preference. Keep the rest of the amplified product in the fridge or on ice for DNA sequencing as described in Subheading 3.2.2. Use a DNA ladder that allows the detection of a fragment of approximately 1,852 bp. Then, run the electrophoresis for about 2 h using 100 V or the necessary to separate the fragments in the electrophoresis system available.
8. Put the gel into a UV-Transilluminator of a Gel Documentation System with UV light. The presence of a fragment of approximately 1,852 bp (Fig. 2) indicates that the amplification ran properly. No other fragments would be detected. You may dispose the gel properly.

#### *3.2.2. HLA-G Promoter Sequencing*

In the previous section, the protocol was given to amplify the HLA-G promoter region by PCR. Once you have it amplified with a verified clean product of approximately 1,852 bp (see Subheading 3.2.1, step 7), you may sequence this PCR product by using the appropriate primers described in Table 3. Alternatively, you may use restriction endonucleases to screen for variability (not within the scope of this chapter). Depending on the sequencer available, the sequencing protocol must be adjusted for each machine and sequencing reagents used. No sequencing protocol is provided in this chapter since it depends on the infrastructure available. Please refer to your sequencer's documentation in order to better adjust a sequencing reaction of the PCR product. In this section, a strategy to evaluate the entire promoter by sequencing using the primers listed in Table 3 is given.

1. To assure a purified product for sequencing, take 10 μL of the PCR product in a separate 0.2 μL PCR tube and add 1 μL of EXO and 1 μL of SAP. Mix the solution by pipetting up and down. Cap the tube and put it on ice before using the thermal cycler.

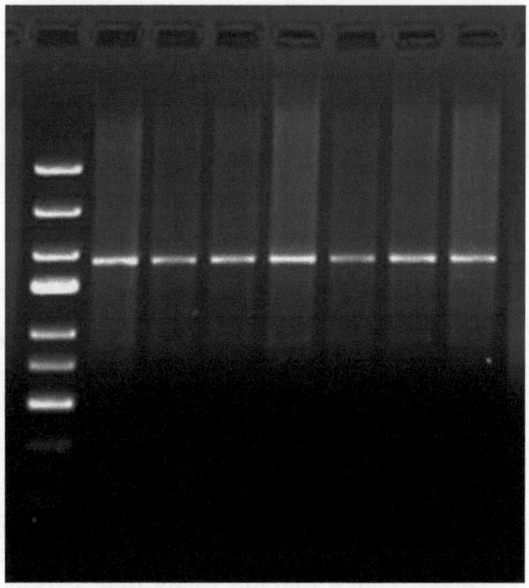

Fig. 2. HLA-G gene promoter amplification products. 1% Agarose gel stained by ethidium bromide. The DNA ladder used was 1 Kb GeneRuler Express (Fermentas). From the heavier to the lighter fragment, the ladder indicates fragments of 5,000, 3,000, 2,000, 1,500, 1,000, 750, 500, 300, and 100 bp. The expected amplification is approximately 1,852 bp.

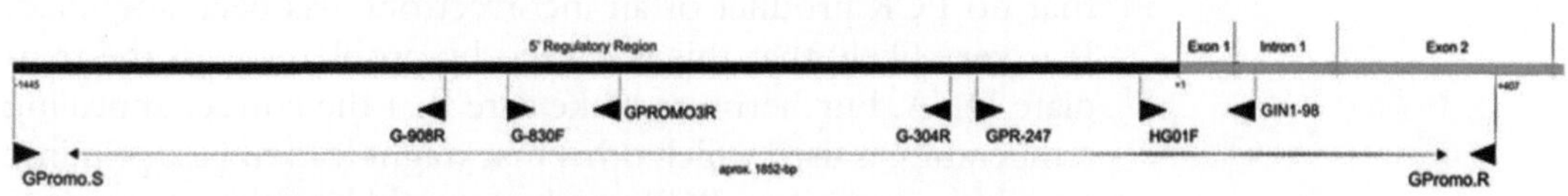


Fig. 3. Primer map used to amplify and sequence the *HLA-G* promoter region.

2. In the thermal cycler, use the following cycling protocol: 37°C for 15 min, then remove from the thermal cycler 80°C for 15 min and keep in freezer or on ice until sequencing.
3. Use the sequencing primers in Table 3 to sequence the HLA-G promoter. Use the sequencing protocol that best suits your sequencer. The location of each primer is given in Table 3. Figure 3 illustrates the position and direction of each primer. Note that, by using all the primers in Table 3 and Fig. 3, it is likely that all sequences of the promoter region will be covered and any variation sites present in this segment will be detected. In addition, these primers are optimized to detect all the 29 known variation sites in the promoter region using a sequencer such as ABI3100 (Applied Biosystems) with 50-cm capillaries.

### 3.3. Analysis of Genotypes and Determination of Haplotypes

1. One strategy to evaluate haplotypes is to use computational inference to obtain haplotypes for each sample by using algorithms such as the PHASE method (15, 16), the EM (Expectation-Maximization) (17, 18), and the ELB (Excoffier-Laval-Balding) (19) algorithms. Please see the further references for information about how to use these and the limitations of the methods (20, 21).

## 4. Notes

1. For the PCR for the coding region you may want to run a control on an electrophoresis gel to confirm that the PCR worked properly. This will mean that you need more than one PCR reaction for each patient because all of the 50 μL (or 30 μL) of PCR product will be needed for further analysis. We suggest this for optimization of DNA concentration as well.
2. We use DNA prepared from EDTA-blood. This is stable and of relative good quality. When, for example, DNA has been extracted from paraffin slices, it is possible that the amount of DNA and/or primer concentration would not be enough or possibly too much.
3. When making more than one gel, it is helpful to prepare them individually. Cooking the gels for too long (which can be necessary when making many gels at once) alters the concentration of the gel when too much TBE evaporates because of the boiling.
4. After visualization of PCR products on the gel, it is possible that no PCR product or an incorrect one has been amplified. It is very likely that this is caused by problems with the template DNA. Furthermore make sure that the correct annealing temperature is used which otherwise might lead to false priming. Possible causes of no PCR products could be either that simply DNA was not added to the mixture or that the DNA was prepared from paraffin slices. In this case, a long enough product cannot be amplified. Suggestions for improvement include simply trying the PCR again making sure to pipette DNA into the PCR mix or measuring the concentration of the DNA to make sure that enough template is present.
5. PSQ manufacturers suggest a maximum of 30 μL PCR product per reaction. We have optimized, and for our purposes, with our DNA templates, 15 μL of PCR product is usually enough. Too much PCR product can also be detrimental for results.
6. Leaving the binding plate to shake for longer than 5 min (manufacturers recommended time) does not make a difference in the results. We have allowed the plate to shake for up to 10 min with no difference in results.
7. The sepharose beads sediment quickly, and when they are at the bottom of the plate, then they are harder to collect with the vacuum prep tool. It is useful to act quickly and gently to collect the maximum amount of beads bound to DNA. If too many beads have been left at the bottom of the plate, it is possible to add a bit (approximately 20 μL) of high purity water, shake for

a minute, and then aspirate one more time. The vacuum filter tool should be left ON at all times in order to not to lose any beads. Be cautious to always hold the filter at the same point, and not to turn it 180° by accident thereby mixing the samples!

## References


1. Carosella ED, Favier B, Rouas-Freiss N, Moreau P, Lemaoult J (2008) Beyond the increasing complexity of the immunomodulatory HLA-G molecule. Blood 111:4862–4870
2. Donadi EA, Castelli EC, Arnaiz-Villena A, Roger M, Rey D, Moreau P (2011) Implications of the polymorphism of HLA-G on its function, regulation, evolution and disease association. Cell Mol Life Sci 68:369–395
3. Robinson J, Waller MJ, Fail SC, Marsh SG (2006) The IMGT/HLA and IPD databases. Hum Mutat 27:1192–1199
4. Castelli EC, Mendes-Junior CT, Deghaide NH, de Albuquerque RS, Muniz YC, Simoes RT, Carosella ED, Moreau P, Donadi EA (2010) The genetic structure of 3′untranslated region of the HLA-G gene: polymorphisms and haplotypes. Genes Immun 11:134–141
5. Castelli EC, Mendes-Junior CT, Donadi EA (2007) HLA-G alleles and HLA-G 14 bp polymorphisms in a Brazilian population. Tissue Antigens 70:62–68
6. Hviid TV (2006) HLA-G in human reproduction: aspects of genetics, function and pregnancy complications. Hum Reprod Update 12:209–232
7. Moreau P, Contu L, Alba F, Lai S, Simoes R, Orru S, Carcassi C, Roger M, Rabreau M, Carosella ED (2008) HLA-G gene polymorphism in human placentas: possible association of G*0106 allele with preeclampsia and miscarriage. Biol Reprod 79:459–467
8. Rizzo R, Hviid TV, Govoni M, Padovan M, Rubini M, Melchiorri L, Stignani M, Carturan S, Grappa MT, Fotinidi M, Ferretti S, Voss A, Laustrup H, Junker P, Trotta F, Baricordi OR (2008) HLA-G genotype and HLA-G expression in systemic lupus erythematosus: HLA-G as a putative susceptibility gene in systemic lupus erythematosus. Tissue Antigens 71: 520–529
9. Sipak-Szmigiel O, Cybulski C, Wokolorczyk D, Lubinski J, Kurzawa R, Baczkowski T, Radwan M, Radwan P, Ronin-Walknowska E (2009) HLA-G polymorphism and in vitro fertilization failure in a Polish population. Tissue Antigens 73:348–352
10. Ober C, Aldrich CL (1997) HLA-G polymorphisms: neutral evolution or novel function? J Reprod Immunol 36:1–21
11. Suarez MB, Morales P, Castro MJ, Fernandez V, Varela P, Alvarez M, Martinez-Laso J, Arnaiz-Villena A (1997) A new HLA-G allele (HLA-G*0105N) and its distribution in the Spanish population. Immunogenetics 45:464–465
12. Tan Z, Shon AM, Ober C (2005) Evidence of balancing selection at the HLA-G promoter region. Hum Mol Genet 14:3619–3628
13. Berger DS, Hogge WA, Barmada MM, Ferrell RE (2010) Comprehensive analysis of HLA-G: implications for recurrent spontaneous abortion. Reprod Sci 17:331–338
14. Rebmann V, van der Ven K, Passler M, Pfeiffer K, Krebs D, Grosse-Wilde H (2001) Association of soluble HLA-G plasma levels with HLA-G alleles. Tissue Antigens 57:15–21
15. Stephens M, Smith NJ, Donnelly P (2001) A new statistical method for haplotype reconstruction from population data. Am J Hum Genet 68:978–989
16. Stephens M, Donnelly P (2003) A comparison of bayesian methods for haplotype reconstruction from population genotype data. Am J Hum Genet 73:1162–1169
17. Excoffier L, Slatkin M (1995) Maximum-likelihood estimation of molecular haplotype frequencies in a diploid population. Mol Biol Evol 12:921–927
18. Excoffier L, Laval G, Schneider S (2005) Arlequin ver. 3.0: an integrated software package for population genetics data analysis. Evol Bioinform Online 1:47–50
19. Excoffier L, Laval G, Balding D (2003) Gametic phase estimation over large genomic regions using an adaptive window approach. Hum Genomics 1:7–19
20. Castelli EC, Mendes-Junior CT, Veiga-Castelli LC, Pereira NF, Petzl-Erler ML, Donadi EA (2010) Evaluation of computational methods for the reconstruction of HLA haplotypes. Tissue Antigens 76:459–466
21. Castelli EC, Mendes-Junior CT, Deghaide NH, de Albuquerque RS, Muniz YC, Simoes

RT, Carosella ED, Moreau P, Donadi EA (2010) The genetic structure of 3′untranslated region of the HLA-G gene: polymorphisms and haplotypes. Genes Immun 11: 134–141

22. Ober C, Aldrich CL, Chervoneva I, Billstrand C, Rahimov F, Gray HL, Hyslop T (2003) Variation in the HLA-G promoter region influences miscarriage rates. Am J Hum Genet 72:1425–1435

# Chapter 8

# Molecular Typing of HLA-E


## Nina Lauterbach, Christina E.M. Voorter, and Marcel G.J. Tilanus



## Abstract

Human leukocyte antigen-E (HLA-E) is a non-classical HLA class I gene that shows a limited degree of polymorphism compared to the classical HLA genes. The HLA-E molecule can bind peptides derived from the leader sequence of various HLA class I alleles and some viral homologues, including CMV. The HLA-E peptide complex can act as a ligand for the CD94/NKG2 receptors expressed on the surface of natural killer cells and T cell subsets. Differences in expression levels between the different HLA-E alleles have been reported and a role for HLA-E polymorphism in stem cell transplantation has been postulated. This chapter focuses on routine technologies for HLA-E typing: the sequence-specific primer-PCR method that uses sequence-specific primers, the PCR sequence-specific oligonucleotides Luminex method, using sequence-specific probes attached to beads and the sequencing-based typing method, where sequencing of the alleles is performed.



**Key words:** Human leukocyte antigen-E, HLA typing method, Sequence-specific primer-PCR, PCR-sequence-specific oligonucleotides, Sequencing-based typing


## 1. Introduction

The human leukocyte antigen-E (HLA-E) gene is located between HLA-A and HLA-C on the short arm of chromosome 6. With only nine alleles encoding three different proteins, HLA-E is the least polymorphic of all MHC class I molecules. Two HLA-E molecules, encoded by HLA-E*01:01 and HLA-E*01:03, exist with about equal frequencies in the population (1, 2). The previously identified HLA-E*01:02 allele was removed from the IMGT/HLA database because the sequence was found identical to HLA-E*01:01:01:01. The allele HLA-E*01:04 has been originally reported in 1 out of 11 Japanese individuals (3), and has not been identified thereafter, even since a population of 50 Japanese


Frank T. Christiansen and Brian D. Tait (eds.), *Immunogenetics: Methods and Applications in Clinical Practice*, Methods in Molecular Biology, vol. 882, DOI 10.1007/978-1-61779-842-9_8, © Springer Science+Business Media New York 2012

individuals has been investigated. It appears very likely that this allele is the result of sequencing artefacts (2). In the remaining 8 alleles, only one non-synonymous substitution is present at position 382, which results in one amino acid difference; an arginine at position 107 in HLA-E*01:01 is replaced by a glycine in HLA-E*01:03 (4). All other nucleotide differences are either located in the non-coding region or are synonymous substitutions. The typing techniques described here have mainly been focused on the non-synonymous substitution, although with sequence-based typing also the synonymous substitutions are identified.

It has been reported that some form of balancing selection is acting on HLA-E to maintain the two alleles (4, 5), implicating that there are functional differences. Indeed, a few studies show in vitro a functional difference between HLA-E*01:01 and HLA-E*01:03 (6–8). Furthermore, studies focusing on the effect of HLA-E polymorphism on stem cell transplantation outcome show a protective role for the HLA-E*01:03 genotype (9–12), albeit that the various inconclusive and contradictive results remain to be resolved and confirmed in larger cohort studies. In Behcet's disease, HLA-E*01:01 seems to be associated with reduced risk (13).

Different HLA-E typing techniques, like sequence-specific primer-PCR (PCR-SSP), RFLP, Taqman and sequencing-based typing (SBT), have been described (1, 2, 9, 13, 14). In this chapter, we describe three different routine methods to identify HLA-E polymorphism in genomic DNA. Method 1, a PCR-SSP method uses two different 5′ primers and a generic 3′primer that distinguish the non-synonymous difference of HLA-E*01:01 and HLA-E*01:03 at amino acid position 107. Method 2, an SSO method is based on the Luminex technology, using different probes for HLA-E*01:01, HLA-E*01:03, and HLA-E*01:04 attached to labelled beads. Method 3 is a direct sequencing method based upon PCR amplification and sequencing with specific primers enabling sequencing of exons 1–5 and the intervening introns. The non-coding differences between HLA-E*01:01:01:01, E*01:01:01:02, and E*01:01:01:03 and between HLA-E*01:03:01:01 and E*01:03:01:02 are located outside this region, whereas all synonymous and non-synonymous substitutions can be detected.

## 2. Materials

### 2.1. PCR-SSP Method

#### 2.1.1. PCR Reaction

1. Optional Biohazard.
2. Thermocycler.
3. Vortex mixer with adjustable speed.
4. Centrifuge with Swing bucket rotor for 96-well microplate.
5. Micropipettes and tips.

6. PCR tubes (Micronics) and caps or seal.
7. Mastermix (MM) for 1,000 reactions (store at –80°C):
   - 1.0 mL 10× PCR buffer II (Perkin Elmer-buffer), (Applied Biosystems).
   - 0.6 mL $MgCl_2$ 25 mM, (Applied Biosystems).
   - 20 μL Each dNTP 100 mM, (Amersham Pharmacia).
   - Optional: 0.1 mL Cresol red 10 mg/mL, (Sigma).
   - 0.5 mL Glycerol (99.5%), ICN.
   - 2.3 mL Aqua Dest (AD) (or 2.4 mL if no cresol red is added).
8. AmpliTaq DNA polymerase (5 Units/μL), (Applied Biosystems). Store at –20°C.
9. HLA-E amplification primers:

| Name | Direction | Sequence 5′-3′ | Location | Position |
|---|---|---|---|---|
| MSSP08079 | Forward | CGAGCTGGGG CCCGACA | Exon 3 | 740–756 |
| MSSP08080 | Forward | CGAGCTGGGG CCCGACG | Exon 3 | 740–756 |
| MSSP08088 | Reverse | TTCCAGGTAGG CTCTCTGG | Exon 3 | 902–920 |

10. Internal control primers (located in the growth hormone gene):

| Name | Direction | Sequence 5′-3′ |
|---|---|---|
| IC1 | Forward | CAGTGCCTTCCCAACCATTCCCTTA |
| IC2 | Reverse | ATCCACTCACGGATTTCTGTTGTGTTTC |

*2.1.2. Agarose Gel Electrophoresis*

1. Agarose electrophoresis grade, (Invitrogen). Store at room temperature (RT).
2. 10× TBE buffer, (Gibco) (dilute with MilliQ to obtain 0.5× TBE-dilution). Store at RT.
3. Ethidium bromide (50 mL, 1% in water), (Fluka Biochemika). Store at 4°C.
4. 50 or 100 bp DNA ladder, (Invitrogen) dilute 50 μL DNA marker with 950 μL aqua dest and 200 μL loading buffer (dissolve in 10 mL AD: 100 mg Orange G, 10 mg SDS, 200 μL 0.5 M EDTA, 500 μL 1 M Tris/HCl pH 8.0, 1 g Ficoll 400, add 6 mL glycerol and water to a final volume of 20 mL). Store at 4°C for maximum 1 year.
5. Geltray and combs.
6. Microgram scale.
7. 50°C Water bath.

8. Gel electrophoresis system, (Biorad).
9. Electrophoresis power supply.
10. UV transilluminator (Geldoc system), (Biorad).

### 2.2. PCR-SSO Method

#### 2.2.1. PCR, Hybridization, and Luminex Bead Reactions

1. HLA-E SSO Luminex kit (One Lambda, not commercially available yet).
   - Denaturation buffer, store at RT.
   - Neutralization buffer, store at RT.
   - Hybridization buffer, store at RT.
   - Wash buffer, store at RT.
   - SAPE stock (100×), store at 4°C.
   - SAPE buffer, store at 4°C.
   - Primer Set D-Mix, store at –30°C (mix should be pink or light purple, when necessary vortex).
   - HLA-E specific amplification primers, store at –30°C.
   - HLA-E SSO beads (including positive and negative control beads), store at –30°C (after thawing store in the dark at 4°C, never re-freeze).
2. Optional: Biohazard.
3. AmpliTaq DNA polymerase (5 Units/μL), (Applied Biosystems). Store at –20°C.
4. 1.5-mL microfuge tubes.
5. PCR tubes (micronics) and caps or seal.
6. Micropipettes and tips.
7. 96-Well, thin walled PCR plate and holder.
8. PCR Thermocycler.
9. Centrifuge
   - Rotor for 1.5-mL microfuge tubes.
   - Swing bucket rotor for 96-well microplate.
10. Vortex mixer with adjustable speed.
11. Luminex fluoranalyser (Luminex Corporation) or Labscan100 (One Lambda).
12. Luminex XMap Sheath fluid.

#### 2.2.2. Optional: Agarose Gel Electrophoresis

See Subheading 2.1.2.

### 2.3. SBT Method

#### 2.3.1. Amplification and Sequencing Reaction

1. Expand High Fidelity PCR kit, containing 10× Expand High Fidelity buffer and Expand High Fidelity enzyme mix, (Roche).
2. dNTP 10 mM each.
3. HLA-E amplification primers:

| Name | Direction | Sequence 5′-3′ | Location | Position |
|---|---|---|---|---|
| E08072 | Forward | CAGCGTCGCCA CGACTCCCGAC | 5′UT | 75–54 |
| E08073 | Reverse | GGCTCGTGTGTGT GGATGG | Intron 5 | 2,219–2,237 |

(Sequences from Paquay et al. (14), see Note 1)

4. HLA-E sequencing primers:

| Name | Direction | Sequence 5′-3′ | Location | Position |
|---|---|---|---|---|
| E08074 | Forward | GAAGGACTC GGGGAG | Intron 1 | 131–145 |
| E08075 | Forward | AGATTCACCCC AAGGCTG | Intron 2 | 549–567 |
| E08076 | Forward | CTAAGTCCA GGCTGGTG | Intron 3 | 1,465–1,481 |
| E08077 | Reverse | AGCCTTGGGG TGAATC | Intron 2 | 551–564 |
| E08078 | Reverse | TCCCTGTTT-CTTCTAC | Intron 3 | 1,062–1,077 |

(Sequences from Paquay et al. (14), see Note 1).

5. ExoSAP-IT, (USB corporation), store at −20°C.
6. BigDye Terminator v1.1 Cycle Sequencing kit (Applied Biosystems) consisting of:
   - 5× BigDye Terminator v1.1/3.1 sequencing buffer, store at 2–8°C.
   - BigDye Terminator v1.1 cycle sequencing mix RR-2500 (BDT), store at temperatures between −15 and −25°C.
7. Montage $SEQ_{96}$ Sequencing Reaction Cleanup kit consisting of injection solution (Millipore) and 96-well SEQ filter plates, (Montáge® life science).
8. 3700/3730 BigDye® Terminator v1.1 Sequencing standard, (Applied Biosystems), store at temperatures between −15 and −25°C.
9. 10× 3730 buffer with EDTA, prepare fresh by adding 16 mL of buffer to 144 mL MilliQ water.
10. Performance optimized polymer (POP-7), (Applied Biosystems).
11. HiDi Formamide, aliquot, freeze-thaw only once, (Applied Biosystems).
12. 96-well Optical Reaction plate with barcode (3730 plate), (Applied Biosystems).
13. 3730 Trayholder, (Applied Biosystems).

14. Plate septa 96 well (Applied Biosystems).
15. Optional: Biohazard.
16. Vortex.
17. Centrifuge with Swing bucket rotor for 96-well microplate.
18. Micropipettes.
19. Pipette tips.
20. 1.5-mL microfuge tubes.
21. PCR tubes (micronics).
22. Thermocycler.
23. 3730 DNA analyzer, (Applied Biosystems).

*2.3.2. Requirements Agarose Gel Electrophoresis*

See Subheading 2.1.2.

## 3. Methods

### 3.1. PCR-SSP

In the HLA-E PCR-SSP approach, two different PCR reactions are used; one positive for HLA-E*01:01 and one positive for HLA-E*01:03. Internal amplification control primers, located in the growth hormone gene, are included to check for any inconsistencies during the PCR. Analysis is performed by agarose gel electrophoresis and by the detection of ethidium bromide-stained fragments.

*3.1.1. Amplification*

1. Prepare the mastermix, the DNA sample and thaw primers (see Note 2).
2. Provide a clean work environment, e.g. a Biohazard and keep the reaction mixes on ice throughout the entire protocol.
3. For each sample, pipette the reaction mix for HLA-E*01:01 and HLA-E*01:03 amplification as described below in two separate PCR tubes (It is most efficient to make reaction mixes before starting, see Notes 3 and 4).

   1× Reaction mix HLA-E*01:01:

| | |
|---|---|
| 4.6 μL | MM |
| 2 pmol | IC1 |
| 2 pmol | IC2 |
| 10 pmol | Forward primer: MSSP08079 |
| 10 pmol | Reverse primer: MSSP08088 |
| Add aqua dest to a final volume of 8 μL | |

1× Reaction mix HLA-E*01:03:

| | |
|---|---|
| 4.6 μL | MM |
| 2 pmol | IC1 |
| 2 pmol | IC2 |
| 10 pmol | Forward primer: MSSP08080 |
| 10 pmol | Reverse primer: MSSP08088 |
| Add aqua dest to a final volume of 8 μL | |

4. Add 100 ng of DNA to each mix and centrifuge the PCR tubes (pulse centrifugation until reaching 200 × *g*).
5. Dilute Taq polymerase with AD to obtain 0.33 Unit/μL and add 1 μL per reaction/tube.
6. Centrifuge the PCR tubes again.
7. Cap or seal the PCR tubes and transfer them to a PCR Thermocycler.
8. Run the PCR program:

| | |
|---|---|
| 2 min-96°C | |
| 10 cycles | 10 s-94°C<br>1 min-65°C |
| 20 cycles | 10 s-94°C<br>50 s-61°C<br>30 s-72°C |
| Hold on 4°C | |

*3.1.2. Electrophoresis*

1. Transfer 200 mL of 0.5% TBE to an Erlenmeyer and add 3 g agarose and mix.
2. Transfer the glass with TBE and agarose to a microwave and boil until the agarose is fully solved (see Note 5).
3. Cool the solvent by holding the glass under cold running water, swirling the glass to obtain an even temperature.
4. Put the glass covered with parafilm in a 50°C water bath for a minimum of 10 min (see Note 6).
5. Add 10 μL ethidium bromide (final concentration 0.5 μg/mL), swirl the glass, and pour the gel solvent in a geltray. Discard the air bubbles and put combs in the gel.
6. Leave the gel for a minimum of 10 min at RT to solidify, followed by approximately 30 min at 4°C.
7. Put sufficient 0.5× TBE buffer in the gel electrophoresis system and add 10 μL ethidium bromide (the gel must be completely covered by buffer).

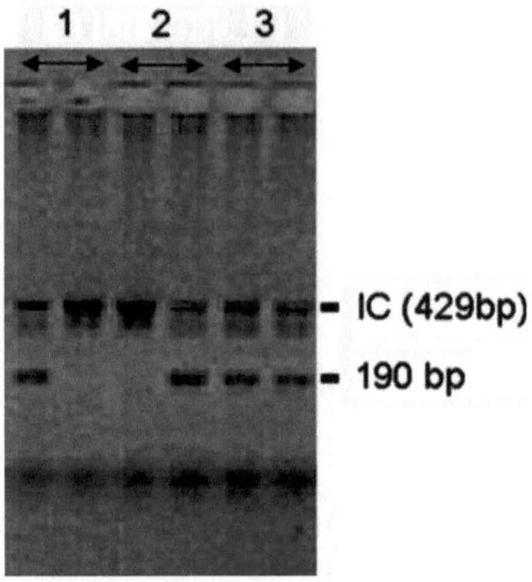


Fig. 1. Example of PCR-SSP reactions for detection of HLA-E*01:01 and HLA-E*01:03 in three samples (see Note 7). The HLA-E-specific PCR product has a fragment length of 190 bp, the internal control is 429 bp. Sample 1 is typed as HLA-E*01:01 homozygous, sample 2 as HLA-E*01:03 homozygous and sample 3 as HLA-E*01:01,01:03 heterozygous.

8. Remove the combs from the geltray and put the geltray in the electrophoresis system.
9. Take the PCR tray out of the thermocycler and centrifuge the tray (pulse centrifugation until reaching 200 × *g*).
10. Load 10 μL of each PCR product in each lane of the gel and 10 μL of 50 bp DNA marker in one lane.
11. Close the electrophoresis lid and run the gel for 36 min at 10 V/cm.
12. Following electrophoresis transfer the gel to a Geldoc system to visualize the ethidium bromide-stained bands under UV-light.

#### 3.1.3. Analysis

1. HLA-E*01:01 and HLA-E*01:03-specific PCR fragments have a length of 190 bp and the internal control fragment has a length of 429 bp. When a specific fragment is visible for only the HLA-E*01:01 mix and negative for the HLA-E*01:03 mix, the sample is typed as HLA-E*01:01 homozygous. A sample is HLA-E*01:03 homozygous, when a specific band is visible for only the HLA-E*01:03 mix and negative for the HLA-E*01:01 mix. When for both mixes the specific fragments are present, the sample is heterozygous, HLA-E*01:01,01:03. An example is shown in Fig. 1.

### 3.2. PCR-SSO

For the SSO method, different probes specific for HLA-E*01:01, *01:03, and *01:04 are bound to fluorescently coded beads, developed in collaboration with Dr J. Lee (One Lambda). HLA-E is amplified using two amplification primers each of which is labelled with biotin. After annealing of the biotinylated DNA amplicon to the beads, the DNA is labelled by addition of streptavidin coated phyco-erythrin. The fluorescence intensity is measured by luminex equipment and analysed manually to determine if the specific probes have bound the complementary DNA and thereby identify if a sample is positive for a certain allele. This method is suitable for large-scale testing and easy to implement in routine luminex typing approaches.

*3.2.1. Amplification*

1. Adjust the concentration of DNA to 20 ng/μL using sterile water.
2. Prepare mastermix (see Note 8) for all reactions:

| Per reaction | 13.8 μL | D-mix* |
|---|---|---|
| | 4.0 μL | HLA-E-specific amplification primers |
| | 0.2 μL | Taq polymerase |
| | 18.0 μL | |
| Add the Taq polymerase immediately before use | | |

*see methods part 2.2.1

3. Pipette 2 μL of DNA onto the bottom of a PCR tube.
4. Mix and centrifuge the MM and aliquot 18 μL into each well containing DNA.
5. Cap or seal and transfer tubes to a PCR Thermocycler.
6. Run PCR program:

| 3 min-96°C | |
|---|---|
| 5 cycles | 20 s-96°C |
| | 20 s-60°C |
| | 20 s-72°C |
| 30 cycles | 10 s-96°C |
| | 15 s-60°C |
| | 20 s-72°C |
| 10 min-72°C | |
| Hold on 4°C | |

7. Amplified DNA is now ready to be tested by hybridization. Optionally, 2–5 μL of the PCR product can be used for analysis by gel electrophoresis. For method, see electrophoresis in Subheading 3.1.2 (see Note 9).

*3.2.2. Denaturation/ Neutralization Procedure*

1. Prepare a crushed ice bath and place a clean 96-well plate in a tray holder.
2. Transfer 5 μL of PCR product into a well of the plate.
3. Add 2.5 μL denaturation buffer per reaction, mix thoroughly, seal or cap the tray and incubate for 10 min at room temperature.
4. Vortex the neutralization buffer, add 5 μL to each reaction, mix thoroughly (notice the colour change to clear or pale yellow) and place the plate on the ice bath.

*3.2.3. Hybridization Procedure*

1. Make sure that the thermocycler has been turned on and is pre-warmed at 60°C.
2. Prepare hybridization mixture by combining 34 μL of hybridization buffer with 4 μL of bead mixture per reaction, see Note 10. Protect the mixture with the fluorescently labelled beads from the light as much as possible.
3. Keep the tray on ice to prevent early annealing. Vortex the hybridization mixture and add 38 μL to each well, mix well by pipetting up and down.
4. Cover tray with tray seal and place PCR plate into the pre-warmed thermocycler.
5. Incubate for 15 min at 60°C.
6. Following incubation, place tray in tray holder, remove seal, and quickly add 100 μL wash buffer to each well.
7. Cover tray with tray seal and centrifuge for 5 min at 1,000–1,300 × *g*.
8. Remove wash buffer by flicking (see Note 11).
9. Repeat the washing step twice.
10. Vortex SAPE stock and prepare 1× SAPE solution during third centrifugation (see Note 12):

    0.5 μL SAPE stock + 49.5 μL SAPE buffer, keep solution in the dark until use.

*3.2.4. Labelling*

1. Add 50 μL of 1× SAPE solution to each well, seal tray, and vortex thoroughly at low speed.
2. Place PCR plate in the pre-warmed thermocycler and incubate for 5 min at 60°C.
3. Following incubation, place tray in holder, remove seal, and quickly add 100 μL wash buffer to each well.
4. Cover tray and centrifuge for 5 min at 1,000–1,300 × *g*.
5. Remove supernatant by flicking.
6. Add 70 μL wash buffer to each well, mix by pipetting, and transfer 80 μL to reading plate.
7. Read the plate in the Luminex apparatus.
8. If tray is not immediately read, keep it in the dark and at 4°C (see Note 13).

*3.2.5. Analysis*

1. The luminex output of one reaction will show the fluorescent intensity (FI) value measured for each bead in the reaction. There are 6 beads present, bead 35 is an internal negative control, no DNA must be bound to this bead. Bead 57 is a positive control, each PCR product must be bound to this bead. Bead 58 contains a probe for HLA-E*01:01, bead 59 for HLA-E*01:03

**Table 1**
**FI values of the various beads and the calculated normalized values**

| Sample | 1 | 2 | 3 |
|---|---|---|---|
| Bead 35 | 14 | 12 | 9 |
| Bead 57 | 3,137 | 3,302 | 3,304 |
| Bead 58 | 2,942 | 100 | 2,414 |
| Normalized value bead 58 | 94 | 3 | 73 |
| Bead 59 | 41 | 2,552 | 2,150 |
| Normalized value bead 59 | 1 | 77 | 65 |
| Bead 60 | 5,184 | 4,965 | 5,314 |
| Normalized value bead 60 | 166 | 151 | 161 |
| Bead 61 | 436 | 415 | 623 |
| Normalized value bead 61 | 14 | 12 | 19 |
| HLA-E typing result | *01:01 | *01:03 | *01:01,01:03 |

Sample 1 is typed as HLA-E*01:01 homozygous, sample 2 HLA-E*01:03 homozygous, and sample 3 heterozygous HLA-E*01:01,01:03

and HLA-E*01:04, bead 60 for HLA-E*01:01 and HLA-E*01:03, and bead 61 for HLA-E*01:04. The measured fluorescence intensity for each bead is an indication of the amount of DNA annealed to the probe. A normalized value can be calculated by [FI (bead)—FI (neg bead)]/[FI (pos bead)–FI (neg bead)] *100. If the normalized value exceeds 30%, the bead is positive. Values below 30% are regarded as negative (see Note 14). Based on the positive and negative reactions, HLA-E typing can be obtained (see Table 1). The FI of the positive control bead must be >1,000 and the FI of the negative control bead must be <100 (see Note 15). Bead counts need to be 100 or greater.

### 3.3. Sequencing-Based Typing

For sequence-based typing, the HLA-E gene is amplified using primers in the 5′ UT region and in intron 5, enabling sequencing of exons 1–5 and the intervening introns. The obtained sequences are analysed using the Lasergene software program, or equivalents, by aligning the sequence of a sample with the known HLA-E alleles. Sequence comparison will enable typing of the alleles HLA-E*01:01:01, 01:03:01, 01:03:02, 01:03:03, 01:03:04, 01:04.

#### 3.3.1. Amplification

1. Provide a clean work environment, e.g. a Biohazard. Keep the reaction mixes on ice throughout the entire protocol.

2. Transfer PCR tubes to a tray and put on ice, calculate the number of reactions needed, and prepare one large batch of mastermix (see Note 16):

| | | |
|---|---|---|
| Per reaction | 5 µL | Expand high fidelity buffer, 10× conc. with 15 mL $MgCl_2$ |
| | 1 µL | Each dNTP (10 mM) |
| | 1 µL | Forward primer E08072 (10 pmol/µL) |
| | 1 µL | Reverse primer E08073 (10 pmol/µL) |
| | 0.75 µL | Expand high fidelity enzyme mix |
| Add aqua dest to a final volume of 48 µL | | |

3. Pipette 48 µL MM/per PCR tube and add 100 ng of DNA.
4. Centrifuge (pulse centrifugation until reaching 200 × *g*).
5. Move the PCR tubes directly to the PCR Thermocycler.
6. Run PCR program:

| | |
|---|---|
| 2 min-94°C | |
| 10 cycles | 15 s-94°C<br>30 s-65°C<br>2 min-72°C |
| 10 cycles | 15 s-94°C<br>30 s-61°C<br>2.5 min-72°C |
| 10 cycles | 15 s-94°C<br>30 s-61°C<br>3.5 min-72°C |
| 7 min-72°C | |
| Hold on 4°C | |

7. After the PCR reaction, 5–10 µL of the PCR products can be checked by agarose gel electrophoresis according to the protocol in Subheading 3.1.2, running the gel for 60 min and using a 100 bp marker. A band with a length of 2.1 kb must be visible.

#### *3.3.2. Purification of the PCR Product*

1. Pipette ExoSAP-IT in a PCR tube (all steps need to be performed on ice) followed by addition of the PCR product (4 µL ExoSAP-IT/10 µL of PCR product), mix well and centrifuge (impulse centrifugation until reaching 200 × *g*).
2. Transfer the PCR tubes to the PCR Thermocycler.
3. Run PCR program:

| | |
|---|---|
| 15 min | 37°C |
| 15 min | 80°C |
| Hold on 4°C (see Note 17) | |

*3.3.3. Sequencing Reaction*

1. In order to perform the sequencing reaction the sequencing (primer) mix has to be made (see Note 18):

| | | |
|---|---|---|
| Per reaction | 1.0 μL | BDT sequencing mix |
| | 1.5 μL | BDT sequencing buffer (5×) |
| | 0.5 μL | Sequencing primer (5 pmol) |
| | 6.0 μL | Aqua Dest |
| | 9.0 μL | |

2. Pipette 9 μL sequencing mix in a new PCR tube on ice and add 1 μL purified PCR product, mix well.
3. Transfer the tubes to a PCR Thermocycler.
4. Run PCR program:

| | |
|---|---|
| 1 min-96°C | |
| 25 cycles | 10 s-96°C<br>5 s-50°C<br>4 min-60°C |
| Hold on 4°C | |

*3.3.4. Purification Following Sequence Reaction*

1. Following the sequencing reaction, purify the products by filtration using a vacuum system.
2. Mix each sequencing reaction product with 20 μL of Millipore buffer (from the Montage $SEQ_{96}$ Sequencing Reaction Cleanup kit) and pipette in a filter plate.
3. Put the filter plate on the vacuum system and extract for 5 min.
4. Add another 40 μL of millipore buffer to the filter plate and extract again until all solution has been extracted (see Note 19).
5. Add 30 μL of millipore buffer, put the filter plate on a vortex, and shake for 10 min at max. 600/min.
6. Transfer 25 μL of the sample to a 3730 plate, add 10 μL of sequencing standard to one well on the same plate (see Note 20) and cover with a septa.
7. Put the plate in the 3730 DNA analyser (or store for maximum 1 day at 4°C) and run the sequencing program (see Note 21).

*3.3.5. Analysis*

1. The sequence output is analysed by the software Lasergene or equivalents (see Note 22). Based upon the A → G nucleotide substitution at position 382 in exon 3 (position refers to cDNA reference sequence IMGT/HLA), HLA-E*01:01 can be distinguished from HLA-E*01:03 and HLA-E*01:04. HLA-E*01:03 can be distinguished from HLA-E*01:04 by the difference at position 532, *01:03 has an A at this position,

whereas *01:04 has a G. HLA-E*01:03:01, *01:03:02, *01:03:03, and *01:03:04 can be identified based upon the nucleotide substitutions at positions 294, 513, and 696.

## 4. Notes

1. The method described by Paquay et al. (14) is the sole proprietary knowledge of Genome Diagnostics BV Utrecht, the Netherlands.

   *PCR-SSP Method*

2. It is most efficient to prepare the master mixes in large amounts for multiple samples and aliquot.
3. Vortex the primers before adding to the mixes.
4. It is most efficient to prepare reaction mixes in larger amounts for multiple samples. Prepared reaction mixes can be stored at –80°C.
5. It is important to boil long enough until all agarose particles are fully dissolved in the TBE buffer and when cooling down to swirl the glass to prevent unequal solidification of the gel.
6. The temperature of the gel mixture must not exceed 60°C when ethidium bromide is added because this high temperature will destroy the ethidium bromide.
7. Very weak or invisible DNA bands (including internal control) can be caused by insufficient mixing of Taq polymerase before adding it to the primer/DNA mixes.

   *PCR-SSO Method*

8. Vortex D-mix and amplification primers before adding to the mix.
9. PCR products can be stored at –80°C to –20°C.
10. Vortex beads well before adding. Once beads are thawed, store beads at 2–8°C and use within 3 months. Do not refreeze bead mixture after thawing.
11. Try to remove (flick) as much wash buffer as possible by inverting the tray and pouring into the waste in one movement. To perform this accurately, training is needed. If you do not succeed in removing all wash buffer at once, you have to repeat the flicking; however, you will have a higher risk of loosing beads. Leaving too much wash buffer can affect your results (see Note 15).
12. Remove the SAPE bottle from storage only when needed, and return immediately to 2–8°C.
13. Prolonged storage of samples (more than 4 h) may result in loss of signal.

14. Since HLA-E*01:04 has never been detected after its initial identification, it has not been possible to check the specificity of the HLA-E*01:04 bead.
15. In case MFI values of the control beads are out of range (too low positive or too high negative control values), we consider it necessary to repeat the procedure. When the MFI value of the positive beads is too low, this could be caused by inadequate PCR amplification, that can be checked by agarose gel electrophoresis. If a correct strong PCR band is observed, the too low positive control value might be caused by insufficient flicking, resulting in a lower concentration of SAPE. A too high negative control value might be due to some contamination. Repeating the reactions with new reagents might be necessary.

*SBT Method*

16. Vortex the primers before adding to the mixes.
17. The purified PCR product can be stored for a maximum of 1 week at 4°C.
18. The amplification primers can also be used as sequencing primers in addition to the described sequencing primers.
19. It is important that all fluid has been extracted; otherwise, it can result in a higher background because the remaining labelled dNTPs could interfere with the sequence analysis.
20. The sequencing standard can be run to check for any inconsistencies during the capillary electrophoresis and analysis procedure.
21. The sequencing reaction products can be analysed by any automated DNA sequencer that is able to detect the Big Dye Terminator-labelled nucleotides.
22. After DNA sequence analysis, the sequences are stored in .AB1 files. DNASTAR software Lasergene contains EDITSEQ, ALIGN, and SEQMAN modules. Individual sequences are selected, these are the sample AB1 files, and HLA-E sequences obtained from the IMGT/HLA database/EBI (www.ebi.ac.uk/imgt/hla) are used as reference. The uploaded reference and sample sequence files are assembled by SEQMAN. From the resulting contig, the nucleotide peaks can be viewed, checked and if necessary adjusted. Extended sequences obtained as displayed in the contig can be used as reference sequence additionally. Lasergene software is a product from DNASTAR, Madison, USA.

## Acknowledgements

The authors thank Jarhow Lee (One Lambda, Los Angeles, USA) for the development of the HLA-E SSO kit and reagents and Els Bielen and Timo Olieslagers for their practical assistance.

## References


1. Antoun A et al (2009) Ethnic variability in human leukocyte antigen-E haplotypes. Tissue Antigens 73(1):39–45
2. Grimsley C et al (2002) Definitive high resolution typing of HLA-E allelic polymorphisms: identifying potential errors in existing allele data. Tissue Antigens 60(3):206–212
3. Ohya K, Kondo K, Mizuno S (1990) Polymorphism in the human class I MHC locus HLA-E in Japanese. Immunogenetics 32(3):205–209
4. Grimsley C, Ober C (1997) Population genetic studies of HLA-E: evidence for selection. Hum Immunol 52(1):33–40
5. Geraghty DE et al (1992) Polymorphism at the HLA-E locus predates most HLA-A and -B polymorphism. Hum Immunol 33(3): 174–184
6. Ulbrecht M et al (1999) Cell surface expression of HLA-E: interaction with human beta2-microglobulin and allelic differences. Eur J Immunol 29(2):537–547
7. Strong RK et al (2003) HLA-E allelic variants. Correlating differential expression, peptide affinities, crystal structures, and thermal stabilities. J Biol Chem 278(7):5082–5090
8. Maier S et al (2000) Implications of HLA-E allele expression and different HLA-E ligand diversity for the regulation of NK cells. Hum Immunol 61(11):1059–1065
9. Tamouza R et al (2005) Association of HLA-E polymorphism with severe bacterial infection and early transplant-related mortality in matched unrelated bone marrow transplantation. Transplantation 80(1):140–144
10. Tamouza R et al (2006) Homozygous status for HLA-E*0103 confers protection from acute graft-versus-host disease and transplant-related mortality in HLA-matched sibling hematopoietic stem cell transplantation. Transplantation 82(11):1436–1440
11. Danzer M et al (2009) Clinical significance of HLA-E*0103 homozygosity on survival after allogeneic hematopoietic stem-cell transplantation. Transplantation 88(4):528–532
12. Ludajic K et al (2009) Association of HLA-E polymorphism with the outcome of hematopoietic stem-cell transplantation with unrelated donors. Transplantation 88(10):1227–1228
13. Park KS et al (2007) HLA-E*0101 and HLA-G*010101 reduce the risk of Behcet's disease. Tissue Antigens 69(2):139–144
14. Paquay MM, Schellekens J, Tilanus MG (2009) A high-throughput Taqman(R) approach for the discrimination of HLA-E alleles. Tissue Antigens 74(6):514–519

# Chapter 9

# Molecular Analysis of Complement Component C4 Gene Copy Number

**Alison S.L. Castley and O. Patricia Martinez**


## Abstract

Classical, alternative, or lectin pathways may activate the complement system cascade. The classical pathway includes the C4 protein and functions in the prevention of immune complex precipitation and in clearance of immune complexes.

Two isotypes of C4—C4A and C4B—are coded by genes located at two loci within the major histocompatibility complex (MHC) on chromosome 6. While these isotypes share over 99% amino acid sequence homology, five nucleotide differences located in exon 26 are responsible for major structural and functional differences between the C4 isotypes.

C4A and C4B are highly polymorphic with over 40 alleles, gene duplications, and "null alleles". C4 genes may be short (14.6 kb) or long (21 kb), due to the absence or presence of an endogenous retroviral sequence—HERV-K(C4)—in intron 9, respectively. The C4 gene copy number (GCN) can vary from 1–3 per haplotype or 2–6 per diploid genome. The variation in GCN leads to a range of C4 plasma protein concentrations among healthy subjects. In subjects with equal numbers of C4 genes, subjects with short genes have C4 plasma levels relatively higher than subjects with long genes.

Variation of the C4 GCN, the gene size (long or short) and the C4 isotypes (C4A and C4B) may also lead to susceptibility to autoimmune disease. Therefore, in subjects with autoimmune disease, a low serum C4 level may be due to ongoing disease activity associated with complement activation and consumption or it may be due to genetic factors. Distinguishing between these will have clinical implications.

Exact determination of GCN can be difficult, at least in part due to the high degree of homology between C4A and C4B and a variety of techniques has been described. This chapter describes a quantitative TaqMan real-time PCR (qPCR) copy number assay, based on our laboratory experience using this assay.


**Key words:** Human complement genes, C4A, C4B, Gene copy number, Real-time PCR

## 1. Introduction

The complement system consists of at least 26 proteins that are expressed constitutively and non-specifically. These proteins participate in a cascade of reactions that need to be activated to function. There are three major pathways for activation of the complement

Frank T. Christiansen and Brian D. Tait (eds.), *Immunogenetics: Methods and Applications in Clinical Practice*, Methods in Molecular Biology, vol. 882, DOI 10.1007/978-1-61779-842-9_9, © Springer Science+Business Media New York 2012

cascade—classical, alternative, and lectin pathways. Different mechanisms or substances activate each of these.

The classical pathway is involved in the prevention of immune complex precipitation and in enhancing binding to CR1 and clearance of immune complexes (1). Homozygous deficiency of components of the classical pathway—C4, C2 and C1—predispose to immune complex-mediated autoimmune disease (2).

The C4 protein is coded by genes located at two loci within the major histocompatibility complex (MHC) on chromosome 6. The length of each of these genes varies depending on the presence or absence of a 6.5 kb endogenous retrovirus insertion—HERV-K(C4)—in intron 9, producing "long" (22 kb) and "short" (14.6 kb) C4 genes (3–7).

The products of these loci—C4A and C4B (8) exhibit an extremely high degree of genomic sequence homology throughout the C4 molecule (9) and share over 99% amino acid sequence (7). Despite this amino acid homology, C4A and C4B are functionally different. C4A binds preferentially to amino groups, such as those found in immune complexes (10), while C4B binds preferentially to acceptor hydroxyl groups found predominantly on the carbohydrates of red blood cell surfaces (11).

C4A and C4B are very polymorphic, with over 40 alleles, including "null alleles" and gene duplications (4, 12). C4 null alleles are defined by the absence of C4 protein in plasma (8, 13, 14). They may be due to gene deletion (4, 15), homo-duplication (16), gene conversion (12), or mutations leading to non-expression.

The variation in gene copy number (GCN) leads to a range of C4 plasma protein concentrations. Uko et al. defined reference ranges for serum C4 concentration in subjects with 0, 1, and 2 C4 null alleles (17) and Rebmann et al. used the C4 plasma concentration to define C4 null alleles and C4A duplications (18). The size of C4 genes seems to determine C4 protein level and activity, with higher C4 protein levels and higher C4 haemolytic activities being detected in subjects with short C4 genes than those with long genes only. A good correlations between the number of long genes with serum levels of C4A, and the number of short genes with serum levels of C4B has also been reported (19–21).

The GCN of C4 and surrounding genes can vary from 1–3 per haplotype (4) or 2–6 per diploid genome, with 60.8% of people with four copies of C4 genes, 27.2% with less than four copies, and 12% with more than four copies (22). Different ancestral haplotypes (AHs) of the MHC carry specific numbers of several genes, including the C4 genes (23).

It has been suggested that variation of the C4 gene copy number, the polymorphism of gene size (long or short) and the C4 isotypes—C4A and C4B—may lead to susceptibility to autoimmune disease. An increased frequency of C4A null alleles in SLE was first reported in 1983 (24). More recently, a variation of 2–6 total C4 GCN has been reported in 1,241 European Americans, with 0–5 C4A and 0–4 C4B isotypes. The risk of SLE significantly increased in subjects with only two copies of C4 and patients with SLE had lower total C4 and C4A genes (OR = 6.514; $P$ = 0.00002) (21). Another study has shown susceptibility to SLE decreased in subjects with five or more total copies of C4 (OR = 0.466; $P$ = 0.016). Both zero copies (OR = 5.267; $P$ = 0.001) and one copy (OR = 1.613; $P$ = 0.022) of C4A were risk factors for SLE, whereas three or more copies of C4A appeared to be protective (OR = 0.574; $P$ = 0.012) (25).

Polymorphism of C4 can be defined by a number of methods, including electrophoretic mobility of the intact protein or its subunits, serologically using the Rodgers (Rg) and Chido (Ch) determinants (26) and by DNA-based methods (27). Exact determination of GCN can be difficult, at least in part due to the high degree of homology between C4A and C4B. Furthermore, the polymorphisms are located in the C4d fragment of the α-chain of the C4 molecule, and only five nucleotide polymorphisms located in exon 26 are responsible for the major structural and functional differences between the C4 isotypes (28).

A number of approaches have been tried to determine the C4 GCN, including counting of fragment numbers following restriction fragment length polymorphism (RFLP) analysis (25), densitometry of products obtained by pulsed field gel electrophoresis (PFGE) and Southern blotting (22), and a multiplex ligation-dependent probe amplification (MLPA) assay combined with isotype-specific ELISAs to determine the level of C4A and C4B (20).

Wu et al. developed quantitative TaqMan real-time PCR (qPCR) assays based on nucleotide sequences specific for the C4A and C4B genes, structural characteristics corresponding to long and short C4 genes, and the breakpoint region of RP-C4-CYP21-TNX (RCCX) modular duplication (29). Using cloned C4 genomic DNA (gDNA) covering six logs of DNA concentrations for calibration and a relative standard curve they described eight HLA haplotypes with single C4 genes in mono-modular RCCX that are associated with multiple autoimmune and infectious diseases and 32 bi-modular, 4 tri-modular, and one quadri-modular RCCX (29).

In this chapter, a qPCR copy number assay based on the method of Wu et al. (29) is described.

In a qPCR, a fluorescence dye is incorporated into the amplified DNA as the PCR proceeds. The dye emits light proportional to the number of amplified copies. The TaqMan dye chemistry is specific and precise for monitoring the kinetics of the amplification process. Quantification of the initial amount of DNA present in the reaction is based on the number of cycles required to reach a threshold ($C_T$), at which the fluorescence is increased significantly and passes an arbitrarily defined value. The greater the initial amount of DNA template, the fewer cycles that are required for the reaction to reach the fluorescence threshold and a smaller $C_T$ observed.

The TaqMan® Copy Number Assay is designed to determine copy number variation within the genome. A duplex PCR of the target gene and a reference sequence known to be present as two copies in a diploid genome is performed. The copy number of the target sequence in a gDNA sample is determined relative to the reference sequence.

The comparative method measures the comparative difference between the target and the reference sequences, and then compares the comparative difference values of test samples to a calibrator sample(s) known to have two copies of the target sequence. The copy number of the target is calculated to be two times the relative quantity.

## 2. Materials

1. Purified patient gDNA at 5 ng/μL (see Notes 1 and 2).
2. C4A TaqMan® Copy Number Assay (100× or 20×—Supplied by Applied Biosystems) (see Notes 3–5).
    (a) Unlabelled, target-specific forward and reverse primers to amplify the C4A gene(s).
    (b) FAM™ dye-labelled TaqMan® MGB probe to detect the C4A sequence.
3. C4B TaqMan® Copy Number Assay (100× or 20×—Supplied by Applied Biosystems) (see Notes 3–5).
    (a) Unlabelled, target-specific forward and reverse primers to amplify the C4B gene(s).
    (b) FAM™ dye-labelled TaqMan® MGB probe to detect the C4B sequence.
4. TaqMan® Copy Number Reference Assay RNase P (Supplied by Applied Biosystems) (see Notes 4–6).
    (a) Two primers to amplify the genomic reference sequence.
    (b) VIC® dye-labelled TAMRA™ probe to detect the genomic reference sequence.
5. TaqMan® Genotyping Master Mix containing AmpliTaq Gold® DNA Polymerase, UP (Ultra-Pure) and dNTPs (Supplied by Applied Biosystems).
6. Applied Biosystems Real-Time PCR Genetic Analyser (i.e. 7900, 7900HT) (purchased from Applied Biosystems).
7. Applied Biosystems CopyCaller™ Software—for post-PCR data analysis of copy number quantitation (Supplied by Applied Biosystems). This is free to download from AB Web site: http://www.appliedbiosystems.com.au (see Note 7).
8. Sterile deionised water (CSL).

9. Adjustable pipettes with aerosol barrier tips (manual or electronic, P10, P20, P100, P200).
10. MicroAmp® Optical 96-Well Reaction Plates (Applied Biosystems).
11. MicroAmp® Optical Adhesive Film or MicroAmp® Optical Caps (Applied Biosystems).
12. Sterile 0.5-mL Eppendorf microcentrifuge tubes (Crown Scientific).
13. Sterile biological safety cabinet.
14. Vortex mixer (Ratek).
15. Plate centrifuge.
16. Separate pre-PCR (an area to set up the C4 reactions) and post-PCR areas (see Note 8).

## 3. Methods

The qPCR reaction occurs in a single tube or well, using universal PCR cycling conditions on an Applied Biosystems Real-Time PCR System. Following amplification, data files containing the sample replicate comparative values for each reporter dye can be exported from the qPCR instrument software and imported into a software analysis tool.

### 3.1. Pre-PCR Set Up

#### 3.1.1. Prepare Genomic DNA

1. Ensure blood has been collected in either ACD or EDTA collection tubes.
2. Extract, purify, and quantify DNA using your usual laboratory methods.
3. Dilute the gDNA. Use sterile deionised water to obtain a concentration of 5 ng/μL (see Notes 1 and 2).
4. Use the diluted gDNA immediately or keep at 4°C for long-term storage.
5. Vortex the diluted gDNA for 5 s before use.

#### 3.1.2. Samples to Be Included

1. Test samples for target copy number assessment.
2. Control samples with known C4 copy number for each C4 assay (see Note 9).
3. A "no template" control (sterile deionised water) used to detect background fluorescence and exclude contamination.
4. For accurate copy number assignment, four replicates of each gDNA test sample, each gDNA control sample and the "no template" control must be set up.

**Table 1**
**Reaction mixture composition – Volume (μL) of reaction mixture components required in a C4 assay**

| | Volume of reagents (μL) | |
|---|---|---|
| | 1 Sample (μL) | Number of reactions[a] |
| C4A or C4B TaqMan® Copy number assay (20×) | 1 | 1 μL × number of reactions |
| TaqMan® Copy number reference assay RNase P (20×) | 1 | 1 μL × number of reactions |
| TaqMan® Genotyping master mix (2×) | 10 | 10 μL × number of reactions |
| Sterile deionised $H_2O$ | 4 | 4 μL × number of reactions |
| Total | 16 | 16 μL × number of reactions |

[a]Number of reactions = 4 × (number of samples + controls[b]) + 2
[b]Samples known to contain 0–4 copies of C4A or C4B (see Note 9). One of these samples, usually the sample containing two copies of C4A or C4B is used as the calibrator sample (see Note 10)

5. A calibrator sample is also required. This is a gDNA sample with known copy number for target of interest—C4A or C4B, depending on the assay being performed (see Note 10).

### *3.2. Prepare PCRs*

1. Calculate the volume of components needed, based on the reaction volume and the number of reactions (see Table 1). Include excess volume to provide for losses that occur during reagent transfers (equivalent to two extra samples). Thus, number of reactions = 4 × [number of samples + controls] + 2.
2. Thaw the TaqMan® Copy Number and TaqMan® Copy Number Reference reagents at room temperature, vortex gently for 5 s and then centrifuge tubes briefly (500 rpm for 10 s).
3. Thoroughly mix the TaqMan® Genotyping Master Mix by flicking and briefly centrifuge (500 rpm for 10 s).
4. Combine the required volumes of reaction components in a microcentrifuge tube (see Table 1). Use separate microcentrifuge tubes for the C4A and for the C4B assays and ensure the tube caps are firmly in place to avoid leakage.
5. Mix the contents thoroughly by flicking or inverting the microcentrifuge tubes, then centrifuge briefly at 500 rpm for 10 s.
6. Pipette 16 μL of reaction mixture into each of the appropriate wells of a MicroAmp® Optical 96-well reaction plate.
7. Briefly vortex the diluted gDNA samples for 5 s (from Subheading 3.1.1, step 5).
8. Using a different pipette tip for each sample, add 4 μL of gDNA (5 ng/μL) and the control samples to the appropriate

replicate wells of the MicroAmp® Optical 96-well reaction plate containing the reaction mixture (see Note 11).

9. Mix the reaction mixture and gDNA by pipetting up and down several times (see Note 12).
10. Seal the reaction plate with optical adhesive film or optical caps, then centrifuge the reaction plate briefly (500 rpm for 10 s).
11. Inspect all the wells to ensure a uniform volume.
12. Run the reactions.

### 3.3. Running the PCRs on the Real-Time Instrument

1. Place the reaction plate on the 7900 qPCR instrument to be used.
2. Under "Instrument" ensure the following parameters are correctly identified on the template.

| Parameter | Setting |
|---|---|
| Run | Standard |
| Reaction plate | 96-Well standard |
| Ramp speed/model | 9600 Emulation |
| Sample volume | 20 μL |

3. Ensure all samples within a C4 copy number assay are uniquely identified and ensure all replicates have the same identifier (see Note 13).
4. Clearly identify the copy number assay for the appropriate wells and omit any unused wells.
5. Run the plate under these conditions:
   (a) Hold at 95°C for 10 min.
   (b) 40 Cycles each of:
      (i) 95°C for 15 s.
      (ii) Followed by 60°C for 60 s.

### 3.4. Post Real-Time PCR Analysis

1. Open the Analysis Settings window of the RT-PCR Instrument software and set:
   (a) Manual $C_T$ Threshold of 0.2.
   (b) Autobaseline—On.
2. Apply settings and close window.
3. Select "Analyse" to analyse experiment and review data.
4. Select the VIC and FAM tabs in the analysis programme individually and make sure that the amplification curves have a distinct exponential amplification phase for (see Figs. 1 and 2):
   (a) Reference Assay (VIC® dye signal) in all samples.
   (b) Copy Number Assay (FAM® dye signal) in most wells.

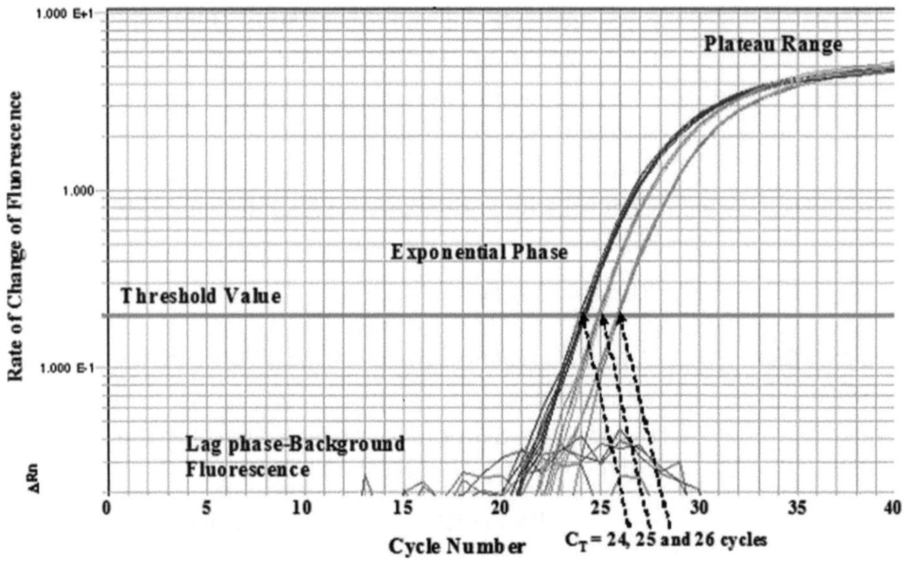


Fig. 1. Principles of the real-time PCR. A fluorescent dye is incorporated into the amplified DNA and emits light proportional to the number of amplified copies. Quantification of the initial amount of target DNA sequence present in the reaction is based on the number of cycles required for the measured fluorescence to reach a given threshold. The number of cycles required to reach that threshold is the $C_T$. The $C_T$ value is highly proportional to the copy number of the target sequence in the template. The greater the copy number present, the fewer cycles of PCR required for the accumulated product to be detected in the PCR process, and the lower the $C_T$ value.

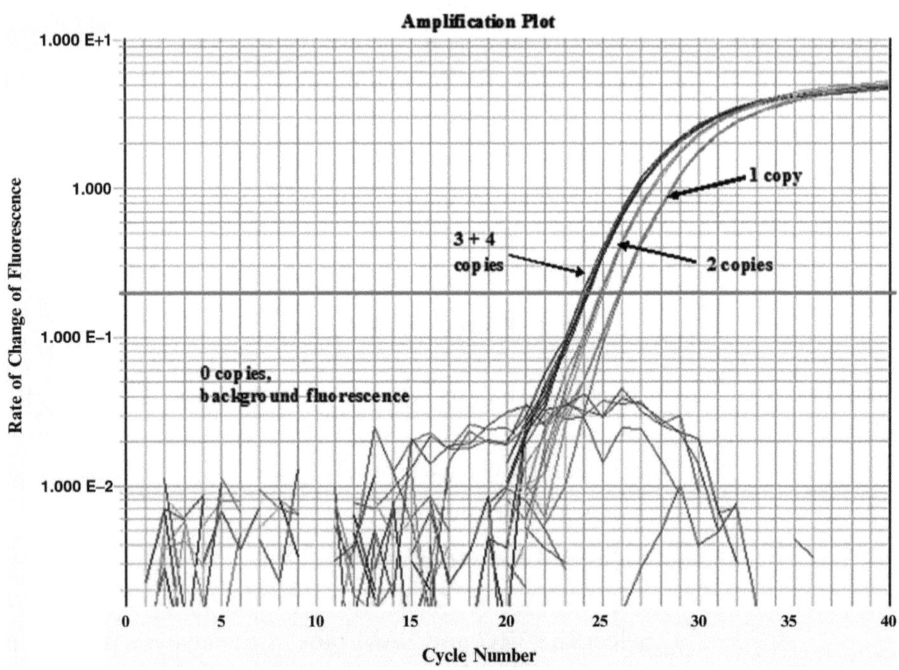


Fig. 2. An amplification profile from a C4B copy number assay from the 7900 (FAM representation). Samples with 1, 2, and 3–4 copy numbers are identified. Zero copy numbers are seen as background fluorescence. The $C_T$ values for samples with one and two C4B copies are 26 and 25 respectively. The $C_T$ value for the sample with three C4B copies is just over 24 and for the sample with four C4B copies is just under 24 (see Figs. 1 and 3).

5. Review the amplification curves for all samples and controls. If there has been a problem with amplification (either no, weak or different shaped amplification curves) review the method (see Notes 14–17).
6. Review the RT-PCR data of replicate samples. Ensure three or more replicates have amplified adequately (see Figs. 1 and 2). Adequate amplification is required for Copy Caller™ analysis.
7. Export results. Export each experiment result or results table to one or more exported RT-PCR files (.txt file).

### 3.5. Utilising CopyCaller™ Software for Final Analysis

1. Open the CopyCaller™ software on the computer.
2. Import the exported (.txt) data into the CopyCaller™ software.
3. Go to "Assay Selection" and highlight one assay at a time. Identify the calibrator sample for use in the analysis go to "Tools"→"Analysis setting" and ensure the 2-copy number calibrator is selected, then "Apply" the parameters.
4. Place a "tick" in the C4 assay you analysed (under "Assay Selection"). The results for the assay should appear.
5. The CopyCaller™ software will assign a copy number to each sample for each assay. The results can have the 0–8 copy numbers (see Fig. 3 and Note 18).

## 4. Notes

1. Patient gDNA must have a UV absorbance A260/A280 ratio greater than 1.7. The ratio of absorption at 260 vs. 280 nm is commonly used to assess protein contamination in solutions.
2. All samples must have the same amplification rate. This is achieved by diluting all gDNA samples to 5 ng/μL. Use the same amount of gDNA for each sample and its replicates to be run in the same assay.
3. If your Taqman® Copy number assay is supplied at 100× concentration, dilute it to 20× with sterile deionised water.
4. To minimise the freeze–thaw cycles of the Taqman® copy number kits and reference kits, sub-aliquot small volumes (15 μL) into small Eppendorf tubes.
5. The Taqman® copy number kits and reference kit should be stored protected from light at −15 to −25°C.
6. The TaqMan® Copy Number Reference RNase P has been optimised for copy number assays by Applied Biosystems. This kit detects the ribonuclease P RNA component H1 (H1RNA) gene (RPPH1) on chromosome 14 and is known to be present as two copies in a diploid genome.

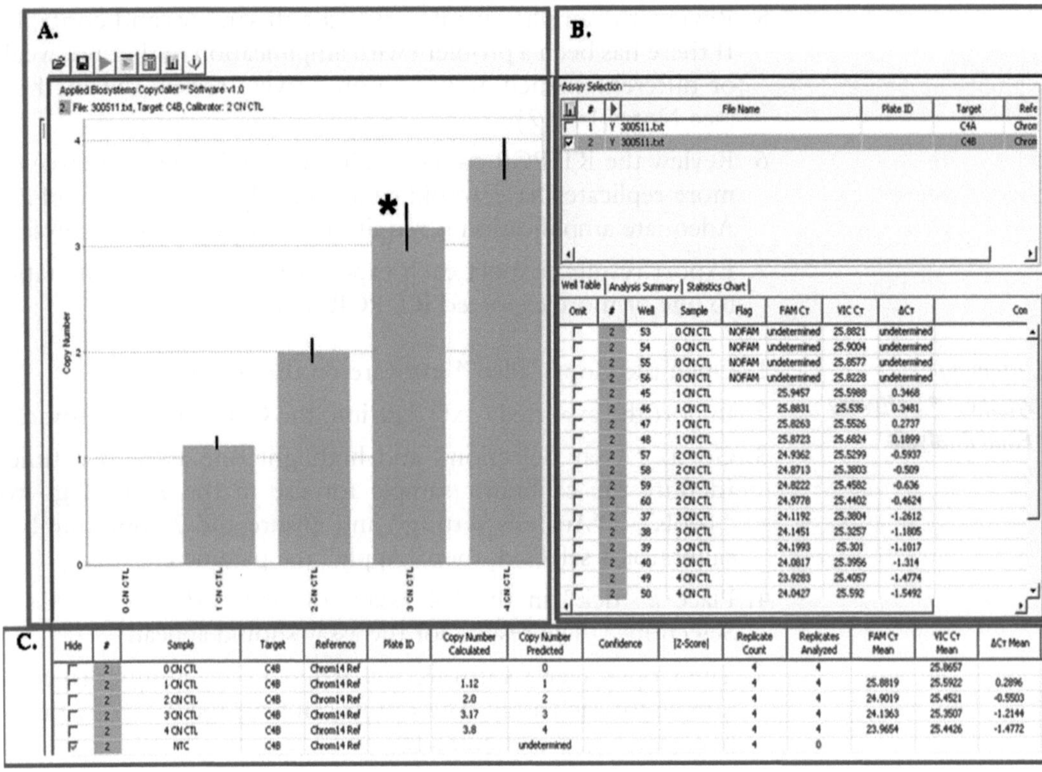


Fig. 3. Results generated by the CopyCaller™ software from the C4B amplification profiles shown in Fig. 2. (**a**) A bar graph of the C4 copy number calculated by the software for each sample from the results shown in (**b**). A copy number range bar (*asterisk*) indicates the minimum and maximum copy number calculated for the replicates of each sample. (**b**) The sample location in the 96-well reaction plate (well), the sample identification (sample), the $C_T$ for FAM (C4) and for VIC (reference sequence) and the difference between the $C_T$ values for C4 and the reference ($\Delta C_T$). For example—wells 57–60 contain replicates of the control that has two copies of C4B (2 CN CTL), with FAM $C_T$ values of 24.9362; 24.8713; 24.8222, and 24.9778. The same samples have VIC $C_T$ values of 25.5299; 25.3803; 25.4582, and 25.4402, respectively. (**c**) The results of the copy number analysis of individual samples. Each *row* shows the combined values of the replicates used to generate the results for a single sample, the expected and the observed copy number for each sample and the mean value of the FAM and VIC $C_T$ for C4 and the reference assay, respectively.

7. To download the Applied Biosystems CopyCaller™ Software, Microsoft Windows® XP Service pack 2 or a later version is required.
8. To avoid contamination of the gDNA, the Taqman® copy number kits and the reference kit are important to have separate areas for PCR reaction set-up (Pre-PCR) and for DNA amplification (Post-PCR).
9. It is important to include gDNA control samples for each C4 copy number assay. Samples with 0–4 copies of C4A and C4B can be purchased from the Coriell Institute for Molecular Research (www.coriell.org). Once you have determined the copy number of C4A and C4B in your in-house gDNA stocks,

these can be used as alternative control samples. The known copy number should always be correctly assigned. The 1–4 copy number controls should always amplify both the C4 assay (FAM) and the reference assay (VIC) control. The 0 copy number controls should amplify only the reference assay (VIC).

10. The calibrator sample is required by the CopyCaller™ software for correct assignment of C4 copy numbers to the samples tested. It is advised to use one of the control samples as the calibrator sample. For the detection of C4A copy numbers, use a gDNA sample with two copies of C4A and for the detection of C4B copy numbers use a gDNA sample with two copies of C4B.
11. To avoid sample mix-up and for ease of identifying samples for analysis, place all replicates of a sample in adjacent wells.
12. To avoid cross-contamination, use a fresh aerosol pipette tip to add and mix each set of replicates. Discard each tip after each set of replicate samples are mixed.
13. Unique identification of all samples for a copy number assay is an important requirement for analysis using the CopyCaller™ software. Ensure all replicates of a sample have the same identifier.
14. If problems with DNA amplification have occurred, ensure that:
    (a) Samples are not contaminated—check the 260/280 ratio and re-extract gDNA if required.
    (b) The gDNA used was at the correct concentration of 5 ng/μL.
    (c) The correct thermal cycling conditions were utilised.
    (d) Reagents have not expired—correct handling, mixing, and storage of reagents are essential.
    (e) There is no inhibitor to the reaction. A serial dilution of the sample can be evaluated to test for this.
    (f) Pipetting techniques are accurate. Use an aerosol-resistant pipette tip and follow appropriate dispensing techniques to prevent bubbles.
    (g) The workspace if free from contaminants. Wear clean gloves and a clean lab coat. Open and close samples and reagents carefully to avoid splashing and clean down work space appropriately.
    (h) For each well the appropriate detector and dye information are selected (FAM for C4 assays and VIC for reference assay).

If all of these have been fulfilled and amplification of the samples continues to fail, the samples may have a polymorphism in the primer- or probe-binding site.

15. The "no template control" should not amplify with either the C4 assays or the reference assay.
16. New batches of C4 TaqMan® Copy Number Assay and TaqMan® Copy Number Reference Assay RNase P should be tested using the control gDNA before routine use.
17. New batches of TaqMan® Genotyping Master Mix should be tested before routine use by running the new batch and the current batch in parallel.
18. The controls utilised in this assay have known C4A and C4B copy numbers (i.e. 0–4 C4 copies). Therefore, the observed copy number for these samples should be the same as the expected copy number for the assay to be valid. All of these should amplify with the reference assay (VIC). All samples, except those with 0 copies of C4, should also amplify with the C4 assay (FAM).

## References


1. Schifferli JA, Ng YC, Peters DK (1986) The role of complement and its receptor in the elimination of immune complexes. N Engl J Med 21:488
2. Lachmann PJ (1987) Heberden Oration 1986. Complement—friend or foe. Br J Rheumatol 26:409–415
3. Prentice HL, Schneider PM, Strominger JL (1986) C4B gene polymorphism detected in a human cosmid clone. Immunogenetics 23: 274
4. Schneider PM, Carroll MC, Alper CA et al (1986) Polymorphism of the human complement C4 and steroid 21-hydroxylase genes: restriction fragment length polymorphisms revealing structural deletions, homoduplications, and size variants. J Clin Invest 78:650
5. Palsdottir A, Fossdal R, Arnason A et al (1987) Heterogeneity of human C4 gene size: a large intron (6.5 kb) is present in all C4A genes and some C4B genes. Immunogenetics 25:299
6. Dangel AW, Mendoza AR, Baker BJ et al (1994) The dichotomous size variation of the human complement C4 genes is mediated by a novel family of endogenous retroviruses, which also establish species-specific genomic patterns among Old World primates. Immunogenetics 40:425
7. Chu X, Rittner C, Schneider PM (1995) Length polymorphism of the human complement component C4 gene is due to an ancient retroviral integration. Exp Clin Immunogenet 12:74
8. Awdeh ZL, Alper CA (1980) Inherited structural polymorphism of the fourth component of human complement. Proc Natl Acad Sci USA 77:3576
9. Ulgiati D, Abraham LJ (1996) Comparative analysis of the C4B1 gene from the HLA-A1, B8, DR3 haplotype. Exp Clin Immunogenet 13:43
10. Law SA, Doods AW, Porter RR (1984) A comparison of the properties of two classes, C4A and C4B, of the human complement component C4. EMBO J 3:1819
11. Isenman DE, Young JR (1984) The molecular basis for the difference in immune hemolysis activity of Chido and Rodgers isotypes of human complement component C4. J Immunol 132: 3019
12. Braun L, Schneider PM, Giles CM et al (1990) Null alleles of human complement C4. Evidence for pseudogenes at the C4A locus and for gene conversion at the C4B locus. J Exp Med 171:129
13. O'Neill GJ, Yang SY, Dupont B (1978) Two HLA-linked loci controlling the fourth component of human complement. Proc Natl Acad Sci USA 75:5165
14. Mauff G, Brenden M, Braun-Stilwell M et al (1990) C4 reference typing report. Complement Inflamm 7:193

15. Carroll MC, Palsdottir A, Belt KT, Porter RR (1985) Deletion of complement C4 and steroid 21-hydroxylase genes in the HLA class III region. EMBO J 4(10):2547
16. Yu CY, Campbell RD (1987) Definitive RFLPs to distinguish between the human complement C4A/C4B isotypes and the major Rodgers/ Chido determinants: application to the study of C4 null alleles. Immunogenetics 25:383
17. Uko G, Christiansen FT, Dawkins RL, McCann VJ (1986) Reference ranges for serum C4 concentrations in subjects with and without C4 null alleles. J Clin Pathol 39:573
18. Rebmann V, Doxiadis I, Kubens BS, Grosse-Wilder H (1992) Quantitation of the human component C4: definition of C4 Q0 alleles and C4A duplications. Vox Sang 62:117
19. Yang Y, Chung EK, Zhou B et al (2003) Diversity in intrinsic strengths of the human complement system: serum C4 protein concentrations correlate with C4 gene size and polygenic variations, haemolytic activities, and body mass index. J Immunol 171(5): 2734–2745
20. Wouters D, van Schouwenburg P, van der Horst A et al (2009) High-throughput analysis of the C4 polymorphism by a combination of MLPA and isotype-specific ELISA's. Mol Immunol 46(4):592
21. Yang Y, Chung EK, Wu YL et al (2007) Gene copy-number variation and associated polymorphisms of complement component C4 in human systemic lupus erythematosus (SLE): low copy number is a risk factor for and high copy number is a protective factor against SLE susceptibility in European Americans. Am J Hum Genet 80: 1037
22. Wu YL, Yang Y, Chung EK et al (2008) Phenotypes, genotypes and disease susceptibility associated with gene copy number variations: complement C4 CNVs in European American healthy subjects and those with systemic lupus erythematosus. Cytogenet Genome Res 123(1–4):131
23. Zhang WJ, Degli-Esposti MA, Cobain TJ et al (1990) Differences in gene copy number carried by different MHC ancestral haplotypes. Quantitation after physical separation of haplotypes by pulsed field gel electrophoresis. J Exp Med 171:2101
24. Christiansen FT, McCluskey J, Dawkins RL et al (1983) Complement allotyping in SLE: association with C4A null. Aust N Z J Med 13:483
25. Bohme JM, Andersson G, Andersson E et al (1985) HLA-DR beta genes vary in number between different DR specificities whereas the number of DQ beta genes is constant. J Immunol 135:2149
26. Giles CM, Uring-Lambert B, Goetz J et al (1988) Antigenic determinants expressed by human C4 allotypes; a study of 325 families provides evidence for the structural antigenic model. Immunogenetics 27:442
27. Schneider PM, Stradmann-Bellinghausen B, Rittner C (1996) Genetic polymorphism of the fourth component of human complement: population study and proposal for a revised nomenclature based on genomic PCR typing of Rodgers and Chido determinants. Eur J Immunogenet 23:335
28. Yu CY, Belt KT, Giles CM et al (1986) Structural basis of the polymorphism of human complement components C4A and C4B: gene size, reactivity and antigenicity. EMBO J 5:2873
29. Wu YL, Savelli SL, Yang Y et al (2007) Sensitive and specific real-time polymerase chain reaction assays to accurately determine copy number variations (CNVs) of human complement C4A, C4B, C4-long, C4-short, and RCCX modules: elucidation of C4 CNVs in 50 consanguineous subjects with defined HLA genotypes. J Immunol 179(5):3012

# Chapter 10

# Genotyping of Single Nucleotide Polymorphisms by 5′ Nuclease Allelic Discrimination

**Mari Malkki and Effie W. Petersdorf**


## Abstract

Real-time quantitative PCR is an efficient method for high-throughput genotyping of single nucleotide polymorphisms (SNPs). In this chapter, we describe the 5′ nuclease allelic discrimination assay for genotyping biallelic SNPs.


**Key words:** Single nucleotide polymorphism, Real-time polymerase chain reaction, TaqMan® chemistry, Reporter dye, Fluorescent label

## 1. Introduction

Single nucleotide polymorphisms (SNPs) are the most common form of human genetic variation (1–8). SNPs are biallelic and occur approximately every 1,000 base pairs (bp) throughout the human genome (1–8). SNPs are powerful markers for mapping genes that cause disease (9–21). Association of SNPs residing within the major histocompatibility complex (MHC) have recently been described for diseases with well-known associations to HLA phenotypes and haplotypes, including rheumatoid arthritis, diabetes, and multiple sclerosis (12–21).

Because of their biallelic nature, SNPs can be readily genotyped using techniques that discriminate any two-way combination of adenine, guanine, cytosine, and thymine nucleotide bases. Among the most robust assays for SNP genotyping, real-time quantitative assays rely on sensitive and specific quantification of amplified DNA or cDNA using polymerase chain reaction (PCR) (22–24). Real-time PCR methods offer a variety of different labels

Frank T. Christiansen and Brian D. Tait (eds.), *Immunogenetics: Methods and Applications in Clinical Practice*, Methods in Molecular Biology, vol. 882, DOI 10.1007/978-1-61779-842-9_10, © Springer Science+Business Media New York 2012

for the detection of genetic variation, including DNA-intercalating agents, such as SYBR® Green (25), fluorogenic probes (26–28), and the widely used TaqMan® chemistry (29, 30).

In this chapter, we describe the real-time 5′-nuclease genotyping assay known as TaqMan® for discriminating between two alleles of a specific SNP. The method may be used for genotyping individual SNPs that reside throughout the human genome. In brief, a wild-type SNP Allele "A" is amplified separately from the alternative Allele "B" using region specific forward and reverse primers and two allele-specific TaqMan® probes designed to target the polymorphism. TaqMan® probes have a fluorescent reporter dye (VIC® specific for allele "A" and 6-carboxyfluorescein [FAM™] specific for allele "B") attached to its 5′ end and a quencher dye (minor groove binder [MGB] or 6-carboxy-tetramethyl-rhodamine [TAMRA]) at its 3′ end. The amplification is performed using a thermal cycler or a real-time PCR system. During amplification each uniquely labeled probe binds preferentially to one of the two alleles of the SNP of interest with different affinity. As amplification proceeds, the Taq polymerase enzyme cleaves the bound probe, and a fluorescent signal is generated. Fluorescent signals are interpreted automatically using sequence detection software dedicated to real-time PCR instrumentation. A fluorescent signal from only the VIC dye indicates homozygosity for Allele "A"; the presence of only FAM dye fluorescence indicates homozygosity for Allele "B," and the presence of both fluorescent signals indicates Allele "A"/ Allele "B" heterozygosity.

## 2. Materials

### 2.1. TaqMan Assay

Supplies needed for performing the TaqMan® assay are as follows:

1. 96-Well optical plates and adhesive optical covers (Applied Biosystems, [ABI]).
2. Splash-free support base for 96-well plates.
3. Plate centrifuge.
4. 10, 200 and 1,000-μL sterile tips.
5. 1–10, 20–200 and 100–1,000-μL single or multiple tip electronic pipets or 10, 20, 200 and 1,000-μL manual pipets.
6. Eppendorf tubes.
7. TaqMan® Universal Master Mix.

### 2.2. Real-Time PCR Instrumentation

ABI 7500 Real-Time PCR system (see Note 1).

### 2.3. Design of Probes and Primers

Currently, over 160,000 inventoried, ready-to-use SNP assays and over 4.5 million predesigned, made-to-order SNPs assays are available from ABI (https://products.appliedbiosystems.com). The particular SNP of interest can be searched by its rs number (http://www.ncbi.nlm.nih.gov/SNP/) from the ABI Web site. ABI 40× or 80× TaqMan® SNP genotyping assays can be ordered for different sample sizes: small scale for 1,500 reactions, medium for 5,000 reactions, and large for 12,000 reactions calculated from 5 μL reaction/sample. The ready-to-use assay mixture is preloaded with (1) the forward and reverse primers for amplification of the polymorphic sequence, and (2) the two allele-specific TaqMan® probes descriptive of the SNP of interest, one labeled with VIC® dye and the other with 6FAM™ dye. Every assay comes with an information file containing details on the chromosomal location of the SNP, allele frequency (only for validated assays) and the nucleotide sequence to which the VIC/FAM reporter dye is linked. Upon delivery, all assays should be protected from light by wrapping the tube in foil. The 40× and 80× assays should be diluted with 1× TE buffer (10 mM Tris–HCl, 1 mM EDTA, pH 8.0) to 20× working mixture for best stability. This assay mixture should be aliquoted in batches to avoid freeze–thaw cycling. Assay should be stored at −15 to −25°C.

For SNPs which do not have ready-made assays available, there are several approaches for the user to design probe and primer sets: (1) use ABI Primer Express Software (see below); (2) use ABI Custom TaqMan® design service; and (3) search of the literature or available databases, such as SNP500Cancer (http://variantgps.nci.nih.gov/cgfseq/pages/snp500.do) for TaqMan® genotyping reagents for the SNP of interest.

Should the user require probes and primers to be designed, the ABI Primer Express software v2.0 provides assay design guidelines developed specifically for quantification assays. The general guidelines are as follows:

1. Import the DNA sequence containing the SNP of interest directly from NCBI dbSNP database (http://www.ncbi.nlm.nih.gov/SNP/).
2. Design forward and reverse amplification primers each with optimal lengths of 20 nucleotides and with matching *Tm* (59°C optimal) within 1°C of each other. Strive for an amplicon length of 75–150 bp. Avoid a guanine residue at the 5′ end of the probe because a G residue adjacent to reporter dye will quench the reporter fluorescent even after cleavage. Target a *Tm* of 65–67°C for each probe and a minimum length of 13 nucleotides. Avoid runs of an identical nucleotide in the probe sequence (especially runs of four or more consecutive Gs

should be avoided). Position the SNP site in the central third of the probe; if this is not possible, then shift the position of SNP site towards the 3′ end of the probe but do not place it in the last two 3′ nucleotides.

## 3. Methods

### 3.1. Preparation of Genomic DNA

Prepare 5–25 ng/μL of DNA in TE buffer (10 mM Tris pH 8.0, 0.1 mM EDTA) or in nuclease-free water. All samples should preferably have the same DNA concentration for genotyping to avoid a wide range of fluorescence activity within a genotype group (see Notes 2 and 3).

### 3.2. Preparation of Probes and SNP Assay Mixture

Dissolve self-designed MGB and TAMRA quenched probes in TE (10 mM Tris–HCl, 1 mM EDTA, pH8.0) or nuclease-free water at 100 μM concentration and the nonlabeled reverse and forward primers in TE (10 mM Tris–HCl, 1 mM EDTA, pH 8.0) at 1,000 μM concentration. To make 20× SNP genotyping assay cocktail containing MGB quencher, use 4 μM for each of the VIC and FAM probe and 18 μM for each of the nonlabeled primer. To make 20× SNP genotyping assay containing TAMRA quencher, use 2 μM for each of the VIC and FAM probe and 14 μM for each of the nonlabeled primer. For example, to make 500 μL of 20× SNP assay mix with MGB quencher use 20 μL each of the VIC and FAM probes, 9 μL each of the nonlabeled primers and 442 μL nuclease-free water.

SNP assays purchased from ABI are ready to use.

### 3.3. TaqMan® Universal PCR Master Mix

This can be purchased from ABI. To avoid PCR contamination from previously amplified material, "carry-over," inclusion of AmpErase® uracil-*N*-glycosylase (UNG) in the buffer is recommended (see Note 4). A single lot of master mix should be used in the same experiment, since lot-to-lot variability can contribute to variation in fluorescence values. The PCR master mix includes a passive reference dye ROX™, which is used to normalize fluorescent signals in individuals wells caused by small differences in PCR reaction mixture volume (see Note 5).

### 3.4. PCR Mixture

For one well, a basic cocktail volume is 3.75 μL containing 2.5 μL 2× Taqman universal PCR master mix, 0.25 μL 20× SNP assay mix, and 1 μL of nuclease-free water. For full 96-well plate this cocktail is made as a 105× mixture to allow for dead volume and pipetting errors as follows: 262.5 μL 2× TaqMan® universal PCR master mix, 26.25 μL 20× SNP assay mix, and 105 μL of nuclease-free water. This cocktail can be scaled up for as many plates as needed.

### 3.5. Amplification of Target Sequence

1. Clean up the working surface with ethanol and water.
2. Label the 96-well optical plate with assay name and plate identifier and put the plate into a PCR splash-free support base (see Note 6).
3. Prepare the PCR mixture for as many plates as needed.
4. Pipet 1.3 μL of individual DNAs into the bottom of wells, changing the tip between every DNA sample. Leave two wells in each plate devoid of template DNA as negative controls; for these wells, add 1.3 μL of water in place of DNA.
5. Add 3.75 μL of PCR master mix onto wall of each well. Change tips if necessary to prevent carry over from well to well.
6. Cover the plate with adhesive optical cover and centrifuge the plates at 1,500 rpm for 1 min to concentrate reagents at the bottom of the wells, and to remove any air bubbles.
7. Place the plate/s in ABI 9700 PCR thermal cycler or 7500 Real-time PCR system (see Note 1). If a real-time machine is used for the amplification step, please follow the manufacturer's instructions for plate setups and use of the machine. For MGB quencher probes, program the following cycling conditions: 2 min 50°C (this step only if UNG containing buffer is used), 10 min 92°C followed by 45 cycles of 30 s 92°C and 1 min 30 s 60°C. For TAMRA quencher probes, recommended conditions are: 2 min 50°C (perform this step only if UNG containing buffer is used), 10 min 95°C followed by 45 cycles of 30 s 95°C and 1 min 30 s 60°C. After cycling, keep plates at 4°C.
8. Read the plates in 7500 Real-Time PCR system using allelic discrimination with automated allele calling settings for the SDS 2.1 software (please refer to manufacturer's instructions) (see Note 7).

## 4. Notes

1. When the Taqman assay for a particular SNP is performed for the first time, it is recommended that a real-time PCR system (such as the ABI 7500 Real-time PCR system) is used to optimize the assay. After optimization, a regular PCR thermocycler, such as the ABI 9700 PCR system, can be used for the amplification step and the real-time PCR machine for the post-PCR data analysis.

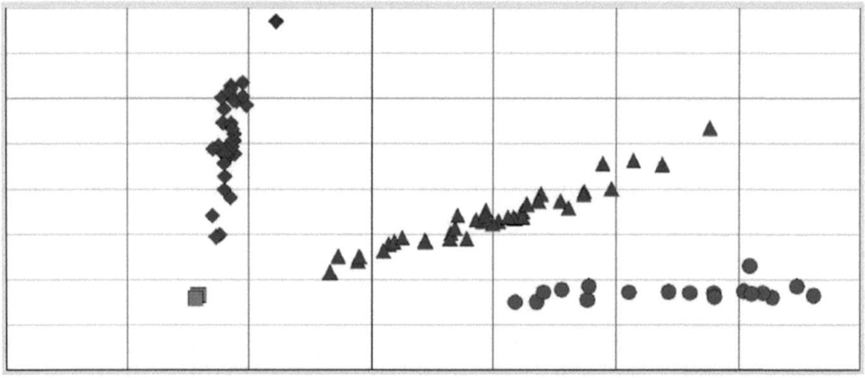

Fig. 1. Example of "trailing" genotype clusters AA (*circle*), AB (*triangle*), and BB (*diamond*). Trailing describes the variation of fluorescence signals among a given genotype that has the appearance of being spread across an imaginary line that extends from the no template control (*square*). This phenomenon is often caused by variability in concentration of individual genomic DNAs.

2. If specific controls for unique SNP genotypes are desired, the user has several resources for verifying whether the SNP of interest has been characterized for a reference cell from the International HapMap Project (http://hapmap.ncbi.nlm.nih.gov/) or the 1000 Human Genomes Project (www.1000genomes.org/). The user may determine whether the cells of interest can be purchased from Coriell Institute for Medical Research (http://ccr.coriell.org/sections/Collections/NHGRI/?SsId=11).
3. The most common cause for trailing of genotype clusters, as illustrated in Fig. 1, is variation in the DNA concentration of the test samples. Trailing may be minimized by accurate measurement of DNA concentration using the picogreen method (following the manufacturer's instructions or by using a standard spectrometer) and use of concentrations of 5–25 ng/mL. Trailing of genotype clustering can also be caused by pipetting error/s, use of expired reagents, the presence of PCR inhibitor in DNA or degraded DNA.
4. TaqMan® Universal PCR Master Mix can be purchased with or without AmpErase® UNG. AmpErase® UNG containing Taqman PCR master mix is recommended for high-throughput PCR applications. AmpErase® UNG can prevent the reamplification of carryover PCR products by removing any uracil incorporated to single- of double-stranded DNA.
5. The fluorescence signal from the passive reference dye ROX™ should be consistent across all wells and, therefore, it serves as an internal fluorescence signal reference to which the reporter dye (FAM and VIC) signal is normalized during data analysis.

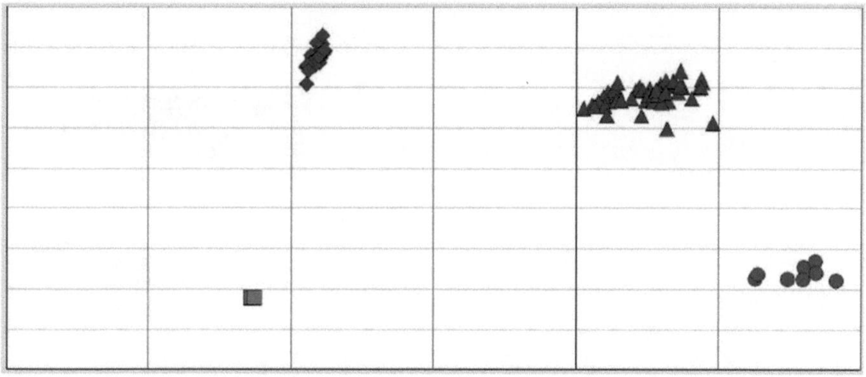

Fig. 2. Example of a good separation of genotype clusters AA (*circle*), AB (*triangle*), and BB (*diamond*). The no template controls (*square*) are distant from any clusters. Samples within a given cluster are close to the center of the cluster and the separation of the three clusters is very clear. Contrast this figure with that shown in Fig. 1.

Signal normalization is necessary to correct for well-to-well non-PCR-related fluorescence signal fluctuations caused by minor differences in concentrations or volume from well-to-well. In the data analysis, the normalized reporter (Rn) is the ratio of the fluorescence intensity of the reporter dye (FAM or VIC) signal to the fluorescence intensity of the passive reference dye signal.

6. Keeping the plate off the work surface prevents dirt getting onto outside of wells. Dirt can get into the real-time machine plate block and cause carryover fluorescence for all plates. Routine background fluorescence check of real-time machine plate block is recommended (please refer to manufacturer's instructions).
7. The vast majority of TaqMan® assays perform well using standard assay and PCR cycling conditions (Fig. 2). However, should modifications be required, it is recommended that for every new assay, the first assay is run on a real-time PCR machine to observe PCR amplification plots (please refer to manufacturer's instructions). An Rn (fluorescence of the reporter dye divided by the fluorescence of a passive reference dye ROX™) vs. PCR amplification cycle number plot and delta Rn (Rn minus baseline) vs. PCR amplification cycle number plot are useful to identify and examine irregularities in amplification; a Ct (threshold cycle) vs. individual well plot is useful to locate outliers in detector data sets and to identify dirty wells in the instrument block.

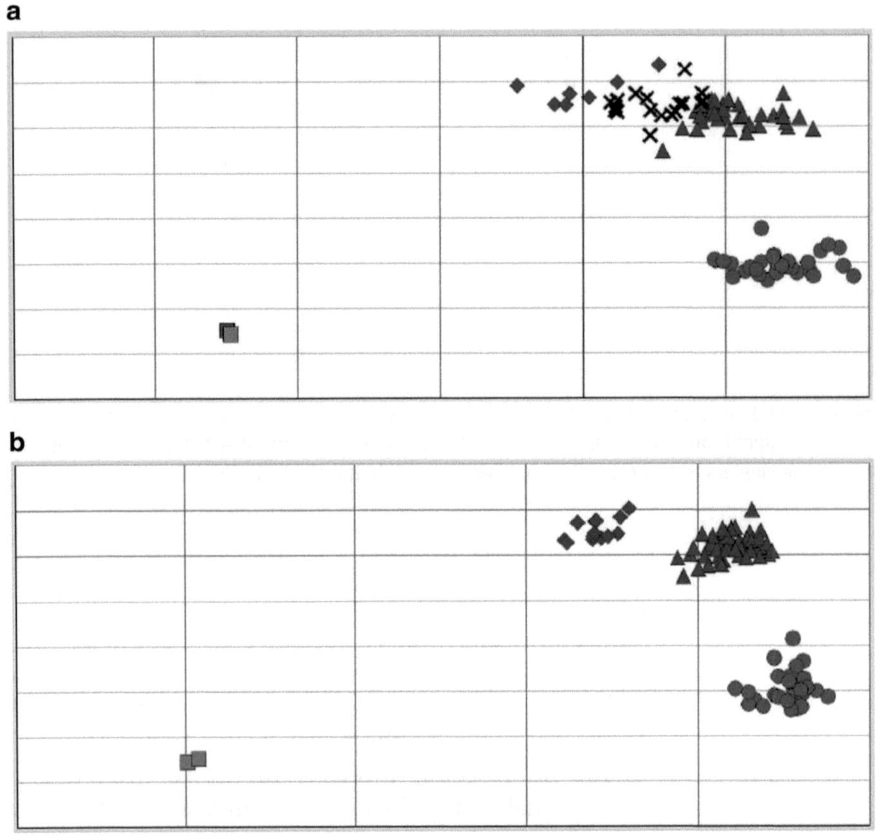


Fig. 3. Example of SNPs assay requiring modification of PCR annealing temperature from 60 to 62°C. (**a**) At 60°C annealing, AB (*triangle*) and BB (*diamond*) clusters are not well separated, (**b**) the same assay with 62°C annealing temperature showing better separation of AB (*triangle*) and BB (*diamond*) clusters.

If assay clustering for AA, AB, and BB genotypes can be discriminated as shown in Fig. 2, the rest of the amplifications for that SNP can be performed using a standard PCR machine followed by real-time PCR machine analysis for post-PCR end-point allelic discrimination plate reads. After amplification, the assay plates can be covered in foil and left at 4°C for few days before doing the end-point reads.

When the genotype clusters are not well separated (Figs. 3 and 4), adjustment of the annealing PCR temperature and/or reducing the number of PCR cycles may help. Start by increasing annealing temperature 1°C at a time from 60 to 61°C and then to 62° as needed (Fig. 3a, b) or decrease it by 1°C from 60 to 59°C (Fig. 4a, b). Although 5 μL reaction volumes are economical, some assays will require 10–25 μL for optimal results.

Failure to achieve clean separation of genotype clusters may indicate the presence of novel polymorphism in the probe sequence and requires sequencing of the target region.

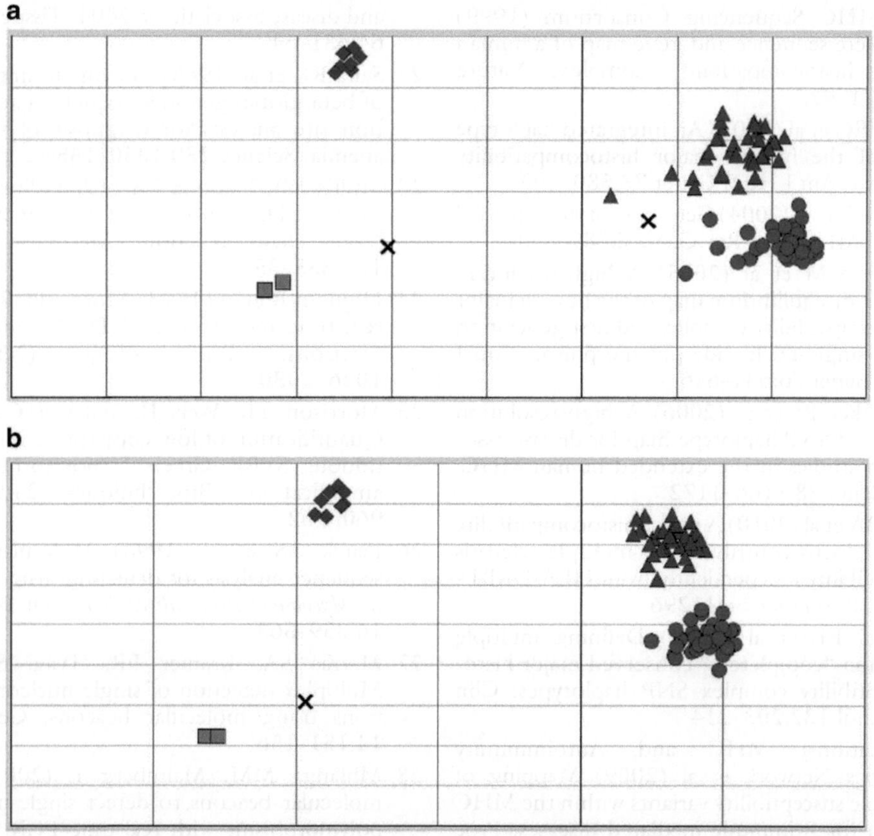


Fig. 4. Example of SNPs assay requiring modification of PCR annealing temperature from 60 to 59°C. (**a**) At 60°C annealing, AB (*triangle*) and AA (*circle*) clusters are not well separated, (**b**) the same assay with 59°C annealing temperature showing better separation of AB (*triangle*) and AA (*circle*) clusters.

## References

1. Kruglyak L (1997) The use of a genetic map of biallelic markers in linkage studies. Nat Genet 17:21–24
2. Wang DG et al (1998) Large-scale identification, mapping, and genotyping of single-nucleotide polymorphisms in the human genome. Science 280:1077–1082
3. Kruglyak L (1999) Prospects for whole-genome linkage disequilibrium mapping of common disease genes. Nat Genet 22:139–144
4. The International SNP Map Working Group (2001) A map of human genome sequence variation containing 1.42 million single nucleotide polymorphisms. Nature 409:928–933
5. Kruglyak L, Nickerson DA (2001) Variation is the spice of life. Nat Genet 27:234–236
6. Sherry ST et al (2001) dbSNP: the NCBI database of genetic variation. Nucleic Acids Res 29:308–311
7. International HapMap 3 Consortium et al (2010) Integrating common and rare genetic variation in diverse human populations. Nature 467:52–58
8. 1000 Genomes Project Consortium et al (2010) A map of human genome variation from population-scale sequencing. Nature 467: 1061–1073
9. Johnson GC et al (2001) Haplotype tagging for the identification of common disease genes. Nat Genet 29:233–237
10. Carlson CS et al (2004) Selecting a maximally informative set of single-nucleotide polymorphisms for association analyses using linkage disequilibrium. Am J Hum Genet 74: 106–120
11. Johnson AD, O'Donnell CJ (2009) An open access database of genome-wide association studies. BMC Med Genet 10:6–23

12. The MHC Sequencing Consortium (1999) Complete sequence and gene map of a human major histocompatibility complex. Nature 401:921–923
13. Walsh EC et al (2001) An integrated haplotype map of the human major histocompatibility complex. Am J Hum Genet 73:580–590
14. Horton R et al (2004) Gene map of the extended human MHC. Nat Rev Genet 5:889–899
15. Miretti MM et al (2005) A high-resolution linkage-disequilibrium map of the human major histocompatibility complex and first generation of tag single-nucleotide polymorphisms. Am J Hum Genet 76:634–646
16. de Bakker PI et al (2006) A high-resolution HLA and SNP haplotype map for disease association studies in the extended human MHC. Nat Genet 38:1166–1172
17. Cree BA et al (2010) A major histocompatibility Class I locus contributes to multiple sclerosis susceptibility independently from HLA-DRB1*15:01. PLoS One 5:e11296
18. Baschal EE et al (2009) Defining multiple common "completely" conserved major histocompatibility complex SNP haplotypes. Clin Immunol 132:203–214
19. International MHC and Autoimmunity Genetics Network et al (2009) Mapping of multiple susceptibility variants within the MHC region for 7 immune-mediated diseases. Proc Natl Acad Sci USA 106(44):18680–18685
20. Valdes AM, Thomson G, Type 1 Diabetes Genetics Consortium (2009) Several loci in the HLA class III region are associated with T1D risk after adjusting for DRB1-DQB1. Diabetes Obes Metab 11(suppl 1):46–52
21. Shiina T, Inoko H, Kulski JK (2004) An update of the HLA genomic region, locus information and disease associations: 2004. Tissue Antigens 64:631–649
22. Saiki RK et al (1985) Enzymatic amplification of beta-globin genomic sequences and restriction site analysis for diagnosis of sickle cell anemia. Science 230:1350–1354
23. Mullis KB, Faloona FA (1987) Specific synthesis of DNA in vitro via a polymerase-catalyzed chain reaction. Methods Enzymol 155:335–350
24. Higuchi R et al (1993) Kinetic PCR analysis: real-time monitoring of DNA amplification reactions. Biotechnology (NY) 11: 1026–1030
25. Morrison TB, Weis JJ, Wittwer CT (1998) Quantification of low-copy transcripts by continuous SYBR Green I monitoring during amplification. Biotechniques 24:954–958; 960; 962
26. Piatek AS et al (1998) Molecular beacon sequence analysis for detecting drug resistance in *Mycobacterium tuberculosis*. Nat Biotechnol 16:359–363
27. Marras SA, Kramer FR, Tyagi S (1999) Multiplex detection of single-nucleotide variations using molecular beacons. Genet Anal 14:151–156
28. Mhlanga MM, Malmberg L (2001) Using molecular beacons to detect single-nucleotide polymorphisms with real-time PCR. Methods 25:463–471
29. Holland PM et al (1991) Detection of specific polymerase chain reaction product by utilizing the 5′—3′ exonuclease activity of *Thermus aquaticus* DNA polymerase. Proc Natl Acad Sci USA 88:7276–7280
30. Heid CA et al (1996) Real time quantitative PCR. Genome Res 6:986–994

# Chapter 11

# High Resolution MICA Genotyping by Sequence-Based Typing (SBT)


## Yizhou Zou and Peter Stastny



## Abstract

We have developed a MICA typing method based on polymerase chain reaction (PCR) sequence-based typing and a computer program that determines the polymorphisms and distinguishes the GCT repeats in exon 5. One PCR amplification was performed to obtain templates of 2.2 kb, including exons 2, 3, 4, and 5 of MICA to be sequenced with two forward and two reverse primers. Overlay of nucleotide sequencing signals resulting from presence of different GCT repeats in exon 5 from two different MICA alleles can be identified by a computer program that analyses the combined signal string containing the 35 bases.



**Key words:** MICA typing, SBT, External domains, Transmembrane region, Computer analysis


## 1. Introduction

The major histocompatibility complex class I chain-related genes A (MICA) are located 46.4 kb centromeric to HLA-B and have been shown to be quite polymorphic, with 65 alleles described so far. It appears that the expression of the MICA gene products is limited mainly to certain epithelial cells, endothelial cells, fibroblasts, and tumor cells (1). MICA genes, although located in the MHC class I region, are structurally quite different from the HLA class I genes and have been reported to be associated with some diseases (2) and with the immune response to transplants (3). Recent studies have shown that the MICA gene products may play a role in the activation of natural killer (NK) cells and other cells that express the NKG2D receptor (4). Because the gut is also one of the major sites of graft-vs.-host disease following bone marrow transplantation, it is of interest that the MIC genes play a role in this process (5). We recently found that organ transplant recipients make antibodies


Frank T. Christiansen and Brian D. Tait (eds.), *Immunogenetics: Methods and Applications in Clinical Practice*, Methods in Molecular Biology, vol. 882, DOI 10.1007/978-1-61779-842-9_11, © Springer Science+Business Media New York 2012

against specific MICA alleles (3) and antibodies against MICA antigens were associated with kidney transplant rejection (6). Some DNA-based typing techniques have previously been described for MICA genes, including sequence-based typing (SBT) (7) and analyses of single strand conformational polymorphisms (SSCP) (8), sequence-specific oligonucleotide probes (SSOP), and sequence-specific primers (SSP) (9). The transmembrane (TM) region of MICA encodes the repeat polymorphism (GCT/Ala), and seven types of repeats have been described as A4, A5, A5.1, A6, A7, A9, and A10. Analysis of the number of repeats has usually been based on the size of the TM fragments determined by a fragment analysis software program following fluorescent PCR amplification (10). In view of the large number of MICA alleles, the typing of the TM region has become more important for resolving ambiguities in MICA allele typing. We have developed a method for analyzing MICA polymorphisms in exons 2–4 and the TM types in exon 5 from the PCR products obtained after generic MICA amplification of exons 2–5 (11). This typing approach uses computerized assignment of polymorphic sites and resolves also the short tandem repeats within the transmembrane region. This method can resolve all of the MICA alleles and performs MICA allele typing without any additional steps.

## 2. Materials

### 2.1. Specimen

1. 5-μL genomic DNA (20 ng/μL) in molecular biology-grade water (see Note 1).

### 2.2. Reagents

1. MICA locus-specific PCR primers (Table 1).
2. High Fidelity Taq (4 U/μL) and 10× PCR buffer with $MgCl_2$.
3. dNTP mix (25 pMol/μL).
4. BigDye® Terminator v3.1 Cycle Sequencing Kit (Applied Biosystems (ABI), Forest, CA, USA).
5. Four sequencing primers: 1F, 2R, 3F, and 4R (Table 1).
6. NaOAc/EDTA buffer.
7. Molecular biology-grade water.
8. Ethanol 99% anhydrous, molecular biology grade.
9. POP-6 (Performance Optimized Polymer) from Applied Biosystems.
10. Hi-Di Formamide from Applied Biosystems.

**Table 1**
**Sequences of primers**

| Use for | Name | Sequences (5′–3′) |
|---|---|---|
| PCR | MICA6823_F | CGTTCTTGTCCCTTTGCCCGTGTGC |
| | MICA9023_R | GATGCTGCCCCATTCCCTTCCCAA |
| Sequencing | 1F | ATTTCCTGCCCCAGGAAGGTTGG |
| | 2R | CAACTCTAGCAGAATTGGAG |
| | 3F | AAGAGAAACAGCCCTGTTCCTCTCC |
| | 4R | GATGCTGCCCCATTCCCTTCCCAA |

### 2.3. Supplies

1. Thin-wall 96-well PCR plates (ISC BioExpress, Kaysville, UT, Cat. T3031-21).
2. Thermal seal sealing films (ISC BioExpress, Cat. T2417-5).
3. Quanti-Marker 100 bp (GeneMate Inc., Kaysville, UT, USA. Cat. QM4-104K).
4. MicroAmp Optical Plate (Applied Biosystems, Part No. N801-0560).
5. Running Buffer, 10× (Applied Biosystems, Part No. 402824).
6. Metal Plate (Applied Biosystems, Cat. MACL09645).
7. MultiScreen®-HV (Millipore, Billerica, MA, USA. Cat. MAHVN4550).
8. Pipette tips for 1–20, 21–200, and 100–1,000 μL.
9. PCR tubes (0.2 thin walled) Applied Biosystems, #N801-0838.
10. Genetic analyzer plate Septa 96-wells Applied Biosystems, #4315933.
11. Genetic analyzer plate Retainer Applied Biosystems, #4317241.
12. Capillary array 50 cm long, Applied Biosystems, #4315930.

### 2.4. Equipment

1. Vertical laminar flow hood.
2. Thermocycler with heated lid and 96-well format.
3. Pipettes, volumes 1–20, 20–200, 100–1,000 μL.
4. Agarose gel apparatus.
5. Gel documentation camera.

6. Electrophoresis power supply.
7. Variable speed vortex.
8. Table top centrifuge (96-well tray holder).
9. ABI 3130 XL Analyzer (16 capillary).
10. Computer and Printer.

## 3. Methods

One set of amplifications was performed for each sample with generic primers (MICA6823-F and MICA9023-R) (see Table 1) to amplify a MICA gene fragment of approximately 2,200 bp including exons 2, 3, 4, and 5. Four sequencing primers (see Table 1, Fig. 1) generate four sequencing fragments for allele-level typing analysis.

### 3.1. DNA Preparation

1. DNA can be isolated from acid-citrate-dextrose (ACD) anticoagulated whole blood, culture cell lines, or buccal epithelial cells. DNA isolation methods vary considerably depending on the starting material. The goal is to prepare high-molecular-weight DNA of sufficient purity to allow HLA and MICA allele-level typing (see Note 1). Preparations of high-quality DNA are critical for amplification of MICA alleles since the length of the amplified fragment is in the range of 2,200 bp. Therefore, a protocol that produces a high-quality DNA preparation should be selected. DNA samples should be of high quality as determined by 260/280 nm absorbance ratios (1.7–2.0). Prepare DNA samples with concentration at 20 ng/μL in water. For example, to make a 100 μL DNA sample at 20 ng/μL from a 100 ng/μL DNA sample, add 20 μL of DNA (100 ng/μL) to 80 μL of water.

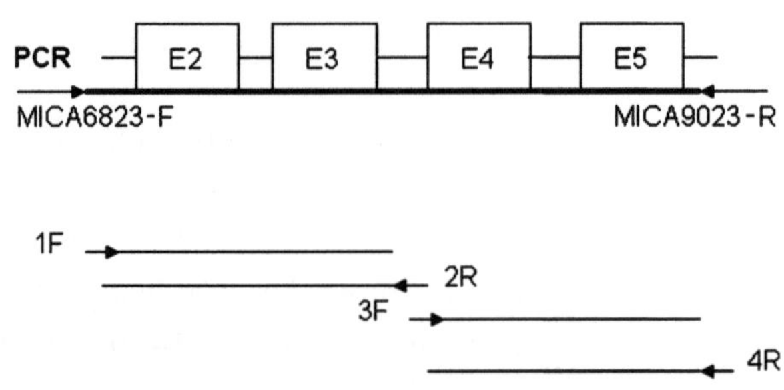


Fig. 1. Strategy for MICA allele-level typing by sequence-based typing (SBT). DNA fragments (2.2 kb) containing the polymorphic sites in exons 2, 3, and 4 and the STR in exon 5 are amplified with the generic MICA-specific primers MICA6823F and MICA9023R. The PCR primer and sequencing locations and their orientation are shown by the *arrows*.

### 3.2. Amplification of MICA Alleles by PCR

1. Primers for MICA allele amplification:
   Forward primer MICA6823-F and reverse primer MICA9023-R are used to amplify a 2,200 bp fragment including exon 2, 3, 4, and 5 of the MICA gene.
2. Prepare the samples for PCR.
   Determine how many DNA samples are to be tested and add positive and negative controls. Calculate as follows:

| | |
|---|---|
| Water | 8.8 μL (*N** + 2) |
| 10× Buffer | 2.0 μL (*N*+2) |
| 2.5 mM dNTP | 2.0 μL (*N*+2) |
| 10 pmol/μL primer 6823_F | 1.0 μL (*N*+2) |
| 10 pmol/μL primer 9023_R | 1.0 μL (*N*+2) |
| 4 U/μL Taq Polymerase | 0.2 μL (*N*+2) |
| 20 ng/μL DNA | 5.0 μL/each |
| Total | 20.0 μL |
| *N** = number of samples + 1 positive control + 1 negative control | |

3. First add 5 μL of DNA samples (20 ng/μL) to PCR tubes separately, then vortex master mix well, spin down briefly, and pipette 15 μL of the PCR master mix into each well.
4. Cap the tube strips and place in pre-warmed thermocycler.
5. Run the following profile (see Note 2).
   MICA locus specific SBT-PCR profile:

| | | |
|---|---|---|
| 1 Cycle | 96°C | 2 min |
| 10 Cycles | 96°C<br>69°C<br>72°C | 30 s<br>50 s<br>90 s |
| 20 Cycles | 96°C<br>67°C<br>72°C | 30 s<br>50 s<br>90 s |
| 1 Cycle | 72°C<br>4°C | 10 min<br>Infinite |

6. Check the PCR products.
   (a) Remove samples from the thermocycler.
   (b) Run the electrophoresis gel (2%) with 4 μL of the PCR product mixed with 4 μL of 2× loading buffer. The gel should be run at 130 V for approximately 20 min.
   (c) To estimate the concentration of the PCR products, compare the bands to the Quanti-Marker 100-bp map. The

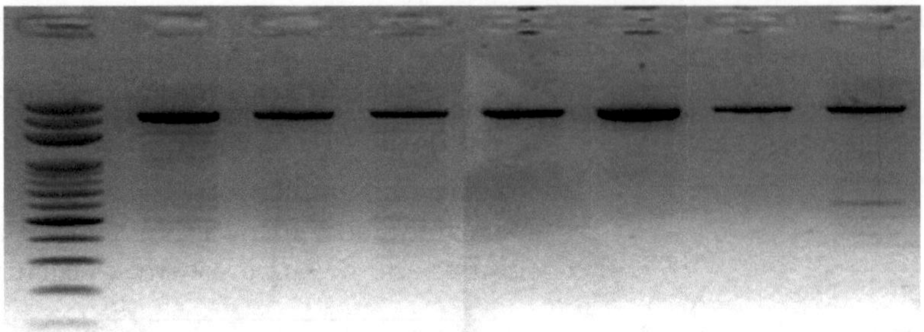

Fig. 2. PCR products of MICA gene amplification. 4 μL of PCR products from DNA samples were loaded to 2% gel for electrophoreses analysis. Bands with molecular weight at 2.2 kb are shown.

map has markers shown at various base pair lengths and various concentrations in ng/band (see Fig. 2, Note 3).

### 3.3. Cleaning the MICA DNA Templates

The PCR products have to be purified before they are used as sequencing templates, because residual PCR primers and nucleotide triphosphates (dNTPs) can interfere with the SBT chemistry resulting in lower data quality. An easy way to perform PCR purification is by using exonuclease I and shrimp alkaline phosphatase (ExoSAP-IT) that will remove unincorporated primers and dNTPs.

1. Take the vial of ExoSAP-IT from the freezer (see Note 4).
2. Add 3.6 μL of ExoSAP-IT to the well containing the PCR products.
3. Seal the purification tray with micro amp full plate covers or caps.
4. Centrifuge at 1,000 × *g* for 30 s.
5. Place in the thermal cycler and run the following profile.

| | |
|---|---|
| 37°C | 30 min |
| 80°C | 15 min |
| 4°C | Infinite |

6. Remove the treated PCR products from the thermocycler.

### 3.4. Preparation for MICA Allele Sequencing

There are four sequencing primers (Table 1) for SBT.

1. Prepare the Sequencing Mix. The following table is for each reaction. To the sequencing plate add 7.25 μL of water, 2 μL of purified PCR product, and 2 μL of primers. Then mix with BigDye and buffer.

Sequencing reaction (15 μL):

| | |
|---|---|
| Water | 7.25 μL (adjustable if more PCR product is needed, see Note 5) |
| PCR product (treated) | 2.0 μL (Adjustable, see Note 6) |
| Sequencing Primer | 2.0 μL (see Note 7) |
| 5× buffer for BigDye | 2.25 μL |
| BigDye | 1.5 μL |
| Total | 15.0 μL |

2. Centrifuge the samples briefly for about 1 min at 800×*g* to remove any bubbles.
3. Put the samples on the thermocycler with the following program. This takes about 1½ h.

| | | |
|---|---|---|
| | 96°C | 1 min |
| 25 cycles | 96°C | 10 s |
| | 50°C | 5 s |
| | 60°C | 2 min |

Keep at 4°C.

4. Following cycle sequencing, the sequencing reaction products have to be purified to remove non-incorporated dye terminators which would otherwise cause sequencing artifacts.

### 3.5. EDTA/NaOAc/Ethanol Precipitation of Cycle-Sequenced Products

After Cycle sequencing is complete, remove plate from thermocycler and place at 4 or −20°C until ready to precipitate. Do not let plate sit in thermocycler overnight (low sample volume leads to easy evaporation). This protocol assumes a 15-μL cycle-sequencing reaction.

1. To each well add 2.5 μL of NaOAc/EDTA (4 part of 3M sodium acetate pH 5.5 plus 1 part of 0.5M EDTA pH 8.0). Mix with pipette tips.
2. Add 25 μL 100% EtOH (from freezer) to each. Mix with pipette tips. Replace sealing tape, seal very well and vortex for 1 min, and incubate at room temperature for 15 min.
3. Centrifuge at 2,500 ×*g* for 30 min.
4. Invert plate onto paper towel and spin at 185 ×*g* for 1 min to dry.
5. Add 50 μL 80% EtOH to each well and mix with pipette tips.
6. Do not vortex and make EtOH fresh to ensure accurate concentration (see Note 8).
7. Centrifuge at 2,500 ×*g* for 15 min.

8. Flick plate contents into sink, invert plate onto paper towel, and spin at 185 ×*g* for 1 min to dry. Start timer immediately.
9. Resuspend samples in 10 μL Hi-Diformamide. Cover plate with sealing tape, vortex thoroughly (15 s), and denature in thermocycler (96°C for 3 min).
10. Centrifuge for 30 s at 1,000 rpm and place it on the support base, specific for each analyzer.
11. Place a full plate over the tray and follow with the 96-well plate retainer.
12. Link tray map to tray ID and click on the green arrow to start the run.
13. The run module for this procedure takes about 90 min for each injection (see Note 9) on the 3130XL ABI Sequencer, when using a 50 cm long capillary array (see Note 10).

#### 3.6. Analysis of Allele-Level Typing by Computer Program

The raw data results are analyzed by the ABI Sequence Analysis program and saved in four electronic files (SampleID_MICA_1F.ab1, SampleID_MICA_2R.ab1, SampleID_MICA_3F.ab1, and SampleID_MICA_4R.ab1). The segments of MICA containing exons 2, 3, 4, and 5 are assembled and the aligned sequences (see Note 11), with MICA*001 as consensus, are analyzed with a program for assignment of MICA alleles (see Note 12, Fig. 3). This software was designed to analyze nucleotide substitutions at polymorphic sites using an updated MICA allele database (see Note 13).

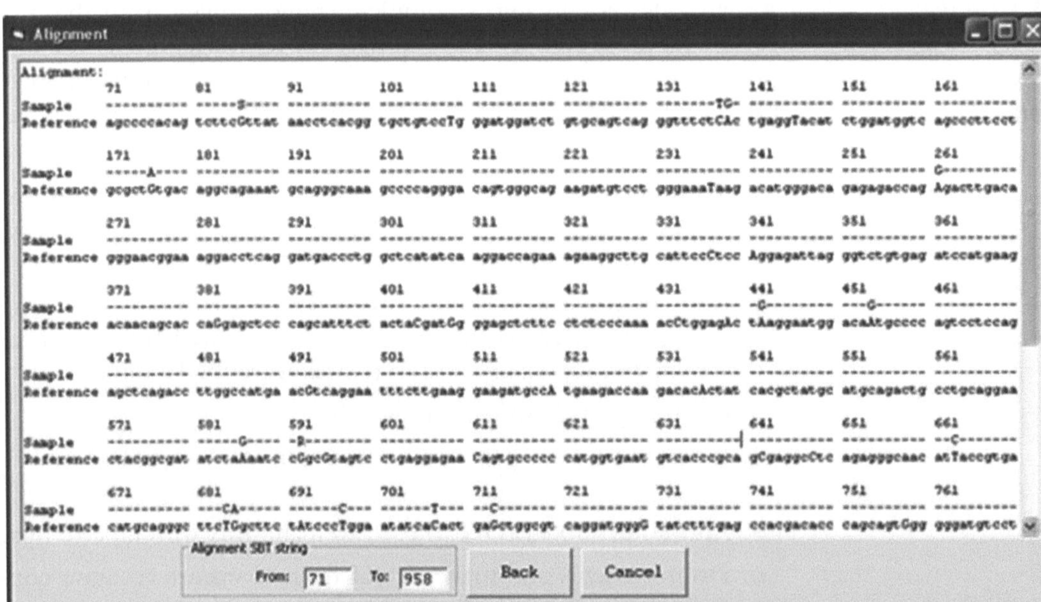


Fig. 3. Alignment of MICA sequences by SBT. This aligned sequence is generated from four sequencing files (see Note 15). Sequences in exon 2, 3, 4, and 5 are assembled as in this alignment window by a computer program. Their intron sequences were removed.

**Table 2**
**Alignment of the STR in the transmembrane region of the MICA genes (5′, 5′–3′)**

| | |
|---|---|
| A4 | GCTGCTGCTGCT*ATTTTTGTTATTATTATTTTCTATGT* |
| A5 | GCTGCTGCTGCTGCT*ATTTTTGTTATTATTATTTTCTA* |
| A5.1 | GCTGCTGGCTGCTGCT*ATTTTTGTTATTATTATTTTCT* |
| A6 | GCTGCTGCTGCTGCTGCT*ATTTTTGTTATTATTATTTT* |
| A7 | GCTGCTGCTGCTGCTGCTGCT*ATTTTTGTTATTATTAT* |
| A9 | GCTGCTGCTGCTGCTGCTGCTGCTGCT*ATTTTTGTTAT* |
| A10 | GCTGCTGCTGCTGCTGCTGCTGCTGCTGCT*ATTTTTGT* |

MICA STR is located in the exon 5 with the different number of "GCT" repeat. MICA allele named by WHO HLA nomenclature is based on the sequences of MICA gene including STR type

Table 2 shows the alignment of the 35 nucleotides containing different STR from (GCT)4 to (GCT)10 in the TM region. Overlay of the sequencing signals may occur due to potentially different number of (GCT) repeats in exon 5 from two different MICA alleles in one sample, and they can be identified using the computer program or manually (see Note 14, Fig. 4).

## 4. Notes

1. Measurement of DNA concentration must be accurate. The integrity of the genomic DNA used is also important to obtain a good yield in the PCR amplification. Always check the electropherogram of each sequencing report to make sure the assignment of nucleotides is correct and there are two positive signals for each assigned heterozygous position. ACD anticoagulant is preferred. Heparin has been shown to inhibit some PCR reactions. Blood samples older than 1 week may produce poor yields and/or poor quality DNA unless they have been stored frozen. One milliliter whole blood has about ten million white cells and yields ~100 μg DNA suitable for ~200 amplification reactions. DNA isolation and PCR set up should be restricted to the pre-PCR area to prevent DNA contamination. The pre-PCR manipulations should be handled in a laminar flow hood. All the reagents should be freshly prepared and/or autoclaved, if appropriate.
2. All Pre-PCR reagents are thawed to room temperature, vortexed, spun, and kept cold until ready to be used. It is better to

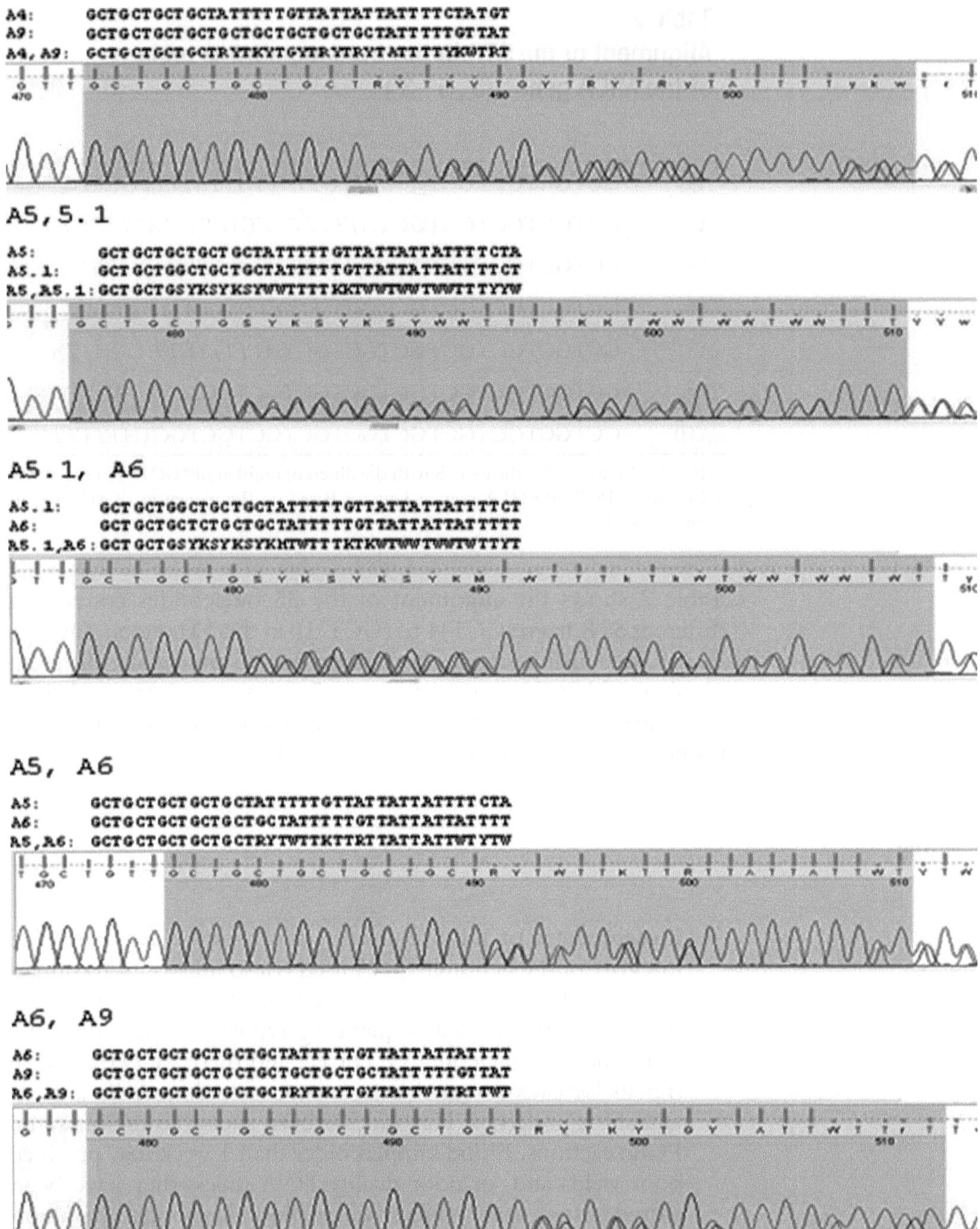


Fig. 4. The combined signals from two different STR types in one sample. Five different sequencing results of the TM polymorphisms are shown with the overlay signals matching the combined TM types from A4/A9, A5/A5.1, A5.1/A6, A5/A6, or A6/A9. Computer typing for MICA TM is based on this algorithm. It is available at this web address: http://www4.utsouthwestern.edu/stastny-lab/download_page.htm.

prepare fresh PCR mixture before testing. Preparation of the positive and negative control of PCR is to monitor the quality of MICA gene application.

3. If some samples failed in PCR, it is likely due to specimen problems. Often adjusting the PCR components, for example, adding more DNA, more Taq polymerase, and/or adding more $Mg^{2+}$, the PCR will overcome this difficulty. Allele drop-out can be caused by mismatch between the primers and target DNA that may present a novel allele differing at the binding sites. Allele drop-out may also occur when a DNA sample with poor quality is used, if this is the reason, the typing will be repeated using a re-purified DNA isolate with optimal quality. Check DNA on a 0.8% agarose gel for DNA sample quality.
4. ExoSAP-IT treated PCR products can stand a "small dilution" sometimes necessary to repeat a given Cycle-Seq reaction (usually 6–8 μL of molecular grade water).
5. Add water, cover the tray, vortex briefly, and spin for 1 min before using it for a new cycle sequencing reaction.
6. Noisy baseline, inappropriate PCR product purification, or poor quality reaction precipitation. Re-purify the sequencing reaction products or purify the PCR products and repeat the sequencing reactions.
7. MICA sequencing primers include four separate primers (1F, 2R, 3F, 4R). The fragments of the sequencing products should be more than 600 bp.
8. Incorrect ethanol precipitation may result in excess salt remaining in the sequence reaction. These salt ions will preferentially inject onto the capillary over the sequence DNA molecules resulting in weak sequence. Be sure to perform the ethanol precipitation correctly and do a well-measured/correct concentration wash step afterwards.
9. Weak signal strength may occur in inappropriate injection time or injection voltage because of variations between instruments. Adjustments of the injection time and/or the injection voltage may be needed to get a signal range from 10 to 2,000 relative fluorescent units.
10. Plates waiting to be run may be stored at −20°C, but probably should be re-denatured before running on the genetic analyzer. Stored plates should be wrapped in foil to protect dyes from light.
11. Novel sequence outside of exon 2–5 will not be detected in this method. Some MICA alleles have the polymorphism in exon 6, which is not part of the segment analyzed in this approach (see Table 3). There are more than 20 groups of

**Table 3**
**Alleles with identical extracellular domains (exons 2, 3, and 4) and their associated transmembrane types (exon 5)**

| Groups[a] | Alleles | TM types |
|---|---|---|
| 1 | MICA002:01 | A9 |
| | MICA020 | A10 |
| | MICA023 | A5.1 |
| | MICA050 | A7 |
| 2 | MICA00801 | A5.1 |
| | MICA027 | A5 |
| | MICA048[b] | A5 |
| 3 | MICA009:01 | A6 |
| | MICA049[b] | A6 |
| 4 | MICA007:01 | A4 |
| | MICA026 | A6 |

[a]Groups of alleles with identical sequences in exons 2, 3, and 4. The differences are either in TM type (group 1, 4) or
[b]Different only in exon 6 (group3) or both (group 2)

known possible ambiguities with random combination of the 65 alleles. Additional testing may be needed to resolve such ambiguities if required. Ambiguous allele assignments can occur when two alleles are present and the composite sequence is identical for more than one combination (*cis/trans* ambiguities).

12. With dye terminator sequencing, the peak incorporation patterns are not completely uniform. For homozygous positions, this is not a problem, but for certain heterozygote positions, one peak may be present at a much lower level than the other. Consequently, the software may not correctly identify these positions as heterozygous sequencing in both orientations. They have to be carefully reviewed and corrected before sending for computer program analysis.
13. Confirm that the allele database utilized is up to date. Web address for the IMGT/HLA database: http://www.ebi.uk/imgt/hla/align.html.
14. In most cases, 3F and 4R sequencing files will be found to have multiple heterozygote positions either due to variation in intron 5 containing 7 or 8T repeats or because the STR types

are different in the two alleles. Those overlaid signals are important and required for successful TM typing by this method.

15. The following file format is suggested when the sequencing files are setup.

    DNASampleName_LocuName_SequencingPrimerName, for example:

    N0123456789_MICA_1F.ab1

    N0123456789_MICA_2R.ab1

    N0123456789_MICA_3F.ab1

    N0123456789_MICA_4R.ab1

    The file names are useful to organize the data by sample and sequencing primers used.

## References


1. Zwirner NW, Fernandez-Vina MA, Stastny P et al (1998) MICA, a new polymorphic HLA-related antigen, is expressed mainly by keratinocytes, endothelial cells, and monocytes. Immunogenetics 47:139–148
2. Stephens HA (2001) MICA and MICB genes: can the enigma of their polymorphism be resolved? Trends Immunol 22:378–385
3. Zwirner NW, Marcos CY, Mirbaha F et al (2000) Identification of MICA as a new polymorphic alloantigen recognized by antibodies in sera of organ transplant recipients. Hum Immunol 61:917–924
4. Cerwenka A, Lanier LL (2003) NKG2D ligands: unconventional MHC class I-like molecules exploited by viruses and cancer. Tissue Antigens 61:335–343
5. Parmar S, Del Lima M, Zou Y et al (2009) Donor-recipient mismatches in MHC class I chain-related gene A in unrelated donor transplantation lead to increased incidence of acute graft-versus-host disease. Blood 114: 2884–2887
6. Zou Y, Stastny P, Süsal C et al (2007) Antibodies against MICA antigens and kidney-transplant rejection. N Engl J Med 357:1293–1300
7. Petersdorf EW, Shuler KB, Longton GM et al (1999) Population study of allelic diversity in the human MHC class I-related MIC-A gene. Immunogenetics 49:605–612
8. Komatsu-Wakui M, Tokunaga K, Ishikawa Y et al (1999) MIC-A polymorphism in Japanese and a MIC-A-MIC-B null haplotype. Immunogenetics 49:620–628
9. Ahmad T, Marshall SE, Mulcahy-Hawes Y et al (2002) High resolution MIC genotyping: design and application to the investigation of inflammatory bowel disease susceptibility. Tissue Antigens 60:164–179
10. Ota M, Katsuyama Y, Mizuki N et al (1997) Trinucleotide repeat polymorphism within exon 5 of the MICA gene (MHC class I chain-related gene A): allele frequency data in the nine population groups Japanese, Northern Han, Hui, Uygur, Kazakhstan, Iranian, Saudi Arabian, Greek and Italian. Tissue Antigens 49:448–454
11. Zou Y, Han M, Wang Z et al (2006) MICA allele-level typing by sequence-based typing with computerized assignment of polymorphic sites and short tandem repeats within the transmembrane region. Hum Immunol 67: 145–151

# Chapter 12

# Standard Methods for the Management of Immunogenetic Data

**Pierre-Antoine Gourraud, Jill A. Hollenbach, Thomas Barnetche, Richard M. Single, and Steven J. Mack**


## Abstract

In this chapter, we outline some basic principles for the consistent management of immunogenetic data. These include the preparation of a single master data file that can serve as the basis for all subsequent analyses, a focus on the quality and homogeneity of the data to be analyzed, the documentation of the coding systems used to represent the data, and the application of nomenclature standards specific for each immunogenetic system being evaluated. The data management principles discussed here are intended to provide a foundation for the data analysis methods detailed in Chaps. 13 and 14. The relationship between the data management and analysis methods covered in these three chapters is illustrated in Fig. 3.

The application of these data management principles is a first step toward consistent and reproducible data analyses. While it may take extra time and effort to apply them, we feel that it is better to take this approach than to assume that low data quality can be compensated for by large sample sizes.

In addition to their relevance for analytical reproducibility, it is important to consider these data management principles from an ethical perspective. The reliability of the data collected and generated as part of a research study should be as important a component of the ethical review of a research application as the security of those data. Finally, in addition to ensuring the integrity of the data from collection to publication, the application of these data management principles will provide a means to foster research integrity and to improve the potential for collaborative data sharing.


**Key words:** Data management, Data standards, High polymorphism, HLA, Immunogenetics, KIR

## 1. Introduction

### *1.1. Avoiding the "Garbage-In Garbage Out" Predicament*

In recent years, large amounts of genetic data have become available to the research community, increasing the potential for new findings in ways that have not previously been possible. The need for standardized data management and statistical analysis increases as more data become available in order to mitigate the variability

Frank T. Christiansen and Brian D. Tait (eds.), *Immunogenetics: Methods and Applications in Clinical Practice*, Methods in Molecular Biology, vol. 882, DOI 10.1007/978-1-61779-842-9_12, 

between individual studies. The difficulty of dealing with heterogeneity between studies is not really new, but it becomes more significant as the amount of accessible data increases.

Sir Arthur Conan Doyle summarized the problem in 1890 in his second novel, "The Sign of Four":

> while the individual man is an insoluble puzzle, in the aggregate he becomes a mathematical certainty. You can, for example, never foretell what any one man will do, but you can say with precision what an average number will be up to. Individuals vary, but percentages remain constant. So says the statistician.

Throughout its history, the field of immunogenetics has provided a continuously changing perspective of individual immunological characteristics. Different levels of information were involved: the source materials level (sera, DNA, RNA, etc.), the experimental level (with the switch from pure serological techniques to a mix of serological and molecular techniques, and the advent of parallel data acquisition instruments), and the analytical level (with development of computer-based data storage and statistical modeling). While immunogenetic data production capacity has clearly advanced significantly, it is not clear that the biostatistical capacity to analyze such quantities of data has developed in a similar manner.

In addition, immunogenetics is distinctive in that it is relevant to both very basic and applied fields of research. Transplantation is the seminal example of gene-based personalized medicine; basic knowledge in molecular anthropology, the history and genetic structure of populations, the genetic components of disease, forensic medicine, and genome evolution all benefit from the progress in immunogenetics. With rivers of data now flowing from high-throughput typing systems, a rigorous statistical approach is needed more than ever to navigate this new immunogenetic sea. In this chapter, we propose some foundational guidelines for the analysis of immunogenetic datasets, focusing on ensuring quality and homogeneity of data in order to escape from the "Garbage-in Garbage-out" predicament. Supplementary materials for this chapter can be found online at http://www.immunogenomics.org/methods.html.

## 2. Data Organization and Storage

### 2.1. Organization of a Master Data File

The "master data file" is the foundation of a quality data analysis. Ideally, a master data file will contain all the data needed for the analysis in a single electronic document, which can be validated, transferred, and exported. While individual software tools may require data to be organized in different ways (i.e., different data

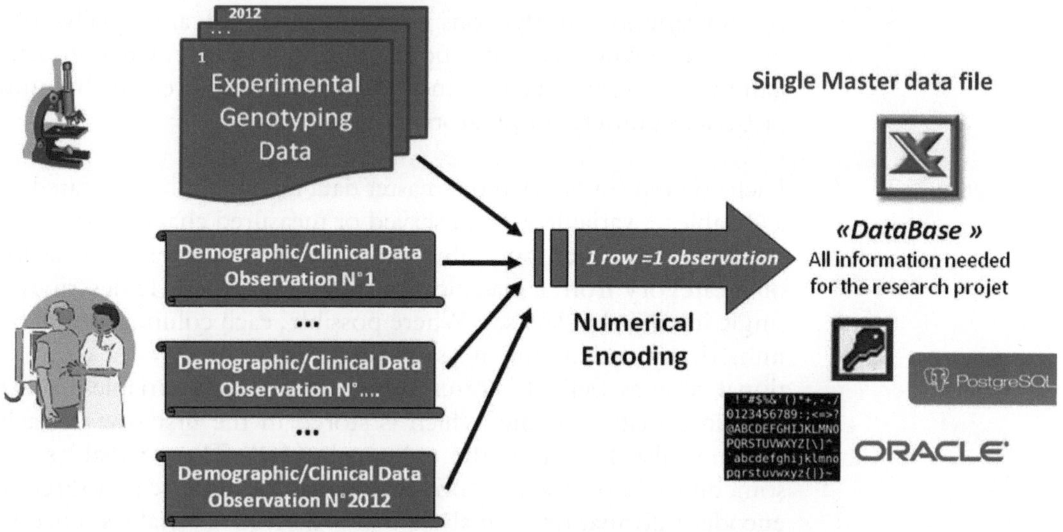


Fig. 1. The benefits of a single master data file. A master data file integrates all data pertinent to a given study in a standard fashion. Genotype and phenotype data that must be compiled for a research project are shown on the *right*. These are all incorporated into a single master data file, which is stored in a database, or as an MS Excel table.

input formats), the master data file should be the source of all data analyzed regardless of the organization of those data. This first step crystallizes all the thought that has been put in the study design and the development of the hypothesis(ses) under investigation. Study design is beyond the focus of this chapter but sample selection, phenotype assessment, and required sample size computations clearly warrant close attention. As shown in Fig. 1, the master data file gathers demographic, phenotypic, and genotypic information; see supplementary Table S1 for a sample master data file.

### 2.2. Characteristics of a Master Data File

A typical master data file consists of (1) a series of rows dedicated to each analytical unit of the study and (2) a series of columns each consisting of either a "primary" or "derived" variable.

#### 2.2.1. Units of Analysis

The master data file is generally structured using a single row dedicated to each analytical unit of the study. The analytical unit is the entity for which the required items of data have been collected and compiled. In general, analytical units are individual subjects, although in some cases the major entity being analyzed in a study is not an individual; for example, a transplantation study may focus on donor/recipient pairs, or an epidemiological study may focus on cases and controls. When nuclear families are analyzed, it may also be more appropriate to consider the nuclear family itself as the analytical unit of the study rather than its constituent members. In these cases, data on more than one individual may be included on a single row of the master data file. Conversely, when the study design involves repeated measures (over time or under different circumstances), observations of a single subject are usually split over several rows. This may be the case for example, when investigating the consistency of a measure between different techniques or between different operators.

*2.2.2. Variables*

Each column (or field) in the master data file should be dedicated to a variable. A variable is an observed or measured characteristic that can have more than one value and to which a numerical measure or a category from a classification can be assigned. It describes a single item in the data set. Where possible, each column should be numerically coded, and missing values must be given a conventional code as well. It is often useful to give each variable a short (but informative) name, which is stored in the first row of each column (also known as the column header). These variables are sometime called "raw" or "primary" variables, because they directly encode information; "analysis" or "derived" variables encode information that can be derived from the raw variables, and can be included in the master data file as well. For example, body mass index (BMI) can be calculated from weight and height variables, but it may be useful to include a calculated BMI in the master data file as well. The master data file may include other variable fields that will contain variable data generated as part of the analyses.

In general, the master data file should be designed to exclude redundancies between fields. At this early stage of the analysis, it is also important to identify the type of the variables being included in the master data file; the two most important variable types are "quantitative" and "qualitative" variables, and the statistical method that will be applied will depend on the type of variable being analyzed.

1. Quantitative variables

   Quantitative variables provide numerical measures of a given characteristic being observed, and can be either "continuous" or "discrete." Continuous quantitative variables have an infinite number of possible values that are not countable, whereas discrete quantitative variables have either a finite number of possible values or a countable number of possible values. For example, in hematopoietic stem cell allogeneic transplantation, the dose of CD34+ cells (e.g., $4.61 \times 10^6$ $kg^{-1}$ of body weight) is a continuous quantitative variable. When these values are rounded (e.g., to $5 \times 10^6$ $kg^{-1}$ of body weight), the variable may be considered as a discrete quantitative variable. In general, mathematical and statistical operations can be carried out on quantitative variables.

2. Qualitative variables

   Qualitative (or categorical) variables allow for classification of individuals based on a characteristic, and can be either "nominal" or "ordinal." Nominal qualitative variables define unordered or non-hierarchical categories, whereas ordinal qualitative variables can be used to order or rank the observations. For example, leukemia subtypes can be defined with a nominal qualitative variable; 1 = acute lymphoblastic leukemia (ALL); 2 = acute myelogenous leukemia (AML), 3 = chronic lymphocytic leukemia (CLL); 4 = chronic myelogenous leukemia (CML), 5 = unclassified leukemia, 999 = data missing, whereas stages of progression to type-1-diabetes (T1D) can be defined with an ordinal qualitative variable; 0 = normal glucose regulation, 1 = impaired fasting glucose, 2 = impaired glucose tolerance, 3 = diabetes mellitus, 999 = data missing. In general, qualitative variables are descriptors and not numbers, and mathematical operations are not appropriate. Instead, qualitative variables are useful for stratifying and dissecting patterns derived from the analysis of quantitative variables.

*2.2.3. Data Dictionary*

In addition to the numerically encoded variables, a master data file should also contain (or be associated with) a dictionary defining each variable and its associated coded values. The minimal items for this data dictionary are the short name of the variable, a detailed description of its content, a specification of the meaning of each associated numerical code, and the code used for missing values. Any additional information or comment that can be useful for a better characterization of the variable has to be mentioned. This effort will ensure sustainability of the data.

Figure 2 shows an example of the data structure in a master data file: numerically encoded data and data dictionary; see

| id | ... | cgend | qage | cleuktyp | ... |
|---|---|---|---|---|---|
| DGU | ... | 1 | 36 | 1 | ... |
| TJH | ... | 0 | 22 | 1 | ... |
| GNK | ... | 1 | 25 | 4 | ... |
| POI | ... | 999 | 45 | 999 | ... |
| DTR | ... | 0 | 63 | 3 | ... |
| ... | ... | 0 | 23 | 2 | ... |

← Numerically encoded master data file

Corresponding dictionary of the variables →

| *Name of the Variable* | *Description of the Variable* | *Type of Variable* | *Coding system* | *Comment* |
|---|---|---|---|---|
| ... | ... | ... | ... | ... |
| **cgend** | Gender of the patient | **Categorial** | 0= female; 1= male; 999 = misisng | |
| **qage** | Age in years at date of exam | **Quantitative continous** | Value in years | |
| **cleuktyp** | Specification of the sub-type of Leukemia for the patient | **Qualitative nominal 4 categories** | (1) Acute lymphoblastic (ALL); (2)Acute myeloid (AML), (3) Chronic lymphocytic (CLL); (4) Chronic myelogenous (CML); (5) Unclassified; (999) Missing | |
| ... | ... | ... | ... | ... |

Fig. 2. Characteristics of a Master Data File and associated Data Dictionary. A data dictionary provides context for the numerically encoded observations recorded in the master data file. Each field (*column*) in the master data file corresponds to a row in the data dictionary, where it is described in a standardized fashion.

supplementary Table S2 for a sample data dictionary for Table S1. Figure 3 presents a "roadmap" to the landscape of statistical techniques; it summarizes the analytical approach: it goes from raw data storage, through analysis of missingness of the data, the use of classical descriptive statistical techniques (both numerical and graphical) to final statistical modeling fueling the interpretation of the data. Figure 3 is also available online as supplementary Figure S1.

### 2.3. Storage of Data

The best way to appropriately organize the data usually requires building a database. Because many research groups do not have the information technology (IT) resources to do so, a spreadsheet application (e.g., Microsoft Excel or its equivalent) is often used instead. Although very easy to use, accidental sorting, deletions, and unintended changes to the data can occur with such spreadsheet applications. For example, when HLA allele names are stored in Excel, it is common for allele names that should be treated as text (e.g., "0101" or "01:01") to be treated as numbers or times (e.g., 101 or 1:01). Such data rearrangements may be difficult to detect and will certainly affect the results of the study. If spreadsheet applications are used to manage allele name data, individual datasets should be stored and transmitted as text-formatted "flat files," and measures should be taken to ensure the validity of allele names prior to analysis.

## 3. Nomenclature Management

The high degree of polymorphism observed for immunogenetic genes and loci, coupled with the structural variation of immune genes, has resulted in regularly updated allele name nomenclatures that keep pace with the growing complexity of these systems, but each nomenclature revision brings with it the potential for confusion when data generated using different nomenclature versions are analyzed together (the so-called immunogenetic tower of Babel) (1). This is a common problem for HLA and KIR genes, alleles, and haplotypes; MHC microsatellites, single nucleotide polymorphism (SNP), copy number variants (CNVs), and small insertion-deletion changes (indels). It is essential that the data in an analysis share a common nomenclature, and that the specific nomenclature version under which a dataset was generated (or validated if the dataset is compiled from multiple sources) is identified in the master data file.

### 3.1. HLA Nomenclature Variation

The HLA nomenclature for allele names has changed considerably over the last several decades. Each allele name contains a string of numbers arranged in "domains" that correspond to polymorphisms at the serological, protein, synonymous nucleotide, noncoding

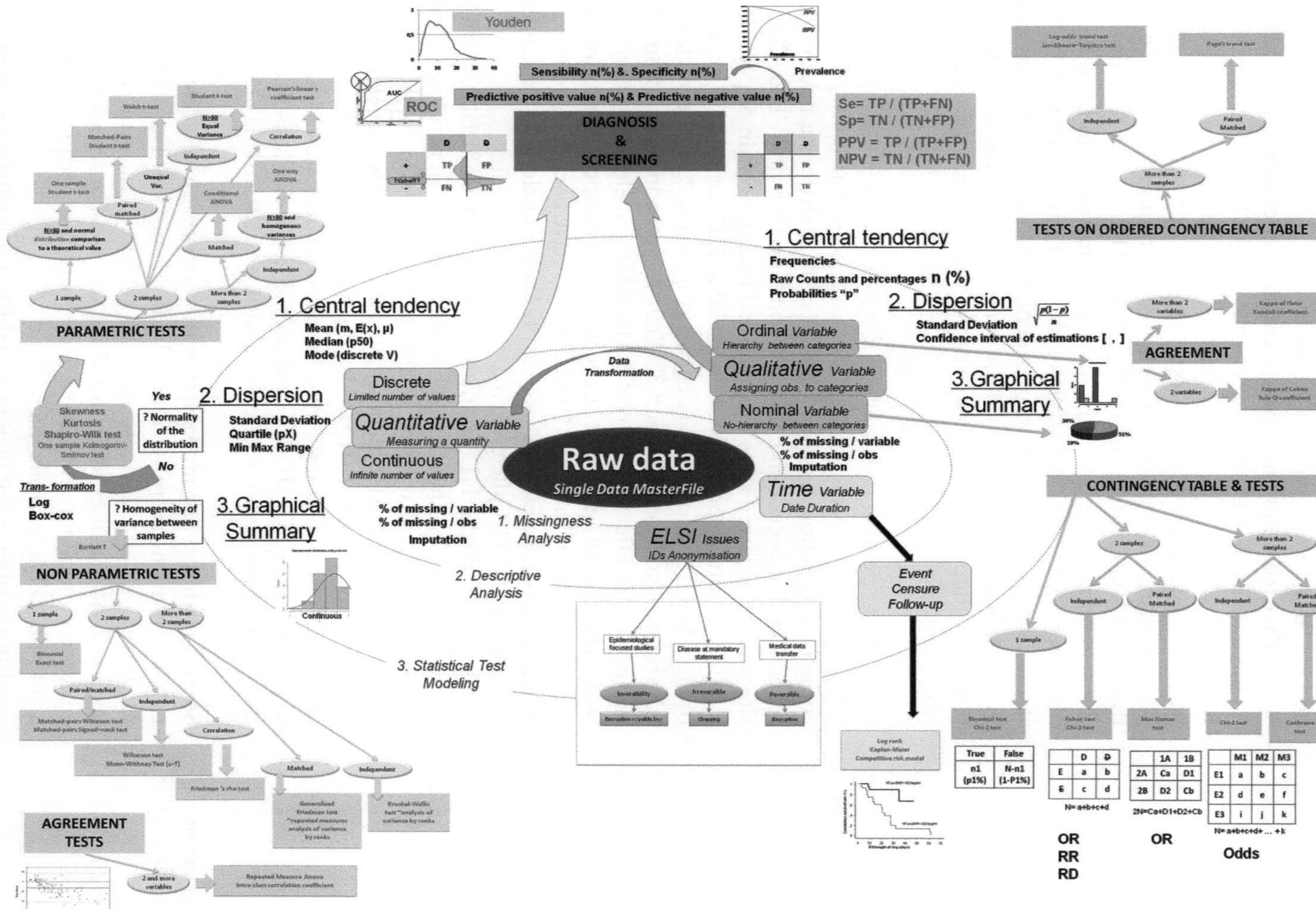


Courtesy of Methodomics Inc.

Fig. 3. A roadmap to the landscape of statistical techniques. This roadmap is a guide summarizing potential approaches to data analysis. Starting with raw data in the center, analyses proceed first through an assessment of missing data, and then the application of classical descriptive statistical techniques (both numerical and graphical), before a set of final statistical tests, specific to the type of data and the hypothesis being tested, and which inform the interpretation of the data, are selected.

nucleotide, and expression levels. The nomenclature has been expanded as new alleles, and new forms of polymorphism have been identified, and the features of three major versions of this nomenclature are outlined in Table 1.

With each improvement to the nomenclature, some allele names have been deleted (2) or changed (e.g., B*1522 changed to B*3543 in 2002 after DNA sequences outside of exons 2 and 3 became available). With the adoption of the current nomenclature version, many allele names have changed in nonobvious ways (e.g., the DPB1*0502 allele changed to *104:01 in order to maintain the sequential order of DPB1 protein sequences), and the locus identifier for HLA-C locus alleles changed from Cw* to C* (3). If the nomenclature version pertinent to a given dataset has not been explicitly identified, it is important to be able to make an educated guess about the likely version under which the data were generated.

#### *3.1.1. Antigen Recognition Sequence Nomenclature*

Rather than treating each allele as distinct, it is often useful to analyze alleles that share the peptide sequences that constitute the antigen recognition sequence (ARS) or that share the nucleotide sequences that encode the ARS as a combined category. The ARS is alternatively referred to as the peptide-binding domain or peptide-binding region (respectively abbreviated as PBD or PBR). The ARS of class II HLA molecules is encoded by exon 2, and the class I ARS is encoded by exons 2 and 3. While the version 2 HLA nomenclature was in effect, allele-codes identifying alleles that share the same ARS encoding exon sequences were developed. For example, the "A*010101g" and "A*02 G1" codes have been used to represent all HLA-A alleles that shared exon 2 and 3 nucleotide sequences with the A*010101 allele (4, 5).

Version 3 of the HLA nomenclature includes official codes for identifying alleles that share an ARS or ARS-encoding exon sequence. Alleles that share an identical ARS are included in a P group (e.g., A*01:01P includes all HLA-A alleles that share the ARS with the A*01:01:01:01 alleles), and alleles that share identical exon 2 or exons 2 and 3 nucleotide sequences are included in a G group (e.g., A*01:01:01G includes all HLA-A alleles that share their exon 2 and exon 3 sequences with A*01:01:01:01) (3).

#### *3.1.2. Nomenclature Conversion Resources*

Several resources are available for the conversion of allele names between nomenclature versions. The ImMunoGeneTics (IMGT)/HLA web site and database provides tables for the conversion of version 2 allele names to version 3 names, and houses a web-based conversion tool for individual allele names at http://www.ebi.ac.uk/imgt/hla/convert_name.html (6).

Entire datasets can be converted from nomenclature version 2 to version 3 using either the Allele Name Translation Tool (ANTT) or Update NomenCLature (UNCL), tools available from the

**Table 1**
**Features of the three nomenclature versions for classical HLA allele names**

| Nomenclature | | Domain size (number of characters) | | | | | |
|---|---|---|---|---|---|---|---|
| Version | Epoch | Serologic[a] | Protein | Synonymous | Noncoding | Expression variants | Examples |
| 1 | 1987–2002 | 2[b] | 2[b] | 1[c] | 2[d] | N[d], L[e] | A*01011 |
| 2 | 2002–2010 | 2 | 2 | 2[f] | 2 | L, N, A[g], C[g], S[g] | A*01010101 A*01010102N |
| 3 | 2010+ | 2 | 2+[g] | 2+[g] | 2+[g] | A, C, N, L, S, Q[h] | A*01:01:01:01 A*01:01:01:02N |

[a]The concept of a serologic specificity does not apply to DPB1 alleles. The first two digits of allele names for unique DPB1 protein sequences have been assigned in numerically (14)
[b]Implemented in 1987 (15)
[c]Implemented in 1990 (16)
[d]Implemented in 1995 (17)
[e]Implemented in 1996 (18)
[f]This domain was expanded to two digits in 2002 (2)
[g]Implemented in 2002 (2)
[h]These domains were explicitly defined as colon-delimited fields in 2010, and can accommodate any number of variants (3)
[i]Implemented in 2010 (3)

immunogenomics data analysis working group (IDAWG) at http://immunogenomics.org/software.html (7). UNCL is a web-based tool, and the ANTT is a locally run tool that can be customized to convert between other nomenclatures and name conventions. Both tools accept data in the form of tab-delimited text files, and generate tab-delimited text files of translated data.

The current version of the Helmberg Sequence COmpilation and Rearrangement Evaluation (SCORE) virtual-DNA analysis database software (8, 9) will convert between version 2 and 3 nomenclatures for allele name data in its database. SCORE will also convert allele names to user-defined nomenclatures.

#### 3.1.3. Allele Name Truncation

Because the polymorphic domains that make up an HLA allele name are arranged in a hierarchical fashion, it is possible to delete domains from the right end of an allele name while retaining important information for analysis. This process of deleting domains is known as truncation (aka right-truncation), and it is important to ensure that truncation has been carried out consistently within a dataset. For example, the full-length A*01:01:01:01 allele name can be truncated to A*01:01:01, A*01:01, and A*01. In some cases, truncation of allele names may be equivalent to applying a P or G group code, but this is not always the case. Depending on the research question being investigated, different levels of truncation may be appropriate (e.g., it may be appropriate to truncate allele names to the peptide level for a study of peptide presentation, but not for a study of allelic diversity and evolution), but all versions of a given allele name must be truncated to the lowest common level for analysis to avoid spurious results.

### 3.2. Microsatellite Nomenclature (14th Workshop)

In general, microsatellite alleles should be identified using both the number of repeats and the fragment size (10). In order to compare the results of several studies, the correspondence between the repeat number and the various fragment lengths (depending on primer pairs used) should be established. This correspondence list must include specific details (e.g., in the form of UniSTS numbers) of the primer pairs used to genotype each microsatellite (http://www.ncbi.nlm.nih.gov/sites/entrez?db=unists). When multiple synonymous names are in use for a given microsatellite allele, the lowest numbered DS6 number should be used as a reference. For example D6S273 should be used to refer to the following synonymous names—142XH6, AFM142xh6, GC378-D6S273. More details can be found on the NCBI's MHC database, "dbMHC" (http://www.ncbi.nlm.nih.gov/projects/gv/mhc/).

### 3.3. Single Nucleotide Polymorphism and Insertion/Deletion Nomenclature

As recently discussed (1), multiple distinct identifiers may exist for a given simple genetic marker (e.g., a SNP or indel), sometimes leading to confusion in the comparison of markers across studies. This is partly due to the fact that the unique reference sequences applied to structurally variable and highly polymorphic

### 3.4. SNPs: RS# and HGVS Nomenclature

regions like the KIR cluster and the MHC region are not appropriate for these markers. One commonly accepted solution to this problem is to use the NCBI's dbSNP reference SNP (RefSNP) accession ID (rs number or rs#) (11). However, because rs numbers are not necessarily stable identifiers across successive dbSNP releases/builds, all references to an rs# should be accompanied by dbSNP build number. For example, rs16375 is not in use anymore in build 130 of dbSNP; rs1704 should be used instead.

Many other possibilities can be used as complementary indications which directly refer to the sequence changes (e.g., rs2306220:A>G). The other acceptable option is to use the Human Genome Variation Society (HGVS) nomenclature (12, 13). For rs16375/rs1704, an accessioned sequence from EBI, GenBank, or DDBJ can be used as the reference sequence NT 007592.14: 20656832insATTTGTTCATGCCT, but many different accessioned genomic or mRNA sequences can be used.

### 3.5. KIR Nomenclature

Ideally, the goal in storing and analyzing KIR data is to have some data representation for each chromosome at every locus. The limitations of the typing technology and the variation in KIR haplotype structure dictate that in many cases the second chromosome will be typed as "unknown" (?). Nevertheless, it is important to have data representation for the full genotype in order to facilitate downstream analyses. Each KIR locus typed can have at least one full genotypic record (more in the case of genotypic ambiguity, which is likely for allelic typing results). When a locus is absent from a given haplotype, this absence must be coded in the data (i.e., as an "absent" allele), and should be denoted as "0."

Where allelic typing is available, a genotype with two alleles represents the simplest case scenario, a heterozygote with the locus present on both haplotypes. However, when we have only one allele detected, e.g., KIR2DL2*002, there are two possible genotypes: "002,002" or "002,0." At present, most typing systems cannot distinguish these. In these cases, the genotype should be treated as ambiguous, i.e., 002,0/002.

For typing data that is strictly presence/absence, the data can be treated as for a biallelic locus: allele "1" = "present" and allele "0" = "absent." If the locus is absent, we have the full genotype 0,0; however for locus present, we have an ambiguous genotype, which may be either "1,0" or "1,1." This can also be represented as an ambiguous genotype : 1,0/1. Because this notation does not consider order, a genotype coding of "0,1" is not used, but would be treated the same as "1,0."

Some KIR loci have particular additional details to consider prior to analyzing data:

1. KIR2DL2/L3:

   KIR2DL2 and KIR2DL3 were formerly treated as separate loci. The alleles were not named in a series; therefore, it is important to distinguish between KIR2DL2 and KIR2DL3 when the data is recorded. In the case of this locus, since all typing systems are able to detect both KIR2DL2 and KIR2DL3 an investigator should always have a full genotype, i.e., no missing data or ambiguity with presence/absence typing.
2. KIR2DL5:

   KIR2DL5 may be either centromeric or telomeric in the KIR cluster, and possibly on both ends. As such, an individual may have four copies of KIR2DL5; at this time there is no way to distinguish these definitively. Many typing systems will simply type for the presence of KIR2DL5; if typed as "absent," there is confirmation of genotypes of 0,0 both centromerically and telomerically. However, a typing of 'present' gives the genotype 1,0/1 on either or both sides of the KIR complex. Some typing systems currently distinguish "KIR2DL5A" and "KIR2DL5B"; all current data suggest that KIR2DL5A corresponds to the telomeric position and that KIR2DL5B corresponds to the centromeric position.
3. KIR2DS3/S5:

   As with KIR2DL5, KIR2DS3/S5 may be either centromeric or telomeric in the KIR complex, and possibly on both ends. As such, an individual may have four copies of the gene. Previously, KIR2DS3 and KIR2DS5 were thought to be different loci, and all current typing systems can distinguish between them. However, an individual who is typed, for example, as positive for both KIR2DS3 and KIR2DS5 in a presence/absence typing system may have these two alleles on either or both sides of the KIR cluster. Some data is emerging that suggests that particular alleles of each of these may be either centromeric or telomeric, but this is not yet confirmed. Presently, the only way to ascertain definitively that an individual has both centromeric and telomeric copies of either KIR2DS3 or KIR2DS5 is the case where we have allelic typing with more than two allele calls for the locus.
4. KIR3DL1/S1:

   As above for KIR2DL2/L3, KIR3DL1 and KIR3DS1 were formerly treated as separate loci. However, it has been recognized for some time that they are allotypes of the same locus, and in this case alleles have been named in a series. As with KIR2DL2/L3, all typing systems minimally detect KIR3DL1 and KIR3DS1, so there should be no missing data/ambiguity in presence/absence typing systems at this locus. If a typing is submitted as, e.g., "3DL1," we know that the genotype is "3DL1,3DL1."

## Acknowledgments

This work was supported by National Institutes of Health (NIH) grants U01AI067068 (JAH, SJM) and U19 AI067152 (PAG) awarded by the National Institute of Allergy and Infectious Diseases (NIAID) and by NIH/NIAID contract AI40076 (RMS). The content is solely the responsibility of the authors and does not necessarily represent the official views of the National Institute of Allergy and Infectious Diseases or the National Institutes of Health.

## Glossary

***Genetic data***

1. Allele: Any of the alternative forms (sets of forms) of DNA sequence at locus. These variants may occur for genes and/or genetic markers.

   Example: B, HLA-DRB1*01:01:01, HLA-A*01, D6S1666 (184).

2. Diplotype: The pair of haplotypes within a given genotype. The chromosomal phase between alleles is always known.

   Example: HLA (A*01 B*08 DR*17, A*26 B*27 DR*17).
   HLA (A*01 B*27 DR*17, A*26 B*08 DR*17).

   When analyzing data for more than one locus, diplotypic data must be distinguished from genotypic data. Because the alleles at different loci in a given genotype can be combined to make many possible haplotype pairs, a genotype must be considered to correspond to multiple diplotypes. Unfortunately, the term "genotype" is sometimes used to refer to a given pair of haplotypes, especially when familial segregation has been studied.

3. Gene: The functional and physical unit of heredity. A gene consists of a DNA segment with a specific sequence. It includes information for the synthesis of mRNA molecules that direct the synthesis of proteins.

   Example: *ABO Glycosyltransferase* gene, *HLA-DRB1* gene, *KIR-2DS3/S5* gene.

4. Genotype: The genetic makeup at one or more loci of an individual. It refers to a set of alleles carried by an individual (regardless of the expression of those alleles). The chromosomal phase (chromosomal identity of alleles at different loci) between alleles may not be known.

Example: HLA-A (1, 2); HLA-B (8, 44); HLA-DRB1 (03, 04).
KIR: KIR (A, A).
Microsatellites: D6S273 (134, 136) D6S273 ( $*(GT)_{19}$, $*(GT)_{20}$).
SNP: RS345336443 (G/G).

5. Haplotype: Set of alleles of contiguous loci. They are usually co-transmitted on a parental chromosome.

   Example: HLA-A*01-B*08-DRB1*03.

6. Locus: Literally, "place" in Latin, it is the specific usual physical location of genes, an individual genetic marker, or set of genetic markers in a genome.

   Example: ABO locus, HLA-DRB locus, KIR-2DS3/S5cen locus, D6S1666 microsatellite locus.

7. Phenotype: The observable expression of alleles as a physical or biochemical trait resulting from the interaction of the genome, the environment, and the experimental settings. In disease studies it may refer to the presence or a manifestation of the disease under study. Disease phenotypes may be reflected in a variety of ways as quantitative or qualitative variables.
   This term may also refer to a set of alleles (expressed or not) detected by a technique. In codominant or heterozygous situations, phenotypes are noted as pairs of data; each pair is specific to a particular gene and locus.

   Example: ABO system: [A]. HLA system: [HLA-A (1, 2); HLA-B (8,44); HLA-DR (3, 4)].

***Phenotypic and demographic data***

1. Admixture: The outcome of interbreeding between members of different populations. An admixed population is generally derived from populations in different geographic regions.
2. Collection site: The location where the sample was collected. This can be identified using latitude and longitude coordinates, or by specifying the country or nation, and city/town/village, or other locale where the collection took place.
3. Complexity: An ordinal variable that represents an estimate of the degree of admixture and population sub-structure in each population sample.

   Example:
   Complexity 1: a population sample collected from a single settlement or group of closely related settlements.
   Complexity 2: a population sample collected from a group of separate but discrete settlements.
   Complexity 3: a population sample collected in a metropolitan area or across an entire nation.
   Complexity 4: an admixed population.

4. Data management methods: The approaches used in storing and processing the data in preparation for analysis. This can

include the formats and programs used to store and edit the data (e.g., a specific spreadsheet program or database system), as well as any modifications that were made to the data between the generation of the data resulting from the typing assay and the inclusion of the data in the master data file. For example, if ambiguities were resolved, the approach used to resolve them should be documented in the data dictionary; if HLA allele data were truncated to a common level, or "binned" into a common sequence category (e.g., treating all alleles that encode the same peptide-binding region as the same allele) this should documented.

5. Ethnicity: A group of individuals (or populations) sharing a common language, culture, or religion, and who are assumed to share a common ancestry. Ethnicity should be distinguished from geography (e.g., "North American" is not an ethnicity), and though ethnicity is often associated with indigenous nationality (e.g., "Irish," "Chinese") qualifiers are often necessary to distinguish ethnicity from nationality (e.g., "Han Chinese").
6. Family: If individuals in the study belong to discrete familial groups, a family ID is qualitative variable identifying membership in a particular pedigree, as well as the relationship to the index case (proband).
7. Geographic region: A specific continental or subcontinental area comprised by multiple nations in which the population is located, or from which the population was derived, if the population is a migrant population. For example, European Americans or European Australians would be assigned to the European region, or to a specific subregion of Europe. Conversely North America would only pertain to Native American/Amerindian/Aleut/Eskimo populations. Populations derived from more than one region (admixed populations) can be assigned to a specific class for the type of admixture (depending on the regions of origin) or included in a single class for all admixed populations. The definitions of each region and admixed class should be defined in the data dictionary.
8. Latitude and longitude: Geographic coordinates that specify specific locations on the surface of the Earth. Latitude and longitude values should be recorded in a decimal format, with minutes and seconds indicated as factions of each degree value. North latitudes and east longitudes should be recorded with positive values, and south latitudes and west longitudes should be recorded with negative values. For example, 35° 20 min south latitude would be recorded as −35.333, and 2° 30 min east longitude should be recorded as 2.5 or +2.5.

10. Population: A group of individuals living in a specific geographic area. More specifically, a population is defined such that all pairs of individual members have the opportunity to mate, and are more likely to mate with each other than with members of other populations. A population should be documented in the data dictionary in terms of the pertinent geographic area and the approximate number of included individuals. Population sample: A unique descriptor for the individuals from a given population that were included in the study. If the study involves multiple sets of individuals (samples) from the same population, each set of individuals should be given a unique name; usually it is sufficient to append the number of individuals to the end of the population name (e.g., antarctica_87, antarctica_207, antarctica_597).
11. Population substructure: A barrier to the opportunity of mating between all pairs of individuals in a population.
12. Proband: The individual under study, primarily used in family-based disease association studies.
13. Status: The status of an individual as affected or unaffected with respect to a disease phenotype, or belonging to a case or a control group.
14. Typing assay: The laboratory method(s) and associated protocols used to generate the data included in the analysis. Many of them are described in this volume. Commonly used molecular methods for HLA and KIR genotyping include sequence-specific priming (SSP), sequence-specific oligo probe (SSO or SSOP), sequence/sequencing-based typing (SBT), matrix-assisted laser desorption/ionization time-of-flight (MALDI-TOF), and reference strand conformation analysis (RSCA). Serology has been used historically for HLA phenotype data generation. When possible, a description of the assay identifying the assay manufacturer and reagent version/lot employed should be included in the data dictionary. Literature citations or references to specific protocols should also be associated with the methods used, especially if multiple distinct methods have been employed in generating the data.

## References


1. Gourraud PA, Feolo M (2010) The Babel Tower revisited: SNPs—Indels—CNVs. Confusion in naming sequence variant always rises from ashes Tissue Antigens 75:199–200
2. Marsh SG, Albert ED, Bodmer WF, Bontrop RE, Dupont B, Erlich HA, Geraghty DE, Hansen JA, Mach B, Mayr WR, Parham P, Petersdorf EW, Sasazuki T, Schreuder GM, Strominger JL, Svejgaard A, Terasaki PI (2002) Nomenclature for factors of the HLA system, 2002. Tissue Antigens 60:407–464
3. Marsh SG, Albert ED, Bodmer WF, Bontrop RE, Dupont B, Erlich HA, Fernández-Viña M, Geraghty DE, Holdsworth R, Hurley CK, Lau M, Lee KW, Mach B, Maiers M, Mayr WR, Müller CR, Parham P, Petersdorf EW, Sasazuki T, Strominger JL, Svejgaard A, Terasaki PI, Tiercy JM, Trowsdale J (2010) Nomenclature

for factors of the HLA system, 2010. Tissue Antigens 75:291–455

4. Cano P, Klitz W, Mack SJ, Maiers M, Marsh SG, Noreen H, Reed EF, Senitzer D, Setterholm M, Smith A, Fernández-Viña M (2007) Common and well-documented HLA alleles: report of the Ad-Hoc committee of the American society for histocompatibility and immunogenetics. Hum Immunol 68: 392–417
5. Robinson J, Mistry K, Marsh SGE (2010) Exon identity and ambiguous typing combinations. Anthony Nolan Research Institute. http://www.ebi.ac.uk/imgt/hla/pdf/ambiguity_v2280.pdf
6. Robinson J, Mistry K, McWilliam H, Lopez R, Parham P, Marsh SG (2011) The IMGT/HLA database. Nucleic Acids Res 39(Database Issue):D1171–D1176
7. Mack SJ, Hollenbach JA (2010) Allele Name Translation Tool and Update NomenCLature: software tools for the automated translation of HLA allele names between successive nomenclatures. Tissue Antigens 75:457–461
8. Helmberg W, Lanzer G, Zahn R, Weinmayr B, Wagner T, Albert E (1998) Virtual DNA analysis—a new tool for combination and standardised evaluation of SSO, SSP and sequencing-based typing results. Tissue Antigens 51: 587–592
9. Helmberg W (2000) Storage and utilization of HLA genomic data—new approaches to HLA typing. Rev Immunogenet 2:468–476
10. Gourraud PA, Cambon-Thomsen A, Dauber EM, Feolo M, Hansen J, Mickelson E, Single RM, Thomsen M, Mayr WR (2007) Nomenclature for HLA microsatellites. Tissue Antigens 69(Suppl 1):210–213
11. Sherry ST, Ward MH, Kholodov M, Baker J, Phan L, Smigielski EM, Sirotkin K (2001) dbSNP: the NCBI database of genetic variation. Nucleic Acids Res 29:308–311
12. den Dunnen JT, Antonarakis SE (2000) Mutation nomenclature extensions and suggestions to describe complex mutations: a discussion. Hum Mut 15:7–12
13. den Dunnen J (2010) Nomenclature for the description of sequence variants. Human Genome Variation Society. http://www.hgvs.org/mutnomen/
14. Bodmer JG, Marsh SGE, Parham P, Erlich HA, Albert E, Bodmer WF, Dupont B, Mach B, Mayr WR, Sasasuki T, Schreuder GMT, Strominger JL, Svejgaard A, Terasaki PI (1990) Nomenclature for factors of the HLA system, 1989. Tissue Antigens 35(1):1990
15. Who Nomenclature Committee (1988) Nomenclature for factors of the HLA system, 1987. Tissue Antigens 32:177–187
16. Bodmer JG, Marsh SG, Albert ED, Bodmer WF, Dupont B, Erlich HA, Mach B, Mayr WR, Parham P, Sasazuki T et al (1991) Nomenclature for factors of the HLA system, 1990. Hum Immunol 31(3):186–194
17. Bodmer JG, Marsh SG, Albert ED, Bodmer WF, Bontrop RE, Charron D, Dupont B, Erlich HA, Mach B, Mayr WR (1995) Nomenclature for factors of the HLA system, 1995. Tissue Antigens 46:1–18
18. Bodmer JG, Marsh SG, Albert ED, Bodmer WF, Bontrop RE, Charron D, Dupont B, Erlich HA, Fauchet R, Mach B, Mayr WR, Parham P, Sasazuki T, Schreuder GM, Strominger JL, Svejgaard A, Terasaki PI (1997) Nomenclature for factors of the HLA system, 1996. Tissue Antigens 49:297–321

# Chapter 13

# Analytical Methods for Immunogenetic Population Data

**Steven J. Mack, Pierre-Antoine Gourraud, Richard M. Single, Glenys Thomson, and Jill A. Hollenbach**

## Abstract

In this chapter, we describe analyses commonly applied to immunogenetic population data, along with software tools that are currently available to perform those analyses. Where possible, we focus on tools that have been developed specifically for the analysis of highly polymorphic immunogenetic data. These analytical methods serve both as a means to examine the appropriateness of a dataset for testing a specific hypothesis, as well as a means of testing hypotheses. Rather than treat this chapter as a protocol for analyzing any population dataset, each researcher and analyst should first consider their data, the possible analyses, and any available tools in light of the hypothesis being tested. The extent to which the data and analyses are appropriate to each other should be determined before any analyses are performed.

**Key words:** Data analysis, Highly polymorphic, HLA, Immunogenetics, KIR, Population study

## 1. Introduction

> The Analytical Engine has no pretensions whatever to originate anything. It can do whatever we know how to order it to perform. It can follow analysis, but it has no power of anticipating any analytical revelations or truths. Its province is to assist us in making available what we are already acquainted with. For, in so distributing and combining the truths and the formulae of analysis, that they may become most easily and rapidly amenable to the mechanical combinations of the engine, the relations and the nature of many subjects in that science are necessarily thrown into new lights, and more profoundly investigated (Ada Augusta, Countess of Lovelace).

While data analysis is a central component of modern genetic and genomic research approaches, most analytical methods have not

Frank T. Christiansen and Brian D. Tait (eds.), *Immunogenetics: Methods and Applications in Clinical Practice*, Methods in Molecular Biology, vol. 882, DOI 10.1007/978-1-61779-842-9_13, © Springer Science+Business Media New York 2012

been developed specifically for immunogenetic data; the high level of polymorphism at the HLA and KIR loci necessitates analytical methods and software tools with the capacity to process 20 or more alleles per locus for many loci. In addition, the extensive linkage disequilibrium (LD) between immunogenetic loci (e.g., covering 3 MB in the MHC) requires the simultaneous computation of association measures between as many as 14 (e.g., in the KIR complex) highly polymorphic loci. Because there is no single tool that can carry out all analyses, and because available tools are not perfect for immunogenetic data, specific concessions must sometimes be made to enable analysis. Researchers and analysts should always remain aware that even when an analytical application is appropriate to the data, analysis can still be confounded by variation in nomenclature and data-resolution (see Chap. 12).

As Ada Lovelace recognized in 1843, analytical tools do not provide new insights or reveal truths; they may allow the implementation of complex methods, but these methods and their assumptions should always be known and understood to the researcher. Therefore, in addition to the discussions in this chapter, researchers should be familiar with the literature describing each method and the manual describing the use of for each analytical tool. No analytical result should be accepted without being presented in the appropriate context.

In general, while some of the analyses described below *can* be performed on paper or in a spreadsheet application, all are best carried out by a dedicated software tool that has been specifically developed with that analysis in mind. This provides a facile means to describe what was done, minimizes error on the part of the analyst, and maximizes reproducibility both by the researcher and by other researchers. Software tools generally run in either a Microsoft Windows, Apple, or Linux/Unix environment (or in a web-browser), but because many tools do not run in all three of these operating systems, we do not recommend one over the others. Researchers should maintain access to all three operating systems in order to take advantage of all available tools.

Many of these calculations are "computationally expensive" in that they are CPU- and memory-intensive. In general, the faster the CPU and the more RAM on a system, the faster an analysis will progress, but contemporary computer systems should be sufficient to the task of running the applications described here. However, care should be taken to ensure that the most recently released version of any application is used for analysis; this will ensure that any known software issues have been addressed. All of the tools that we describe here are free, so there is no reason to rely on an outdated version. Finally, many of the analyses described here have been implemented as functions and packages written in R, the language and environment for statistical computing (1). While we recommend specific R packages for analysis, and generally recommend using the R language, a tutorial on R programming is beyond the scope of this chapter.

In the sections that follow, we may discuss one particular software tool or application in the context of a given analysis. Relationships between analytical methods and some available tools are summarized in Table 1. However, this table is not intended to be comprehensive; there are many more possible analyses than those described here, and there are many more tools available than are discussed. For example, the compilation of genetic analysis software at http://www.nslij-genetics.org/soft/ (2) includes 520 applications. Finally, supplementary population datasets (derived from the master data set included in the supplementary materials for Chap. 12) and associated files are available online at http://www.immunogenomics.org/methods.html; these datasets demonstrate input formats and were used to generate the example figures and tables associated with each analysis.

## 2. Data Reporting

The verification of published findings through independent replication is a core element of scientific research. Whereas replication is often interpreted to pertain primarily to the generation of experimental data, it is equally important that analyses of those data be replicated. To facilitate replication of analytical outcomes, the data analyzed must be reported in an accurate and thorough manner. Data described in the body of an immunogenetic paper should be presented as both raw allele counts and the allele frequencies calculated from them; this will allow other investigators to perform additional analyses (using counts) and will permit easy identification of the extent of differences in frequencies. In addition, all alleles, genotypes, and haplotypes (including rare variants) should be made available, either within the body of the paper or as supplementary material.

## 3. Analyses

### 3.1. Calculation of Gene (Allele) Frequencies

1. Direct Counting

   With the advent of molecular typing techniques, the need to estimate gene (allele) frequencies (GF) from phenotype data has diminished. In most cases, gene frequencies for HLA data can be obtained via direct counting, where the number of observations for a given allele is divided by the number of chromosomes ($2n$, where $n$ = sample size) under study.

**Table 1**
**Matrix of population genetic analyses and available software tools**

| Analysis | General statistical software (e.g., SAS) | MS Excel | GenAlEx[a] | PyPop[b] | Arlequin[c] | EstiHaplo[d] | PHYLIP[e] | Structure[f] | CLUTO[g] | PLINK[h] | R package[i] | GenePop[j] |
|---|---|---|---|---|---|---|---|---|---|---|---|---|
| Carrier frequency estimation | + | + | ++ | – | | – | – | – | | – | | |
| Hardy–Weinberg | – | – | + | +++ | ++ | – | – | – | | + | | ++ |
| Haplotype estimation | – | – | + | +++ | ++ | +++ | – | – | +++ | + | haplo.stats ++ | |
| Linkage disequilibrium | – | – | | +++ | ++ | – | – | – | +++ | + | | ++ |
| Measures of selection | – | – | ++ | +++ | ++ | – | – | – | – | – | | |
| Measurement of genetic differentiation | – | – | ++ | – | ++ | – | ++ | ++ | +++ | – | ++ | ++ |
| Principal component analysis | – | – | ++ | – | | – | – | – | – | – | ++ | |
| Phylogenetic analysis | – | – | | – | – | – | ++ | + | +++ | – | ++ | |
| Population structure analysis | – | – | | – | ++ | – | – | ++ | +++ | – | | |

– = analysis is not possible with that tool; + = analysis is possible, but the tool is not recommended for this analysis; ++ = analysis is possible with this tool; +++ = this tool has been optimized for the analysis of immunogenetic data

[a]http://www.anu.edu.au/BoZo/GenAlEx/

[b]http://www.pypop.org

[c]http://cmpg.unibe.ch/software/arlequin3/

[d]http://www.methodomics.com/estihaplo

[e]http://evolution.genetics.washington.edu/phylip.html

[f]http://pritch.bsd.uchicago.edu/structure.html

[g]http://glaros.dtc.umn.edu/gkhome/views/cluto/

[h]http://pngu.mgh.harvard.edu/~purcell/plink/

[i]http://www.r-project.org/

[j]http://genepop.curtin.edu.au/

The PyPop (python for population genomics) application (3) can be used to calculate allele frequencies in this manner. Supplementary Tables S1, S2, S3, and S4 are PyPop-formatted synthetic genotype data files for four populations. Supplementary Table S5 is a PyPop configuration file specific for these data. Further examples of PyPop-formatted HLA allele-frequency data and configuration files, developed by Solberg et al. (4), can be found at http://www.pypop.org/popdata. These calculations are also easily accomplished directly from a Microsoft Excel spreadsheet via the Genetic Analysis in Excel (GenAlEx) Excel add-on (5).

2. Estimation from carrier frequencies

   Direct counting cannot be used for all immunogenetic data. A notable exception remains for the KIR loci, where much of the available data have been generated on a presence/absence basis for many KIR loci, yielding phenotypes for which only carrier frequencies (CF, the presence of 1 or two of the considered allele) can be obtained by direct counting. In these cases, it is necessary to estimate gene frequencies. This can be done with the assumption that the population under study is in Hardy–Weinberg equilibrium (HWE) (see the final equation in step 3). The most simple equation is given by:

$$\mathrm{GF} = 1 - \sqrt{1 - \mathrm{CF}}.$$

   However, Lynch and Milligan (6) have shown that this provides a downwardly biased estimate and suggest that a better estimate is obtained by:

$$\mathrm{GF} = 1 - (x^{1/2}(1 - (\mathrm{var}(x) / 8x^2))^{-1}).$$

   where $x = 1-\mathrm{CF}$, and $\mathrm{var}(x) = x(1-x)/N$, where $N$ is the number of sampled individuals.

   Table 2 presents gene frequencies estimated using each of these methods (formula a and formula b) in comparison to frequencies calculated by direct counting.

3. Confidence intervals

   Any estimated GF^ should be accompanied by a confidence interval (CI), a range of values that reveals the precision of the estimated frequency. The likelihood that the CI includes the actual population GF is given by the confidence level (usually, a 95% chance). For GF estimated from a sample of size $n$, the CI has a lower bound of:

$$\hat{\mathrm{GF}} - \varepsilon\sqrt{(\mathrm{GF}(1 - \mathrm{GF}) / n)}.$$

   And an upper bound of:

$$\hat{\mathrm{GF}} + \varepsilon\sqrt{(\mathrm{GF}(1 - \mathrm{GF}) / n)},$$

**Table 2**
**Comparison of methods for determining gene frequencies for present/absent data**

| | | | Gene frequency estimate from carrier frequency | | Direct counting[a] | |
|---|---|---|---|---|---|---|
| **Locus** | **Count** | **Carrier frequency** | **Formula a** | **Formula b** | **Count** | **Gene frequency** |
| Present | 109 | 0.4225 | 0.2401 | 0.2398 | 62 | 0.2403 |
| Absent | 243 | 0.9419 | 0.7589 | 0.7570 | 196 | 0.7597 |
| Total[b] | 352 | 1.3643 | 0.9989 | 0.9968 | 258 | 1 |

[a]Assuming a molecular method that can distinguish homozygotes from heterozygotes
[b]$2n = 258$

where ε invokes the Normal distribution to determine the probability of the CI associated with the estimated GF. For a 95% CI, ε is 1.96, and for a 99% CI, ε is 2.576. $\sqrt{(\mathrm{GF}(1-\mathrm{GF})/n)}$ is an approximation of the standard error of the estimated GF.

### 3.2. Hardy–Weinberg Testing

The Hardy–Weinberg (HW) principle provides a useful model for primary quality control (QC) verification of the integrity of genotype data, as genotyping errors may result in both individual genotype deviations and overall deviations from HW equilibrium (HWE) (see Note 1). In addition, HW testing is also useful for detecting sampling errors (see below) in population samples. Confidence in the accuracy of Hardy–Weinberg testing is therefore crucial for confidence in subsequent analyses, as many analytical methods (e.g., LD and haplotype estimation, Ewens–Watterson analyses of selection) are predicated on an assumption of HWE in the data set. In a Hardy–Weinberg test, observed genotype counts are compared to those expected under Hardy–Weinberg equilibrium proportions (HWEP), as calculated by generating a table of all possible genotypes, using an appropriate statistical method. The relationship between the allele and genotype frequencies under HWEP is given as:

$$f(A_i A_i) = p_i^2$$

and

$$f(A_i A_j) = 2p_i p_j,$$

where $p_i$ is the allele frequency of $A_i$. and $p_j$ is the allele frequency of $A_j$. When a population is in HWE, there will not be a significant departure from these allele and genotype frequencies and there will be no change in allele frequencies between generations.

Tests of *overall* locus-level HWEP compute a $p$-value to estimate the significance of observed deviations across all genotypes. Significant deviation of observed genotype counts from expected HWEP can result from factors that include sampling errors (the sampling of admixed, stratified, or some other form of blended populations), inbreeding or other nonrandom mating, natural selection, and genotyping errors. Tests for deviation from HWEP have low power, and significant deviation from HWEP is *not* common. Genotyping errors (e.g., failure to detect a specific allele, resulting in an excess of homozygotes) are the first consideration when significant deviations from HWEP are detected (especially when such deviations are detected only at a single locus in a multilocus analysis), rather than the operation of selection, admixture, or nonrandom mating, unless the sample is suspected to be from an unusual population.

1. Chi-square testing

   Hardy–Weinberg testing can be particularly challenging for highly polymorphic datasets. Historically, the chi-square test has been the standard approach for testing fit to HWEP at the overall locus-level (regardless of the level of polymorphism at that locus). However, this test can lead to false acceptance or rejection of the null hypothesis when individual expected genotype counts in the table of all possible genotypes are small or close to zero (also known as, "sparse cells" in the table of all genotypes, as represented by the shaded cells with low numbers of expected genotypes in the upper half of Fig. 1). Sparse cells can be problematic because the minimum number of observed genotypes must be 1, while the minimum number of *expected* genotypes will be the square of the frequency of the rarest allele. It is not unusual for 30–40 or more alleles to be observed at the highly polymorphic HLA loci, with a wide range of frequencies, resulting in many such sparse cells. As a result, the ratio of observed to expected ($O/E$) genotypes can be as large as 100 or 1000 for rare genotypes in large populations with no actual HWEP deviation, while the $O/E$ ratio for common genotypes will usually be much smaller (usually between 0.2 and 5), even in cases of actual deviation from HWEP. Three approaches can be taken to increase the accuracy of Hardy–Weinberg tests of immunogenetic data; (1) rare alleles can be "lumped" together in a combined class (as in the lower half of Fig. 1) for the chi-square test to be effective; (2) a complete enumeration of all possible tables of all possible genotypes (an exact test) can be undertaken, or (3) approximations to such complete enumerations can be made via resampling.

No Allele "Lumping"

| Allele | Count | Frequency |
|---|---|---|
| **1** | 12 | 0.29 |
| **2** | 10 | 0.24 |
| **3** | 9 | 0.21 |
| **4** | 5 | 0.12 |
| **5** | 2 | 0.05 |
| **6** | 2 | 0.05 |
| **7** | 1 | 0.02 |
| **8** | 1 | 0.02 |
| Total | 42 | 1 |

Number of Each Genotype Expected

| | **1** | **2** | **3** | **4** | **5** | **6** | **7** | **8** |
|---|---|---|---|---|---|---|---|---|
| **1** | 3.43 | | | | | | | |
| **2** | 5.71 | 2.38 | | | | | | |
| **3** | 5.14 | 4.29 | 1.93 | | | | | |
| **4** | 2.86 | 2.38 | 2.14 | 0.60 | | | | |
| **5** | 1.14 | 0.95 | 0.86 | 0.48 | 0.10 | | | |
| **6** | 1.14 | 0.95 | 0.86 | 0.48 | 0.19 | 0.10 | | |
| **7** | 0.57 | 0.48 | 0.43 | 0.24 | 0.10 | 0.10 | 0.02 | |
| **8** | 0.57 | 0.48 | 0.43 | 0.24 | 0.10 | 0.10 | 0.05 | 0.02 |

Alleles 5-8 "Lumped"

| Allele | Count | Frequency |
|---|---|---|
| **1** | 12 | 0.29 |
| **2** | 10 | 0.24 |
| **3** | 9 | 0.21 |
| **4** | 5 | 0.12 |
| **5-8** | 6 | 0.14 |
| Total | 42 | 1 |

Number of Each Genotype Expected

| | **1** | **2** | **3** | **4** | **5-8** |
|---|---|---|---|---|---|
| **1** | 3.43 | | | | |
| **2** | 5.71 | 2.38 | | | |
| **3** | 5.14 | 4.29 | 1.93 | | |
| **4** | 2.86 | 2.38 | 2.14 | 0.60 | |
| **5-8** | 3.43 | 2.86 | 2.57 | 1.43 | 0.86 |

Fig. 1. Sparse cells and the "lumping" of alleles into combined classes. The effect of creating a combined, "lumped" allele class on expected genotype counts is illustrated in the upper and lower halves. In the upper half, expected genotype counts are calculated for all eight alleles; the expected counts for the ten genotypes comprising alleles 5, 6, 7, and 8 (*shaded*) are much less than 1. In the lower half, alleles 5–8 have been lumped into the "5–8" allele class, and no genotype in the table has an expected count less than 0.6.

2. Exact tests

   An exact test for HWEP was developed by Louis and Dempster (7). This test generated all possible tables of genotypes (based on observed allele frequencies) when the sample size and allele frequencies are held constant in accordance with the exact distribution. The *p*-value was given by the cumulative conditional probability of obtaining a table of genotypes (with sample size and allele frequencies equal to the observed sample) with a conditional probability less than or equal to that of the genotypes in the observed sample (8, 9). This test provides the exact *p*-value for every sample and it does not require input parameters that may affect the result. However, the number of possible tables of genotypes grows exponentially as either the sample size ($n$) or the number of distinct alleles ($k$) increases, reducing the feasibility of this test when $n$ and $k$ are large.

3. Resampling approximations

   Resampling *approximations* to complete enumeration of all possible tables were developed for data sets with larger numbers of alleles, where the *asymptotic* chi-square test may be particularly problematic and *exact* tests with complete enumeration were not possible (10–13). While these *approximation* or resampling tests are often erroneously referred to as "exact" tests, they do not perform a true exhaustive search for all possible tables of genotypes. These methods generally use the Monte Carlo (MC) simulation method to approximate to the exact *p*-value and, therefore, represent an acceptable alternative to the *exact* test.

Guo and Thompson (10) developed the first conventional MC test of HWEP based on Levene's conditional sampling distribution and also proposed a MC test that uses a finite and irreducible Markov Chain (MCMC) (14) to randomly generate tables of all possible genotypes. In these MC-based tests, the *p*-value is given by the fraction of randomly generated tables with a conditional probability less than or equal to the conditional probability of the observed genotypes. Resampling MC and MCMC tests perform very favorably when compared to the *exact* test and always outperform the chi-square test. However, the MCMC method may fail to approximate to the exact *p*-value in a few cases, and the MC test is preferred in cases where the *exact* test cannot be performed.

Chi-square tests, and MC and MCMC resampling approximations of the exact test are performed by PyPop, which has been designed specifically for the analysis of highly polymorphic immunogenetic data. For the chi-square test, PyPop automatically creates combined categories of rare alleles based on a user-defined "lumping" threshold, with a default value of 5.

4. Hardy–Weinberg testing of individual genotypes

   Chen et al. (15) measured the goodness of fit of individual genotypes to expected HWEP in MC approximations of the exact test by comparing disequilibrium coefficients (16, 17). PyPop calculates two measures (Chen and Diff) of the goodness of fit of individual genotypes when the MC or MCMC test is implemented. In cases when locus-level deviations from HWEP are detected, these individual genotype tests may help identify the specific genotypes contributing to the deviation, but should be considered only when the number of expected genotypes is at least 1. As noted above, large p-values may result when a genotype with an expected count much less than 1 is observed once or twice; researchers should avoid making analytical inferences on the basis of these *p*-values.

### 3.3. Haplotype Estimation

Estimated haplotypes and haplotype frequencies play a central role in most genetic studies. Haplotype-level analyses are important to studies of the etiology of human disease, selective forces acting on populations, and optimal sizes for bone-marrow donor registries (BMDRs). Associations between markers and disease loci that are not evident with a single-marker locus may be identified in multilocus marker analyses using estimated haplotype frequencies (HFs). The design of studies and the recruitment of the samples are dependent on the possibility of identifying haplotypes by segregation analysis in families or estimating haplotypes from population samples of phase-unknown unrelated individuals (18). Haplotypes are used for disease association mapping, QTL mapping, and even imputing underlying genetic markers (19).

The term "haplotype" now includes any set of genetic polymorphisms (i.e., all DNA sequence variation including deletion/insertions) at contiguous loci. Except when recombination occurs, these neighboring genetic polymorphisms are cotransmitted by a single parental chromosome. Haplotypes may be represented as blocks of DNA sequence variants (e.g., SNP haplotype blocks), or groups of sequence variants can be abstracted into an allelic nomenclature at the level of a functional locus, as in the HLA and KIR systems.

#### 3.3.1. Expectation-Maximization Algorithm

Early work on the estimation of haplotype frequencies from unrelated genotype data was based on the expectation-maximization (EM) algorithm with the assumption of HWEP at the locus-level (20–24). Later work refined, explored, and extended aspects of the algorithm (25–30). Application to haplotypes of SNPs (31–33) and Bayesian methods (34, 35) are commonly used. It remains unclear whether the Bayesian algorithms perform better than maximum likelihood implemented in EM algorithm (35).

Haplotypes can be estimated using a number of software tools, for example, in a standard implementation of the Expectation-Maximization (EM) algorithm in the haplo.stats package for R, the open source language, and environment for statistical computing (1). Although there is a great desire within the immunogenetic community for applications capable of analyzing very large (>million individuals) data sets, available HF and LD estimation software are generally limited in their capacity to a few thousands of individuals. For example, precompiled versions of PyPop are currently limited to 7 loci and 5,000 individuals when it comes to estimating haplotypes and calculating LD values. In contrast, haplo.stats can accommodate very large datasets, depending on the number of alleles at each locus; for example, haplo.stats estimates haplotypes for 240,000 individuals over four loci with an average of 25.5 alleles per locus, or 60,000 individuals over 50 loci with the same mean number of alleles. Supplementary Table S6 is a haplo.stats-formatted version of the synthetic genotype data in Supplementary Tables S1–S4. The "master data file" described in Chap. 12 of this volume (Chap. 12 Supplementary Table S1) can also serve as a haplo.stats input file.

Population-level haplotype frequencies are estimated via EM using simultaneous maximum-likelihood estimation of $n$-locus haplotype frequencies. The expectation step determines the expected number of copies for each haplotype contributing to a given genotype. For a three locus haplotype, this is calculated as:

$$E[n_{abc} \mid P_i] = 2 f_{abc} S f_{abc} \;/\; P_r (P_i),$$

where $S$ is the number of ambiguous haplotypes in $P_i$, $E[n_{abc}|P_i]$ is the expected number of copies of haplotype $H_{abc}$ within $P_i$, and $f_{abc}$ is the frequency of each other possible haplotype $H_{abc}$ to form the genotype of frequency $P_i$. The maximization step determines new estimates for $f_{abc}$ for the next iteration of the algorithm. At each iteration, the estimations globally improve.

### 3.3.2. Challenges to the Use of Estimated Haplotypes

1. Rare estimated haplotypes

   The performance of haplotype frequency estimation algorithms is sensitive to various aspects of the population under study (35). Estimated frequencies for rare haplotypes ($n = 1$ or 2 in a dataset), which incorporate low-frequency alleles, are often incorrect, even when the EM algorithm finds the global maximum likelihood (27, 36, 37). The accuracy of haplotype estimates is critical for association and candidate gene studies, fine-mapping of disease genes, and for microsatellite, SNP, and protein level variation, and the presence or absence of specific low-frequency alleles and haplotypes must inform the robustness of associations. Analytical inferences should not be made on the basis of these rare haplotypes.

2. Haplotype estimation for immunogenetic data

   The diversity and complexity of Immunogenetic data poses additional challenges for haplotype estimation. Over the past 30 years, the Immunogenetic community has seen an exponential increase of the number of HLA alleles leading to regular nomenclature revisions, and this phenomenon now extends to the KIR genes (38). In both the MHC and KIR regions we have: heterogeneity of typing resolution, heterogeneity of typing techniques, heterogeneity of allele nomenclatures, continual discovery of new alleles, large numbers of allele per loci (roughly >50), and high haplotype diversity (roughly >1,000). In addition, KIR and HLA data are very sensitive to ethnic background diversity. The potential for population substructure is particularly relevant for immunogenetic data due to the fact that MHC and KIR genes can reflect both the selective and demographic histories of populations. These issues are exacerbated in BMDRs where sample sizes for specific research questions are often very large (>100,000).

   Little is known about the behavior of estimated haplotypes in the extreme situations described above for the HLA and KIR regions and little attention has been paid to the biases affecting haplotype frequency estimation. The frequency of the alleles, the sample size of the dataset, the various levels of missing information, and the various levels of linkage disequilibrium surely influence the accuracy of the estimation. Haplotype frequency estimations are primarily affected by sampling fluctuation. In HLA and KIR, it is highly likely that the sample sizes are usually too small to cover the extent of the haplotype diversity. As a result, the haplotype frequencies and linkage disequilibrium between alleles are overestimated; such a bias would occur even if the chromosome phase was known.

3. HF Estimation for KIR

Because some KIR genes are present *only* on certain haplotypes, the space of possible KIR haplotypes excludes some locus combinations that *could* be generated from the observed genotypic data. The EM algorithm for estimating KIR HFs must be modified to account for this reduced combinatorial space, e.g., using an a priori list of known/possible haplotypes to constrain the EM algorithm (39, 40). The user-designated a priori haplotype list is said to span a set of observed genotypes if each observed genotype can be generated from at least one pair of haplotypes in the list. If the list does not span the observed genotypes, the resulting estimates must be carefully interpreted.

Several recent KIR HF estimation studies have noted shortcomings in the use of such constraints, imposed by the need to specify predefined haplotype patterns (Fig. 2). Yoo et al. (40) found that accuracy measures related to haplotype identification were particularly low for fewer than 200 individuals and sug-

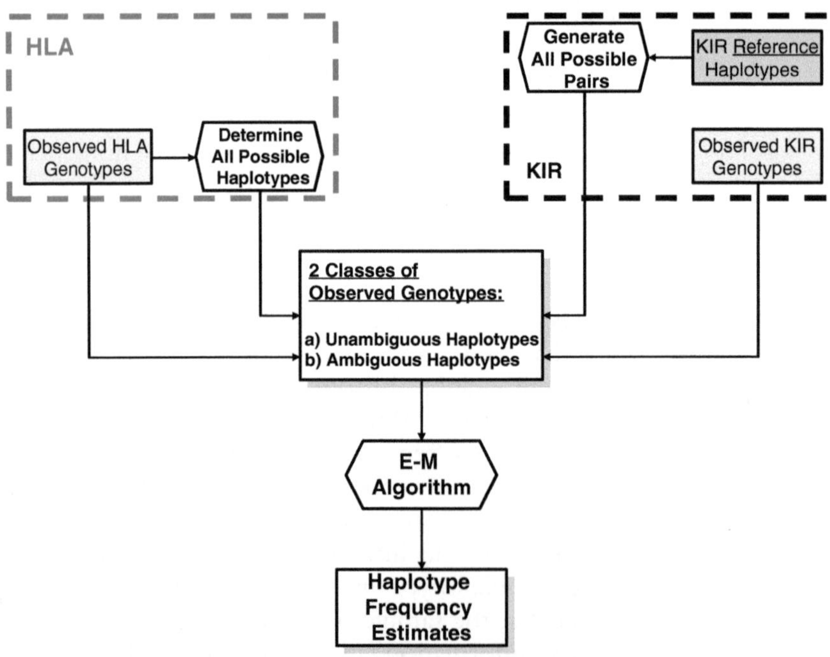


Fig. 2. Overview of HLA haplotype estimation and KIR haplotype estimation strategies. The EM algorithm for estimating KIR haplotype frequencies (HFs) can be modified from the standard approach applied to HLA genotypes (*upper-left box*) to account for a reduced combinatorial space using a set of reference haplotypes as an a priori list of known/possible haplotypes to constrain the algorithm (*upper-right box*).

gested that more than 500 individuals would provide acceptable estimation accuracy. In describing their HAPLO-IHP software, Yoo et al. noted that unusual haplotypes incompatible with constraints may be incorrectly rejected. When the a priori list of user-defined haplotypes does not span the observed genotypes, haplotypes that may not exist are "constructed" in an attempt to satisfy user-defined haplotype patterns.

### 3.4. Measures of Linkage Disequilibrium

Linkage disequilibrium is defined as the nonrandom association of alleles at two loci. High levels of LD combined with high levels of polymorphism are the defining characteristic of immunogenetic loci. Measurement of LD provides a means to assess the degree to which pairs of alleles are likely to be observed on the same haplotype and has important implications in analyzing immunogenetic data for population and disease association studies.

#### 3.4.1. Haplotype-Level LD statistics

1. $D_{ij}$ and $D'_{ij}$

   Pairwise disequilibrium statistics can be calculated for each haplotype for polymorphic loci:

   $$D_{ij} = x_{ij} - p_i \times q_j,$$

   where $x_{ij}$ is the estimated haplotype frequency (see previous section) and $p_i$ and $q_j$ are the *i*th and *j*th allele frequencies at the two loci. In order to account for differing allele frequencies at the loci, a normalized disequilibrium value can be used (41). This is given by:

   $$D'_{ij} = D_{ij} / D_{\max},$$

   where $D_{\max}$ is the lesser of $p_i q_j$ and $(1-p_i)(1-q_j)$, when $D_{ij}$ is <0 and $p_i(1-p_i)$ and $q_j(1-q_j)$, when $D_{ij}$ is >0.

2. $r^2$

   The $r^2$ measure is another means of normalizing $D_{ij}$ to account for differing allele frequencies. This is the square of the correlation coefficient ($r$) between the alleles at the $p$ and $q$ loci (42). Because $r$ is given as:

   $$r = (D_{ij} / p_i \times q_j(1-p_i)(1-q_j))^{1/2},$$

   $r^2$ is therefore given as:

   $$r^2 = D_{ij}^2 / (p_i \times q_j(1-p_i)(1-q_j)),$$

#### 3.4.2. Global LD Statistics

For loci with more than two alleles, global LD statistics extend the haplotype-level statistics to account for all possible combinations of alleles at each locus (43).

1. $W_n$

   $W_n$ is a multiallelic extension of the correlation measure $r$. The chi-square value for testing the significance of LD can be written as $W/(2N)$ where:

$$W = (\sum \sum D_{ij} / p_i \times q_j)^{1/2},$$

and $p_i$ and $q_j$ are the observed allele frequencies at each of the two loci having $k$ and $l$ alleles, respectively. $W_n$, or Cramer's V statistic, is a normalized value that addresses differing numbers of alleles at the two loci (44, 45).

$$W_n = W / \sqrt{(\min(k, l) - 1)}.$$

The values of $W_n$ fall between 0 and 1, and the significance of the overall disequilibrium is assessed using the abovementioned chi-square test. It should be noted that the $W_n$ measure is always symmetric with respect to two loci, whereas the number of alleles reported at each locus can differ considerably. It is therefore important not to overinterpret values of $W_n$ for locus pairs with highly asymmetric numbers of alleles. Finally, for biallelic loci, $W_n$ is equivalent to $r$.

2. $D'$

$D'$ is a second global disequilibrium statistic, which sums the absolute value of normalized $D_{ij}$ values over all haplotypes, weighted by the frequencies of the alleles in each haplotype (46). As with $W_n$, $D'$ values fall between 0 (equilibrium) and 1 (linkage). This is given as:

$$D' = \Sigma\Sigma p_i \times q_j \mid D'_{ij} \mid,$$

PyPop calculates $D_{ij}$, $D'_{ij}$, $D'$ and $W_n$ values.

#### 3.4.3. Graphical Representation of LD Patterns

The interpretation of LD values between many markers can be facilitated through the graphical representation of LD patterns. Compared to a tabular presentation of LD values, such visual representations facilitate the identification of patterns and interesting subsets of the data. So-called "heat maps" are a common means of representing pairwise LD values across markers, as a half-matrix in which the strength of the LD (e.g., the log of the *p*-value) is represented by a color scale. However, most of the software tools developed for graphical LD presentations represent biallelic markers and can therefore only represent average LD between multiallelic loci. Popular software tools for this purpose include graphical overview of linkage disequilibrium (GOLD) (47), Haploview (48), MIDAS (49), and various packages in R (e.g., LDHeatmap (50)). While PyPop does not generate graphical LD representations, PyPop-generated LD data can be imported directly to R. To our knowledge, only MIDAS will simultaneously represent the interallelic component of LD.

### 3.5. Measurement of Selection

1. Ewens–Watterson homozygosity statistic

The expected proportion of homozygotes under Hardy–Weinberg, for an observed value of $k$ and a given sample size ($n$), is used as a measure of the allele-frequency distribution and compared to the distribution expected under the neutral model for the same values of $k$ and $n$ (51). Allele-frequency distributions are used to calculate Watterson's homozygosity F statistic (52). This is given by:

$$F = \sum p_i^2,$$

where $p_i$ is the frequency of the $i$th allele at a locus. The homozygosity test can be accomplished using the exact test described by Slatkin (53, 54). For given values of $n$ and $k$, all possible configurations of alleles are listed (each configuration is a distinct way of distributing the $n$ sampled genes into $k$ allelic categories). The probability of obtaining a particular configuration can be computed under the null hypothesis of neutrality using the Ewens sampling formula (51). The homozygosity value of each configuration along with its probability gives the sampling distribution for F under neutrality. This distribution is used to find the probability of obtaining homozygosity values equal to or larger than that observed, for a test of positive selection, by examining how many configurations result in homozygosities greater than this observed value (53). Similarly, a test of balancing selection is based on the probability of obtaining a homozygosity value as small as or smaller than the observed value. Significant $p$-values reject the null hypothesis that the sample came from a population that is undergoing neutral evolution.

2. Normalized deviate of homozygosity

   Homozygosity values calculated for different values of $n$ and $k$ can be directly compared by calculating the normalized deviate of homozygosity ($F_{nd}$) (55). This is given by:

$$F_{nd} = (F_{obs} - F_{exp}) / \sqrt{\text{var}(F_{exp})},$$

   where $F_{obs}$ is the homozygosity value calculated for an observed frequency distribution, $F_{exp}$ is the mean homozygosity expected under the neutral model. While $F_{nd}$ is a normalized deviate (similar to a $z$-score), the sampling distribution for $F_{nd}$ is not normally distributed, so that $p$-values cannot be inferred from a given $F_{nd}$ value using traditional parametric methods. Statistical significance for an $F_{nd}$ value is given by the significance of the corresponding $F_{obs}$ value.

   The normalized deviate of homozygosity can also be used to characterize homozygosity values that deviate significantly from the null hypothesis in terms of modes of evolution. $F_{nd}$ values significantly lower than 0 result from allele-frequency distributions that are more "even" than expected and are consistent with the action of balancing selection. $F_{nd}$ values significantly higher than 0 result from allele-frequency distributions that are more skewed than expected toward specific alleles and are consistent with either directional selection or an extreme demographic effect.

In addition, because $F_{nd}$ is equal to 0 under the null hypothesis, a paired sign test (56) can be used to compare multiple $F_{nd}$ values against the expectation of neutrality.

PyPop calculates $F$ and $F_{nd}$ values.

### 3.6. Measures of Genetic Diversity

1. Heterozygosity

   The level of genetic diversity at a given locus is dependent upon the allele frequencies of the marker and the number of alleles observed in the sample. Within a given population, variation may be described by the heterozygosity ($H$), which ranges between 0 and 1:

$$H = 1 - \Sigma p_i^2,$$

   where $p_i$ is the frequency of the $i$th allele. For a population in HWE, this is the probability that a random individual in the population is a heterozygote. Heterozygosity will be maximized when all alleles are at an equal frequency.

2. Polymorphism information content

   The polymorphism information content (PIC) value is an additional statistic based on allele frequencies at a locus that describes the ability of a marker to differentiate individuals within a population (57):

$$\text{PIC} = 2\Sigma\Sigma p_i \times p_j(1 - p_i \times p_j),$$

   where $p_i$ is the frequency of the $i$th allele, and $p_j$ is the frequency of the $(i+1)$th allele. This is the probability that one of two individuals in a randomly mating population is a heterozygote and that the other is a different genotype. As with heterozygosity (H), PIC is maximized when all alleles are at equal frequency. The values of H and PIC are very similar at high heterozygosities, but PIC will never exceed H and its values are less than H when heterozygosity is low.

### 3.7. Measures of Genetic Differentiation

The measures below are used to quantify genetic variation within and between populations and to determine subdivisions (subpopulations) of a single source (total population).

1. $F_{ST}$

   $F_{ST}$ values quantify levels of population differentiation by assessing the proportion of genetic variance in subpopulations relative to the total genetic variance (58). $F_{ST}$ can be calculated based on a partitioning of heterozygosity:

$$F_{ST} = (H_t - H_S) / H_t,$$

where $H_t$ is the heterozygosity of the total population, and $H_s$ is the average heterozygosity of the subpopulations. Nei (59) has shown that this can be expressed in terms of allele frequencies:

$$F_{ST} = \Sigma\text{var}(p_i) / \Sigma\text{var}(1 - p_i),$$

where $p_i$ is the allele frequency of the *i*th allele in the total population and var($p_i$) is the variance of the *i*th allele over subpopulations. $F_{ST}$ is a qualitative measure, and Wright (60) has suggested guidelines for interpretation of these values:

0–0.05 indicates little genetic differentiation between subpopulations

0.05–0.15 indicates moderate genetic differentiation between subpopulations

0.15–0.25 indicates great genetic differentiation between subpopulations

0.25 and above indicates very great genetic differentiation between subpopulations

It has been shown that there is good concordance between $F_{ST}$ and average divergence times within and between subpopulations, given neutral loci and assuming the infinite alleles mutation model (61). $F_{ST}$ has been traditionally applied to data such as those obtained for allozyme variation. This measure may lose some power when applied to loci with a relatively high mutation rate, as has been suggested for microsatellite loci. Several different methods have been applied to estimate mutation rates for microsatellites (62, 63) and rates ranging from $10^{-3}$ to $10^{-5}$ have been reported.

2. $R_{ST}$

Additional measures related to $F_{ST}$ have been described for application to microsatellite data. Slatkin (64) introduced $R_{ST}$, which has similar properties to $F_{ST}$, but assumes a stepwise mutation process, as well as a relatively high mutation rate. It is calculated as:

$$R_{ST} = (S - S_w) / S,$$

where $S_w$ is the sum over all loci of twice the weighted mean of the within population variances, $V(A)$ and $V(B)$, and $S$ is the sum over all loci of twice the variance of the combined populations, $V(A+B)$. In computer simulations, it was demonstrated that $R_{ST}$ may provide a relatively more unbiased estimate of coalescence times compared to $F_{ST}$.

3. Population-pairwise $F_{ST}$

The degree of differentiation between pairs of populations (population-pairwise $F_{ST}$) can be used to investigate the existence of population structure (64–66). In accounting for small differences in subpopulation sample sizes, the population-pairwise $F_{ST}$ calculation may result in small negative pairwise $F_{ST}$ values; it is common practice to treat these negative values as being equivalent to zero. Pairwise standardized $F_{ST}$ values ( $F_{ST'}$ values) are generated using Hedrick's method of dividing each value by the maximum population-pairwise $F_{ST}$ value (67), allowing comparison of genetic differentiation between loci with different mutation rates and between populations with different effective sizes. For $n$ subpopulations, this population-pairwise approach results in a matrix of $n(n-1)$ $F_{ST}$ or $F_{ST'}$ values.

Arlequin will calculate $F_{ST}$ and population-pairwise $F_{ST}$ values. Supplementary Table S7 includes Arlequin-formatted genotype data for the synthetic datasets discussed in this chapter.

### 3.8. Graphical Representations of Genetic Difference Data

There are a variety of methods for representing genetic difference data between subpopulations in a graphical (as opposed to tabular) format. In many cases, the graphical representation can be applied independently of the measure of differentiation, so that multiple different genetic differentiation measures can be compared using the same graphical representation and multiple graphical representations can be applied to the same genetic differentiation measure. Because the graphical representation usually depends on an additional analysis, we describe some of the commonly used representations here as individual analyses.

In general, these representations should not necessarily be thought of as providing the definitive answer to a question so much as they serve as aids for the interpretation of genetic differentiation data that may be too complex to present in a tabular format (as with LD values). As Ada Lovelace noted, "the Analytical Engine has no pretensions whatever to *originate* anything." The results of these methods should always be interpreted critically, and the researcher who uses these methods should develop a set of criteria for accepting or rejecting the results of a method *before* using that method. Overinterpretation of any of these representations should be avoided when there is no obvious historical, functional, or biological basis for them.

1. Principal component analysis

   Principal component analysis (PCA) is used for dimensionality reduction in a data set, identifying those elements that contribute most to its variance, and is particularly useful as an exploratory tool in a complex data set (68). For the representation of genetic differentiation analyses, it is common to present the results of a PCA via multidimensional scaling (MDS), where each range for a given component is presented along a corresponding MDS axis (69, 70). Each data-element (a population or an individual) is represented by its position relative to each axis. This MDS approach allows the comparison of similarities and differences between populations, or the individuals that they comprise. For a 2D PCA MDS plot, distribution of points along the primary ($x$) axis will correspond to the greatest amount of variation in genetic distances in the data set (the first principal component); distribution along the $y$-axis corresponds to the next highest degree of the remaining variation that is not correlated with the $x$-axis (the second principal component). Because there can be many more than two principal components (as long as there remains variation that is not correlated with higher order components), comparisons can be related with multiple 2D PCA plots, representing the intersection of different components, or with multiple 3D visualizations. However, increasingly smaller percentages of the variance are represented by the higher numbered components, and these are usually not presented. In some cases, it may be necessary to present multiple plots for the same components. For example, when some populations display extensive genetic differentiation relative to others, it is often difficult to illustrate the differences between populations with relatively low degrees of differentiation; the PCA for these latter populations can be presented in a MDS plot with a smaller scale.

As noted above, PCA can be used to investigate differentiation between sampled individuals or between populations. The PCA-mediated comparison of individuals in multiple populations is in essence a population structure analysis, which is described below. For population-level analyses, genetic distances are first calculated in a pairwise fashion (e.g., as population-pairwise $F_{ST}$ values) between populations, and PCA is performed to assess the variation in distance between populations. PCA MDS analysis is available in a wide variety of statistical software applications (e.g., GenAlEx, and R packages). A population-level PCA would proceed via the following steps:

(i) Calculate allele or haplotype frequencies in a set of subpopulations.
(ii) Use a differentiation measure to generate a genetic distance matrix for the subpopulations.
(iii) Calculate the principal components from the distance matrix.
(iv) Generate a (series of) MDS figure(s) representing two or three of the principal components.

A 2D population-level PCA MDS plot generated in GenAlEx for the synthetic datasets discussed in this chapter is presented in Fig. 3. GenAlEx formatted data are included in Supplementary Table S8. (see Note 2).

2. Population structure analysis

Population substructure and population admixture can be directly investigated by estimating the likelihood that a given genotype belongs to a specific population. Likelihood values

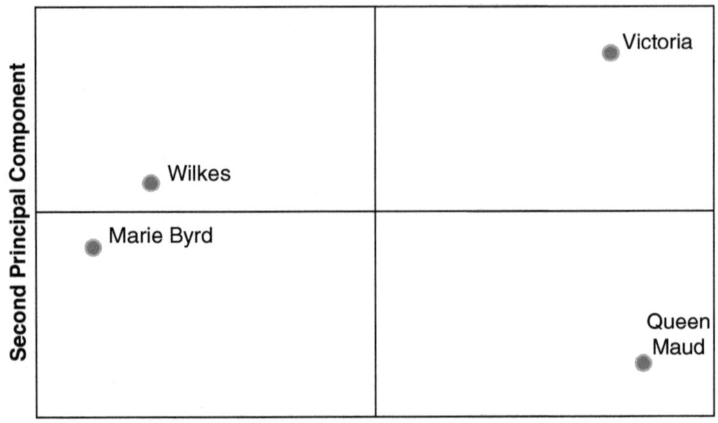


Fig. 3. Population-level principal component analysis multidimensional scaling plot generated using the supplementary data. Population-level principal component (PC) analysis of the synthetic data in Supplemental Table S8. The internal axes represent values of 0.0 for each component. The first PC in this plot represents 70% of the variance in these data, and the second PC represents 26%. Higher order PCs describe only 4% of the variance and do not need to be presented.

can be calculated based on HWEP, allele frequencies, and LD (if available) and are used to assign individual genotypes to specific groups or clusters, which can range from individual populations to geographic regions. As with phylogenetic trees, these clustering results can be displayed using multiple graphical representations. A 2D individual-level PCA plot generated in GenAlEx for the synthetic datasets discussed in this chapter is presented in Fig. 4.

While there are many clustering tools available, the most widely used is Structure (71, 72), which Rosenberg et al. (73) used to cluster the populations of the CEPH Human Genetic Diversity Panel, largely by geographic origin, on the basis of genotype data for a genome-wide set of 377 microsatellites. Structure iteratively resamples individuals into a number of user-defined clusters (K) and calculates the likelihood for each organization via Bayesian inference from expected HWEPs. In addition, other types of clustering analyses can also be carried out with Arlequin, CLUTO (74), and various R packages.

Supplementary Table S9 contains Structure-formatted genotype data for the synthetic datasets discussed in this chapter. Figure 5 includes structure plots generated with these synthetic datasets for $K=2$ and 4 (see Note 3).

3. Phylogenetic analysis

A phylogenetic tree (aka dendrogram) is a branching representation of the evolutionary history between populations, individuals, or gene/protein sequences (taxa) based upon similarities and differences in some characteristic (for our purposes, immunogenetic allele and haplotype frequencies) shared by all taxa.

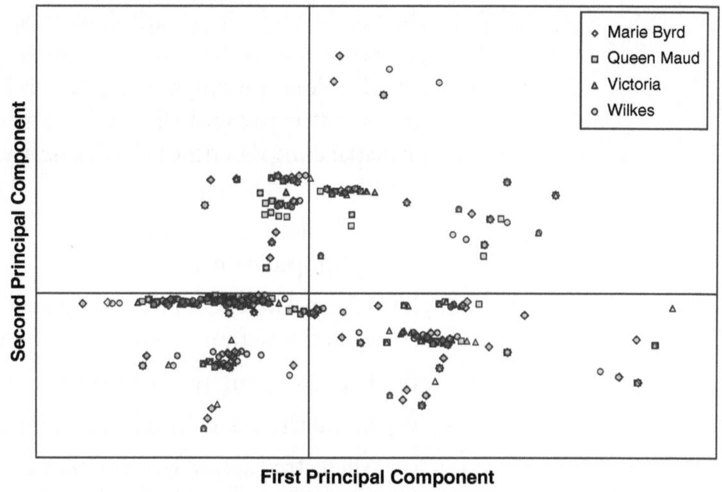


Fig. 4. Individual-level principal component analysis multidimensional scaling plot generated using the supplementary data. Individual-level principal component (PC) analysis of the synthetic data in Supplemental Table S8. The internal axes represent values of 0.0 for each component. The first PC in this plot represents 21% of the variance in these data, and the second PC represents 19%. Because higher order PCs describe 60% of the variance (evident from the extensive clustering of individuals in the second PC dimension), additional PC dimensions should be presented.

Fig. 5. Structure bar plot generated using the supplementary data. Structure analysis of the synthetic data in Supplementary Table S9 with the number of clusters (K) set to 2 or 4. Vertical bars represent each individual included in the analysis, and each tone (or color in the electronic version) indicates the extent to which that individual's genotype is derived from one of the K clusters, with each tone (or color) corresponding to a cluster. Because of the low number of loci and the extensive sharing of alleles between populations, very few individuals are assigned to a single cluster (tone/color). However, the relative relatedness of each population can be inferred from the tone/color compositions of their constituents.

Trees generated using gene or protein sequences (sequence trees) often allow inferences regarding the relative "age" of sequence variants and the inference of ancestral sequences. We do not discuss sequence trees here. Trees generated using population-level allele-frequency data (population trees) can represent relative degrees of shared ancestry between populations. Where sequence trees can be interpreted as gene genealogies, population trees should be considered as graphs of the general trends in relationships between modern populations, which can change in ways (e.g., admixture, splitting, fusion, bottlenecks, etc.) that nucleotide and protein sequences cannot. In particular, the relationships represented by population trees are generally representative of the first (and sometimes second) principal components of the frequency data used to generate them. Population trees are generated via the following general steps.

(i) Calculate allele or haplotype frequencies in a set of subpopulations.

(ii) Use a differentiation measure to generate an estimated genetic distance matrix for the subpopulations.

(iii) Calculate the tree topology from the distance matrix.

(iv) Generate a tree figure representing that tree topology.

Allele-frequency-based genetic distance calculations do not take the sequence relationships between individual alleles into account, so that all alleles are considered to be equidistant from each other; for many immunogenetic alleles (e.g., those that diverged prior to the radiation of human populations from Africa), this should not be an issue, but when populations display large differences in frequency for alleles or haplotypes that have been relatively recently generated (e.g., DRB1*08:02:01 and DRB1*08:07), genetic distances may be overestimated, resulting in very large branch lengths. Similarly, alleles that may be reported differently depending on the typing method used (e.g., DRB1*14:01:01 and DRB1*14:54) may result in similar overestimates. In these cases, the datasets should be reviewed for consistency in the level of resolution of typing, and alternate names for what is potentially the same allele should be binned into a common category (e.g., DRB1*14:01:01G). Finally, trees including isolated populations with low values of $k$, in which a few alleles are subject to genetic drift, may suffer similar problems. It is oftentimes useful to establish threshold for sample size (e.g., $2n>49$) and $k$ (e.g., >5) to exclude populations that are too small or display too few alleles.

In general, phylogenies can be drawn as either "rooted" or "unrooted" trees, as illustrated in Fig. 6; rooted trees identify a common ancestor for all of the taxa, giving the tree directionality from root to twigs. We recommend presenting population trees constructed using immunogenetic allele and haplotype frequencies as unrooted, as it is difficult to know exactly how or where to place the root. For example, the influence of low values of k on branch lengths (discussed above) raises questions about the effectiveness and appropriateness of midpoint rooting. Similarly, because these trees are based on frequency distributions, the lack of a nonhuman population sharing allelic and haplotypic diversity with human populations makes outgroup rooting difficult.

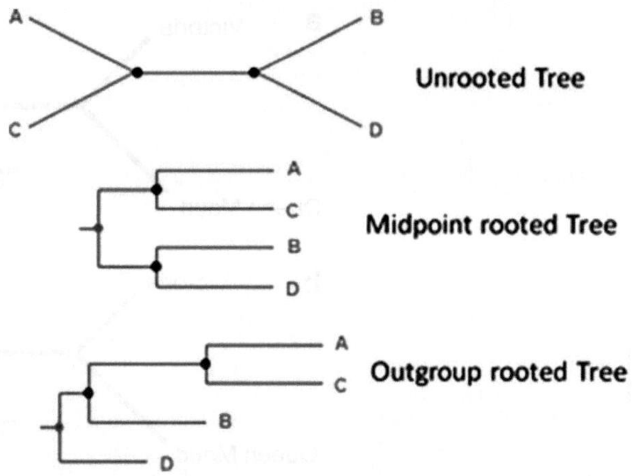


Fig. 6. Examples of phylogenetic trees. Three representations of the same phylogeny for four taxa (A–D). *Black dots* indicate nodes in each tree. The branches between each taxon and the nearest node are known as "twigs" or "leaves". *Grey dots* in the rooted trees indicate the position of the root node. Taxa A and C are more similar to each other than either is to taxon B or D, and taxa B and C are more similar to each other than either is to taxon A or D. In the unrooted tree and the midpoint rooted tree, A and C are in one clade, and B and D are in a second clade. In the outgroup rooted tree, A, B, and C are in a single clade, to the exclusion of D.

PHYLIP

The PHYLogeny Inference Package (PHYLIP) (75, 76) is a software suite of applications for building phylogenetic trees using a variety of methods. Supplementary Table S10 is a PHYLIP GENDIST-formatted allele-frequency data file for the synthetic population datasets analyzed in this chapter. Figure 7 includes a pair of unrooted Neighbor-Joining (NJ) (77) trees generated using the data included in Supplementary Tables S7 and S10.

The tree in Fig. 7a is based on Nei's standard genetic distances (SGD) (78) calculated in PHYLIP, whereas the tree in Fig. 7b is based on population-pairwise $F_{ST}$ values calculated in Arlequin. A genetic distance scale should be included with every tree.

Steps (ii)–(iv) outlined above were carried out with PHYLIP to generate Fig. 7a using the GENDIST (for step ii.), NEIGHBOR (for step iii.), and DRAWTREE (for step iv) programs to draw unrooted NJ trees based on Nei's Standard Genetic Distances. Figure 7b was generated using the same procedure for steps (iii) and (iv), but steps (i) and (ii) were carried out using Arlequin to generate population-pairwise $F_{ST}$ values.

PHYLIP's GENDIST estimates genetic distance with three different measures—Nei's SGD, Cavalli-Sforza's chord distance (79), and Reynold's genetic distance (65)—and each measure is based on implicit assumptions that may not always apply to immunogenetic data. For example, all three measures assume that population differentiation derives from genetic drift, yet the HLA loci have been shown to be under balancing selection in numerous studies (4, 80, 81).

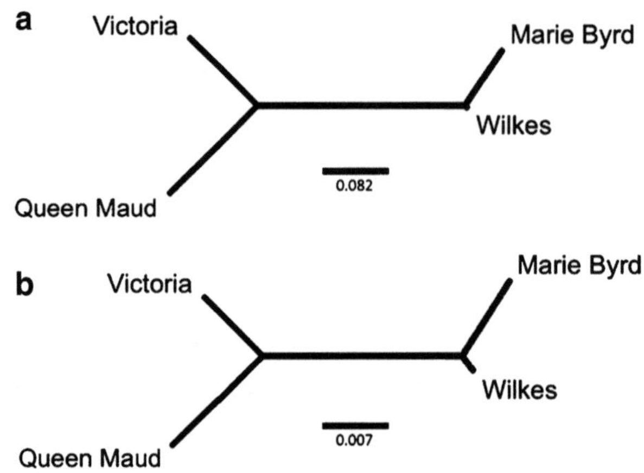


Fig. 7. Phylogenetic trees generated using the supplementary data. (**a**) Unrooted neighbor-joining tree generated in PHYLIP using Nei's standard genetic distances (included in Supplemental Table S10) generated for the synthetic data in Supplementary Tables S1–S4. Inset bar shows a genetic distance of 0.082. (**b**). Unrooted neighbor-joining tree generated in PHYLIP using population-pairwise $F_{ST}$ distances generated in Arlequin for the synthetic data in Supplementary Table S7. *Inset bar* shows a population-pairwise $F_{ST}$ distance of 0.007.

Nei's SGD assumes that new alleles arise by neutral mutation, and that the mutation rate is equal across all loci; again, the latter assumption clearly does not hold for HLA loci, where there are many more class I alleles than class II alleles, and where many HLA-B alleles are observed to be restricted to specific regions of the world, whereas most HLA-DQA1 and DQB1 alleles are observed in all populations (82).

However, the Cavalli-Sforza and Reynolds distance models assume no mutation; frequency differences between populations are assumed to be the result of genetic drift alone. This assumption of no mutation seems even a further departure from observed immunogenetic biology than the assumption of locus-identical neutral mutation, as unique HLA alleles are observed on a regular basis (83), and natural selection appears to have favored novel HLA allele variants over older variants in North and South American populations (84, 85).

Clearly, none of these models applies perfectly to immunogenetic data. Our empirical experience has been that HLA gene-trees conform best to expectations when generated using Nei's SGD; this distance estimate includes a mutational component, which clearly applies to HLA data.

PHYLIP's NEIGHBOR (see Note 4) builds trees with either of two clustering methods—NJ and Unweighted Pair Group Method with Arithmetic Mean (UPGMA) (86, 87). For the purposes of this discussion, the primary difference between these methods is the assumption of the rate of evolution. The NJ method does not assume a regular stochastic evolutionary rate (i.e., a molecular clock), while the UPGMA method does. This difference means that NJ trees are inherently unrooted (and should be drawn as such), while UPGMA trees are inherently rooted. The assumption of a molecular clock in the UPGMA method makes these trees particularly ill-suited for building immunogenetic gene-frequency trees, as exonic immunogenetic allelic differentiation does not conform to a molecular clock model; for the HLA loci, different modes of evolution are in effect for introns, non-ARS-encoding exon sequences, and ARS-encoding exon sequences (85, 88, 89).

*For the generation of immunogenetic gene-frequency trees in PHYLIP, we recommend building NJ trees with Nei's SGD.*

4. Criteria for rejection or acceptance of trees

   As discussed above, it is important to develop criteria for the purpose of evaluating trees prior to analysis. Sequence trees can be evaluated via bootstrapping (90, 91), in which a population of trees is generated by resampling subsets of the primary data. The topologies of the resulting trees are compared and each branch in the consensus tree is evaluated based on degree of sharing of topological features across the population of trees.

   For sequence trees, resampled datasets are generated by randomly sampling and duplicating subsets of nucleotide or peptide positions, but resampled gene-tree datasets are generated by randomly sampling and duplicating entire loci; therefore bootstrapping cannot be used to evaluate gene-trees constructed for single loci, and bootstrapping performs poorly for gene-trees constructed with a small number of loci. For example, gene-trees constructed using two loci will yield bootstrap values of 0.0, 0.5, or 1.0.

   Studies of population relationships at non-MHC loci have generally shown a close correlation between genetics and geography, so that populations tend to share similar allele frequencies with their neighbors on a local level (92, 93). Therefore, it is not unreasonable to expect that most populations will be represented as being more closely related to their neighbors (populations in the same global region) than to nonneighboring populations in gene-trees, and that most relationships in a tree will corroborate geographic, historical, anthropologic, and linguistic evidence. Mack and Erlich (94) proposed that HLA gene-trees be rejected as invalid if more than 6% of the intraregional population relationships in that tree do not meet this expectation. This criterion is necessarily conservative; if a tree meets no expectations, it is difficult to say which relationships are genuine, and which might be spurious. Trees such as these may reveal more about the diversification of the loci investigated than than they do about population relationships. Finally, population relationships, however unexpected, that are repeatedly observed in trees derived from different markers, clearly merit serious consideration as reflecting actual relationships rather than as a spurious artifact of the tree-building process.

## 4. Notes

1. For the most part, publications that use HW testing in this manner, including this chapter, share a common approach: regardless of the method, all attempt to detect a statistically significant difference between the observed genotype frequencies and those expected under HWEP; these expected frequencies derive from a Null hypothesis ($H_0$) that assumes the HW model is true. While much effort has gone into the development of these statistical methods, the approach itself is rarely questioned. Perhaps, rather than evaluating data on the basis of a failure to detect statistically significant HW deviations, it should be demonstrated that any detected departure from HWE is below a critical threshold, allowing one to assume that the HW model still applies.

   The field of bioequivalence clinical trials has shown that classical difference testing may not be optimal for assessing absence of association when dealing with the modest effects that characterize departure from the HW model in genetic epidemiology studies. Whereas difference testing returns the probability of observing a difference by chance, equivalency testing returns the probability of observing a lack of departure (or a modest departure) by chance. Equivalence testing is often implemented as two one-sided tests: one returns the probability of observing a lack of difference if the actual departure is positive (e.g., homozygote excess), and the other returns the probability of a lack of difference if the actual departure is respectively negative (heterozygote excess). In the future, a more natural approach to the HW testing may better quantify the extent to which data do not depart from HWEP.

2. To generate a population-level PCA plot using GenAlEx, population allele frequencies are calculated and a genetic distance matrix is derived from the frequency distributions for each locus. In this case Nei's unbiased genetic distances (95) were used, but Nei's standard genetic distances (78) can also be used. The PCA is based on the genetic distance between population groups. For a PCA plot at the individual level (see Fig. 4), a matrix of genetic distances is computed from the raw genotype data, and the PCA plot is generated from the between-individual distance matrix.

3. When creating a Structure project with this file, indicate the number of individuals (694), the ploidy of the data (2, diploid), the number of loci (2), the value provided for missing data (−1), the presence of a header row of marker names, the special format for the file including all data for each individual on a single line, the inclusion of a column for the sample ID of each sampled individual, and the inclusion of a column identifying the population origin for each sampled individual. Then, create a parameter set that defines the ancestry model (admixture), the allele-frequency model (independent), and the run-length in terms of the length of Burnin Period (50,000), and the number of Monte Carlo Markov Chain (MCMC) reps after Burnin (50,000). For other datasets, these last two values will need to be determined empirically, by observing the number of reps necessary for the alpha-value to converge. To start a Structure run, specify the number of clusters (K) assumed for the data (2 or 4). Group the resulting Bar Plot by population ID to generate results similar to those in Fig. 5. Because Structure clustering is accomplished via Bayesian inference, Structure should be run multiple times for datasets that include large numbers of individuals at many markers, and the results compared for overall trends.
4. When using NEIGHBOR, researchers should always use the Jumble (J) option to randomize the input order of taxa.

## Acknowledgments

This work was supported by National Institutes of Health (NIH) grants U01AI067068 (JAH, SJM) and U19 AI067152 (PAG) awarded by the National Institute of Allergy and Infectious Diseases (NIAID) and by NIH/NIAID contract AI40076 (RMS, GT). The content is solely the responsibility of the authors and does not necessarily represent the official views of the National Institute of Allergy and Infectious Diseases or the National Institutes of Health.

## References

1. R Core Development Team (2008) R: A language and environment for statistical computing. R Foundation for Statistical Computing, Vienna, Austria
2. Li W, Hu Z, Jiang W (2010) An alphabetic list of genetic analysis software. North Shore LIJ Research Institute. http://www.nslij-genetics.org/soft/. Accessed 7 Oct 2010
3. Lancaster AK, Single RM, Solberg OD, Nelson MP, Thomson G (2007) PyPop update—a software pipeline for large-scale multilocus population genomics. Tissue Antigens 69(s1):192–197
4. Solberg OD, Mack SJ, Lancaster AK, Single RM, Tsai Y, Sanchez-Mazas A, Thomson G (2008) Balancing selection and heterogeneity across the classical human leukocyte antigen

loci: a meta-analytic review of 497 population studies. Hum Immunol 69(7):443–464

5. Peakall R, Smouse PE (2006) GENALEX 6: genetic analysis in Excel. Population genetic software for teaching and research. Mol Ecol Notes 6:288–295
6. Lynch M, Milligan BG (1994) Analysis of population genetic structure with RAPD markers. Mol Ecol 3:91–99
7. Louis EJ, Dempster ER (1987) An exact test for Hardy-Weinberg and multiple alleles. Biometrics 43(4):805–811
8. Levene H (1949) On a matching problem arising in genetics. Ann Math Stat 20(1):91–94
9. Emigh TH (1980) A comparison of tests for Hardy-Weinberg equilibrium. Biometrics 36(4):627–642
10. Guo SW, Thompson EA (1992) Performing the exact test of Hardy-Weinberg proportion for multiple alleles. Biometrics 48(2): 361–372
11. Huber M, Chen Y, Dinwoodie I, Dobra A, Nicholas M (2006) Monte Carlo algorithms for Hardy-Weinberg proportions. Biometrics 62:49–53
12. Yuan A, Bonney GE (2003) Exact test of Hardy-Weinberg equilibrium by Markov chain Monte Carlo. Math Med Biol 20:327–340
13. Ebrahimi N, Bilgili D (2007) A new method of testing for Hardy-Weinberg equilibrium and ordering populations. J Genet 86:1–7
14. Metropolis N, Rosenbluth AW, Rosenbluth MN, Teller AH, Teller E (1953) Equations of state calculations by fast computing machines. J Chem Phys 21:1087–1092
15. Chen JJ, Hollenbach JA, Trachtenberg EA, Just JJ, Carrington M, Rønningen KS, Begovich A, King MC, McWeeney SK, Mack SJ, Erlich HA, Thomson G (1999) Hardy-Weinberg testing for HLA class II (DRB1, DQA1, DQB1 and DPB1) loci in 26 human ethnic groups. Tissue Antigens 54:533–542
16. Hernández JL, Weir BS (1989) A disequilibrium coefficient approach to Hardy-Weinberg testing. Biometrics 45(1):53–70
17. Chen JJ, Thomson G (1999) The variance for the disequilibrium coefficient in the individual Hardy-Weinberg test. Biometrics 55:1269–1272
18. Barnetche T, Gourraud PA, Cambon-Thomsen A (2005) Strategies in analysis of the genetic component of multifactorial diseases; biostatistical aspects. Transpl Immunol 14(3–4): 255–266
19. Guan Y, Stephens M (2008) Practical issues in imputation-based association mapping. PLoS Genet 4(12):e1000279
20. Piazza A (1975) Haplotypes and linkage disequilibria from three-locus phenotypes. In: Kissmeyer-Nielsen F (ed) Histocompatibility testing. Munskgaard, Copenhagen, pp 923–927
21. Dempster AP, Laird NM, Rubin DB (1977) Maximum likelihood from incomplete data via the EM algorithm. J R Stat Soc 39:1–38
22. Ott J (1977) Counting methods (EM algorithm) in human pedigree analysis: linkage and segregation analysis. Ann Hum Genet 40:443–454
23. Yasuda N (1978) Estimation of haplotype frequency and linkage disequilibrium parameter in the HLA system. Tissue Antigens 12:315–322
24. Morton NE, Simpson SP, Lew R, Yee S (1983) Estimation of haplotype frequencies. Tissue Antigens 22(4):257–262
25. Hawley ME, Kidd KK (1995) HAPLO: a program using the EM algorithm to estimate the frequencies of multisite haplotypes. J Hered 86:409–411
26. Long JC, Williams RC, Urbanek M (1995) An E-M algorithm and testing strategy for multiple-locus haplotypes. Am J Hum Genet 56:799–810
27. Fallin D, Schork NJ (2000) Accuracy of haplotype frequency estimation for biallelic loci, via the expectation-maximization algorithm for unphased diploid genotype data. Am J Hum Genet 67:947–959
28. Tishkoff SA, Pakstis AJ, Ruano G, Kidd KK (2000) The accuracy of statistical methods for estimation of haplotype frequencies: an example from the CD4 locus. Am J Hum Genet 67:518–522
29. Kirk KM, Cardon LR (2002) The impact of genotyping error on haplotype reconstruction and frequency estimation. Eur J Hum Genet 10:616–622
30. Single RM, Meyer D, Hollenbeck J, Nelson M, Noble JA, Erlich HA, Thomson G (2002) Haplotype frequency estimation in patient populations: the effect of departures from Hardy-Weinberg proportions and collapsing over a locus in the HLA region. Gen Epidemiol 22:186–195
31. Stephens M, Smith NJ, Donnelly P (2001) A new statistical method for haplotype reconstruction from population data. Am J Hum Genet 68:978–989
32. Niu T, Qin ZS, Xu X, Liu JS (2002) Bayesian haplotype inference for multiple linked single-nucleotide polymorphisms. Am J Hum Genet 70:157–169
33. Qin ZS, Niu T, Liu JS (2002) Partition-ligation-expectationmaximization algorithm for haplotype inference with singlenucleotide

polymorphisms. Am J Hum Genet 71: 1242–1247

34. Stephens M, Donnelly P (2003) A comparison of Bayesian methods for haplotype reconstruction from population genotype data. Am J Hum Genet 73:1162–1169
35. Niu T (2004) Algorithms for inferring haplotypes. Genet Epidemiol 27(4):334–347
36. Slatkin M, Excoffier L (1996) Testing for linkage disequilibrium in genotypic data using the Expectation-Maximization algorithm. Heredity 76:377–383
37. Tishkoff SA, Kidd KK (2004) Implications of biogeography of human populations for 'race' and medicine. Nat Genet 36(Suppl 11):S21–S27
38. Robinson J, Waller MJ, Fail SC, Marsh SG (2006) The IMGT/HLA and IPD databases. Hum Mutat 27:1192–1199
39. Gourraud PA, Gagne K, Bignon JD, Cambon-Thomsen A, Middleton D (2007) Preliminary analysis of a KIR haplotype estimation algorithm: a simulation study. Tissue Antigens 69(Suppl 1):96–100
40. Yoo YJ, Tang J, Kaslow RA, Zhang K (2007) Haplotype inference for present-absent genotype data using previously identified haplotypes and haplotype patterns. Bioinformatics 23(18):2399–2406
41. Lewontin RC (1964) The interaction of selection and linkage. I. General considerations; heterotic models. Genetics 49:49–67
42. Hill WG, Robertson A (1968) Linkage disequilibrium in finite populations. Theor Appl Genet (Der Ziichter) 38:226–231
43. Klitz W, Stephen JC, Grote M, Carrington M (1995) Discordant patterns of linkage disequilibrium of the peptide transporter loci within the HLA class II region. Am J Hum Genetics 57:1436–1444
44. Cramer H (1946) Mathematical methods of statistics. Princeton University Press, Princeton, NJ
45. Cohen J (1988) Statistical power analysis for the behavioral sciences. Erlbaum, Hillsdale, NJ
46. Hedrick PW (1987) Gametic disequilibrium measures: proceed with caution. Genetics 117(2):331–341
47. Abecasis GR, Cookson WO (2000) GOLD-graphical overview of linkage disequilibrium. Bioinformatics 16:182–183
48. Barrett JC, Fry B, Maller J, Daly MJ (2005) Haploview: analysis and visualization of LD and haplotype maps. Bioinformatics 21(2):263–265
49. Gaunt TR, Rodriguez S, Zapata C, Day IN (2006) MIDAS: software for analysis and visualisation of interallelic disequilibrium between multiallelic markers. BMC Bioinformatics 7:227–237
50. Shin J-H, Blay S, McNeney B, Graham J (2006) LDheatmap: an R function for graphical display of pairwise linkage disequilibria between single nucleotide polymorphisms. J Stat Soft 16 Code Snippet 3
51. Ewens WJ (1972) The sampling theory of selectively neutral alleles. Theor Popul Biol 3(1):87–112
52. Watterson G (1978) The homozygosity test of neutrality. Genetics 88:405–417
53. Slatkin M (1994) An exact test for neutrality based on the Ewens sampling distribution. Genet Res 64:71–74
54. Slatkin M (1996) A correction to the exact test based on the Ewens sampling distribution. Genet Res 68:259–260
55. Salamon H, Klitz W, Easteal S, Gao X, Erlich HA, Fernandez-Vina M, Trachtenberg EA (1999) Evolution of HLA class II molecules: allelic and amino acid site variability across populations. Genetics 152:393–400
56. Conover W (1980) Practical nonparametric statistics. Wiley, New York
57. Chakravarti A (1991) Information content of the Cen tre d'Etude du Polymorphisme Humain (CEPH) family structures for linkage studies. Hum Genet 87:721–724
58. Wright S (1951) The genetic structure of populations. Ann Eugen 15:323–354
59. Nei M (1977) F-statistics and analysis of gene diversity in subdivided populations. Ann Hum Genet 41:225–233
60. Wright S (1978) Evolution and the genetics of populations, vol 4. The University of Chicago Press, Chicago, Variability Within and Among Natural Populations
61. Slatkin M (1991) Inbreeding coefficients and coalescence times. Genet Res 58:167–175
62. Weber JL, Wong C (1993) Mutation of human short tandem repeats. Hum Mol Genet 2(8):1123–1128
63. Gyapay G, Morissette J, Vignal A, Dib C, Fizames C, Millasseau P, Marc S, Bernardi G, Lathrop M, Weissenbach J (1994) The 1993–1994 Genethon human genetic linkage map. Nat Genet 7:246–339
64. Slatkin M (1995) A measure of population subdivision based on microsatellite allele frequencies. Genetics 139:457–462
65. Reynolds J, Weir BS, Cockerham CC (1983) Estimation for the coancestry coefficient: basis for a short-term genetic distance. Genetics 105:767–779

66. Weir BS, Cockerham CC (1984) Estimating F-statistics for the analysis of population structure. Evolution 38:1358–1370
67. Hedrick PW (2005) A standardized genetic differentiation measure. Evolution 59:1633–1638
68. Pearson K (1901) "On lines and planes of closest fit to systems of points in space" (PDF). Phil Mag 2(6):559–572
69. Cox TF, Cox MAA (2001) Multidimensional Scaling, 2nd edn. Chapman and Hall, Boca Raton, FL
70. Borg I, Groenen P (2005) Modern multidimensional scaling: theory and applications, 2nd edn. Springer, New York
71. Pritchard JK, Stephens M, Donnelly P (2000) Inference of population structure using multilocus genotype data. Genetics 155(2):945–959
72. Hubisz MJ, Falush D, Stephens M, Pritchard JK (2009) Inferring weak population structure with the assistance of sample group information. Mol Ecol Resour 9(5):1322–1332
73. Rosenberg NA, Pritchard JK, Weber JL, Cann HM, Kidd KK, Zhivotovsky LA, Feldman MW (2002) Genetic structure of human populations. Science 298(5602):2381–2385
74. Karypis G. (2002) CLUTO: a clustering toolkit. Technical Report 02-017. University of Minnesota, Minneapolis, MN
75. Felsenstein J (1989) PHYLIP—Phylogeny Inference Package (Version 3.2). Cladistics 5:164–166
76. Felsenstein, J. (2005) PHYLIP (Phylogeny Inference Package) version 3.6 (Distributed by the author). Department of Genome Sciences, University of Washington, Seattle
77. Saitou N, Nei M (1987) The neighbor-joining method: a new method for reconstructing phylogenetic trees. Mol Biol Evol 4(4):406–425
78. Nei M (1972) Genetic distance between populations. Am Nat 106:283–292
79. Cavalli-Sforza LL, Edwards AFW (1967) Phylogenetic analysis: models and estimation procedures. Am J Hum Genet 19:233–257
80. Hughes AL, Nei M (1988) Pattern of nucleotide substitution at MHC class I loci reveals overdominant selection. Nature 335:167–170
81. Hughes AL, Yeager M (1998) Natural selection at major histocompatibility complex loci of vertebrates. Ann Rev Genet 32:415–435
82. Sanchez-Mazas A, Fernandez-Viña M, Middleton D, Hollenbach JA, Buhler S, Di D, Rajalingam R, Dugoujon JM, Mack SJ, Thorsby E (2011) Immunogenetics as a tool in anthropological studies. Immunology 133(2):143–164
83. Middleton D, Gonzalez F, Fernandez-Vina M, Tiercy JM, Marsh SG, Aubrey M, Bicalho MG, Canossi A, Carter V, Cate S, Guerini FR, Loiseau P, Martinetti M, Moraes ME, Morales V, Perasaari J, Setterholm M, Sprague M, Tavoularis S, Torres M, Vidal S, Witt C, Wohlwend G, Yang KL (2009) A bioinformatics approach to ascertaining the rarity of HLA alleles. Tissue Antigens 74:480–485
84. Cadavid LF, Watkins DI (1997) Heirs of the jaguar and the anaconda: HLA, conquest and disease in the indigenous populations of the Americas. Tissue Antigens 6:702–711
85. Erlich HA, Mack SJ, Bergström T, Gyllensten UB (1997) HLA class II alleles in Amerindian populations: implications for the evolution of HLA polymorphism and the colonization of the Americas. Hereditas 127(1–2):19–24
86. Sokal R, Michener C (1958) A statistical method for evaluating systematic relationships. Univ Kansas Sci Bull 38:1409–1438
87. Murtagh F (1984) Complexities of hierarchic clustering algorithms: the state of the art. Comput Stat Quart 1:101–113
88. Bergström TF, Josefsson A, Erlich HA, Gyllensten UB (1997) Analysis of intron sequences at the class II HLA-DRB1 locus: implications for the age of allelic diversity. Hereditas 127(1–2):1–5
89. Bergström TF, Josefsson A, Erlich HA, Gyllensten U (1998) Recent origin of HLA-DRB1 alleles and implications for human evolution. Nat Genet 18(3):237–242
90. Felsenstein J (1985) Confidence limits on phylogenies: an approach using the bootstrap. Evolution 39:783–791
91. Penny D, Hendry MD (1985) Testing methods of evolutionary tree construction. Cladistics 1:266–278
92. Cavalli-Sforza LL, Menozzi P, Piazza A (1994) The history and geography of human genes. Princeton University Press, Pinceton, NJ
93. Cavalli-Sforza LL, Feldman MW (2003) The application of molecular genetic approaches to the study of human evolution. Nat Genet 33:266–275
94. Mack SJ, Erlich HA (2007) Population relationships as inferred from classical HLA genes. 13th International histocompatibility workshop anthropology/human genetic diversity joint report. In: Hansen JA (ed) Immunobiology of the human MHC: Proceedings of the 13th international histocompatibility workshop and conference, vol I. IHWG, Seattle, pp. 747–757
95. Nei M (1978) Estimation of average heterozygosity and genetic distance from a small number of individuals. Genetics 89:583–590

# Chapter 14

# Analytical Methods for Disease Association Studies with Immunogenetic Data

**Jill A. Hollenbach, Steven J. Mack, Glenys Thomson, and Pierre-Antoine Gourraud**

**Abstract**

Disease association studies involving highly polymorphic immunogenetic data may involve analyses at one or many units of analysis, including amino acid, allele, genotype and haplotype levels, as well as consideration of gene–gene or gene–environment interactions. The selection of the appropriate statistical tests is critical and will be dependent on the nature of the dataset (e.g., case-control vs. family data) as well as the specific research hypotheses being tested. This paper describes the various study and analysis categories used for such analyses, including the advantages and limitations of such techniques.

**Key words:** HLA, KIR, Immunogenetic, Data analysis, Disease association, Case-control, Family

## 1. Introduction

> Statistics may be defined as "a body of methods for making wise decisions in the face of uncertainty."
>
> W.A. Wallis

There is no shortage of statistical methods and tools available for the analysis of genetic data; in disease association studies these provide the results upon which we draw inferences about human health, and often influence the direction of future research, clinical protocols, and public health policy. However, just as Wallis suggested statistics assist us in making wise decisions in an uncertain world, it is also imperative that we first *make wise decisions about*

Frank T. Christiansen and Brian D. Tait (eds.), *Immunogenetics: Methods and Applications in Clinical Practice*, Methods in Molecular Biology, vol. 882, DOI 10.1007/978-1-61779-842-9_14, © Springer Science+Business Media New York 2012

*how we apply statistical methods.* Unless utilized properly, statistics can provide misleading results in disease association studies, consuming precious resources and often leading investigators down blind alleys.

The human leukocyte antigen (HLA) loci serve as a model for the study of genetic variation in human health and disease (1). Their critical role in disease predisposition in a variety of autoimmune, infectious diseases and cancers (2–25), as well as transplant outcomes, has long been recognized. Likewise, a role for the killer cell immunoglobulin-like receptors (KIR) loci and their HLA ligands in autoimmune diseases (26–29) and infectious diseases (HIV and Hepatitis C (30, 31)) as well as solid organ and hematopoietic stem cell transplantation (32–34) and pregnancy (35, 36) is now established. However, the high levels of polymorphism associated with these loci mean that particular care must be taken when analyzing data for disease association studies, in order to avoid confounding results. In this chapter, we discuss the appropriate application of common statistical methods in the analysis of highly polymorphic immunogenetic data. While most of these analyses can be undertaken with either customized or commercial computer software, no *existing* programs, either individually, or in aggregate, can handle the breadth and complexity of the analyses needed to detect primary and secondary disease genes in polymorphic immunogenetic regions. The complex linkage disequilibrium (LD) patterns common to many immunogenetic data are a major complicating factor in deciphering specific *causal* genetic variants. Further, many analysis programs do not work with the high degree of polymorphism found in some regions, for example HLA, while others only allow a limited number of highly polymorphic loci to be evaluated.

The effects of environmental factors, age of onset and gender-specific effects, undetected heterogeneity of disease, gene–gene and gene–environment interactions further complicate our attempts to detect predisposing (PRE) genes for complex diseases. We thus strongly recommend a multistrategy approach using a variety of complementary methods. The data should be studied carefully to understand differences in significance obtained from different methods. There is no "best practice" for the types of analyses needed for these projects. The power of different methods will vary depending on the specific genetic and environmental features of the disease under consideration; for most complex diseases this involves many unknown factors. Although we must rely heavily on computers, in the final analysis of multiple effects in a genetic region and/or interaction or independent effects between unlinked genes, manipulation of the data by the individual investigator must play a crucial role.

## 2. Study and Analysis Categories

### 2.1. Case-Control Studies

Case-control studies are a critical, population-based tool for epidemiological studies, including genetic association studies. These studies generally involve samples of unrelated individuals with the (disease) phenotype of interest and a corresponding control sample of unrelated, unaffected (or randomly ascertained) individuals drawn from the same (ethnic and preferably geographic) population. While a discussion of study design, including power calculations and sample size considerations is out of the scope of this chapter, a general recommendation in immunogenetic studies is to have a minimum of 200 chromosomes (100 individuals) in each of the case and control cohorts, although much larger sample sizes are preferable. Among the advantages of case-control studies is elimination of the necessity to collect data from family members, which is often logistically difficult and costly. However, case-control studies can be very sensitive to population stratification within the sample cohorts, a particularly important issue in immunogenetic data, where allele frequency distributions can vary considerably between human ethnic groups. If the samples are not collected with scrupulous attention to homogeneity of ancestry background, investigators run the risk of misinterpreting genetic difference between cases and controls. In these cases, heterogeneity between cases and controls due to allele frequency differences related to population stratification may be mistaken for association with a particular locus.

Population analyses, including calculations of gene (allele) frequencies, tests for fit to expectations under Hardy–Weinberg Equilibrium (HWE), and estimations of haplotype frequencies, are the first step in any study involving immunogenetic data, and will provide additional means to assess any underlying population substructure, as well as additional units of analysis on which association analyses will be performed. These calculations are detailed in Chap. 13. Many computer software programs are available to perform such calculations on genetic data, but as mentioned in Chap. 13, care must be taken to utilize tools either specifically designed for immunogenetic data (e.g., the PYPOP analytical package (http://www.pypop.org)) or those that are able to handle the high levels of polymorphism characteristic of these loci.

#### 2.1.1. Contingency Tables

1. Basic construction and analysis of contingency tables, with particular attention to sparse cells.

   A contingency table, or cross-tabulation, is used to test the difference, or independence, of frequency distributions for categorical variables. Tests for heterogeneity between specific groups (e.g., cases and controls) for immunogenetic data can be performed using contingency table testing and a standard Chi-square ($\chi^2$) measure. Software implementations of contingency table analyses are available through a variety of commercial packages (e.g., SAS (37), SPSS (38), GraphPad Prism (http://www.grahpad.com)); through open source statistical software packages (e.g., the "chisq.test" function in the R language for statistical computing (39)); and various online calculators (e.g., http://www.physics.csbsju.edu/stats/contingency_NROW_NCOLUMN_forqm.html).

A contingency table is always constructed utilizing raw *counts*, rather than frequency data. The preferred approach in this type of analysis for highly polymorphic immunogenetic data is to first examine heterogeneity in overall allele frequency distributions in cases vs. controls for a particular locus, using a $2 \times k$ row by column ($r \times c$) contingency table. Analyses of these data historically relied on series of $2 \times 2$ tests for each allele observed due to the presence of untyped (the so-called blank) alleles; due to the often high frequencies of blanks in initial studies, allele counts and frequencies could not easily be calculated. As described in Chap. 13, the widespread use of DNA typing in most immunogenetic studies now allows for direct ascertainment of allele frequencies.

Analysis based on a series of $2 \times 2$ tests requires corrections for multiple comparisons (usually utilizing the Bonferroni method), with a correction factor minimally equivalent to the number of alleles tested. However, when significance of the association of all individual alleles is assessed with the a priori knowledge of *overall* heterogeneity at the locus, it is not necessary to correct for multiple comparisons in subsequent $2 \times 2$ tests intended to identify the allele(s) with significant contributions to the overall deviation at the locus. An example of a $2 \times k$ contingency table is given in Table 1 and a related $2 \times 2$ table for one allele is given in Table 2.

Rare alleles pose a particular challenge in traditional association tests in disease studies that use the $\chi^2$ test for goodness-of-fit. Although the $\chi^2$ test has been the standard approach for testing fit at the overall locus-level, this test can lead to false acceptance or rejection of the null hypothesis when the expected genotype counts in a contingency table are small (aka, "sparse cells"), as discussed in Chap. 13 with regard to Hardy–Weinberg (HW) testing; the $\chi^2$ test is *inappropriate* if any expected count is less than one or if the expected count is less than five in more than 20% of all cells in a contingency table. It is not unusual for 30 or more alleles to be observed at the HLA loci for example, with a wide range of frequencies, resulting in many sparse cells. Although Yates' correction for continuity is sometimes applied to account for numerous sparse cells, this

**Table 1**
**A 2×k contingency table for case-control data**

| Allele | Case (count) | Control (count) | Row total |
|---|---|---|---|
| 0101 | 75 | 29 | 104 |
| 0102 | 5 | 5 | 10 |
| 0301 | 59 | 56 | 115 |
| 0401 | 6 | 15 | 21 |
| 0701 | 9 | 25 | 34 |
| 0701 | 6 | 11 | 17 |
| 0801 | 73 | 39 | 112 |
| 1101 | 39 | 35 | 74 |
| 1103 | 9 | 4 | 13 |
| 1104 | 40 | 24 | 64 |
| Binned | 33 | 25 | 57 |
| *Total* | *354* | *268* | *622* |

**Table 2**
**A 2×2 contingency table for allele 0101**

| Allele | Case (count) | Control (count) | Row total |
|---|---|---|---|
| 0101 | 75 | 29 | 104 |
| Others (*not* 0101) | 279 | 239 | 517 |
| *Total* | *354* | *268* | *622* |

may be overly conservative, and the preferred method is to combine low frequency alleles into a single category, often referred to as the "binned" category (Table 1). A conservative (and recommended) approach is to combine alleles with an expected value of less than five in cases or controls into the binned category prior to calculation of the $\chi^2$ statistic. The $\chi^2$ statistic for a contingency table analysis of case-control data for a genetic association is calculated as:

$$\chi^2 = \sum \frac{(O_i - E_i)^2}{E_i},$$

where

$O_i$ = the observed count of allele $i$

$E_i$ = the expected count of allele $i$

And the derived values are summed over all cells in the tables. The expected count for each cell in the $r \times c$ table is calculated as

$$\frac{(\mathit{row}\text{ total allele } i) \times (\text{column total})}{2n},$$

where

Column total = sum of the counts in the column
Row total = number observations of allele $i$ in all subjects
$n$ = number individuals (cases + controls)
$2n$ = number chromosomes (cases + controls)

The degrees of freedom (df) for the goodness of fit $\chi^2$ analysis are calculated from the number of alleles with expected values in cases and controls of five or greater, plus the combined category, −1 (i.e., $k-1$). A $p$-value is obtained by comparing the test statistic to the $\chi^2$ distribution for the appropriate degrees of freedom.

In the example given in Table 1, we obtain a value of $\chi^2 = 39.71$, with df = 10. This indicated significant differences between cases and controls at the overall locus level, with $p < 0.001$. In the example in Table 2 for a $2 \times 2$ table for an individual allele, $\chi^2 = 11.88$, df = 1, $p < 0.001$.

These analyses can be performed at the allele level, as shown in the example, as well as for genotypes and haplotypes. In a haplotype-level analysis, population-level haplotype frequencies are first estimated (see Chap. 13) and the frequency estimates are converted to counts based on the sample size. Particular care must be taken when working with estimated haplotypes to combine the many rare types that are typically estimated, as well as to not over-interpret the data.

Summary: Basic steps for contingency table analysis in case-control studies with immunogenetic data

(a) Construct a $2 \times k$ table of allele (or genotype or haplotype) counts for cases and controls (see Table 1 example).
(b) Combine all alleles with expected values of four or less in cases or controls into a common "binned" category.
(c) Calculate the $\chi^2$ test statistic for the table and assess significance.
(d) If results are significant at the *overall locus level*, perform additional testing using $2 \times 2$ contingency tables for each allele (expected counts of five or more only) against all other alleles.

2. Relative Predispositional Effects (RPE).

While contingency table testing will reveal whether the overall allele frequency distributions at a locus differ significantly between cases and controls, identifying all allele(s) that contribute significantly to these differences can be difficult. The RPE method can be used to identify all heterogeneity in disease risk at the primary disease gene; alleles, haplotypes, or genotypes with the strongest predisposing (PRE) or protective (PRO) effects are sequentially removed from the analysis until no further heterogeneity in risk effects is seen. Determining the order in which haplotypes, genotypes or alleles are sequentially removed requires interplay between the contribution to the $\chi^2$ heterogeneity test, the ORs (see below) or Patient/Control (*P/C*) ratio (40) and the control frequencies of the allele, haplotype, or genotype. In the simplest application of this method, the allele with the greatest contribution to the overall $\chi^2$ values is removed, and the test statistic is recomputed, with degrees of freedom correspondingly reduced by one. If the new $\chi^2$ is found to be statistically significant at the test level, the process is repeated, with each subsequent analysis involving the removal of the greatest contributor to the overall $\chi^2$ from the previous analysis, until the test statistic is no longer found to be significant. In some cases more than one allele can be removed at a time, for example, where there are two PRE alleles with strong effects or a PRE and PRO allele when prior evidence has validated both as significant and strong effects.

The application of the RPE method to HLA data for juvenile idiopathic arthritis (JIA) (41, 42) is summarized in Table 3. The effect of individual alleles is indicated as either predisposing, neutral, or intermediate (INT) or protective. Rare alleles which cannot be placed into one of these categories either by the RPE method or all pairwise comparisons below have no effect given. Significant *p*-values for these comparisons are shaded gray.

The overall analysis of the complete dataset shows considerable heterogeneity in risk ($p<1.1E-27$). DRB1*0801 (PRE), DRB1*1501, and DRB1*0701 (PRO) are the strongest effects (the set of alleles labeled 1 in column 1). Repeat analysis after the removal of these three alleles still gives a highly significant result ($p<4.1E-10$), with DRB1*1104 (PRE) and DRB1*0401 (PRO) as the strongest effects (set labeled 2 in column 1). Note that a strong argument could be made for deleting these alleles also at the previous round, but this does not alter the outcome. With the removal of these strong effects, there is only minimal evidence of remaining risk heterogeneity ($p<0.02$), with DRB1*1103 ($p<0.01$) (PRE) and DRB1*0103 ($p<0.02$) (PRO) the strongest effects

**Table 3**
**JIA-OP HLA-DRB1 allele data ranked by odds ratio (OR)**

| RPE[a] | A[b] | B[c] | DRB1 | Patient | Control | Chi-square ($\chi^2$) | *p*-Value[d] | Effect | OR | CI[e] | CI[e] |
|---|---|---|---|---|---|---|---|---|---|---|---|
| | | Ix | *1103 | 12 | 1 | 6.80 | 0.009 | PRE | 9.40 | 1.22 | 72.49 |
| 1 | I | Ix | *0801 | 102 | 13 | 48.61 | 3.1E−12 | PRE | 6.90 | 3.83 | 12.43 |
| 2 | I | Ix | *1104 | 57 | 11 | 20.71 | 5.3E−06 | PRE | 4.26 | 2.21 | 8.20 |
| | | | *0403 | 9 | 3 | 1.68 | 0.20 | | 2.33 | 0.63 | 8.65 |
| 3 | II | IIx | *1301 | 90 | 38 | 9.99 | 0.002 | INT | 1.95 | 1.31 | 2.90 |
| | | IIx | *0102 | 9 | 5 | 0.35 | 0.55 | INT | 1.39 | 0.46 | 4.18 |
| | II | IIx | *1101 | 60 | 36 | 1.42 | 0.23 | INT | 1.31 | 0.85 | 2.02 |
| | | IIx | *0901 | 9 | 6 | 0.08 | 0.78 | INT | 1.16 | 0.41 | 3.28 |
| | II | IIx | *0101 | 74 | 50 | 0.52 | 0.47 | INT | 1.16 | 0.79 | 1.69 |
| | II | IIx | *0301 | 89 | 61 | 0.50 | 0.48 | INT | 1.14 | 0.81 | 1.62 |
| | | IIx | *1201 | 10 | 8 | 0.006 | 0.94 | INT | 0.96 | 0.38 | 2.46 |
| | II | IIx | *1302 | 28 | 23 | 0.05 | 0.82 | | 0.94 | 0.53 | 1.64 |
| | | | *1303 | 10 | 9 | 0.11 | 0.74 | | 0.86 | 0.34 | 2.12 |
| | | | Binned[f] | 27 | 27 | 0.92 | 0.34 | | 0.76 | 0.44 | 1.31 |
| | | | *1601 | 6 | 8 | 1.05 | 0.30 | | 0.58 | 0.20 | 1.67 |
| | | | *1401 | 11 | 18 | 4.05 | 0.04 | | 0.46 | 0.22 | 0.99 |
| | | | *1502 | 5 | 10 | 3.26 | 0.07 | | 0.38 | 0.13 | 1.12 |
| | III | IIIx | *0404 | 7 | 16 | 6.34 | 0.01 | PRO | 0.33 | 0.14 | 0.81 |
| 1 | III | IIIx | *1501 | 38 | 80 | 28.24 | 1.1E−07 | PRO | 0.33 | 0.22 | 0.49 |
| 1 | III | IIIx | *0701 | 30 | 65 | 23.92 | 1.0E−06 | PRO | 0.33 | 0.21 | 0.51 |
| 2 | III | IIIx | *0401 | 21 | 47 | 18.10 | 2.1E−05 | PRO | 0.33 | 0.19 | 0.55 |
| 3 | | IIIx | *0103 | 4 | 11 | 5.42 | 0.02 | PRO | 0.28 | 0.09 | 0.87 |
| | | | *Total* | *708* | *546* | *182.1* | 1.1E−27 | PRO | | | |

[a] *Numbers* denote the order of removal due to largest effect(s) in the relative predispositional effect (RPE) analysis

[b] Set A: Based on pairwise allele comparisons, the common alleles are divided into mutually exclusive, and significantly different, predisposing (PRE) (I), neutral (intermediate (INT)) (II), and protective (PRO) (III) categories for use later in amino acid comparisons (described below)

[c] Set B: The sets I, II, and III above are expanded (indicated by Ix, IIx, and IIIx) to include rare alleles, while excluding those alleles which do not clearly fall into one of the three risk categories

[d] The individual *p*-values are biased as the assumption of a 1 df $\chi^2$ is incorrect, and conservative; the *p*-values can be used however for a relative ranking of the allelic effects

[e] The upper and lower 95% confidence intervals (CIs) for the odds ratio (OR) are given (see below)

[f] The binned category consists of all alleles with an expected value <5 under the $\chi^2$ test of heterogeneity of patient and control allele counts

(set labeled 3 in column 1). Note that these latter *p*-values would not be significant with corrections for multiple comparisons of either the overall tests, or those for individual alleles. Notwithstanding, we mention these results, since our principal aim is to detect heterogeneity that may be relevant to detecting additional disease genes in a genetic region or identifying the causal amino acids in the *primary* disease gene.

3. Conditional Haplotype Method (CHM).

   With immunogenetic disease associations, the high level of LD between many of the genes means that multiple disease associations are often observed; some of these may indicate a causative genetic factor, and others may be due to LD with this causative factor. In order to account for LD within a genetic region, stratification by the disease-associated alleles using the CHM can be employed (43). We stress that it is important to identify *all* heterogeneity in disease risk at the *primary* disease PRE gene, *including* relatively weak effects, before proceeding with conditional analyses to detect *secondary* genetic effects. Otherwise, spurious results may be seen resulting from heterogeneity in relative risk effects at the primary disease gene at the allele, haplotype, or genotype levels. If all genes directly involved in disease susceptibility have been identified, then the relative frequencies of alleles at the other loci on high-risk haplotypes should be the same in cases and controls; similarly for INT and PRO haplotypes. While fit to these expectations does not exclude the possibility that other genes in the genetic complex are involved in disease, lack of fit unequivocally shows that all disease-PRE genes in the region have *not* been identified.

   For the CHM, we denote the primary disease locus by *A* (or the primary plus secondary loci that have been identified), that is, all putative disease PRE loci in the region, and alleles or haplotypes thereof by *Ai*, $i = 1,2,\ldots,iA$, and a linked marker locus by *B*, with alleles *Bk*, $k = 1,2,\ldots,kB$, then, under the null that the *A* locus defines all disease predisposition in the region:

   $$f_{\text{pat}}(Ai - Bk) / f_{\text{pat}}(Ai - Bl) = f_{\text{con}}(Ai - Bk) / f_{\text{con}}(Ai - Bl),$$

   where $f_{\text{pat}}(\cdot)$ and $f_{\text{con}}(\cdot)$ represent patient and control frequencies. That is, although the frequencies of the haplotypes *Ai*–*Bk* and *Ai*–*Bl* will differ between patients and controls, the relative frequency of their ratios will be the same in patients and controls, for each *Ai*.

   Inequality of these relative frequencies in patients and controls is expected if the allele or SNP or haplotypes thereof under study ***does not include all*** genes involved in the disease process and in LD with the marker loci. While fit to these expectations does not exclude the possibility that other genes in the region are involved in disease, lack of fit unequivocally shows that all disease-PRE genes in the region have *not* been identified (provided that stratification effects have not produced spurious results).

4. Amino acid-level analyses.

   In some cases, the analytical challenges posed by rare alleles can be avoided by analyzing the data at the amino-acid level. Immunogenomic studies have generally focused on allele- and locus-level polymorphisms, considering individual amino-acid or nucleotide polymorphisms only as they pertain to specific hypotheses. However, HW, LD, association, and selective neutrality analyses can be performed entirely at the amino-acid level, considering each amino-acid polymorphism independently of the others that constitute an allele sequence. The issues surrounding rare alleles are attenuated in these analyses, as the level of polymorphism at any individual amino-acid position is not as high as at the allele or locus level. However, variation in the number of variants at each amino-position poses challenges for LD estimates and attempts to correlate statistics between positions.

5. Sequence feature variant type analysis.

   Recently, a novel approach to genetic association analyses has been developed by subdividing genes/proteins into biologically relevant structural (e.g., beta-strand 1) and functional (e.g., peptide binding site) sequence features (SFs), and their "alleles," called variant types (VTs) (44). In SFVT analyses, association tests are performed on the VTs of these biologically relevant SFs.

#### 2.1.2. Odds Ratios and Relative Risk

Odds ratios (OR) are used in disease association studies as means to describe the strength of association between two variables, and reflect the ratio of odds of an outcome (e.g., disease) occurring in one group (e.g., individuals *with* allele *a*) to the odds of it occurring in another group (individuals *without* allele *a*). Relative risk (RR) is a related but different measure that describes the risk of having the outcome of interest relative to exposure (e.g., positive or negative for allele *a*). In case-control studies, the OR is the preferred measure, due in part to its use in logistic regression (see next section), allowing a more ready comparison of results derived from different methods. Another important advantage to the OR is that it is by its mathematical nature invertible, i.e., the OR for predisposition to disease is the direct inverse of the OR for protection; this is extremely important in terms of immunogenetic studies, where alleles may be associated in either a PRO or PRE role. It is not unusual to find both PRO and PRE alleles in a given disease study for a given locus; the ability to invert ORs allows more direct

**Table 4**
**Generic 2 × 2 table**

| Allele | Case (count) | Control (count) |
|---|---|---|
| Y | a | b |
| *Not* Y | c | d |

comparison of the relative strengths of predisposition vs. protection. In contrast, RR is not invertible. RR is more applicable to prospective studies, but for retrospective studies OR is preferred.

1. Calculation of OR and RR.

   Both OR and RR are calculated for each allele of interest in a 2 × 2 table. The OR is a simple cross-product of a 2 × 2 table. A generic example is given in Table 4.

   The OR for Table 4 is given by:

$$\mathrm{OR} = \frac{ad}{bc}.$$

   The RR is given by

$$\mathrm{RR} = \frac{a/(a+b)}{c/(c+d)}.$$

   For the example given in Table 2, OR = 2.22 and RR = 1.34.

2. Confidence intervals.

   Values for OR and RR are only meaningful when presented in terms of a corresponding confidence interval (CI). A confidence interval provides a likely range of values for an estimate of a particular parameter within a particular level of significance. The standard probability level is generally set at 95%, meaning that there will be a 95% chance that the value of interest (here, the OR or RR) will fall within that range. For OR and RR, a CI that includes one is not considered statistically significant, as the null hypothesis in this test is OR or RR = 1.

   Derivation of the CI is approached in a variety of ways, most of which require the use of computer software, and may include resampling (bootstrap), likelihood or other statistical methods. A full discussion of these methods is not possible here, and their application will ultimately depend on the type of data and analytical methods and software used by the investigator. Most statistical software packages compute basic CIs

**Table 5**
**Example of input variables for logistic regression analysis**

| Independent variable (HLA or KIR)[a,b] | Dependent variable (disease status)[c] | Covariable | | | |
|---|---|---|---|---|---|
| | | Risk factor: *smoking (yes/no)*-Binary[d] | Risk factor: *smoking (years)*-Quantitative[e] | Risk factor: *smoking (duration)*-Ordinal[f] | Genetic: *snp*-Categorical[g] |
| 0101,0401 | 0 | 1 | 15.8 | 1 | 1 |
| 0401,0501 | 0 | 1 | 10 | 2 | 2 |
| 0301,0401 | 1 | 1 | 2.5 | 3 | 3 |
| 0101,0501 | 1 | 0 | 1 | 2 | 4 |

[a]Data can be analyzed at the allele, genotype, haplotype, or other user-defined level
[b]User will need to specify the genetic model, e.g., recessive, codominant, etc.
[c]By convention, 0 = control; 1 = case
[d]Here, risk factor (smoking) is analyzed as present or absent. 0 = nonsmoker, 1 = smoker
[e]Here, risk factor (smoking) is analyzed as a continuous quantitative variable, number of years smoked
[f]Here, risk factor (smoking) is analyzed as an ordered discrete variable, number of years smoked categorized 1 = 0–5 years; 2 = 6–10 years; 3 = 11–20 years; 4 = more than 20 years
[g]Here, SNP data categorized by genotype, e.g., 1 = AG; 2 = AT; 3 = GG; 4 = GT

according to Clopper and Pearson (45), often known as the "exact" method.

#### 2.1.3. Logistic Regression

Analysis using logistic regression can also be used in case-control studies. Logistic regression is a form of *generalized linear modeling* for data with a dichotomous, or binary, outcome variable, such as case-control data where the outcome is either "affected" or "unaffected." Among its advantages, logistic regression provides a means to develop association models that include the contribution of both quantitative and qualitative covariables, which can involve cumbersome stratification procedures in contingency table testing; logistic regression is a critical tool in the analysis of complex multivariate datasets. Example of potential types of input variables for a logistic regression analysis with immunogenetic data are given in Table 5. Attention must be paid to how both quantitative and qualitative variables are coded, because interpretation of the ORs can greatly vary. For example in Table 5, including number of years smoking as a covariate will provide a single OR associated with each increment of 1 year of smoking and assumes that the risk increment is fully proportional to years smoking. This model may not make sense, so in some cases it is more appropriate to recode quantitative variables as binary (e.g., smoking yes/no in Table 5) or discrete, ordinal (e.g., smoking duration, Table 5), rather than continuous, variables.

A disadvantage of logistic regression analysis is a tendency to overestimate Ors (46) in sample sizes <500, possibly leading to erroneous conclusions. Therefore, as with any statistical method, care must be taken in both the application and interpretation of results in logistic regression analyses. In addition, it is important that the data be reported in a manner that allows readers to reanalyze the data (see below, data reporting).

Logistic regression analysis is always performed using computer software. While many commercial (e.g., SAS, SPSS, STATA) and free (e.g., PLINK (47)) software packages can be used .for logistic regression, many are not suitable for polymorphic immunogenetic data. For example, PLINK performs logistic regression for SNP or copy number variant(CNV) data and will not handle the level of polymorphism typical of HLA or KIR data. HLA or KIR data may be recorded for conditional analysis of SNP or CNV data in PLINK, but this will depend on the specific research question. There are also several packages and standard functions for the R language (e.g., the "glm" function in the base package) that can perform logistic regression, but extreme care must be taken in the coding of immunogenetic data, as many of these functions are not designed to handle high levels of polymorphism.

A regression analysis produces a model that includes all of the variables that are useful in predicting the (dichotomous) outcome variable. Logistic regression provides an OR for each variable involved in predicting outcome, and can be particularly useful in immunogenetic studies that must account for a number of cofactors in assessing associations. Several options are available in building the most parsimonious model, i.e., the one explaining the maximum of the variance with the minimal number of variables. A backward stepwise approach can be particularly productive in an exploratory analysis; independent variables are removed from the full model and the fit of the new model is tested at each step. This procedure allows the investigator to eliminate noncontributing variables and build a more parsimonious model. A forward stepwise approach can be more robust when large numbers of variables are studied. In this procedure, the most significant variables are successively added to an empty model, until the addition of variables does not contribute to significantly increase the variance explained by the model.

### 2.2. Family-Based Studies

Family studies have long been the bread and butter of genetic epidemiology. Family studies provide a means to assess genetic linkage and/or association by testing within a nuclear family.

#### 2.2.1. Pedigree Types in Family Studies

The simplest type of family study involves (1) "trios," sets of "simplex" families consisting of a proband (an individual with the disease phenotype of interest) and both of the proband's parents (Fig. 1a). Additional family collections may include (2) multiplex sib pairs (MSP) pedigrees with two or more affected siblings (Fig. 1c), (3) multiplex parent child (MPC), with one affected parent and child (Fig. 1b) and (4) multiplex parent sibs (MPS) with at

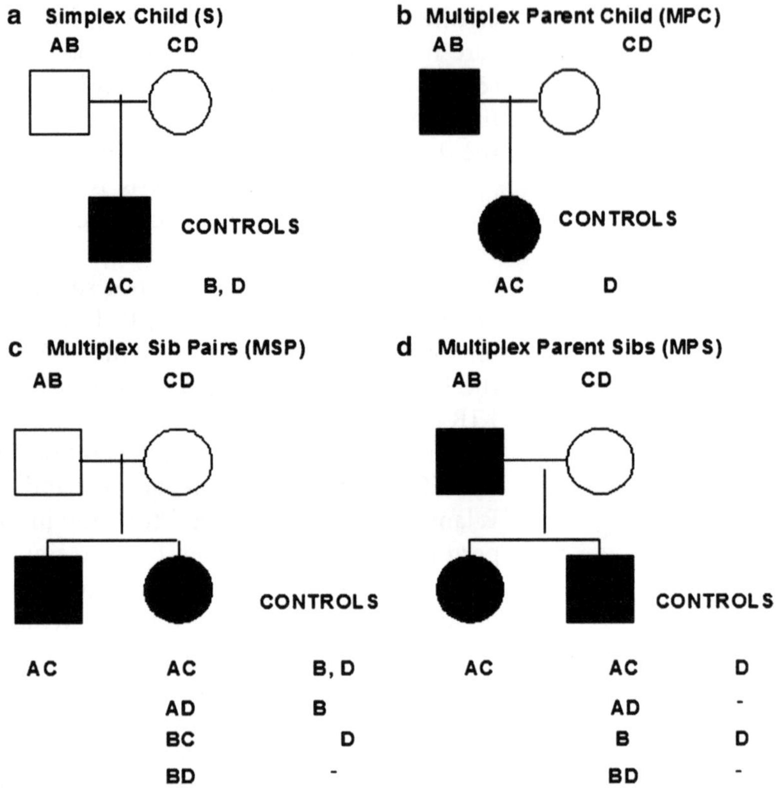


Fig. 1. The four family-based ascertainment schemes are selected in the presence of at least: (**a**) one affected child (S), (**b**) one affected child and one affected parent (multiplex parent child (MPC)), (**c**) two affected sibs (multiplex sib pairs (MSP)), and (**d**) two affected sibs and one affected parent (multiplex parent sibs (MPS)). As noted in the text, additional family members (parent or sib) may be affected within each of these schemes; they occur with frequencies expected under the disease model and are retained in analyses. For the MSP and MPS ascertainment schemes, using the ordered notation of Thomson (55) the first affected sib ascertained is always denoted by genotype AC, with the four possible genotypes for the second affected sib listed.

least one affected parent and two or more affected siblings (Fig. 1d). The type of analyses available will depend on the nature of the pedigrees collected.

#### 2.2.2. Affected Sib Pair Method

When considering related individuals, the loci linked to disease susceptibility are expected to be found in the region of the genome inherited from the same ancestors. Affected sib pair methods can be used in the study of HLA-associated diseases. Deviations from the Mendelian random expectations of 25, 50, and 25% that two affected sibs will on average share 2, 1, and 0 parental chromosomes in common identical by descent (IBD) suggest a disease PRE gene in the region. Several statistics can be used, a goodness-of-fit $\chi^2$ is commonly used and tests the null hypothesis of the absence of linkage with the disease locus.

#### *2.2.3. Transmission Disequilibrium Test and Affected Family-Based Controls*

Originally developed as a test for genetic linkage, the Transmission Disequilibrium Test (TDT) is applicable as an association test as well, since it always tests a compound hypothesis of linkage and association: only linked markers that are associated with disease can give a significant result. The fundamental basis for the TDT involves the likelihood that if a marker is linked to disease, there will be a bias in transmission from parents to the affected individual. In the TDT test, only parents who are heterozygous for the marker of interest are considered. The TDT test has the advantage of being robust with respect to population structure, thereby sidestepping the possible pitfall of population stratification often encountered in case-control studies. The TDT test looks at deviations from the expected 50:50 ratio of transmitted and nontransmitted alleles from parents heterozygous for the marker alleles.

The use of nuclear family data (two parents and their children) to estimate control marker allele frequencies (and similarly haplotype frequencies) was introduced, with application to HLA data, by Rubinstein et al. (48), and Falk and Rubinstein (49). In families ascertained for the presence of at least one affected child, termed S (simplex) pedigrees (also referred to as *trio* families), the two parental marker alleles *not* transmitted to the affected child (the proband) are used as population (control) alleles (see Fig. 1a). These are referred to as affected family-based controls (AFBACs). This matched design for patient (parental transmitted) and "control" (parental nontransmitted) marker alleles avoids ethnic confounding in the case of a stratified population (50–52).

Field (53) and Thomson (54)—extended this AFBAC approach to nuclear pedigrees ascertained for the presence of at least two affected sibs, termed MSP pedigrees (although referred to then as MS pedigrees, for multiplex sibs); using the alleles from both parents that are *never* transmitted to either sib in the affected sib pair as the "control" population (Fig. 1c). Additionally, MPC and MPS ascertainment schemes were considered: these extend the S and MSP ascertainment schemes to also include at least one affected parent. The non- or never-transmitted alleles, respectively, from the *unaffected* parent form the respective AFBAC populations (Fig. 1b, d). Similar extensions apply to other ascertainment schemes, e.g., with ascertainment based on the presence of at least three affected sibs in a nuclear family, the AFBACs are the parental alleles *never* transmitted to any of the three affected sibs.

AFBAC is similar to the TDT in that it examines the transmission of marker alleles in family trios. The AFBAC method has often mistakenly been equated to a heterogeneity test of association of patient and AFBAC frequencies. The AFBAC method per se is for obtaining an unbiased estimate of marker allele frequencies, and does not refer to any specific test of association/linkage. The TDT is the appropriate statistical test to apply. However, note that in the case of a homogenous population sample, the results from a TDT and contingency table analysis will be very similar. Here, all non-transmitted parental alleles are considered, regardless of whether the parents are homozygous or heterozygous.

Statistical tests to apply to the AFBAC data (alleles or haplotypes) are as follows (55):

(a) Equality of AFBAC maternal and paternal frequencies (a significant difference may imply a maternal/fetal interaction effect, in which case only the paternal AFBACs should be used).

(b) Test for equality of AFBAC frequencies with control marker frequencies available from any other sources, e.g., population data, other disease studies, and AFBACs ascertained under different criteria. With case/control data, one must be careful to understand the ascertainment scheme for the controls, i.e., whether it is from a random *or* nondiseased population. For rare diseases, there will be little difference, but for common diseases this is not the case.

(c) Test for multiplicative structure of the paternal transmitted and nontransmitted alleles for S ascertainment, with appropriate modifications for other ascertainment schemes, and similarly for the maternal alleles. A significant difference in the latter case may reflect a maternal/fetal interaction effect.

(d) Test for a multiplicative structure of the paternal nontransmitted alleles and the child's genotype for S ascertainment, with appropriate modifications for other ascertainment schemes, and similarly for the maternal alleles. A significant difference in the latter case may reflect a maternal/fetal interaction effect.

(e) Test for fit to HWP of the AFBAC genotypes created, with S ascertainment, from the maternal and paternal nontransmitted alleles in each family. For MS ascertainment, only the families where both sibs share the same two parental alleles (AC) (Fig. 1c) are used in this test. A significant deviation from HWP may reflect a maternal/fetal interaction effect.

**Table 6**
**Potential units of analysis for killer cell immunoglobulin-like receptors (KIR) data in disease association**

| Analytical unit | Examples |
|---|---|
| KIR ligands | HLA-C1 carrier; HLA-C1 homozygous; HLA-C2 carrier; HLA-C2 homozygous; HLA-Bw4 carrier; HLA-Bw4 homozygous; HLA-Bw6 carrier; HLA-Bw6 homozygous; HLA-Bw4_Thr80 carrier; HLA-Bw4_Ile80 carrier |
| KIR genes | KIR2DL1; KIR2DP1; KIR2DL2; KIR2DL3; KIR2DL5; KIR3DL1; KIR2DS1; KIR2DS2; KIR2DS3; KIR2DS4; KIR2DS5; KIR3DS1 |
| KIR diplotypes | AA; AA (with no activating); AB; BB; centromeric AA; telomeric AA; centromeric AB; telomeric AB; centromeric BB; telomeric BB |
| KIR haplotypes | A; B; B variants |
| KIR and ligands | KIR2DL1 with HLA-C2; KIR2DL1 without HLA-C2; KIR2DL2 with HLA-C1; KIR2DL2 without HLA-C1; KIR2DL3 with HLA-C1; KIR2DL3 without HLA-C1; KIR3DL1 with HLA-Bw4; KIR3DL1 with HLA-Bw4_Ile80; KIR3DL1 with HLA-Bw4 homozygous; KIR2DL3 with HLA-C1; KIR3DS1 with HLA-Bw4; KIR3DS1 with HLA-Bw4_Ile80; KIR3DS1 with HLA-Bw4 homozygous |

## 3. KIR Data: Special Considerations

While KIR data are in many ways typical of immunogenetic data, with high levels of polymorphism and linkage disequilibrium through the region, as well as a clear history of extensive recombination and gene conversion events, the limitations of most typing techniques mean that in many cases investigators will have to deal with large amounts of missing data. Likewise, most typing techniques cannot detect or distinguish between loci that may be duplicated on a KIR haplotype. In addition, the relationship between the KIR and their HLA ligands dictates consideration of interaction effects between these two important polymorphic regions when analyzing for disease associations. Table 6 illustrates potential units of analysis in disease association studies with KIR data. This list is by no means exhaustive, and the ultimate choice of analyses performed should be determined by the specific research hypotheses being tested in the study.

Issues specific to the analysis of KIR data for disease association studies include:

1. *Treatment of presence/absence or gene-content typing data.* As allele level KIR genotyping improves, datasets will contain a mixture of gene-content and allele level typing data. Analysis of KIR data at the gene-content level may at times be more robust than at the allele level, or vice-versa. In gene-content

data analyses, allele frequencies must be estimated using expected frequencies under Hardy–Weinberg Equilibrium Proportions (HWEP) or phenotype frequencies. Allele- and locus-level experimental data can be compared to published allele-level KIR typing datasets.

2. *Incorporation of HLA interaction effects.* It is not clear how best to model the KIR interaction with its HLA ligand; analyses could define HLA at a broad functional level or use molecular (HLA allele) designations. Current research depends almost exclusively on broad designations, but recent work suggests some crossover in HLA-C-group KIR ligand specificity. We will assess the impact of HLA-ligand definition using both broad designations and allelic designations for HLA ligands using published data and model.
3. *Controlling for other HLA associations.* Many disease associations with KIR also show strong HLA associations (e.g., autoimmune disorders). Accounting for primary HLA associations while accounting for HLA's function as a KIR ligand involves consideration of the extensive linkage disequilibrium throughout the HLA region.
4. *The use of estimated haplotypes vs. the standard A/A and B/x designations.*
5. *The treatment of haplotypic data.* It is unclear how chromosomal location should be considered for otherwise identical loci (e.g., KIR2DS3), and there are no standards for (locus level) CNV.

## 4. Data Reporting

A basic premise in scientific research involves the necessity of replication of studies. Although this is usually taken to mean replication of the laboratory findings, it is important that data analyses be replicated as well. In order to facilitate replication of analytical outcomes, it is imperative that there be a careful and thorough reporting of data. For immunogenetic studies, the data should be listed as both raw counts and frequencies; this will allow other investigators to perform additional analyses (using counts) as well as meta-analysis. We recommend the authors provide either within the body of the paper or as supplemental material, a list of all alleles, haplotypes and genotypes, including rare variants.

## Acknowledgments

This work was supported by National Institutes of Health (NIH) grants U01AI067068 (JAH, SJM) and U19AI067152 (PAG) awarded by the National Institute of Allergy and Infectious Diseases (NIAID) and 1R01DK061722 (JAH) awarded by the National Institute of Diabetes and Digestive and Kidney Diseases (NIDDK). The content is solely the responsibility of the authors and does not necessarily represent the official views of the National Institutes of Health.

## Glossary

**Bonferroni correction** The most commonly used method of correcting for multiple comparisons. Generally, the test significance level is divided by the number of comparisons made in the study, thereby increasing the overall stringency of the significance testing.

**Confidence interval** A likely range of values for an estimate of a particular parameter within a particular level of significance.

**Contingency table** Also known as a *cross-tabulation*. A $2 \times n$ table used to analyze heterogeneity between two sets of observations of two or more categorical variables.

**Genetic association** The occurrence within a population, greater than that expected by chance, of a genetic trait with a particular phenotype.

**Logistic regression** A statistical method to determine which in a set of independent variables has a predictive relationship to a binary-dependent outcome variable.

**Multiple comparisons** Also know as *multiple testing*. Performing a statistical test multiple times in the same analysis, thereby increasing the number of chances that the null hypothesis will be incorrectly rejected, leading to false positive associations.

**Odds ratio** The ratio of odds of an outcome occurring in one group to the odds of it occurring in another group.

**Population stratification** Also referred to as *population substructure*. Allele frequency differences between subpopulations within a study population due to ancestry differences or selection biases.

**Relative risk** A measure that describes the risk of having the outcome of interest relative to exposure.

**Yates correction for continuity** An adjustment to the $\chi^2$ test statistic performed by subtracting 0.5 from the (O-E) value for each cell in a contingency table. The purpose of this correction is to account for sparse cells in the table which may introduce discontinuity with regard to the $\chi^2$ distribution.

## References


1. Vandiedonck C, Knight JC (2009) The human major histocompatibility complex as a paradigm in genomics research. Brief Funct Genomic Proteomic 8(5):379–394
2. Mather KA, President M, Eastel S, Hollenbach J, Klitz W, Huttley G, Thomson G (2007) Long distance linkage disequilibrium between HLA microsatellites in two human populations. In: Hansen JA (ed) Immunobiology of the human MHC: proceedings of the 13th international histocompatibility workshop and congress. IHWG Press, Seattle
3. Ann B, Begovich WK, Steiner LL, Grams S, Suraj-Baker V, Hollenbach J, Trachtenberg E, Louie L, Zimmerman PA, Hill AVS, Stoneking M, Sasazuki T, Rickards O, Titanji VPK, Konenkov VI, Sartakova ML (1999) HLA DQ hapotypes in 15 different populations. In: Kasahara M (ed) Major histocompatibility complex: evolution, structure and function. Springer, Tokyo
4. Petzel-Erler ML, Gorodezky C, Layrisse Z, Klitz W, Fainboim L, Vullo C, Bodmer J, Egea E, Navarrete C, Infante E, Alaez C, Olivo A, Debaz H, Bautista N, de la Rosa G, Vazquez MN, Navarro JL, Pujol MJ, Duran C, Schafhauser C, Faucz FR, Janzen M, Maciag P, Boldt ABW, Souza PSA, Probst CM, da Silva GF, Makhatadze N, Dominguez E, Montagnani S, Matos M, Martinez A, Herrera F, Hollenbach J, Thomson G, Pando M, Satz L, Larriba J, Fernandez G, Pesoa SA, Borosky A, Garavito G, Angel L, Brown J, Llop E (1997) Anthropology component report for region Latin-America: Amerindian and admixed populations. In: Charron D (ed) Genetic diversity of HLA: functional and medical implications. EDK Press, Paris
5. Trachtenberg EA, Hayes E, Hollenbach JA, Keyeaux G, Bernal J, Klitz W (1997) HLA class II variation and linkage disequilibrium in nine Amerindian and three African American tribes from Columbia. Results of expedicion humana. In: Charron D (ed) Genetic diversity of HLA: functional and medical implications. EDK Press, Paris
6. Trachtenberg E, Vinson M, Hayes E, Hsu YM, Houtchens K, Erlich H, Klitz W, Hsia Y, Hollenbach J (2007) HLA class I (A, B, C) and class II (DRB1, DQA1, DQB1, DPB1) alleles and haplotypes in the Han from southern China. Tissue Antigens 70:455–463
7. Begovich AB, Moonsamy PV, Mack SJ, Barcellos LF, Steiner LL, Grams S, Suraj-Baker V, Hollenbach J, Trachtenberg E, Louie L, Zimmerman P, Hill AV, Stoneking M, Sasazuki T, Konenkov VI, Sartakova ML, Titanji VP, Rickards O, Klitz W (2001) Genetic variability and linkage disequilibrium within the HLA-DP region: analysis of 15 different populations. Tissue Antigens 57:424–439
8. Bergstrom TF, Engkvist H, Erlandsson R, Josefsson A, Mack SJ, Erlich HA, Gyllensten U (1999) Tracing the origin of HLA-DRB1 alleles by microsatellite polymorphism. Am J Hum Genet 64:1709–1718
9. Bergstrom TF, Mack SJ, Gyllensten U, Ehrlich HA (2000) Evolution of HLA-DRB loci, DRB1 lineages, and alleles: analyses of intron-1 and -2 sequences. In: Kasahara M (ed) Major histocompatibility complex: evolution, structure and function. Springer, Tokyo
10. Crawford MH, Reddy BM, Martinez-Laso J, Mack SJ, Erlich HA (2001) Genetic variation among the Golla pastoral caste subdivisions of Andhra Pradesh, India, according to the HLA system. Hum Immunol 62:1031–1041
11. Ellis JM, Mack SJ, Leke RF, Quakyi I, Johnson AH, Hurley CK (2000) Diversity is demonstrated in class I HLA-A and HLA-B alleles in Cameroon, Africa: description of HLA-A*03012, *2612, *3006 and HLA-B*1403, *4016, *4703. Tissue Antigens 56:291–302
12. Erlich HA, Mack SJ, Bergstrom T, Gyllensten UB (1997) HLA class II alleles in Amerindian populations: implications for the evolution of HLA polymorphism and the colonization of the Americas. Hereditas 127:19–24
13. Hildesheim A, Apple RJ, Chen CJ, Wang SS, Cheng YJ, Klitz W, Mack SJ, Chen IH, Hsu MM, Yang CS, Brinton LA, Levine PH, Erlich HA (2002) Association of HLA class I and II alleles and extended haplotypes with nasopharyngeal carcinoma in Taiwan. J Natl Cancer Inst 94:1780–1789
14. Johansson A, Ingman M, Mack SJ, Erlich H, Gyllensten U (2008) Genetic origin of the Swedish Sami inferred from HLA class I and class II allele frequencies. Eur J Hum Genet 16:1341–1349
15. Leffell MS, Fallin MD, Erlich HA, Fernandez-Vijna M, Hildebrand WH, Mack SJ, Zachary AA (2002) HLA antigens, alleles and haplotypes among the Yup'ik Alaska natives: report of the ASHI Minority Workshops, Part II. Hum Immunol 63:614–625
16. Mack SJ, Bugawan TL, Moonsamy PV, Erlich JA, Trachtenberg EA, Paik YK, Begovich AB, Saha N, Beck HP, Stoneking M, Erlich HA (2000) Evolution of Pacific/Asian populations inferred from HLA class II allele frequency distributions. Tissue Antigens 55:383–400

17. Mack SJ, Erlich HA (1998) HLA class II polymorphism in the Ticuna of Brazil: evolutionary implications of the DRB1*0807 allele. Tissue Antigens 51:41–50
18. Mack SJ, Tu B, Lazaro A, Yang R, Lancaster AK, Cao K, Ng J, Hurley CK (2009) HLA-A, -B, -C, and -DRB1 allele and haplotype frequencies distinguish Eastern European Americans from the general European American population. Tissue Antigens 73:17–32
19. MacKenzie J, Perry J, Ford AM, Jarrett RF, Greaves M (1999) JC and BK virus sequences are not detectable in leukaemic samples from children with common acute lymphoblastic leukaemia. Br J Cancer 81:898–899
20. Meyer D, Single RM, Mack SJ, Erlich HA, Thomson G (2006) Signatures of demographic history and natural selection in the human major histocompatibility complex loci. Genetics 173:2121–2142
21. Solberg OD, Mack SJ, Lancaster AK, Single RM, Tsai Y, Sanchez-Mazas A, Thomson G (2008) Balancing selection and heterogeneity across the classical human leukocyte antigen loci: a meta-analytic review of 497 population studies. Hum Immunol 69:443–464
22. Tang TF, Hou L, Chen M, Belle I, Mack S, Lancaster A, Ho GY, Hwang WY, Alsagoff F, Ng J, Hurley CK (2007) HLA haplotypes in Singapore: a study of mothers and their cord blood units. Hum Immunol 68:430–438
23. Tu B, Mack SJ, Lazaro A, Lancaster A, Thomson G, Cao K, Chen M, Ling G, Hartzman R, Ng J, Hurley CK (2007) HLA-A, -B, -C, -DRB1 allele and haplotype frequencies in an African American population. Tissue Antigens 69:73–85
24. Cao K, Hollenbach J, Shi X, Shi W, Chopek M, Fernandez-Vina MA (2001) Analysis of the frequencies of HLA-A, B, and C alleles and haplotypes in the five major ethnic groups of the United States reveals high levels of diversity in these loci and contrasting distribution patterns in these populations. Hum Immunol 62:1009–1030
25. Hollenbach JA, Thomson G, Cao K, Fernandez-Vina M, Erlich HA, Bugawan TL, Winkler C, Winter M, Klitz W (2001) HLA diversity, differentiation, and haplotype evolution in Mesoamerican Natives. Hum Immunol 62: 378–390
26. Khakoo SI, Chloe LT, Martin MP, Brooks CR, Gao X, Astemborski J, Cheng J, Goedert JJ, Vlahov D, Hilgartner M, Cox S, Little AM, Alexander GJ, Cramp ME, O'Brien S, Rosenberg WMC, Thomas DL, Carrington M (2004) HLA and NK cell inhibitory receptor genes in resolving hepatitis C virus infection. Science 305:872–874
27. Williams AP, Bateman AR, Khakoo SI (2005) Hanging in the balance. KIR and their role in disease. Mol Interv 5:226–240
28. Li Y, Zhang T, Ho C, Orange JS, Douglas SD, Ho WZ (2004) Natural killer cells inhibit hepatitis C virus expression. J Leukoc Biol 76:1171–1179
29. Hollenbach JA, Ladner MB, Saeteurn K, Taylor KD, Mei L, Haritunians T, McGovern DPB, Erlich HA, Rotter JI, Trachtenberg EA (2009) Susceptibility to Crohn's disease is mediated by KIR2DL2/KIR2DL3 heterozygosity and the HLA-C ligand. Immunogenetics 61(10): 663–671
30. Gaudieri S, Desantis D, McKinnon E, Moore C, Nolan D, Witt CS, Mallal SA, Christiansen FT (2005) Killer immunoglobulin-like receptors and HLA act both independently and synergistically to modify HIV disease progression. Genes Immun 6:683–690
31. Khakoo SI, Carrington M (2006) KIR and disease: a model system or system of models? Immunol Rev 214:186–201
32. Kunert K, Seiler M, Mashreghi MF, Klippert K, Schonemann C, Neumann K, Pratschke J, Reinke P, Volk HD, Kotsch K (2007) KIR/HLA ligand incompatibility in kidney transplantation. Transplantation 84:1527–1533
33. Gedil MA, Steiner NK, Hurley CK (2007) KIR3DL2: diversity in a hematopoietic stem cell transplant population. Tissue Antigens 70: 228–232
34. Sun JY, Gaidulis L, Dagis A, Palmer J, Rodriguez R, Miller MM, Forman SJ, Senitzer D (2005) Killer Ig-like receptor (KIR) compatibility plays a role in the prevalence of acute GVHD in unrelated hematopoietic cell transplants for AML. Bone Marrow Transplant 36:525–530
35. Lanier LL (1999) Natural killer cells fertile with receptors for HLA-G? Proc Natl Acad Sci USA 96:5343–5345
36. Moffett A, Hiby SE (2007) How does the maternal immune system contribute to the development of pre-eclampsia? Placenta 28 (suppl A):S51–S56
37. Hu LP, Tao LX (2009) (Statistical analysis using SAS software package for data of RxC contingency table (part two)]. Zhong Xi Yi Jie He Xue Bao 7:878–882
38. Horstmann GA (1988) [Product of the month: SPSS statistical package for the sciences]. Radiologe 28:438–439
39. R Development Core Team (2008) R: a language and environment for statistical computing. R Foundation for Statistical Computing, Vienna
40. Thomson G, Valdes AM, Noble JA, Kockum I, Grote MN, Najman J, Erlich HA et al (2007)

Relative predispositional effects of HLA class II DRB1-DQB1 haplotypes and genotypes on type 1 diabetes: a meta-analysis. Tissue Antigens 70:110–127

41. Hollenbach JA, Thompson SD, Bugawan TL, Ryan M, Sudman M, Marion M, Langefeld CD, Thomson G, Erlich HA, Glass DN (2010) Juvenile idiopathic arthritis and HLA class I and class II interactions and age-at-onset effects. Arthritis Rheum 62:1781–1791
42. Thomson G, Marthandan N, Hollenbach JA, Mack SJ, Erlich HA, Single RM, Waller MJ, Marsh SG, Guidry PA, Karp DR, Scheuermann RH, Thompson SD, Glass DN, Helmberg W (2010) Sequence feature variant type (SFVT) analysis of the HLA genetic association in juvenile idiopathic arthritis. Pac Symp Biocomput:359–370
43. Thomson G, Valdes AM (2007) Conditional genotype analysis: detecting secondary disease loci in linkage disequilibrium with a primary disease locus. BMC Proc 1(suppl 1):S163
44. Thomson G, Marthandan N, Hollenbach JA, Mack SJ, Erlich HA, Single RM, Waller MJ, Marsh SGE, Guidry PA, Karp DR, Scheuermann RH, Thompson SD, Glass DB, Helmberg W (2009) Sequence feature variant type (SFVT) analysis of the HLA genetic association in juvenile idiopathic arthritis. Proceedings of the 2010 pacific society of biocomputing conference. Pac Symp Biocomput:359–370
45. Clopper CJ, Pearson ES (1934) The use of confidence or fiducial limits illustrated in the case of the binomial. Biometrika 26: 404–413
46. Nemes S, Jonasson JM, Genell A, Steineck G (2009) Bias in odds ratios by logistic regression modelling and sample size. BMC Med Res Methodol 9:56
47. Purcell S, Neale B, Todd-Brown K, Thomas L, Ferreira MA, Bender D, Maller J, Sklar P, de Bakker PI, Daly MJ, Sham PC (2007) PLINK: a tool set for whole-genome association and population-based linkage analyses. Am J Hum Genet 81:559–575
48. Rubinstein P, Walker M, Carpenter C, Carrier C, Krassner J, Falk C, Ginsberg F (1981) Genetics of HLA disease associations: the use of the haplotype relative risk (HRR) and the "haplo-delta" (Dh) estimates in juvenile diabetes from three racial groups. Hum Immunol 3: 384
49. Falk CT, Rubinstein P (1987) Haplotype relative risk: an easy reliable way to construct a proper control sample for risk calculations. Ann Hum Genet 51:227–233
50. Khoury MJ, Beaty TH (1994) Applications of the case-control method in genetic epidemiology. Epidemiol Rev 16:134–150
51. Schaid DJ, Sommer SS (1994) Comparison of statistics for candidate-gene association studies using cases and parents. Am J Hum Genet 55:402–409
52. Thomson G (1995) Mapping disease genes: family-based association studies. Am J Hum Genet 57:487–498
53. Field LL (1991) Non-HLA region genes in insulin dependent diabetes mellitus. Baillieres Clin Endocrinol Metab 5:413–438
54. Thomson G (1993) AGFAP method: applicability under different ascertainment schemes and a parental contributions test. Genet Epidemiol 10:289–310
55. Thomson G (1995) Analysis of complex human genetic traits: an ordered-notation method and new tests for mode of inheritance. Am J Hum Genet 57:474–486

# Chapter 15

# Impact of HLA Matching and HLA Antibodies in Organ Transplantation: A Collaborative Transplant Study View

**Caner Süsal and Gerhard Opelz**


## Abstract

The Collaborative Transplant Study (CTS) was initiated in 1982 in Heidelberg, Germany, and originated from the need to gain further insight into the complex problems and risks involved in human organ transplantation. Currently, more than 400 transplant centers in 45 countries are contributing to this voluntary international effort, and from the beginning of the study, the impact on graft outcome of immunological factors, such as matching for HLA antigens and allosensitization to HLA and non-HLA antigens, have been areas of interest. Herein, we summarize the recent findings from the CTS on these two topics.


**Key words:** HLA matching, HLA antibodies, Crossmatch, Kidney transplantation, Liver transplantation, Heart transplantation

## 1. Introduction

With graft survival rates steadily improving during recent years, there is debate whether organs should be allocated according to compatibility for HLA, or whether HLA matching should be ignored and kidneys from deceased donors should be transplanted locally with the shortest possible cold ischemia time. For example, in a survey of transplantations in which one kidney was shipped and the other was transplanted locally, Mange et al. found that the shipment of deceased-donor kidneys was associated with an increased risk of graft failure during the first posttransplant year (1). This result, however, might not necessarily be a result of longer ischemia but could be due to a better physiological quality of donor organs retrieved and transplanted locally. Results from the Collaborative Transplant Study (CTS) (2) indicate that short cold ischemia does not eliminate the effect of HLA matching and argue for continued kidney exchange efforts for achieving better HLA

Frank T. Christiansen and Brian D. Tait (eds.), *Immunogenetics: Methods and Applications in Clinical Practice*, Methods in Molecular Biology, vol. 882, DOI 10.1007/978-1-61779-842-9_15, © Springer Science+Business Media New York 2012

compatibility (3, 4). Recent CTS work has focused on factors other than graft survival and showed that better HLA matching in renal transplantation is associated with the administration of lower dosages of immunosuppressive agents (5) and a lower incidence of side effects of immunosuppression, such as non-Hodgkin lymphoma and hip fractures (5, 6). Others have shown that better HLA matching is associated with lower grade sensitization if a patient lost a kidney graft and is relisted for a retransplant (7). A recent CTS analysis indicated that HLA matching might also improve the currently poor long-term outcome in lung transplantation (8).

## 2. HLA Matching in Kidney Transplantation

### *2.1. HLA Matching, Cold Ischemia Time and Graft Outcome in Kidney Transplantation*

In a comparative analysis of more than 130,000 deceased-donor kidney transplantations performed during two successive decades (1985–1994 and 1995–2004), we were able to demonstrate that—in spite of improvements in immunosuppression and a significant decline in the length of ischemic preservation—the effect of HLA matching on the survival rate of kidney transplants from deceased donors continues to be influential (4). While numerically the percent improvement in graft survival through HLA matching was smaller in recent years, the relative contribution of HLA mismatches to the fraction of graft failures remained nearly unchanged (Fig. 1). The main difference between the results obtained in the comparative analysis of two decades was an improvement in the overall graft survival rate. However, when 3 HLA-A + B + DR mismatches were taken as reference, transplants with no HLA mismatches showed a relative risk (RR) of failure of 0.76 (95% confidence interval [CI] 0.71–0.80) among transplants performed 1985–1994 and 0.83 (CI 0.77–0.89) in the decade 1995–2004, and likewise the increased risk of failure associated with six mismatches changed only little, from 1.23 (CI 1.14–1.32) in 1985–1994 to 1.16 (CI 1.05–1.27) in 1995–2004. Analysis of transplants performed from 2000 to 2004, during which most recipients presumably received "modern" immunosuppressive treatment, continued to show a strong and statistically significant HLA matching effect.

In a separate analysis, cold ischemia up to 18 h was found not to be detrimental for graft outcome, and short cold ischemia did not eliminate the effect of HLA matching (3). These findings altogether indicated that an abandonment of HLA matching in exchange for transplanting with short ischemia times would be detrimental to clinical kidney transplantation. For practical/logistical reasons, we recommend emphasis on the avoidance of poorly matched grafts (4, 5 or 6 HLA-A + B + DR mismatches) which is feasible even in programs with relatively short transplant waiting lists.

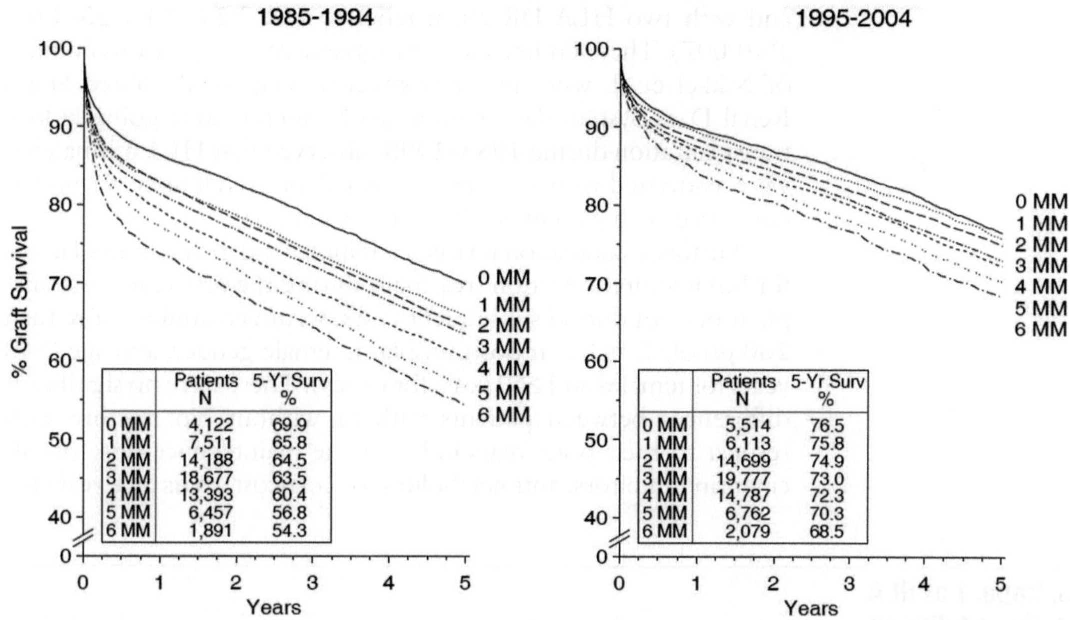


Fig. 1. Graft survival rates in relation to the number of HLA-A, -B, -DR mismatches for transplants performed between 1985 and 1994 (*left*) and between 1995 and 2004 (*right*). Transplants from deceased donors were analyzed. Numbers of mismatched HLA antigens (MM) and numbers of patients studied are indicated together with graft survival rates in percent observed at 5 years posttransplant. The association of HLA matching with graft survival was statistically significant in both decades (weighted regression $P<0.001$). Reproduced from ref. (4) with permission from Wolters Kluwer Health.

### 2.2. Impact of HLA Mismatching on Incidence of Posttransplant Non-Hodgkin Lymphoma After Kidney Transplantation

Posttransplant non-Hodgkin lymphoma is a rare but serious complication after organ transplantation which is associated with high mortality. In a recent analysis of more than 150,000 deceased-donor kidney transplant recipients reported to the CTS study, we found that one and two HLA-DR mismatches were a significant risk factor for posttransplant non-Hodgkin lymphoma, particularly for the location kidney and central nervous system, whereas two HLA-B mismatches increased the risk for the development of lymphoma of the kidney (5). An independent analysis of some 9,000 pediatric kidney transplant recipients showed that two HLA-DR mismatches were associated with a twofold higher risk of developing non-Hodgkin lymphoma, which led us to conclude that two HLA-DR mismatches should be avoided altogether in pediatric renal transplantation (9).

### 2.3. Association of Mismatches for HLA-DR with Incidence of Posttransplant Hip Fracture in Kidney Transplant Recipients

Bone fractures are a frequent complication after kidney transplantation for which various predisposing factors, such as older age, female gender, diabetes (10–12), extended duration of ESRD disease, (11, 13) and prolonged pretransplant dialysis (10, 11), have been identified. Analysis of some 20,000 kidney transplant recipients reported to CTS showed that there was a significant association between the number of HLA-DR mismatches and the occurrence of osteoporosis within 5 years after transplantation (6). Importantly, the risk of hip fracture increased for grafts with one HLA-DR mismatch to a hazard ratio (HR) of 1.85 (95% CI 1.18–2.89, $P=0.007$)

and with two HLA-DR mismatches to HR 2.24 (CI 1.25–4.02, $P=0.007$). These findings were in agreement with previous findings of Nikkel et al. who, in a retrospective analysis of United States Renal Data System data from 68,814 patients undergoing kidney transplantation during 1988–1998, observed that HLA mismatches were associated with a 9% increase in risk of overall bone fracture as compared with patients with no mismatch (10).

Further examination revealed additional independent risk factors for hip fracture: rejection treatment during the first year posttransplant but not during subsequent years, serum creatinine more than 260 μmol/L at 1 year posttransplant, female gender, and age (≥40 years for females and ≥60 years for males). There were no significant differences between patients with or without hip fracture with respect to their body mass index or the maintenance dose of calcineurin inhibitors, antimetabolites, or corticosteroids at 1 year (6).

## 3. Impact of HLA Compatibility on Lung Transplant Survival

The impact of HLA compatibility on graft survival was examined in some 8,000 deceased-donor lung transplants performed during 1989–2009 and reported to CTS (8). While graft survival rates showed a stepwise decrease as the combined number of HLA-A + B + DR mismatches increased from one to six, it was striking that lung transplants with "perfect" matches, that is zero HLA mismatches, showed an extremely poor outcome with half of all grafts failing during the first year. It thus appears that compatibility at all three HLA loci represents a particular constellation that can override the beneficial effect of HLA matching in terms of ameliorating immunologic rejection, probably by increasing the risk of severe lung transplant damage due to HLA-restricted immune phenomena. Donor lung preservation for up to 12 h was not associated with inferior graft survival vs. shorter preservation times, thereby providing a window for efforts at HLA matching. These results indicate that it may be appropriate to consider HLA matching of donor lungs within restricted geographical areas to achieve a moderate level of matching in order to help to improve the current poor long-term outcomes after lung transplantation.

## 4. HLA Matching and Presensitization in Organ Transplantation

### *4.1. Poor HLA Match in Previous Transplant as a Cause of Presensitization*

Meier-Kriesche et al., who examined some 16,000 renal transplant candidates in the USA that were relisted after loss of a primary kidney transplant, found that with increasing numbers of HLA mismatches of the first transplant there was a significant increase in panel reactive antibody (PRA) at relisting (7). Only 10% of the patients became sensitized after failure of a 0 HLA-A, -B-mismatched transplant, whereas the proportion rose up to 37% with increasing HLA mismatches. Because high PRA is associated with prolonged waiting times, the authors concluded that many patients are negatively impacted from poor HLA matching of their first kidney transplant when needing a second transplant.

### 4.2. Pronounced Impact of HLA Matching in Patients with High Alloreactivity

In the CTS study, we continue to observe a pronounced influence of HLA matching on graft outcome in patients with pretransplant HLA antibodies or high serum levels of the T-cell activation marker sCD30 (14–16), indicating that presensitization at the B- and T-cell level influences the impact of HLA compatibility. In patients without HLA antibodies and low sCD30, HLA mismatches have only a modest influence on graft outcome, suggesting that these patients can tolerate relatively poorly matched organs. It follows that particular attention to HLA matching should be paid in sensitized patients with increased B- and/or T-cell alloreactivity.

Altogether, data from the CTS as well as other transplant registries indicate that kidney exchange programs for the purpose of achieving better HLA matches continue to be meaningful. We believe that at a time when the shortage of donor organs is the predominant issue in discussions on how to provide patients with end-stage renal failure with optimal access to renal transplantation, the transplant community would be ill advised to eliminate HLA matching, a factor that significantly reduces the rate of allograft failure, severe side effects of immunosuppressive agents, and sensitization.

### 4.3. Presensitization as a Major Problem in Organ Transplantation

Although graft survival rates improved greatly during the last 25 years, sensitization of the recipient at the B-cell level still represents a major problem in kidney transplantation. Dependent on the antibody detection method, approximately 20–40% of patients on the kidney transplant waiting list possess serum alloantibodies prior to transplantation, a phenomenon called presensitization. Mainly three events can lead to presensitization: blood transfusion, pregnancy, and previous transplantation. Although there are great individual variations, generally the probability that a patient will develop antibodies increases with the frequency of exposure to foreign antigen. According to older literature, 15–25% of women develop antibodies after the first pregnancy and this rate increases to 50–60% after the second pregnancy. Lymphocytotoxic B-cell reactivity was detectable in 20% of waiting list patients who were treated with 1 blood transfusion, 40% after 10 transfusions, and 70% after 20 transfusions (17). Using an ELISA screening assay, we found HLA antibodies of the IgG isotype in 17% of patients waiting for a first transplant, 64% for a second, 84% for a third, and 92% for a fourth graft. Using the more sensitive Luminex technology, El-Awar et al. reported that almost all patients waiting for a regraft had HLA antibodies of the IgG, IgM, or IgA isotypes in their serum (18). At our own center, retransplant recipients currently make up 14% of the kidney waiting list.

An additional critical issue is antibody development against allogeneic antigen systems on graft endothelium other than HLA that are not necessarily detected in routine antibody testing. The influence of high PRA on graft outcome in transplants between HLA-identical siblings (19), the anti-MICA reactivity in eluates from rejected kidney allografts described by Zou et al. (20), the report by Terasaki and Ozawa who found that lymphocytotoxicity correlated better with graft outcome than solid phase flow cytometry or ELISA (which exclude non-HLA reactivity) (21), the recent results by Breimer et al. who observed, in the absence of HLA antibodies, significantly more rejections in patients with a positive flow cytometric endothelial crossmatch (22), and the work by Reinsmoen et al. who found a strong association between the presence of high antibody binding to Angiotensin type 1 receptor and antibody-mediated rejection in recipients whose sera did not contain antibody to donor HLA or MICA (23), all indicate that antibodies directed against non-HLA antigens are important. In our Heidelberg algorithm for transplantation of broadly sensitized high risk patients, we use additional measures, such as peritransplant apheresis, to reduce such presumed undetected antibody activity below clinically relevant threshold levels (24).

### 4.4. Disadvantages Associated with Presensitization

Presensitized kidney recipients have two major disadvantages: (a) they are less likely to receive a transplant due to a high number of HLA antigens defined as unacceptable because they would cause a positive pretransplant crossmatch; positive crossmatches occur especially if the antibodies are directed against a wide range of HLA specificities (high panel reactive antibodies [PRA]); (b) they reject their grafts more readily even if the pretransplant crossmatch is negative, possibly due to the presence of weak donor-specific antibodies that were overlooked in the crossmatch test. Alternatively, it has been suggested that high PRA reactivity may be an indicator of a generally high responder status against foreign alloantigens. It is an important task of the HLA laboratory to identify a suitable donor against whom the recipient is not sensitized.

According to Fuggle and Martin, presensitized patients remain, dependent on the grade of PRA, two or three times longer on the waiting list than nonsensitized patients (25). Actual data from the CTS indicate that, despite recent developments in the management of presensitized patients, patients who are positive in cytotoxic PRA testing as well as patients who are negative in cytotoxic PRA testing but positive in ELISA testing for HLA class I antibodies continue to show an inferior graft outcome (2, 26).

Positive crossmatches in the complement-dependent lymphocytotoxic test were shown in the 1960s to be associated with hyperacute rejection (27) so that performance of a lymphocytotoxic crossmatch prior to transplantation has become a standard method for reducing antibody-mediated damage and improving graft outcome in kidney transplantation. Because heart and liver grafts cannot be cold-stored as long as the kidney, it is still a matter of debate whether crossmatching in heart and liver transplantation is useful. Last year, we analyzed the relationship of positive lymphocytotoxic T-cell and B-cell crossmatches and flow-cytometric crossmatches with transplant survival in kidney, heart, and liver transplants from deceased donors reported to CTS (28). These results are described below.

## 5. Analysis of Positive Kidney, Heart, and Liver Transplant Crossmatches Reported to the Collaborative Transplant Study

Currently, with improved methods of immunosuppression, desensitization, and antibody detection, some "weak" positive crossmatch reactions are no longer considered a contraindication at some centers. Virtual crossmatches gained ground (29) and consequently the mandatory performance of a pretransplant crossmatch is not anymore an iron rule. Sometimes, a crossmatch test performed after the transplant operation unexpectedly can turn out positive. For these reasons, a number of kidney transplantations were performed and reported to the CTS despite a positive crossmatch against donor T lymphocyte targets. On the other hand, positive crossmatches against B-cell targets have generally not been considered a contraindication to transplantation because investigators disagreed on the clinical relevance of this test (30–33). Some 20 years ago, flow cytometry crossmatching was introduced and claimed to be superior to the lymphocytotoxicity assay because of higher technical sensitivity (34). Others claimed that the flow crossmatch excludes too many patients from transplantation based on false positive results (35). Therefore, at some centers, complement-dependent lymphocytotoxic crossmatching and flow cytometry crossmatching was performed in parallel, and the flow crossmatch was not necessarily considered the determining test. This resulted in positive flow crossmatches reported to CTS. In this manner, over the years a sizable number of positive crossmatch kidney transplants were recorded in the CTS database and became available for analysis. Most heart and liver transplants reported to CTS are done without a pretransplant crossmatch test. At some centers, crossmatches are performed retrospectively for study purposes, and the results have been compiled in the CTS database.

Our analysis showed that, overall, high rates of hyperacute rejection were not observed with any type of positive crossmatch or type of organ transplant (28), probably because immunosuppressive treatment has improved. When first kidney transplant recipients were analyzed, positive lymphocytotoxic T-cell crossmatches were associated with significantly decreased graft survival in the period between 1990 and 1999, but not from 2000 to 2007, suggesting that special selection and treatment measures may have been effectively developed and applied in recent years. Positive B-cell crossmatches were associated with inferior graft outcome during both time intervals.

When kidney retransplants were analyzed, the percentage of positive crossmatches was approximately twice as high as compared to the fraction of positive crossmatches in first transplants, emphasizing the sensitizing effect of first graft rejection. The effect of positive T-cell or B-cell crossmatches on graft survival was markedly stronger in retransplants as compared with first grafts, and the effect was fairly consistent in the two time periods. Positive flow crossmatches were not associated with statistically inferior outcomes, neither in first nor in retransplants, suggesting that antibody reactivity detectable with the sensitive flow technology is often so weak that current immunosuppressive regimens are sufficient for preventing antibody-mediated rejection. Alternatively, special preconditioning and immunosuppressive treatment methods may have prevented graft rejections in these patients. The impact of a positive T- and B-cell cytotoxic and flow cytometric crossmatch on kidney graft survival in transplantations performed between 1995 and 2008 is shown in Fig. 2.

In the analysis of heart transplants, the fraction of positive T-cell crossmatches was approximately eight times higher, and that of positive B-cell crossmatches approximately two times higher than that in kidney transplants. Interestingly, both T-cell and B-cell crossmatches were associated with significantly lower heart transplant outcome in the recent time period from 2000 to 2007, as compared to the earlier 1990–1999 period, conceivably because induction treatment for prevention of graft rejection with potent antibody agents (OKT3 or ATG) has become less common due to the well recognized increased risk of posttransplantation lymphoma associated with such treatment (36–38).

In liver transplantation, the fraction of positive crossmatches was even higher than that in heart transplants during the first time period (1990–1999) and similar during the recent time period (2000–2007). Positive T-cell crossmatches in liver transplantation were statistically significantly associated with impaired graft survival, especially during the recent analysis period (2000–2007). Positive B-cell crossmatches did not show a significant association with outcome.

That the majority of heart and liver transplants continue to be done without a pretransplant crossmatch test is probably related to the fact that immediate hyperacute graft rejection is rarely observed and that the impact of a positive crossmatch is therefore not obvious.

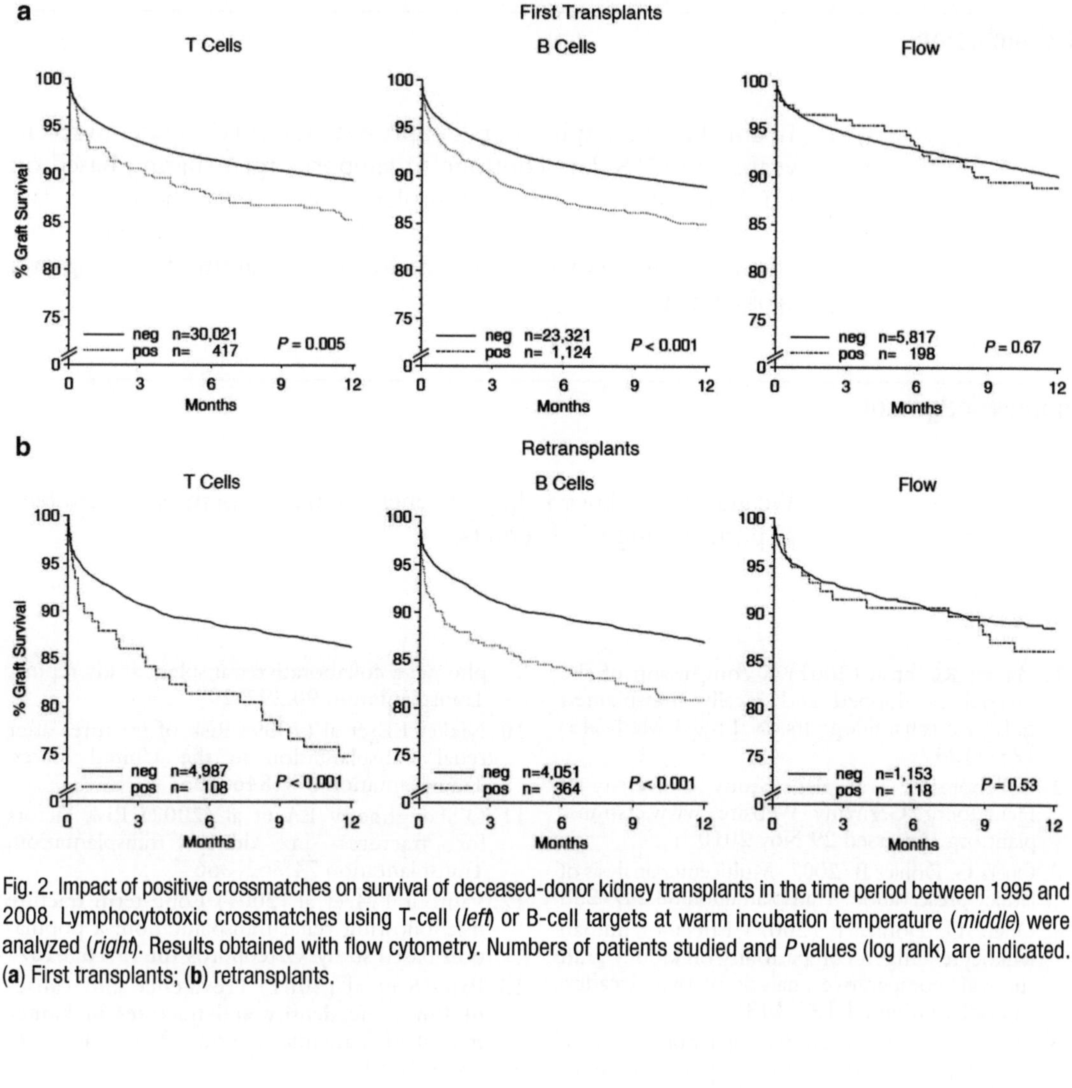


Fig. 2. Impact of positive crossmatches on survival of deceased-donor kidney transplants in the time period between 1995 and 2008. Lymphocytotoxic crossmatches using T-cell (*left*) or B-cell targets at warm incubation temperature (*middle*) were analyzed (*right*). Results obtained with flow cytometry. Numbers of patients studied and *P* values (log rank) are indicated. (**a**) First transplants; (**b**) retransplants.

Posttransplantation follow-up, however, shows a progressive graft loss rate in crossmatch-positive recipients during the first 3 months. The CTS results strongly argue for the performance of pretransplantation T-cell crossmatches in heart and liver transplantation. Because the crossmatch test can be performed in the period between declaration of brain death and removal of the donor organ, prolonged organ preservation times can usually be avoided. However, in the case of a positive crossmatch finding, a crossmatch-negative back-up patient needs to be selected for transplantation, a procedure that requires logistical preparations. Pretransplantation characterization of the recipient's alloantibodies and subsequent virtual crossmatching are further approaches for reducing the number of positive crossmatch results in heart and liver transplantation.

## 6. Conclusion

In conclusion, despite overall improved graft survival rates in recent years, the CTS data continue to support organ sharing based on HLA matching in kidney transplantation. Furthermore, the data suggest that, similar to kidney transplant recipients, end-stage heart and liver patients would benefit from HLA antibody testing and crossmatching.

## Acknowledgments

We gratefully acknowledge the generous support of the staff members at participating CTS centers.

### References

1. Mange KC et al (2001) A comparison of the survival of shipped and locally transplanted cadaveric renal allografts. N Engl J Med 345: 1237–1242
2. Collaborative Transplant Study, University of Heidelberg, Germany, Website. www.ctstransplant.org. Accessed 29 Nov 2010
3. Opelz G, Döhler B (2007) Multicenter analysis of kidney preservation. Transplantation 83:247–253
4. Opelz G, Döhler B (2007) Effect of human leukocyte antigen compatibility on kidney graft survival: comparative analysis of two decades. Transplantation 84:137–143
5. Opelz G, Döhler B (2010) Impact of HLA mismatching on incidence of posttransplant non-Hodgkin lymphoma after kidney transplantation. Transplantation 89:567–572
6. Opelz G, Döhler B (2010) Association of mismatches for HLA-DR with incidence of posttransplant hip fracture in kidney transplant recipients. Transplantation 91:65–69
7. Meier-Kriesche HU et al (2009) A lifetime versus a graft life approach redefines the importance of HLA matching in kidney transplant patients. Transplantation 88:23–29
8. Opelz G et al (2010) Impact of HLA compatibility on lung transplant survival and evidence for an HLA restriction phenomenon: a collaborative transplant study report. Transplantation 90:912–927
9. Opelz G, Döhler B (2010) Pediatric kidney transplantation: analysis of donor age, HLA match, and posttransplant non-Hodgkin lymphoma: a collaborative transplant study report. Transplantation 90:292–297
10. Nikkel LE et al (2009) Risk of fractures after renal transplantation in the United States. Transplantation 87:1846–1851
11. O'Shaughnessy EA et al (2002) Risk factors for fractures in kidney transplantation. Transplantation 74:362–366
12. Vautour LM et al (2004) Long-term fracture risk following renal transplantation: a population-based study. Osteoporos Int 15:160–167
13. Patel S et al (2001) Prevalence and causes of low bone density and fractures in kidney transplant patients. J Bone Miner Res 16: 1863–1870
14. Opelz G et al (1999) HLA compatibility and organ transplant survival. Collaborative Transplant Study. Rev Immunogenet 1:334–342
15. Süsal C, Pelzl S, Opelz G (2003) Strong human leukocyte antigen matching effect in nonsensitized kidney recipients with high pretransplant soluble CD30. Transplantation 76:1231–1232
16. Süsal C, Döhler B, Opelz G (2009) Presensitized kidney graft recipients with HLA class I and II antibodies are at increased risk for graft failure: a Collaborative Transplant Study report. Hum Immunol 70:569–573
17. Opelz G et al (1981) Lymphocytotoxic antibody responses to transfusions in potential kidney transplant recipients. Transplantation 32: 177–183
18. El-Awar N et al (2002) Almost all patients who are waiting for a regraft of a kidney transplant

have anti-HLA antibodies. Transplant Proc 34:2531–2532

19. Opelz G, Collaborative Transplant Study (2005) Non-HLA transplantation immunity revealed by lymphocytotoxic antibodies. Lancet 365:1570–1576
20. Zou Y et al (2006) Detection of anti-MICA antibodies in patients awaiting kidney transplantation, during the post-transplant course, and in eluates from rejected kidney allografts by Luminex flow cytometry. Hum Immunol 67: 230–237
21. Terasaki PI, Ozawa M (2005) Predictive value of HLA antibodies and serum creatinine in chronic rejection: results of a 2-year prospective trial. Transplantation 80:1194–1197
22. Breimer ME et al (2009) Multicenter evaluation of a novel endothelial cell crossmatch test in kidney transplantation. Transplantation 87: 549–556
23. Reinsmoen NL et al (2010) Anti-angiotensin type 1 receptor antibodies associated with antibody mediated rejection in donor HLA antibody negative patients. Transplantation 90: 1473–1477
24. Morath C et al (2010) An integrative approach for the transplantation of high-risk sensitized patients. Transplantation 90:645–653
25. Fuggle SV, Martin S (2008) Tools for human leukocyte antigen antibody detection and their application to transplanting sensitized patients. Transplantation 86:384–390
26. Süsal C, Döhler B, Opelz G (2009) Presensitized kidney graft recipients with HLA class I and II antibodies are at increased risk for graft failure: a Collaborative Transplant Study report. Hum Immunol 70:569–573
27. Patel R, Terasaki PI (1969) Significance of the positive crossmatch test in kidney transplantation. N Engl J Med 280:735–739
28. Opelz G, Döhler B, Süsal C (2009) Analysis of positive kidney, heart, and liver transplant crossmatches reported to the Collaborative Transplant Study. Hum Immunol 70:627–630
29. Bingaman AW et al (2008) A virtual crossmatch protocol significantly increases access of highly sensitized patients to deceased donor kidney transplantation. Transplantation 86:1864–1868
30. Ettenger RB et al (1979) Long-term cadaver allograft survival in the recipient with a positive B lymphocyte crossmatch. Transplantation 27:315–318
31. Hourmant M et al (1990) Effect of positive crossmatch against donor B lymphocytes in kidney transplantation: a prospective one center study. Clin Transpl 301–309
32. Bryan CF et al (2007) Renal graft survival is not influenced by a positive flow B-cell crossmatch. Clin Transpl 21:72–79
33. Magee CC et al (2008) Renal transplantation in patients with positive lymphocytotoxicity crossmatches: one center's experience. Transplantation 86:96–103
34. Kerman RH et al (1990) Improved graft survival for flow cytometry and antihuman globulin crossmatch-negative retransplant recipients. Transplantation 49:52–56
35. Christiaans MH et al (1996) No advantage of flow cytometry crossmatch over complement dependent cytotoxicity in immunologically well-documented renal allograft recipients. Transplantation 62:1341–1347
36. Swinnen LJ et al (1990) Increased incidence of lymphoproliferative disorder after immunosuppression with the monoclonal antibody OKT3 in cardiac-transplant recipients. N Engl J Med 323:1723–1728
37. Opelz G, Henderson R (1993) Incidence of non-Hodgkin lymphoma in kidney and heart transplant recipients. Lancet 342:1514–1516
38. Opelz G, Döhler B (2004) Lymphomas after solid organ transplantation: a Collaborative Transplant Study report. Am J Transplant 24:222–230

Chapter 16

# Screening for Antibodies Against MICA by Luminex Flow Cytometry

Yizhou Zou and Peter Stastny

## Abstract

Antibodies against MICA have been found in organ transplant recipients and were found to be associated with decreased survival of kidney allografts. The MICA antibody screening assay is a Luminex-based solid phase immunoassay designed to detect IgG antibodies binding to beads pre-coated with recombinant preparations of MICA alleles. These beads coated with soluble MICA recombinant proteins including 11 common alleles have been produced in our laboratory and similar preparations have been available from commercial sources. Here, we describe the procedure of MICA antibody screening with a prepared kit, in which all the reagents were optimized and standardized. We also review how to document the quality of single MICA antigen beads using MICA-specific monoclonal antibodies, as well as quality control of the procedure and data analysis.

**Key words:** Single antigen MICA beads, Antibodies, Luminex, MICA epitopes, Positive and negative control sera

## 1. Introduction

To test for antibodies against MICA antigens (1), pre-diluted positive and negative control sera and patient sera are added to the appropriate wells, allowing any antibodies against MICA to bind to the corresponding beads having attached to MICA recombinant glycoproteins (2). Any unbound antibody is washed away. A PE-labeled anti-human IgG antibody is added. A second incubation allows the PE-labeled anti-IgG antibody to bind to any anti-MICA (IgG) antibodies that have become attached to the bound MICA antigens on the beads. Next, any unbound anti-IgG is washed away. As in other Luminex-based immunoassays (3), beads with different single antigens can be distinguished by their color and the specific MICA antibody signal is measured in a Luminex

Frank T. Christiansen and Brian D. Tait (eds.), *Immunogenetics: Methods and Applications in Clinical Practice*, Methods in Molecular Biology, vol. 882, DOI 10.1007/978-1-61779-842-9_16, © Springer Science+Business Media New York 2012

flow cytometry system (4). This PE signal mean fluoresce intensity (MFI) is proportional within a range to the amount of MICA antibody that is bound. The bead mixture and the goat anti-human IgG-PE are light sensitive and should be stored in the dark. All reactions occur at room temperature and in the dark. Store serum aliquots, wash buffer, and bead mixture on ice until used.

## 2. Materials

1. Serum Samples.
   Freshly obtained serum is the specimen of choice. A sterile clotted blood sample with no anticoagulant is preferred (see Note 1). The following reagents are calculated for 25 tests:
2. Bead Mixture: (500 μL): We use a mixture of 11 beads coated with single MICA glycoproteins and two control beads. The storage buffer is optimized and the preparation is ready for testing human sera. Do not dilute or concentrate these beads. Protect the beads from light by keeping exposure to light to a minimum. It is possible to store at 2–8°C in the dark for 4 weeks or to store them at −80°C in the dark for 6 months. Ensure the beads are resuspended before dispensing.
3. Sample Dilution Buffer 5× (500 μL): This sample dilution buffer is used to reduce the background signals with human serum. The sample dilution buffer must be diluted to a working solution (1×) with 2 mL of PBS pH = 7.4 containing 0.05% Tween-20 (prepared by user) and can be stored at 2–8°C.
4. Positive Control Serum (40 μL ready to use): This serum or serum mixture is obtained by combining sera which contain MICA-specific antibodies to all the MICA antigens on the beads. Store at 2–8°C (see Note 1) (5). Negative Control Serum (40 μL ready to use): This serum is obtained from an individual known to have no antibodies against MICA antigens. Store at 2–8°C (see Note 2).
5. Secondary Antibody-PE: (20 μL) Goat anti-Human IgG conjugated to phycoerythrin in PBS. Must be diluted by adding appropriate amount of sample dilution buffer (1×) before use (we use 1,630 μL). Store at 2–8°C (see Note 3).
6. Wash Solution: 0.05% Tween-20/PBS (PBST): Not provided in the kit and should be prepared by the user.
7. Luminex beads with recombinant MICA antigens (Table 1) in the storage buffer (0.05% Tween-20/PBS plus 0.05% Azide).
8. Luminex 100 System (Luminex, Austin, TX).

**Table 1**
**Luminex beads and MICA antigens attached to them (see Note 4)**

| Luminex bead ID | Antigens |
|---|---|
| #02 | Negative control (see Note 5) |
| #03 | Positive control (see Note 5) |
| #04 | rMICA*001 |
| #06 | rMICA*002 |
| #11 | rMICA*004 |
| #17 | rMICA*006 |
| #19 | rMICA*007 |
| #24 | rMICA*008 |
| #26 | rMICA*009 |
| #32 | rMICA*012 |
| #34 | rMICA*017 |
| #41 | rMICA*018 |
| #43 | rMICA*019 |

9. Whatman 96-well Plate (Whatman Inc., Piscataway NJ, Cat # 7701-2250).
10. Thermowell Sealing Tape (Corning Inc., Corning NY, Cat# 6569).
11. Eppendorf pipette and tips (Eppendorf, Hauppauge NY).

## 3. Methods

### *3.1. The Microbead Assay for MICA Antibody Detection*

1. Collect serum samples to be tested and centrifuge the samples for 10 min at 1,300 × *g* (see Note 6).
2. Prepare working solution (1×) from sample dilution buffer (5×, 500 μL) in a new tube by adding 2 mL of PBS pH7.4, 05% tween-20 (prepared by user).
3. Add 25 μL of the working solution (1×) to each well that is going to be used for the assay in a 96-well black Whatman tray. Save remaining buffer for the secondary antibody dilution.
4. Add 15 μL of each centrifuged serum sample to each appropriately assigned well and mix with the preloaded working solution 1× (see Note 7). Cover the plate with Thermowell sealing

tape to prevent the entry of light and allow this mixture to incubate for 20 min at room temperature, shaking it at 150 rpm in a desk-shaking machine at room temperature.

5. While this mixture is incubating, prepare the bead mixture by resuspending the beads and mixing them well by vortexing at room temperature.
6. Add 20 μL of bead mixture to each well and mix by pipetting.
7. Cover the plate with Thermowell sealing tape (to restrict light and for further sample mixing) and shake the plate at 150 rpm for 40 min as step 4 (first incubation).
8. During the first incubation prepare the appropriate volume of wash solution (0.05% tween-20/PBS, 100 mL).
9. After the first incubation is complete, remove the tray from the rotator, and gently remove the cover tape from the tray (make sure that the suspension does not spill to other wells of the tray. Also, remove any bubbles that have been formed over the wells by blotting the top of the tray with a paper towel; do not overturn the tray at this point).
10. Add 120 μL of the prepared wash solution (PBST) to each well, cover with sealing tape and vortex well.
11. Centrifuge the tray for 5 min at 1,300 ×*g*.
12. After centrifugation, gently remove the sealing tape, invert and flick the tray. While still overturned, blot onto several paper towels. Tap the tray gently to remove excess wash solution (flicking involves throwing the supernatant out of the washed tray without disturbing the pelleted immune complexes formed by the Luminex beads). Once the tray has been flicked and returned to upright position, do not invert the tray for a second time before blotting, as this will cause the beads to be flushed out onto the paper towel (if this has occurred repeat steps 10 and 11 before blotting).
13. Repeat steps 10–12 three times using 180 μL of wash solution for a total of at least four washes (see Note 8).
14. During the final washing step, prepare the secondary antibody. Mix well.
15. Add 60 μL of the secondary antibody solution into each well; cover with sealing tape and vortex the tray. Place the tray on the shaker at 150 rpm for a 30-min incubation.
16. After the final wash is flicked out of the tray, resuspend the contents of the well in 60 μL of PBS 1×.
17. Proceed to the Luminex flow cytometry according to the instruction from manufacturer. Bead information for a Luminex template file is provided in Table 1.

18. Determine MICA antibodies and specificities by a computer program or by manual calculation using the method given in Table 2.

### 3.2. Quality Controls

1. Positive control and negative control sera should be included with each test. The MFI values of each bead with the control sera indicate if the test is valid (see Note 9).
2. Different reagent lots in kits must never be mixed.
3. Monoclonal antibodies against MICA can be used to assess conjugation of MICA antigens to the beads.

Current lot Luminex beads are coated with 11 preparations of single MICA antigens, including MICA*001, *002, *004, *006, *007, *008, *009, *012, *017, *018, and MICA*019, representing

**Table 2**
**Data analysis form for Luminex**

| | | Negative control | | Positive control | | Sample MFI | | | Assignment | | |
|---|---|---|---|---|---|---|---|---|---|---|---|
| Bead ID | MICA antigen | MFI ref. | MFI raw (1) | MFI ref. | MFI raw (2) | Raw (3) | Adjusted (4) | Cutoff value suggested | Score (5) | ± (7) | Note |
| 02 | Negative Ctrl | 188 | | 44 | | | | 1,339 | | | |
| 03 | Positive Ctrl | 22,934 | | 21,436 | | | | 4,000 | | | |
| 04 | MICA*001 | 99 | | 10,975 | | | | 985 | | | |
| 06 | MICA*002 | 69 | | 10,149 | | | | 958 | | | |
| 11 | MICA*004 | 271 | | 12,319 | | | | 1,092 | | | |
| 17 | MICA*006 | 151 | | 12,830 | | | | 1,183 | | | |
| 19 | MICA*007 | 264 | | 15,730 | | | | 1,106 | | | |
| 24 | MICA*008 | 133 | | 13,314 | | | | 1,205 | | | |
| 26 | MICA*009 | 96 | | 6,152 | | | | 1,072 | | | |
| 32 | MICA*012 | 119 | | 7,038 | | | | 905 | | | |
| 34 | MICA*017 | 62 | | 8,849 | | | | 938 | | | |
| 41 | MICA*018 | 103 | | 8,067 | | | | 913 | | | |
| 43 | MICA*019 | 280 | | 16,914 | | | | 1,237 | | | |

(1) = MFI raw data of negative control serum tested
(2) = MFI raw data of positive control serum tested
(3) = MFI raw of sample serum tested
(4) = (3)—the smallest one of raw (3), the smallest one usually is the raw data generated from the negative control beads if not, find the smallest one generated from 11 single antigen beads. Adjusted MFI is the value after background removed. Cutoff value listed is used as reference that was calculated from 20 normal serum testing for each single antigen beads
(5) = score by 0-invalid; 1-negative; 2-doubt; 4-weak positive; 6-positive; 8-strong positive

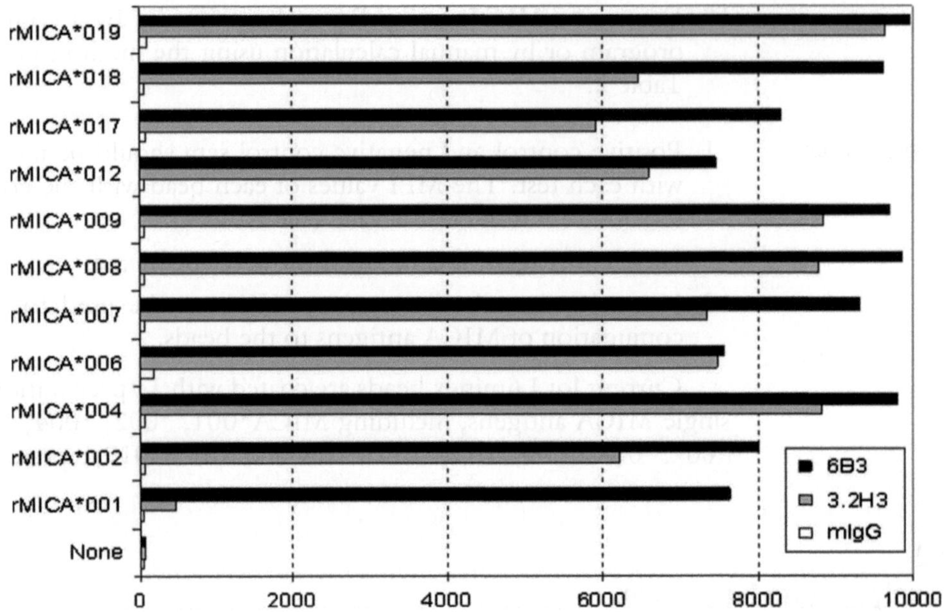


Fig. 1. Reaction of single MICA antigen beads with MICA-specific monoclonal antibodies. The beads were tested with mAb 6B3 (*black bars*) or 3.2H3 (*gray bars*) or normal mouse IgG (mIgG, *open bars*) on 11 single antigen beads named as rMICA*001,*002, *004, *006, *007, *008, *009, *012, *017, *018, and *019. Results are given as mean fluorescence intensities (MFI).

the 11 most common MICA alleles. All of these beads give strong signals with the monomorphic MICA-specific monoclonal antibody 6B3, which is a monoclonal antibody recognizing native MICA proteins. All are positive also with 3.2H3, except for MICA*001, which is known not to be recognized by this antibody. The mean fluorescence intensities vary between 6,000 and 10,000. Normal mouse IgG and beads without antigen show very low background (Fig. 1).

### 3.3. Analysis of Results

1. Data files are generated with the bead numbers and their median fluorescence intensities (MFI) in spreadsheet format. The raw MFI data obtained by Luminex flow cytometry are converted to the relative amounts of MICA antibodies by subtracting the background. The threshold is determined for each bead using the means of the relative amount plus threefold SD of IgG binding in serum from normal subjects ($n > 20$) as shown in Table 3. Based on the relative amount of each MICA allele-specific antibody and the threshold for each antigen bead (see Note 10), scores are assigned as follows: 1 = negative; 2 = doubtful, ≥threshold and < threshold + 600; 4 = weak positive, ≥threshold + 600 and < threshold + 1,800; 6 = positive, ≥threshold + 1,800 and < threshold + 5,400; 8 = _ strong positive, ≥threshold + 5,400.

**Table 3**
**Threshold values above which results are considered positive (score ≥ 4)**

| Luminex bead ID | | MFI after removing background |
|---|---|---|
| #02 | Negative control | 1339 |
| #03 | Positive control | 4000 |
| #04 | rMICA*001 | 985 |
| #06 | rMICA*002 | 958 |
| #11 | rMICA*004 | 1092 |
| #17 | rMICA*006 | 1183 |
| #19 | rMICA*007 | 1106 |
| #24 | rMICA*008 | 1205 |
| #26 | rMICA*009 | 1072 |
| #32 | rMICA*012 | 905 |
| #34 | rMICA*017 | 938 |
| #41 | rMICA*018 | 913 |
| #43 | rMICA*019 | 1237 |

2. MFI generated by each bead with a tested serum minus background signal is used to interpret the results using the threshold values suggested above. To do this, first we find the lowest MFI value among the negative control beads and the 11 antigen beads for a given serum. Then subtract this smallest number from each of the 13 raw MFI values obtained. Finally, the remaining MFI is used to compare to the threshold values given in Table 3. Sera with an MFI greater than the threshold value are considered positive.

### 3.4. Common Serologic Patterns of Antibodies Against MICA

1. There are 14 common serologic patterns of human antibodies against MICA antigens as demonstrated by their differential absorption/reactivity (5). Among these, two broad serologic patterns of antibodies against MICA groups (MICA-G1 and MICA-G2, Table 4) are most frequently detected in transplant recipients. The next frequent serologic patterns of MICA antibodies are MICA-G3, G4, and G5. Those antibodies might react with public epitopes of MICA antigens. Five serologic patterns of MICA antibodies (ID6-10, Table 4) may react with MICA epitopes that recognize shared epitopes among small groups of MICA alleles. Four serologic patterns of MICA antibodies (ID11-14, Table 4) that react with a single MICA allele are less frequently found in patient sera (see Note 11).

**Table 4**
**Common serologic patterns of antibodies against MICA**

| ID | Pattern | Reaction with single antigens of MICA | | | | | | | | | | |
|---|---|---|---|---|---|---|---|---|---|---|---|---|
| | | *001 | *002 | *004 | *006 | *007 | *008 | *009 | *012 | *017 | *018 | *019 |
| 1 | MICA-G1 | + | + | | | + | | | + | + | + | |
| 2 | MICA-G2 | | | + | + | | + | + | | | | + |
| 3 | MICA-G3 | + | | + | + | + | + | + | + | | + | + |
| 4 | MICA-G4 | + | + | + | + | + | | + | + | + | + | |
| 5 | MICA-G5 | + | | | | + | | | + | | + | |
| 6 | MICA-0217 | | + | | | | | | | + | | |
| 7 | MICA-469 | | | + | + | | | | + | | | |
| 8 | MICA-0819 | | | | | | + | | | | | |
| 9 | MICA-46919 | | | + | + | | | + | | | | + |
| 10 | MICA-11218 | + | | | | | | | + | | + | |
| 11 | MICA-01 | + | | | | | | | | | | |
| 12 | MICA-04 | | | + | | | | | | | | |
| 13 | MICA-06 | | | | + | | | | | | | |
| 14 | MICA-12 | | | | | | | | + | | | |

## 4. Notes

1. Serum should be separated from red cells when stored or shipped. Microbial contaminated, hemolyzed, lipemic, or heat inactivated sera may give inconsistent test results and should be avoided.
   (a) Re-calcified plasma can also be used.
   (b) Unacceptable serum specimens.
      i. Serum exposed to excessive heat or repeated freeze–thaw cycles.
      ii. Specimens with bacterial or fungal contamination.
      iii. Specimens containing visible aggregates and/or fibrin.

   Preclear these specimens by centrifugation at 1,300 × *g* for 10 min. Positive control serum produces a high MFI with each bead.

2. Negative control serum gives a low MFI with all beads except the positive control beads.
3. Since the fluorescence of diluted Ab2-PE may change with time, make dilution immediately before use. The optimal concentration of Ab2-PE was determined by titration. It will be different with each new batch of second antibody or new kit lot.
4. MICA single antigen beads were developed in our laboratory. Commercial MICA single antigen beads are available from Tepnel (6) and One Lambda (3). Validation of each kit of beads is needed before use in testing. Serum exchange, parallel testing, and antibody absorption studies are useful to determine the sensitivity, specificity, and stability of the MICA antibody test kit.
5. Positive control beads (#03) were pre-coated with the purified normal human IgG. Negative control beads (#02) were prepared in the same way as other beads, but no antigen was added. High MFI reactivity with bead #03 indicates that the appropriate anti-human IgG secondary antibody was added to each of the positive control sera, negative control serum, and patient serum assay wells.
6. If there are suspended particles on the surface of the serum after centrifugation, do not include the suspended particles when adding serum samples for testing.
7. Pipetting accuracy is important, since dilution of patient serum is performed as part of the assay. Do not pipet 15 μL patient serum with a 200-μL pipetting device.
8. Complete washing is important and necessary before you add the secondary antibodies. A common error when using the assay is incomplete washing. This could result in a low MFI in the positive control beads, and could cause false negative results.
9. The positive control serum supplied in the kit should give a high MFI for each of the antigen beads. The negative control serum in the kit should not give an MFI of more than 1,000 except the MFI from positive control (beads #03).
10. Each laboratory should determine thresholds for positive tests similar to the methods described here for defining cutoff values.
11. A few patient sera will exhibit high background binding. They may require special treatment in order to lower the background nonspecific binding so that the assay can be correctly interpreted. Antibody absorption and elution can be used to resolve questionable results in most cases.

## References


1. Bahram S, Bresnahan M, Geraghty DE et al (1994) A second lineage of mammalian major histocompatibility complex class I genes. Proc Natl Acad Sci 91:6259–6263
2. Zou Y, Heinemann FM, Grosse-Wilde H et al (2006) Detection of anti-MICA antibodies in patients awaiting kidney transplantation, during the post-transplant course, and in eluates from rejected kidney allografts by Luminex flow cytometry. Hum Immunol 67: 230–237
3. Terasaki PI, Ozawa M, Castro R (2007) Four-year follow-up of a prospective trial of HLA and MICA antibodies on kidney graft survival. Am J Transplant 7:408–415
4. Zou Y, Stastny P, Süsal C et al (2007) Antibodies against MICA antigens and kidney-transplant rejection. N Engl J Med 357:1293–1300
5. Zou Y, Qin Z, Silveus A et al (2009) Polymorphisms of MICA recognized by human alloantibodies. Immunogenetics 61:91–100
6. Duquesnoy RJ, Mostecki J, Hariharan J et al (2008) Structurally based epitope analysis of major histocompatibility complex class I-related chain A (MICA) antibody specificity patterns. Hum Immunol 69:826–832

# Chapter 17

# HLA Antibody Detection and Characterization by Solid Phase Immunoassays: Methods and Pitfalls

**Andrea A. Zachary, Renato M. Vega, Donna P. Lucas, and Mary S. Leffell**

## Abstract

Solid phase immunoassays for the detection and characterization of HLA-specific antibodies provide greatly increased sensitivity, specificity, and time and reagent efficiency, compared to the traditionally used cell-based methods. Testing is performed using commercially available test kits. The assays are of two general types: enzyme-linked immunosorbent assays and multianalyte bead. The types vary in both sensitivity and equipment requirements.

While these assays afford great improvement over the cell-based assays, they can be confounded by interference from substances within the serum that result in high background reactivity. The high sensitivity of the assays also makes them more susceptible to environmental factors and operator variability. The user must be aware of the capabilities of the various formats, the factors that can affect test results, and lot to lot variability of any single product. Knowledge of the characteristics of each product and thorough and accurate analysis of the results are essential to the utility of these assays.

**Key words:** Enzyme-linked immunosorbent assays, HLA antibody, HLA phenotype panel, Luminex®, Multianalyte bead assays, Pooled antigen panel, Single antigen panel, Solid phase immunoassays

## 1. Introduction

For more than 30 years, detection and characterization of HLA-specific antibodies (HLA-Ab) were performed using cell-based methods. These methods were hampered by the requirement for a sufficient quantity of viable lymphocytes, low specificity, and prior to the use of flow cytometry, low sensitivity. Isolation of soluble HLA antigens was achieved in the mid 1970s (1), but it was 20 more years before there was success in maintaining the native conformation of soluble HLA molecules following fixation to a solid phase (2, 3). The development of solid phase immunoassays (SPI)

Frank T. Christiansen and Brian D. Tait (eds.), *Immunogenetics: Methods and Applications in Clinical Practice*, Methods in Molecular Biology, vol. 882, DOI 10.1007/978-1-61779-842-9_17, © Springer Science+Business Media New York 2012

for HLA-Ab provided enormous advantages for both HLA-Ab testing for transplantation and the investigation of serologically defined HLA epitopes. Testing by SPI reduces reactivity of antibodies to non-HLA antigens, thereby increasing specificity, increases sensitivity significantly, provides evaluation of antibody strength on a continuous scale facilitating manual analysis and determination of specificity, and can be partially or fully automated. Further advantages are that SPI are available as kits from several manufacturers, allowing laboratories to avoid the laborious task of preparing tests and providing some measure of consistency among laboratories. However, optimizing utility of these assays requires thorough and ongoing quality control. As of this writing, kits are available for the characterization of antigens encoded by antigens of the HLA-A, -B, -C, -DRB1, -DRB3-5, -DQA, -DQB, -DPA, -DPB, and MICA loci. Collectively, these kits test for antibodies to most, but not all, HLA antigens which would be impossible given the polymorphism of the HLA system. Additionally, many of the kits provide the allele identity of the target molecule.

This chapter will discuss the types of assays commercially available, the test procedures, manufacturer-provided materials and reagents and those that must be provided by the laboratory, advantages and disadvantages of the various tests available, test capabilities, problems with and shortcomings of the various tests, and clinical applications. Manufacturers provide detailed instructions for performance of their tests, and therefore, descriptions of the assays provided here will be somewhat generic. Specific information not included here can be found at the web sites of the various manufacturers which are listed below in alphabetical order. Note: since manufacturers may introduce new products or platforms or modify existing ones, web sites should be checked for such changes before deciding to use a particular system.

GEN-PROBE: http://www.gen-probe.com/products-services/
ONE LAMBDA: http://www.onelambda.com

### 1.1. Commercially Available Assays

#### 1.1.1. Formats

Kits for the detection and characterization of HLA-Ab are available in three formats: pooled HLA antigens, panels of individual HLA phenotypes, and panels of single HLA antigens (4, 5). Pooled antigen kits, as the name implies, consist of a pool or mixture of various HLA antigens and generally include the most common HLA specificities found in several racial groups. The pools may be derived through isolation of antigens from the cells of hundreds of individuals or by mixing antigens prepared in transfected cell lines or baculovirus systems. The pools may be comprised of class I (cI) antigens only, class II (cII) only, or a mixture of cI and cII if the platform used can distinguish the individual antigen classes in a mixture. Phenotype panels are comprised of an array of individual cI or cII phenotypes while single antigen panels have the HLA antigens present as individual, purified antigens.

The pooled antigen test provides a rapid and cost-efficient system for determining the presence or absence of HLA-Ab. This test does not determine specificity. However, it does provide an indication of relative strength and breadth of antibody making it useful when monitoring sequential sera from a patient (4). Phenotype panels provide an opportunity to determine antibody specificity and strength. These panels frequently include a phenotype that includes two or more antigens of a potential donor, enhancing the ability to assess the collective strength of the antibodies against that donor. Further, each antigen is almost always present in multiple phenotypes providing a safeguard if one phenotype fails to react properly. Sera reactive with more than 95% of the panel may make it difficult to determine, conclusively, the presence of an antibody to antigens represented by a limited number of phenotypes. However, because the phenotypes that all bear the target of an antibody cluster together when the reactions are listed in descending order of strength, many antibody specificities can be identified in very broadly reactive sera. Single antigen panels permit identification of antibodies that may be masked by other antibodies or react poorly in phenotype panels. Further, since these panels often include multiple alleles within an antigen group, it is easier to detect antibodies reactive with only some alleles within an antigen group. Although single antigen panels have the ability to detect most, if not all, HLA-Ab present in a serum, there are several things to be considered. It is difficult to assess the collective strength of multiple antibodies in a serum as it has been shown that the collective strength of the antibodies is not equivalent to the sum of the strengths of reactivities with the individual antigens (6). Further, the failure of one antigen may not be recognized which may result in the failure to detect antibody to that antigen. As expected, the overall sensitivities of the assays increase with the amount of individual antigen on each bead, so that the order of sensitivity is single antigens > phenoytpes > pooled antigens.

*1.1.2. Assay Types, Matrices, and Platforms*

Two general types of assays are available, multiplex or multianalyte bead assays and enzyme-linked immunosorbent assays (ELISA) (4, 5, 7). For both types of assay, commercial kits provide the matrix with bound soluble HLA antigens. The bead assays are performed on either a conventional flow cytometer or a Luminex® fluoroanalyzer, depending on the kit. In these assays, polystyrene beads are impregnated with fluorescent dyes and beads bearing different pools of antigens, phenotypes, or single antigens are differentiated by the fluorescence of the bead. After incubation with control or test sera, a fluorochrome-labeled anti-human globulin is added to detect beads that have antibody bound. When tested in a conventional flow cytometer, beads of different fluorescence are identified on the

FL2 channel while the intensity of fluorescence is read on the FL1 channel. Multiplex beads for use with the Luminex® platform are incorporated with different combinations of ten dilutions of each of two different dyes to yield 100 different beads. The Luminex® fluoroanalyzer has two lasers: one of which identifies the bead and the other identifies beads with bound antiglobulin. In both assays, different levels of reactivity can be used to approximate relative antibody strength. Depending on the assay format and manufacturer, these assays utilize 10–20 μL of test serum per test.

ELISA are performed on either microtiter or microtest plastic plates. The procedure is comparable to that for the bead assays except that the antiglobulin is bound to an enzyme and test reactions are detected colorimetrically after addition of a color-producing substrate. The required serum volume is approximately 300 μL. In general and depending on the cutoff value used for positivity, the bead-based assays are more sensitive than are the ELISA (8–10).

The antiglobulin reagent provided with all assays is specific for human IgG. It is possible to use reagents specific for other classes of immunoglobulin and for IgG subclasses (11); however, the titer and specificity of those reagents must be verified by the user. Assays have also been developed for the detection of the C4d and C1q components of complement (12–14). However, in our experience, the values obtained for IgG subclasses and C4d may be low (15) and may be more applicable to determining relative quantities.

## 2. Materials

### 2.1. Bead-Based Assays

*Materials Provided* (see Note 1)

1. Analysis software.
2. Beads with bound HLA antigens (see Note 2).
3. Fluorochrome-labeled antiglobulin (varies among manufacturers).
4. Negative control serum (varies among manufacturers).
5. Positive control serum (varies among manufacturers).
6. Wash buffer.

*Materials Required But Not Provided*

1. Adhesive plate sealers.
2. Instrument: flow cytometer or Luminex® fluoroanalyzer, depending on kit.
3. Sheath fluid.

4. Calibration beads.
5. Microcentrifuge.
6. Microfuge tubes.
7. Millipore filter plates or microtiter plates.
8. Multiscreen vacuum manifold (kit dependent).
9. Plate holder for centrifuge.
10. Rotator or plate shaker.
11. Various adjustable and multichannel pipettes.
12. Vortex mixer.
13. Computer.

### 2.2. Conventional ELISA

*Materials Provided*

1. Microtest plates or well strips for use in microtiter plates, preloaded with HLA molecules (see Note 3).
2. Enzyme-conjugated anti-human IgG.
3. Antibody diluent.
4. Colorimetric enzyme substrate (varies among manufacturers, see Note 4).
5. Substrate buffer (varies among manufacturers).
6. Control sera (varies among manufacturers).
7. Plate sealers.
8. Stop reagent.
9. Wash buffer.

*Materials Required But Not Provided*

1. 37°C water bath or incubator.
2. Deionized water.
3. Tubes for sample and reagent dilution.
4. Microplate washer (optional).
5. Adjustable pipetors and Multichannel pipetor with tips.
6. Plate reader with appropriate filters.†

† Adapted for microtest plates when necessary.

## 3. Methods

### 3.1. Sample Preparation (See Notes 5–7)

1. Obtain blood samples in tubes without anticoagulant.
2. Separate and centrifuge serum to remove aggregates. Do not use sera that are lipemic, hemolyzed, microbially contaminated, or heat-inactivated.

3. Store sera at 4–8°C for up to 48 h or below 35°C for longer periods. Serum to be stored longer at 4–8°C should have sodium azide added to a final concentration of 0.1% to prevent microbial growth.

### 3.2. Bead-Based Assays

*Generic Procedure* (see Note 1).

1. Reagents such as wash solution and PE-IgG must be thoroughly mixed prior to use.
2. Pre-wet wells (when using filter plates on the Luminex platform only).
3. Add serum and beads. Manufacturers specify volumes of each. Bead suspensions should be mixed well periodically to assure even dispersion of the beads (see Note 2).
4. Incubate 30 min on a shaking platform to allow specific binding of antibody, when present, to bead-bound antigen. Shaking is necessary to prevent beads from settling which will reduce contact with antibody (see Note 8).
5. Discard supernatant fluid (see Note 9).
6. Wash beads (number of washes is manufacturer specific) to remove unbound immunoglobulin (see Note 10).
7. Discard supernatant fluid and add labeled antiglobulin reagent.
8. Incubate 30 min on a shaking platform.
9. Wash to remove unbound antiglobulin and resuspend beads (see Note 10).
10. For delayed acquisition with a flow cytometer, add a fixing solution.
11. Acquire beads (see Notes 11–17).
12. Perform analysis using manufacturer-provided software. Total time needed for procedure is approximately 4 h excluding data review and analysis. Times will vary depending on the use of robotic fluid handling systems, operator experience, and number of samples tested.
13. In addition to control sera, bead sets have built in control beads.

### 3.3. Conventional ELISA

*Generic Procedure* (see Note 3)

1. Dilute all reagents and sera according to manufacturer's instructions. Include a negative serum with each run to establish background reactivity.
2. Pre-wet test wells, let stand, aspirate fluid. This will rehydrate the bound antigens.
3. Add pre-diluted test and control serum to wells of microtest trays or microtiter strips (see Note 4).

4. Cover tray and incubate 30–45 min at 37°C (GenProbe) or 1 h at 20–25°C (One Lambda) (see Note 18).
5. Remove liquid from wells and wash three times to remove any unbound immunoglobulin (see Note 19).
6. Add conjugated antiglobulin reagent.
7. Cover tray and incubate 30–45 min at 37° (GenProbe) or 40 min at 20–25°C (One Lambda).
8. Remove liquid from wells and wash to remove unbound antiglobulin (see Note 20).
9. Add enzyme substrate (see Note 21).
10. Incubate in the dark 30 min at 20–25°C (GenProbe) or 10–15 min at 37°C (One Lambda) to allow the reaction to equilibrate (see Note 22).
11. Add stop reagent in the same sequence as for substrate. Trays may be stored in the dark for 30 (GenProbe) or 60 min (One Lambda) (see Note 23).
12. Read absorbance (optical density) at 405–410 nm (GenProbe) or 630 nm (One Lambda) (see Note 24).
13. Perform analysis using manufacturer-provided software or manually utilizing recording sheets provided with kit. The percent PRA is calculated by dividing the number of positive HLA-Ab-containing wells by the total number of antigen preparations in the panel. The cutoff value for positivity is calculated as a percentage of the range of reactivity of the provided serum control (SC) tested in the positive wells minus the non-specific background of the test serum (or antibody diluent) tested in the blank wells (One Lambda) or two times the OD value of the mean of the negative control wells (GenProbe). The assignment of antibody specificity is aided by ranking the reactions with test sera in descending order of strength.

Total time needed for procedure is approximately 4 h excluding data review and analysis. Times will vary depending on the use of robotic fluid handling systems, operator experience, and number of samples tested.

## 4. Notes

1. GenProbe reagents are provided together in a kit and are lot-specific. One Lambda reagents are sold individually. GenProbe pooled antigen and phenotype panels must be stored at 4°C. GenProbe single antigen beads must be stored at −80°C and can be refrozen up to six times. One Lambda single antigen,

pooled antigen, and phenotype beads must be stored at −65°C. They can be frozen only once, but they may be stored at 4°C up to 3 months.

2. Beads should be kept in suspension by periodic mixing on a Vortex mixer while being added to tubes or wells.
3. Reagents and trays should be stored according to manufacturer's instructions. Trays and microwell strips/plates should be protected from moisture.
4. Be careful not to touch the well bottom. Change pipet tips regularly to avoid cross contamination.
5. Substances inherent in the serum or external agents such as therapeutic antibodies may interfere with test results. We have shown that low values for the internal positive control (approximately <8,500 MFI for single antigen panels and <12,000 MFI for phenotype panels) or high values for the internal negative control (approximately >150 MFI for all negative controls or >500 MFI for any one control for panels with multiple negative controls, or >200 MFI for panels with a single negative control) indicate test interference that may result in reduced values with HLA targets and that may alter the specificities detected (16). Substances inherent in the serum may include high levels of IgM, immune complexes, and antibody to plastic, among others. There are two commercial bead-bound products for the reduction of background in Luminex® assays: SeraClean™ from GenProbe and Adsorb Out™ from One Lambda, Inc. For both products, the beads are added to a serum known to have high background reactivity, incubated, and then removed, ideally with whatever is causing high background bound to the beads. The results are variable and are probably affected by the amount and nature of interfering factors. Also, it is not possible to know if this process also reduces or dilutes HLA-Ab. We have shown that hypotonic dialysis, dialyzing serum against distilled water, is effective in eliminating or substantially reducing high background in nearly all cases. This procedure is based on the differing solubilities of IgM and IgG in distilled water which results in the precipitation of IgM but not IgG. It is possible that this procedure also eliminates some immune complexes. Dithiothreitol (DTT), a reducing agent, has been reported to reduce background in sera tested on single antigen beads (17), but in our experience it actually increases reactivity with the negative control and is not as effective as hypotonic dialysis in restoring normal reactivity to test sera in the Luminex® assay. Interestingly, we have found that sera tested on glass microchips often do not display the high background that they exhibit with a plastic matrix. Low positive and/or high negative controls indicate that reactivity with antigen-bearing beads

has been compromised and accurate interpretation of the results requires some treatment of the serum.

6. Therapeutic agents may also result in test interference. Agents shown to impact test results include Thymoglobulin, high dose IVIg, Eculizumab, and Bortezomib (18, 19). Thymoglobulin is a polyclonal rabbit serum and can thus be removed by absorbing the serum with beads coated with an anti-rabbit immunoglobulin. We have shown that hypotonic dialysis also resolves some or all of the interference caused by Eculizumab and Bortezomib.
7. Groups of patients, defined by the type of transplant, may demonstrate, on average, different levels of background or test interference.
8. All incubations should be performed in the dark at 20–25°C. Beads and fluorochrome-labeled antiglobulin are light sensitive and extended exposure may cause photo-bleaching. These reagents should be protected from light as much as possible.
9. When using filter plates, the vacuum pressure should be no greater than that required to aspirate samples. If using a vacuum manifold, do not exceed 100 mmHg. High vacuum pressure may cause beads to be crushed (misshaped) resulting in bead failures.
10. Insufficient washing may produce false negative reactions due to blocking of the antiglobulin by residual immunoglobulin in the wells. Inconsistent washing may yield inconsistent test bead and control reactivity.
11. Instruments for bead analysis should be calibrated daily or before each run if daily runs are not performed.
12. Bead acquisition should occur within the manufacturer's specified time frame.
13. Unusually high acquisition times (>20 s/sample) may be indicative of addition of incorrect bead volumes (concentrations). This may result in false negative or weak test bead reactivity.
14. If using a filter plate and one or more test wells appear clogged, scratch the plastic dimple underneath test well.
15. Low bead counts may be a result of instrument clogs and/or instrument out of calibrated range. Possible solutions are to sonicate the sample probe and/or re-calibrate instrument.
16. Inclusion of one or more well-characterized sera in a test run can provide an indication of when test sensitivity is unacceptable.
17. There is no serum control for Luminex assays; however, high positive control bead values (>20,000 MFI) and low negative

control bead values (<50 MFI), with unusually low test bead values (<100 MFI) (together) may indicate that serum was not added to the assay.

18. Test plates must be covered during incubations to prevent evaporation.
19. Inadequate washing before addition of antiglobulin will result in reduced specific reactivity due to blocking of the antiglobulin reagent by residual immunoglobulin.
20. Inadequate washing before addition of substrate will increase non-specific reactivity due to reactivity between free conjugated antiglobulin and substrate.
21. Colorimetric enzyme substrate and substrate buffer are light sensitive and should be mixed immediately prior to use.
22. Time and temperature of the substrate incubation are critical and failure to adhere to manufacturer's specifications may lead to increased background.
23. Optimal reactivity requires that stopping solution be added at the required time.
24. Plate readers should be calibrated according to manufacturer's recommendations or whenever problems arise. If trays are stored for rereading, OD values will diminish over time.

## 5. Data Analysis and Interpretation

Analysis software is available for all products and the manufacturers also provide calculations for performing analyses manually. The initial calculations performed by the software are to determine positivity and negativity. These calculations take into account the overall reactivity of the assay as determined from the negative control bead(s) and background noise due to individual bead variability. The values for background noise are lot specific. Also, different assays within and between manufacturers may yield different negative and positive control bead values. Thresholds for positivity can be altered by the user. The software can also perform analyses to determine specificity, correlation coefficients, chi-squared values, two-by-two analysis data for each specificity, and values normalized for antigen density. The analysis software can: provide customized reports designed by the user and lot-specific updates for background noise; allow the user to view all data for a particular patient; search by sample, patient, or test run; and generate single patient or batch reports in a variety of document formats.

Specificities may be analyzed by antigen, allele, or cross-reactive antigen groups.

We have found that computer-generated interpretation of results is not sufficient for accurate specificity assignment and that all results should be examined manually. Attention must be paid to controls. Very low negative controls may result in low test values being scored by computer analysis as positive. Low positive controls (MFI < 12,000) or high negative controls (MFI > 400) may indicate the presence of interfering factors that may result in reduced test serum values and incorrect specificity determination (this will be discussed further in Subheading 7).

When using a phenotype panel and listing reactions in descending order of strength, phenotypes bearing a common target antigen will be clustered together when the test serum contains antibody to that antigen. This can provide two types of information. First, the strongest reacting phenotypes often contain two or more antigens that are targets of antibodies in the serum, providing an estimate of the collective strength of those antibodies. Second, the test scores of these clustered phenotypes may be low and interpreted as negative by the computer but the non-random assortment of antigens strongly suggests the presence of low-level antibody.

Certain beads or wells may give consistently high results with negative control serum or consistently low or negative results with specific antibody. This information should be taken into account when assigning specificity.

Both the alpha and beta chain of HLA-DQ and HLA-DP molecules are polymorphic and interpretation of positive reactions with DQ or DP molecules should take into account the possibility of specificity to either chain. It may be possible to identify antibody directed to antigens on the alpha chain by the clustering of antigens with a common alpha chain. Greater assurance of that specificity is provided by a positive reaction with a molecule comprised of the suspect alpha chain and a beta chain found in the serum donor's own phenotype. Additionally, a serologic epitope may depend on the combination of certain alpha and beta chains (20). Specificity for this type of epitope may be difficult to define with certainty if the panel contains only one representation of that alpha-beta combination. Further confirmation may be obtained by performing a crossmatch with cells bearing the target molecule. However, this would require that the antibody is strong enough to yield a positive reaction and that the serum does not contain antibodies to other antigens on the target phenotype.

There is a maximum amount of antibody that can bind to targets. For sera that contain more antibody than can be bound to the target, the relative strength of the antibody cannot be assessed accurately. In such cases, tests of diluted serum may yield better information about antibody strength, but the user is advised to note any manufacturer's cautions or recommendations about interpreting data from serum diluted beyond the manufacturer's recommendations and to interpret data from such dilutions with caution.

## 6. Quality Control

Each lot of kits should be tested with human serum from a healthy, non-sensitized male or a pool of sera from such individuals. The serum should be known to lack HLA-Ab and should give unquestionable negative reactions with all or nearly all targets, individual beads, or wells (except the internal positive control if one is included in the kit). Higher than expected reactions with any target may indicate the likelihood of non-specific reactivity and/or higher than expected reaction strength with that target in the presence of antibody specific for the target. Reactivity with the negative control serum also provides information about the different background reactivities of the targets, although this should be accounted for by the manufacturer's software.

Each new lot of kits should be tested with several sera containing different, well-characterized, HLA-Ab to check the sensitivity and specificity of the lot.

Each run should include positive and negative control sera to determine the validity of the run.

Ongoing monitoring of each target should be performed to assess the possibility of inappropriately low reaction strength or increased background. The data should also be used to evaluate lot-to-lot differences in reaction strength.

Positive and negative control targets should be monitored for consistency and level of reactivity.

Whenever new targets are introduced into a new lot, their reactivity should be evaluated with antibody specific for the HLA antigen(s) of that target.

## 7. Technical Issues

Variability exists among formats, among platforms, among similar products from different manufacturers, between lots of the same product from the same manufacturer, between tests run on different days, and between tests run by different technologists. We have already noted that specificity and sensitivity are greater for single antigen panels than for phenotype panels and for phenotype panels than for pooled antigen panels. Not surprisingly, single antigen panels appear to be less robust than do phenotype panels. This may be due in part to the higher amounts of individual antigen in the single antigen panels. If one antigen in a phenotype is susceptible to losing its native conformation, the impact on reaction strength may be buffered, to some extent by other antigens in the phenotype. However, the effect will be more obvious when the affected antigen is the only target. Further, the increased sensitivity of the single antigen panel may make it more susceptible to environmental variables. In phenotype panels, the effect of distortion of one antigen is greater when that antigen is in the homozygous state or when the amount of that antigen has been increased above normal by the manufacturer.

As noted earlier, we and others have observed differences in sensitivity and in susceptibility to background among the different platforms.

The single antigen products from different manufacturers differ both in the panel composition and in the sensitivity and specificity of the reactions with different antigens; therefore, use of more than one product can provide complementary information. While use of more than one manufacturer's kit may be cost prohibitive, the cost may be offset by the improved information obtained from using more than one kit, particularly when accurate assessment of antibody strength is critical.

We and others have observed significant differences in the sensitivity of different lots of the same product. Recently, we documented mean increases in sensitivity between consecutive lots of a single antigen multiplex bead kit of 5,500 MFI for the A locus and 2,400 MFI for the B locus, representing a 125–275% increase in reactivity *(unpublished data)*. On the one hand, this increased sensitivity could be beneficial if the specificity is high; but on the other hand, this is a serious problem when monitoring sequential samples from a single patient. The problem is exacerbated if the laboratory is unaware of this change until it becomes apparent after extended use of the product.

Day-to-day and tech-to-tech variability is inevitable for serologic assays but can lead to incorrect interpretation of antibody strength. After introducing a robotic liquid handling system into the laboratory, we performed an analysis of the variability between sequential duplicate tests with the pooled antigen format performed by a single technologist compared to duplicate tests performed using the robotic device. We tested sera with different strengths of reactivity. The variability in reaction strength for the technologist-performed assays was 7.9–22.8 compared to only 4.9–6.6% for the robotic-assisted liquid handling assays (21). Run-to-run variability must be accounted for when interpreting results. An example is given in Fig. 1, which shows the strength of HLA-Abs from sequential serum specimens from the same patient plotted against the strength of the positive control. The left side of the plot shows an unmistakable increase in HLA-Abs with a much more limited change in the reaction strength of the positive control. However, beginning with week 6, the HLA-Ab strength and that of the positive control are parallel suggesting that apparent changes in the HLA-Ab strength most likely reflect day-to-day differences in test sensitivity. Correct interpretation of changes in

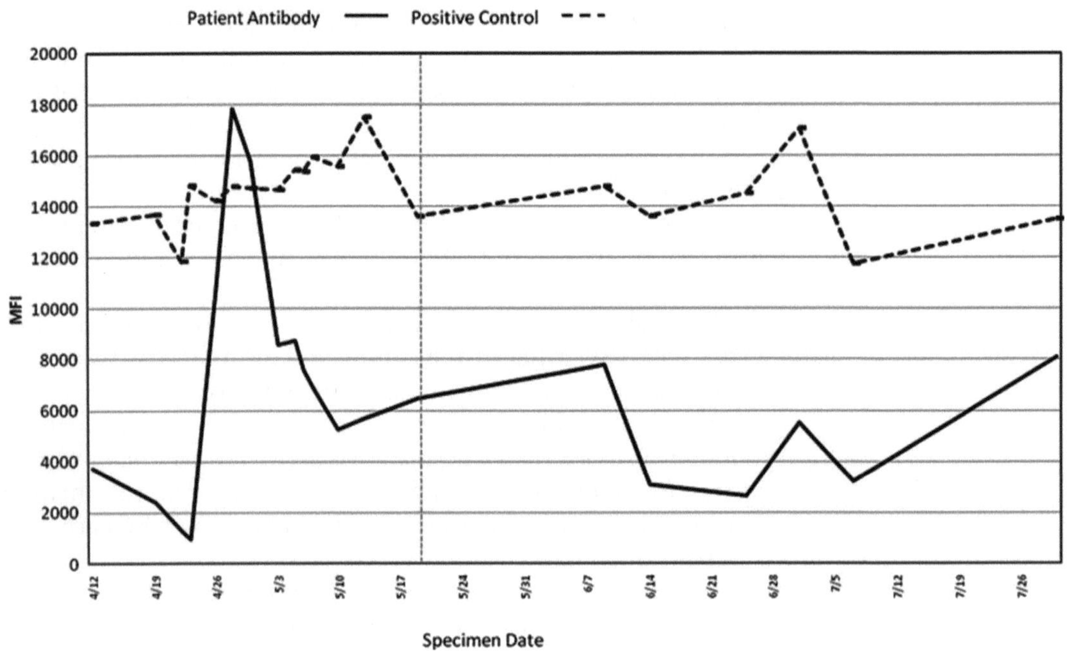


Fig. 1. Test serum vs. positive control. Run-to-run variability must be accounted for when interpreting results of HLA antibody testing. The strength of HLA-Abs from sequential serum specimens from the same patient is plotted against the strength of the positive control. The *left* side of the plot shows an unmistakable increase in HLA-Abs with a much more limited change in the reaction strength of the positive control. However, beginning with week 6 (*dotted vertical line*), the HLA-Ab strength and that of the positive control are parallel suggesting that apparent changes in the HLA-Ab strength most likely reflect day-to-day differences in test sensitivity.

HLA-Ab is critical when these data are used to determine clinical treatment.

The amount and condition of antigen is known to vary among the different HLA antigens (22). Distortion of the HLA target will yield a false positive reaction with antibody reactive with a non-native epitope resulting from the distortion of the molecule and will yield reactions that are incorrectly negative or weaker than expected with antibody to a native HLA epitope that is lost.

Differing amounts of antigen will yield different reaction strengths with a fixed amount of antibody. The amounts of Cw, DQ, and possibly DP antigens are known to be increased above that of other antigens in some kits (6). This enhances the ability to detect antibodies to these antigens, but the reaction strength cannot be considered comparable to that for other antigens, given the same amounts of antibody.

If the target bead or well is not completely coated with antigen or a blocking agent, immune complexes and immunoglobulin can adhere nonspecifically to the matrix or to the capture antibody if a capture antibody is used. This could lead to a false positive reaction. While one might anticipate that the reaction strength would be low, this may not be the only source of non-specific binding.

## 8. Applications

The development and use of SPI for HLA-Ab has provided a significant benefit for transplantation and for further identification of serologic epitopes. The more specific characterization of HLA-Ab has enhanced their detection. Applied prior to transplant, this information permits the identification of antibodies that are likely to yield crossmatch tests positive at different sensitivity levels such as cytotoxicity and flow cytometry. In turn, this permits calculation of the percentage of the donor population with which a patient will have a positive crossmatch (23). In the United States, this is utilized by the United Network for Organ Sharing (UNOS), the administrator of the National Organ Procurement and Transplantation Network. Using allele and haplotype frequencies for HLA-A, -B, -DRB1, and -DQB antigens from thousands of donors from four racial groups, UNOS has established a program for calculating this percentage, referred to as the calculated PRA (CPRA). An online program is maintained by UNOS and can be accessed at http://optn.transplant.hrsa.gov/resources/professionalResources.asp?index=78. Transplant programs are required to test patient sera using at least one SPI and enter unacceptable antigens from which the patient's CPRA is determined and incorporated into the allocation algorithm. Use of the CPRA has decreased the incidence of failure to transplant the intended recipient because of a positive crossmatch by 83% (24). Even without the elegant CPRA calculations, this would not have been possible without the more precise recognition of HLA-Ab made possible by SPI.

The assessment of HLA-Ab strength and specificity by SPI can also be used to perform a virtual crossmatch which has multiple applications (6, 25–31). Prior to transplantation, the virtual crossmatch based on SPI results permits procurement of organs with minimal permissible cold ischemia times, such as hearts and lungs, from a broader geographic area than does using data from cytotoxicity tests. The virtual crossmatch can expedite the process of paired donation among multiple transplant centers by eliminating the need for testing geographically distant donors who would have a positive crossmatch. The virtual crossmatch is also useful for monitoring patients following transplantation when cell-based crossmatch tests are not possible because of the presence of humanized or chimeric lymphocyte reactive therapeutic antibodies (4).

SPI are invaluable to desensitization programs. Reinsmoen et al. (32) have correlated the results of crossmatch tests with those of SPI and determined a maximum antibody strength that permits successful transplantation in patients being desensitized with high-dose IVIg. In our program, the course of donor-specific antibody (DSA), assessed by SPI prior to transplant is used to measure treatment efficacy and, in turn, adjust the treatment when indicated (33).

Post-transplant monitoring is essential since desensitized patients are at higher risk for antibody-mediated rejection (AMR) and SPI allows for rapid detection of changes in DSA strength and of the development of new DSA.

As has been shown by several groups, post-transplant monitoring of DSA, particularly in patients at higher risk for AMR, provides an opportunity for early intervention when DSA appears or increases in strength (34–40). SPI tests are more rapid and more sensitive and specific than are cell-based assays. With cell-based assays, the presence of DSA was often not detected until nephrectomy of a failed graft. This may have been due to adsorption of DSA onto the graft, reducing circulating levels of DSA below that detectable in the cell-based assays. However, SPI can detect very low levels of circulating DSA in the presence of an allograft. We have shown (41, 42) that DSA is always detected when renal biopsies are positive for C4d but that not all patients with circulating DSA have C4d positive biopsies. Thus, early detection of DSA may be a surrogate for the more invasive biopsy. We have also shown that pro-inflammatory events can cause increases in the breadth and/or strength of HLA-Ab (43). Again, early detection of these changes can be clinically relevant to patients awaiting deceased donor transplantation and to patients already transplanted.

An unresolved issue is the level of DSA that is clinically relevant. It has been shown that increased episodes of AMR are associated with DSA levels detectable by ELISA but not with levels detectable only by bead-based assays (9, 44). However, the risk incurred with DSA present only at levels detected by the most sensitive assays is one of current debate, with numerous reports both supporting (27, 45, 46) and questioning (26, 47–49) a negative impact associated with low-level antibodies. Since any amount of DSA indicates sensitization, there is a risk of a clinically relevant increase in the DSA level; therefore, monitoring of such patients is appropriate. The frequency of DSA among transplanted patients was not discernible in the era of cell-based assays. Terasaki has shown that dysfunction of renal grafts may not occur for months after the development of DSA (50). Thus, the clinical conundrum is when to intervene. SPI assessment of DSA is providing valuable information about the effects of antibodies of different strengths and different specificities and is likely to yield information that will lead to improved graft outcomes.

SPI tests of HLA-Ab combined with determination of HLA alleles have provided information about epitopes shared among alleles and have provided the opportunity to identify antibodies to an antigen that appears to be identical in a donor-recipient pair, but which is encoded by different alleles in the donor and recipient (51–53). Using SPI one can also identify antibodies to the alpha chains of DQ and DP antigens. This information is useful to determining the epitope composition of different HLA antigens and to reconcile crossmatch results that would otherwise appear anomalous (20).

## 9. Considerations and Recommendations

The review of the capabilities and shortcomings of various formats and platforms suggests that complete and accurate information about a patient's HLA-Abs is best obtained with the use of more than one assay. While this may appear to be cost prohibitive, by customizing the use of multiple assays according to the antibodies of a patient, we have been able to maintain test costs in the lowest quartile of independent US laboratories.

There has been much recent discussion about two issues surrounding SPI: results reporting and standardization. There is interest in having some quantitative measure of sensitization using test values expressed as MFIs or OD ratios. As we have noted above, the values are affected by several factors, including: the antibody specificity, with antibodies to enhanced antigens yielding higher values; by the format used, with higher values obtained with single antigen panels than with phenotype panels; by the sensitivity of the particular lot of reagents used; by the presence of interference causing high background and reduced test values; and by the day-to-day variability inherent in serologic assays. All of these factors must be taken into consideration for a meaningful interpretation of the test results. The trend of DSA and the crossmatch reactivity that would be predicted from the SPI results are likely to be more meaningful clinically. However, this implies that thorough and accurate analysis of the test results by the laboratory scientist and technologist is absolutely necessary to providing such meaningful interpretation.

Standardization of test results would be extremely useful for interpreting data from different laboratories. However, there are several hurdles to overcome to achieve this goal. Most importantly, at present there are no reference sera with known amounts of antibody to use as standards. Monoclonal antibodies are not representative of the polyclonal nature of antibodies present in most patients and even mixtures of such antibodies would not replicate the nature of patient's sera which contains other factors that could affect test results. Second, while some laboratories treat sera to remove interfering factors, at present this is not done universally. Third, the high degree of sensitivity of SPI and its susceptibility to variability suggests that standardization might only be achieved by considering ranges of test values. Fourth, standardization cannot be readily achieved until manufacturer-provided kits are standardized from lot to lot. The question is, how much of a problem is this. A perusal of the literature reveals that multiple variations of the cytotoxicity crossmatch have been used. Differences in incubation times and temperatures, the use of an antiglobulin, the source and specificity of the antiglobulin, and the ratio of cells to serum can have a significant impact on test sensitivity. These same factors will affect the results of flow cytometric crossmatch tests. Further, with flow cytometric testing, there has been no standardization of the cytometers used, the antiglobulin reagent used, the reading scale, or the threshold for positivity. The only data normalization has been with the use of ratios or molecules of equivalent soluble fluorochromes. In fact, there are many publications of the results of allogeneic crossmatch results without results of autologous crossmatches which, when positive, would affect the interpretation of the allogeneic crossmatch. To date, this has not been raised publicly as an issue as has standardization of SPI. We believe that the more important practice is to have results standardized and correlated with clinical outcomes within a transplant program. However, this does not eliminate the need for appropriate testing and accurate test interpretation, nor does it preclude longer term efforts to achieve some standardization in test reporting by inclusion of criteria for the definition of clinically relevant antibodies. Despite the above noted issues, the development and use of SPI for testing HLA-Abs has had a very significant impact that has improved the care of transplant patients, our knowledge of the immunogenicity of HLA antigens, and is likely to lead to increased understanding of the humoral response to HLA antigens.

## References

1. Oh SK et al (1975) Soluble HL-A antigens in serum. I. Isolation and purification. Eur J Immunol 5:161–166
2. Buelow R et al (1995) Detection of panel-reactive anti-HLA class I antibodies by enzyme-linked immunosorbent assay or lymphocytotoxicity. Results of a blinded, controlled multicenter study. Hum Immunol 44:1–11
3. Zachary AA et al (1995) Evaluation of HLA antibodies with the PRA-STAT test. An ELISA test using soluble HLA class I molecules. Transplantation 60:1600–1606
4. Zachary AA, Leffell MS (2008) Detecting and monitoring human leukocyte antigen-specific antibodies. Hum Immunol 69:591–604
5. Tait BD (2009) Solid phase assays for HLA antibody detection in clinical transplantation. Curr Opin Immunol 21:573–577
6. Zachary AA et al (2009) Using real data for a virtual crossmatch. Hum Immunol 70:574–579
7. Fuggle SV, Martin S (2008) Tools for human leukocyte antigen antibody detection and their application to transplanting sensitized patients. Transplantation 86:384–390
8. Zeevi A, Girnita A, Duquesnoy R (2006) HLA antibody analysis: sensitivity, specificity and clinical significance in solid organ transplantation. Immunol Res 36:255–264
9. Phelan D et al (2009) Living donor renal transplantation in the presence of donor-specific human leukocyte antigen antibody detected by solid-phase assay. Hum Immunol 70:584–588
10. Leffell MS, Montgomery RA, Zachary AA (2005) The changing role of antibody testing in transplantation. Clin Transpl 259–271
11. Bartel G et al (2007) Determinants of the complement-fixing ability of recipient presensitization against HLA antigens. Transplantation 83:727–733
12. Smith JD et al (2007) C4d fixing, Luminex binding antibodies—a new tool for prediction of graft failure after heart transplantation. Am J Transplant 7:2809–2815
13. Wahrmann M et al (2009) Clinical relevance of preformed C4d-fixing and non-C4d-fixing HLA single antigen reactivity in renal allograft recipients. Transpl Int 22:982–989
14. Chin C et al (2011) Clinical usefulness of a novel C1q assay to detect immunoglobulin G

antibodies capable of fixing complement in sensitized pediatric heart transplant patients. J Heart Lung Transplant 30(2):158–163

15. Lucas DP et al (2010) Effect of desensitization on DSA strength and C4D deposition. Transplantation 90:96
16. Zachary AA et al (2009) Naturally occurring interference in Luminex assays for HLA-specific antibodies: characteristics and resolution. Hum Immunol 70:496–501
17. Kosmoliaptsis V et al (2010) Improved Luminex-based human leukocyte antigen-specific antibody screening using dithiothreitol-treated sera. Hum Immunol 71:45–49
18. Houp J et al (2010) Considerations in interpreting solid phase antibody data. Hum Immunol 71:s18
19. Lucas DP (2007) Removal of interfering substances from sera and cells for screening and crossmatch. In: Rosenberg JC (ed) ASHI laboratory manual, 4.2 edn. Mt. Laurel, New Jersey. American Society for Histocompatibility and Immunogenetics
20. Tambur AR et al (2010) The complexity of human leukocyte antigen (HLA)-DQ antibodies and its effect on virtual crossmatching. Transplantation 90(10):1117–1124
21. Vega RM et al (2008) Laboratory automation: coming of age. Hum Immunol 69:s105
22. Warner P (2009) Nebulous humors: defining alloantibodies in the 21st century. Hum Immunol 70:623–626
23. Zachary AA, Braun WE (1985) Calculation of a predictive value for transplantation. Transplantation 39:316–318
24. Cecka JM et al (2010) Calculated PRA: initial results show benefits for sensitized patients and a reduction in positive crossmatches. Am J Transplant 11:719–724
25. Stehlik J et al (2009) Utility of virtual crossmatch in sensitized patients awaiting heart transplantation. J Heart Lung Transplant 28:1129–1134
26. Ferrari P et al (2010) Virtual crossmatch approach to maximize matching in paired kidney donation. Am J Transplant 11:272–278
27. Morris GP et al (2010) Virtual crossmatch by identification of donor-specific anti-human leukocyte antigen antibodies by solid-phase immunoassay: a 30-month analysis in living donor kidney transplantation. Hum Immunol 71:268–273
28. Amico P et al (2009) Utility of the virtual crossmatch in solid organ transplantation. Curr Opin Organ Transplant 14:656–661
29. Tambur AR et al (2008) Tailoring antibody testing and how to use it in the calculated panel reactive antibody era: the Northwestern University experience. Transplantation 86:1052–1059
30. Bingaman AW et al (2008) A virtual crossmatch protocol significantly increases access of highly sensitized patients to deceased donor kidney transplantation. Transplantation 86:1864–1868
31. Appel JZ 3rd et al (2006) Role of flow cytometry to define unacceptable HLA antigens in lung transplant recipients with HLA-specific antibodies. Transplantation 81:1049–1057
32. Reinsmoen NL et al (2008) Acceptable donor-specific antibody levels allowing for successful deceased and living donor kidney transplantation after desensitization therapy. Transplantation 86:820–825
33. Leffell MS, Zachary AA (2009) The role of the histocompatibility laboratory in desensitization for transplantation. Curr Opin Organ Transplant 14:398–402
34. Leffell MS, Zachary AA (2010) Antiallograft antibodies: relevance, detection, and monitoring. Curr Opin Organ Transplant 15:2–7
35. Riethmüller S et al (2010) Donor-specific antibody levels and three generations of crossmatches to predict antibody-mediated rejection in kidney transplantation. Transplantation 90:160–167
36. Hachem RR et al (2010) Anti-human leukocyte antigen antibodies and preemptive antibody-directed therapy after lung transplantation. J Heart Lung Transplant 29:973–980
37. Zeevi A et al (2009) Emerging role of donor-specific anti-human leukocyte antigen antibody determination for clinical management after solid organ transplantation. Hum Immunol 70:645–650
38. Everly MJ, Terasaki PI (2009) Monitoring and treating post transplant human leukocyte antigen antibodies. Hum Immunol 70:655–659
39. Piazza A et al (2006) Post-transplant donor-specific antibody production and graft outcome in kidney transplantation: results of sixteen-year monitoring by flow cytometry. Clin Transpl 323–336
40. Reinsmoen NL, Nelson K, Zeevi A (2004) Anti-HLA antibody analysis and crossmatching in heart and lung transplantation. Transpl Immunol 13:63–71
41. Kraus ES et al (2009) Subclinical rejection in stable positive crossmatch kidney transplant patients: incidence and correlations. Am J Transplant 9:1826–1834

42. Zachary AA et al (2003) Specific and durable elimination of antibody to donor HLA antigens in renal-transplant patients. Transplantation 76:1519–1525
43. Locke JE et al (2009) Proinflammatory events are associated with significant increases in breadth and strength of HLA-specific antibody. Am J Transplant 9:2136–2139
44. Zachary AA, Leffell MS (2010) Barriers to successful transplantation of the sensitized patient. Expert Rev Clin Immunol 6:449–460
45. Verghese PS et al (2010) Impaired graft survival in pediatric renal transplant recipients with donor-specific antibodies detected by solid phase assays. Pediatr Transplant 14:730–734
46. Gibney EM et al (2006) Detection of donor-specific antibodies using HLA-coated microspheres: another tool for kidney risk stratification. Nephrol Dial Transplant 21:2625–2629
47. Leffell MS, Zachary AA (2010) Anti-allograft antibodies: some are harmful, some can be overcome, and some may be beneficial. Discov Med 9:478–484
48. Bielmann D et al (2007) Pretransplant risk assessment in renal allograft recipients using virtual crossmatching. Am J Transplant 7:626–632
49. Aubert V et al (2009) Low levels of human leukocyte antigen donor-specific antibodies detected by solid phase assay before transplantation are frequently clinically irrelevant. Hum Immunol 70:580–583
50. Terasaki PI, Cai J (2008) Human leukocyte antigen antibodies and chronic rejection: from association to causation. Transplantation 86:377–383
51. El-Awar N et al (2009) Epitopes of HLA-A, B, C, DR, DQ, DP, and MICA antigens. Clin Transpl 295–321
52. Cano P, Fernández-Viña M (2009) Two sequence dimorphisms of DPB1 define the immunodominant serologic epitopes of HLA-DP. Hum Immunol 70:836–843
53. Marrari M et al (2010) Human monoclonal antibody reactivity with human leukocyte antigen class I epitopes defined by pairs of mismatched eplets and self-eplets. Transplantation 90(12):1468–1472

# Chapter 18

# Detection and Characterisation of Alloreactive T Cells

Mandvi Bharadwaj, Nicole A. Mifsud, and James McCluskey

## Abstract

T cell alloreactivity is responsible for much of the morbidity and mortality associated with tissue transplantation and graft versus host disease. Immunoassays for ex vivo monitoring and quantitation of alloreactive T cells are being increasingly utilised to provide valuable information for individualised clinical management of transplant recipients. Here we describe detailed methodologies for both traditional and novel assays utilised for the detection, quantitation, and functional characterisation of alloreactive T cells and highlight the key advantages and disadvantages of each system.

**Key words:** Allogeneic, Alloreactivity, $^{51}$Cr release assay, Enzyme-linked immunospot, Graft versus host disease, Intracellular cytokine staining, T cells, T cell receptors, Tetramer staining

## 1. Introduction

αβ T cell receptors (TCR) conventionally respond to foreign peptide antigens bound to polymorphic molecules encoded by self major histocompatibility complex (MHC) genes. However, some T cells can also respond to non-self (allogeneic or allo) peptide-MHC (pMHC) molecules resulting in alloreactivity. T cell allorecognition is thus defined as the ability of a T cell to recognise allogeneic MHC molecules, i.e. non-self but from the same species. Alloreactive T cells play a central role in graft rejection and graft versus host disease (GVHD) (1).

Historically, $^{51}$Cr release assays were specifically developed as a simple and highly sensitive in vitro assay system to measure the cytolytic activity of alloreactive T cells (2) expanded in response to stimulation with donor allogeneic lymphocytes, in mixed lymphocyte cultures. However, the mixed lymphocyte culture only permitted a qualitative analysis that confirmed the presence of

Frank T. Christiansen and Brian D. Tait (eds.), *Immunogenetics: Methods and Applications in Clinical Practice*, Methods in Molecular Biology, vol. 882, DOI 10.1007/978-1-61779-842-9_18, © Springer Science+Business Media New York 2012

alloreactive T cells, giving no information on their frequency within the culture. Subsequent development of limiting dilution analysis (LDA) (3), wherein multiple replicates of serially diluted effector cells (patient peripheral blood mononuclear cells [PBMC)) are co-incubated with allogeneic stimulators (allogeneic PBMC or target cells) for a minimum of 7 days before being analysed in a $^{51}$Cr release assay (2), was a significant advance, facilitating quantification of the frequency of specific T cells participating in an immune response (4–6). A comprehensive description of the LDA is detailed in a recent review (7). This technique was later adopted for assessing the in vitro potential of allogeneic mismatches to generate GVHD or allograft rejection (8).

Technological advance in the past 2 decades has enabled the development of other novel approaches that cannot only detect, but also quantify and characterise alloreactive T cells based on phenotypic and functional differences in T cell subsets, thus providing the scientist/clinician with a wide spectrum of immunoassays. Indeed these are being increasingly utilised for ex vivo monitoring and quantitation of alloreactive T cells to aid the modulation of immunosuppressive therapy post-organ transplant. The following chapter provides detailed methods for the traditional as well as some more recent assays utilised for the detection and characterisation of alloreactive T cells, and highlights the advantages and disadvantages of each system.

### 1.1. $^{51}$Chromium (Cr) Release Assays

Despite the increasing reluctance to utilise radioactive assay systems, more than 4 decades after it was first developed, the $^{51}$Cr release assay is still considered as the gold standard for measuring the cytolytic efficiency of CD8$^{+}$ T cells for both alloreactivity (8, 9) and anti-viral T cell responses (10, 11). Host PBMCs or alloreactive T cells proliferating in an LDA or mixed lymphocyte culture are co-incubated with $^{51}$Cr labelled, allogeneic stimulators (targets), and the $^{51}$Cr released in the culture medium is measured after 4–5 h. This provides a measurement of the specific lysis of the $^{51}$Cr labelled targets by the alloreactive T cells. Whilst a direct correlation has been demonstrated between precursor frequencies determined by an LDA and clinical data on prediction and outcomes of GVHD (12–15), there are also reports suggesting that the enumeration of allo-specific T cell precursor frequencies by an LDA may not correlate with human transplant outcomes (16–18). Furthermore, studies based on anti-viral T cells in Epstein–Barr virus (EBV), Influenza virus, and Lymphocytic Choriomeningitis virus infection have highlighted inherent biological and technical problems associated with the LDA (12, 19–22). Overall, the LDA may only assess the precursor frequency of a single dominant alloantigen rather than accurately reflecting the complexity of the alloresponse generated by all of the mismatched HLA antigens.

### 1.2. Enzyme-Linked Immunospot Assay

The enzyme-linked immunospot (ELISPOT) assay provides a methodology for the detection and quantitation of activated T cells (11, 22–25) on the basis of cytokine secreted by each cell. Briefly, wells of specialized ELISPOT plates are coated with a primary antibody specific for the cytokine of interest; T cells (PBMCs, purified T cell subsets or in vitro expanded T cells) are added to the wells and co-cultured with a stimulus (24) (e.g. allogeneic PBMCs, target cells, antigenic peptide, or a mitogen) for a relevant time period (24–48 h). During the incubation period, activated T cells locally secrete cytokines that are captured by the primary antibody. A secondary biotinylated antibody is subsequently applied for the specific detection of the secreted cytokine followed by an enzyme-conjugated Streptavidin. Finally, a substrate relevant for the enzyme (conjugated to Streptavidin) is added and the enzyme converts the substrate into an insoluble coloured product that forms a discrete spot (see Fig. 1) at the location of the secreting cell. Enumeration of these spots provides the frequency of the relevant T cells. As very low frequency T cells (one cell in 100,000), secreting a wide array of cytokines can be analysed, this technique therefore has a broad range of clinical applications including vaccine trials (26) and immune tracking for T cells in infectious disease (11), cancer (27), autoimmunity (28), and transplantation (29, 30). The ELISPOT assay has various advantages over the $^{51}$Cr release assay, including (1) non-radioactive quantitation of activated T cells, (2) ex vivo analysis (independent of clonal expansion), (3) less labour intensive, (4) shorter assay time, and (5) increased sensitivity. The recent development of the Fluorospot technique (31), which utilises fluorescent detection in lieu of enzymatic detection, has facilitated the simultaneous detection of two cytokines in a single test, allowing differentiation of cells with alternative cytokine profiles as

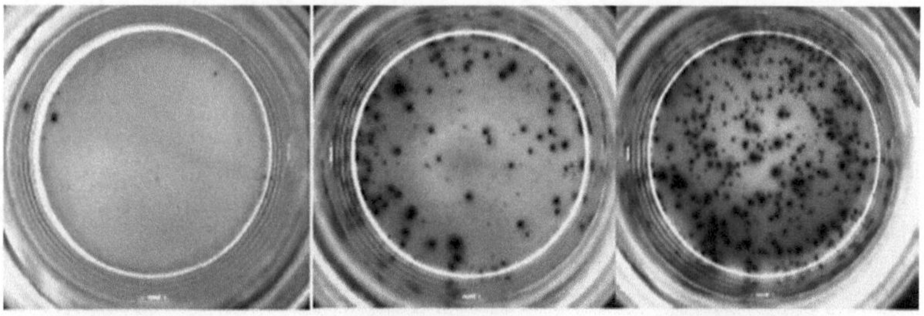


Fig. 1. Figure shows pictures of three wells of an enzyme-linked immunospot (ELISPOT) plate containing the negative control (responders alone), test (responders + allogeneic stimulators), and a positive control (responders + viral peptide or phytohaemagglutinin). The *dark spots* in the wells represent cytokine secreting cells. All samples should be tested in triplicate and analysed under a constant setting on the ELISPOT reader.

well as the co-expression of two cytokines by a single cell (31). However, as the measurement of the number of spots generated by each cytokine secreting T cell is assisted by computerised imaging equipment, the user-defined options including size, gradient, and intensity thresholds can introduce a degree of subjectivity in the analysis of the assay and interpretation of results. This can however be resolved by using appropriate controls and keeping the settings of the ELISPOT/Fluorospot reader consistent for each assay.

### 1.3. Peptide/MHC Tetramer Staining

The design and application of soluble MHC tetrameric complexes for investigating anti-viral $CD8^+$ T cells was first described in 1996 (32). Subsequently, tetrameric complexes have revolutionised the quantitation and dissection of antigen-specific T cell responses (32–35). The generation of pMHC tetramers is described in a number of publications (7, 23, 32). The HLA/$\beta_2$m/peptide tetrameric complex is conjugated to a fluorochrome of interest, such as phycoerythrin (PE), fluorescein isothiocyanate (FITC), or allophycocyanin (A-PC), and used as a staining reagent for flow cytometry. MHC class I tetramers have been extensively used for the detection of antigen-specific $CD8^+$ T cells in both viral infections (10) and alloreactive conditions (9). However, more recently the development of MHC class II tetramers (36–38) have further advanced the analysis of $CD4^+$ T cells in the fields of autoimmunity (39–41), tumour antigens (42), and virology (43).

It is noteworthy that $CD8^+$ T cell frequencies quantitated by tetramer staining have been shown to be higher than those detected by conventional cytotoxicity assays (44). This is probably due to the ability of tetramers to detect different T cell phenotypes including naïve, memory, and effector cells and the tendency for memory T cells to undergo apoptosis upon activation (activation-induced cell death) resulting in a loss of reactive T cells in culture (45). Compared to the traditional assays, the pMHC complexes (1) are quantitative and sensitive (1:50,000), (2) do not involve radioactivity, (3) require minimal material (blood, tissue), (4) are a fast approach, (5) permit batch processing for large numbers, (6) can be used in combination with other cell surface antibodies used for T cell phenotyping (10, 19, 26, 32, 46, 47), and (7) do not kill the T cells allowing the cells to be sorted for use in other assays (such as ELISPOT and intracellular cytokine staining [ICS]). Recent studies investigating the antiviral T cells (10) and/or cross-reactive virus-specific T cells recognising specific HLA alloantigens have demonstrated the power in combining both pMHC tetramers and the ICS assay (10, 48, 49) (described below). The only major limitation of this assay is that both the peptide epitope and MHC-restriction elements must be known for the detection of specific T cells.

### 1.4. Intracellular Cytokine Staining

The activation of T cells initiates the production of cytokines that can be detected and quantitated using ICS (7, 50, 51). Briefly, T cells are activated through co-incubation with a stimulus for a total of 6 h. An inhibitor of intracellular transport is added after the first 2 h to arrest the transport of newly synthesised proteins, including cytokines, from the endoplasmic reticulum into the Golgi. Post-incubation, the T cells are stained with a cocktail of specific monoclonal antibodies (mAbs) for cell surface phenotyping. The T cells are then paraformaldehyde fixed, permeabilised in mild detergent, and stained with anti-cytokine antibodies. Phenotypic analysis is facilitated by flow cytometry.

The T cell frequencies detected by ICS have been shown to correlate with frequencies obtained by pMHC tetramers in HIV patients (52) and with ELISPOT in an Influenza study of healthy individuals (53). Conversely, no correlation was demonstrated between the frequencies detected by ICS and pMHC tetramers in a metastatic melanoma study (54), and the enumeration of EBV-specific T cells and alloreactive T cells by ICS yielded higher frequencies than that obtained by the LDA-based $^{51}$Cr release assay (55). Notwithstanding the discrepancies in the frequency of T cells enumerated by the different assay systems, ICS has been used for the detection of cytokine producing CD4$^{+}$ T cells in the peripheral blood of individuals with HIV (56) and quantification of activated allo-specific CD8$^{+}$ T cells in healthy controls (9, 57) and solid organ transplant recipients (58). It has various advantages over the other assays described above, including (1) analysis of large numbers of cells, (2) multiparameter analysis using combinations of intracellular and cell surface antibodies, (3) parallel measurement of T cell cytokine profiles, and (4) measurement of cytotoxic potential using a degranulation marker.

## 2. Materials

All consumables and reagents should be sterile unless otherwise specified.

### 2.1. Isolation of PBMC and In Vitro Expansion of Allogeneic CD8$^{+}$ T Cells

1. Polypropylene tubes: 50 and 10 mL.
2. Polystyrene tubes: 30 mL (V-bottom).
3. Serological pipettes: 10 and 25 mL.
4. Polypropylene 1 mL transfer pipettes.
5. Glass Pasteur pipettes.
6. Pipette tips: 0.5–10, 10–200, and 200–1,000 μL.
7. Cell culture plates: 6-well, 12-well, 24-well, 48-well, and 96-well (U-bottom).

8. RPMI (Culture/assay media): RPMI 1640 media (Gibco-Invitrogen Corporation, USA) supplemented with 150 μM Non-essential Amino Acids (Gibco-Invitrogen Corporation, USA), 7.5 mM HEPES (MP Biomedicals, Eschwege, Germany), 150 μg/mL Streptomycin sulphate (Sigma, MO, USA), 150 U/mL Benzyl-penicillin (CSL, Australia), 2 mM L-glutamine (MP Biomedicals, Eschwege, Germany), and 76 μM 2-mercaptoethanol (Sigma, MO, USA). Should be stored at 2–8°C.
9. Foetal calf/bovine serum (FCS or FBS, heat inactivated for 30 min at 56°C, Millipore).
10. RF10: RPMI (supplemented with antibiotics, non-essential amino acids, and glutamine, as described in step 8) supplemented with 10% heat inactivated FCS/FBS (as described in step 9).
11. Human recombinant Interleukin-2 (IL-2) (Cetus Corporation, Emeryville, CA). This should be stored at −20°C in small aliquots to prevent frequent freeze thawing.
12. RF10 + 20 U/mL of IL-2: RF10 supplemented with human recombinant IL-2 to achieve a final concentration of 20 U/mL. (Medium containing IL-2 should be made fresh but can be stored overnight at 4°C for up to 24 h).
13. Ficoll-Paque PLUS (GE Healthcare), stored at room temperature in the dark.
14. Irrigation water (Baxter), stored at room temperature.
15. Phosphate Buffered Saline (PBS, Life Technologies), stored at room temperature.
16. Trypan Blue (Sigma) dilute to 0.2% in PBS, stored at room temperature.
17. Biohazard class II cabinet.
18. Centrifuge.
19. Aspirator.
20. Pipette gun.
21. Pipettes: 0.5–10, 10–200, and 200–1,000 μL.
22. Bright field microscope (cell counting).
23. Haemocytometer (cell counting).
24. Incubator: 37°C, 5% $CO_2$.
25. Centrifuge.
26. Gamma irradiator.
27. Vortex.

### 2.2. Dissection and Quantitation of the Alloreactive CD8+ T Cell Response

#### 2.2.1. $^{51}Cr$ Release Assays

1. Polypropylene tube: 10 mL.
2. Syringe: 1 mL.
3. Pipette tips: 0.5–10, 10–200, and 200–1,000 μL.
4. Cell culture plate: 96-well (U-bottom).
5. RPMI and RF10: as described in Subheading 2.1 (steps 8 and 10).
6. 200 mM peptide, stored at −20°C.
7. $Na^{51}CrO_4$ as the $^{51}Cr$ stock solution (stored in a lead shielded box in a room dedicated to radioisotopes) (Perkin Elmer, USA).
8. Triton X-100 (Sigma).
9. LumaPlate-96 containing scintillant (Packard Biosciences-Perkin Elmer, USA).
10. Plastic plate sealers.
11. Radiation badge.
12. Laminar flow or Biohazard class II cabinet.
13. Centrifuge.
14. Pipettes: 0.5–10, 10–200, and 200–1,000 μL.
15. Multichannel pipette: 10–200 μL.
16. Bright field microscope (cell counting).
17. Haemocytometer (cell counting).
18. Incubator: 37°C, 5% $CO_2$.
19. Lead lined Esky to transport labelled targets.
20. Top count plate reader (Top count Microplate; Packard Instrument Co, Meriden, CT).
21. Biohazard bag and containers for low level and high level "hot-waste".
22. Geiger-Müller counter.

#### 2.2.2. ELISPOT Assay

1. Polypropylene tubes: 1.5 and 10 mL.
2. Serological pipettes: 10 mL.
3. Pipette tips: 0.5–10, 10–200, and 200–1,000 μL.
4. Reagent reservoirs.
5. Aluminium foil.
6. Capture mAb: Anti-IFN-γ (suggested clone l-DIK, anti-IFN-γ mouse IgGl 1 mg/mL, from Mabtech) (see Note 1).
7. Detection mAb: Anti-IFN-γ-biotin (suggested clone 7-B6-1-biotin anti-IFN-γ mouse IgG1-1 mg/mL from Mabtech).

8. Multiscreen plates (0.45 ~ 1 m) from Millipore Australia Pty. Ltd (Sterile; 10 plates) (see Note 1).
9. Streptavidin-alkaline phosphatase (Lyophilized powder, 1 mg protein, Sigma; resuspended in 1 mL of sterile $H_2O$).
10. 5-bromo-4-chloro-3-indolyl phosphate/Nitro blue tetrazolium (BCIP/NBT) tablet- SigmaFast™ (Sigma).
11. PBS.
12. PBS + 5% FCS.
13. PBS + 0.05% Tween 20 (PBST) (Sigma).
14. 0.1 M sodium bicarbonate ($NaHCO_3$), pH 9.6.
15. 1 mg/mL of Phytohaemagglutinin (PHA).
16. Stock solutions of 200 μM peptides stored at −20°C.
17. RPMI and RF10: as described in Subheading 2.1 (steps 8 and 10).
18. Biohazard class II cabinet.
19. Centrifuge.
20. Pipettes: 0.5–10, 10–200, and 200–1,000 μL.
21. Multichannel pipette: 10–200 μL.
22. Bright field microscope (cell counting).
23. Haemocytometer (cell counting).
24. Incubator: 37°C, 5% $CO_2$.
25. ELISPOT reader (AID Autoimmun Diagnostika GmbH, Germany).

*2.2.3. Intracellular Cytokine Staining*

1. Cell culture plates: 96-well (U-bottom).
2. Polypropylene tubes: 1.5 and 10 mL.
3. Polystyrene tube: 5 mL (non-sterile).
4. Glass Pasteur pipettes.
5. Serological pipettes: 10 mL.
6. Pipette tips: 0.5–10, 10–200, and 200–1,000 μL.
7. Reagent reservoirs.
8. Aluminium foil.
9. RPMI and RF10, RF10 + 20 U/mL IL-2: as described in Subheading 2.1 (steps 8, 10, and 12).
10. Geneticin (G418, Life Technologies).
11. Hygromycin B (Life Technologies).
12. 200 μM peptide, stored at −20°C.
13. Monoclonal antibodies, stored at +2 to 8°C (see Note 2 and Table 2).
14. Tetramers, stored at +2 to 8°C (see Note 3 and Table 3).

15. 500 μg/mL Monensin (Sigma), stored at +2 to 8°C.
16. 10 μg/mL Brefeldin A (Sigma), reconstituted in 100% methanol and stored at −20°C.
17. 16% Paraformaldehyde (ProSciTech), stored at room temperature. Prior to use in assay, dilute to 1% final concentration in PBS. Mix well and store at +2 to 8°C.
18. 1% Saponin (Sigma), stored at room temperature. Dissolve 0.5 g Saponin in 50 mL Milli-Q water. Mix well and filter through 0.22-μm disc filter. Prior to use in assay, dilute to 0.3% final concentration in PBS. Mix well and store at room temperature.
19. PBS, stored at room temperature.
20. Biohazard class II cabinet.
21. Centrifuge.
22. Incubator: 37°C, 5% $CO_2$.
23. Aspirator.
24. Pipette gun.
25. Pipettes: 0.5–10, 10–200, and 200–1,000 μL. Multichannel: 5–50 and 200–1,000 μL.
26. Bright field microscope (cell counting).
27. Haemocytometer (cell counting).
28. Flow cytometer for FACS.
29. Flow Cytometric software: CellQuest™ (Becton Dickinson), FlowJo (Treestar Inc., Ashland, OR) (see Note 4).

*2.2.4. Tetramer Staining*

1. Cell culture plates: 96-well (U-bottom).
2. Polypropylene tubes: 1.5 and 10 mL.
3. Polystyrene tube: 5 mL (non-sterile).
4. Glass Pasteur pipettes.
5. Pipette tips: 0.5–10, 10–200, and 200–1,000 μL.
6. Aluminium foil.
7. RPMI, stored at +2 to 8°C.
8. RPMI and RF10, RF10+20 U/mL IL-2: as described in Subheading 2.1 (steps 8, 10, and 12).
9. Geneticin (G418, Life Technologies).
10. Hygromycin B (Life Technologies).
11. 200 μM peptide, stored at −20°C.
12. Monoclonal antibodies stored at +2 to 8°C (see Note 2 and Table 2).
13. Tetramers, stored at +2 to 8°C (see Note 3 and Table 3).
14. Biohazard class II cabinet.
15. Centrifuge.

16. Incubator: 37°C, 5% $CO_2$.
17. Pipette gun.
18. Bright field microscope (cell counting).
19. Haemocytometer (cell counting).
20. Pipettes: 0.5–10, 10–200, and 200–1,000 μL. 8-channel: 5–50 and 200–1,000 μL.
21. Flow cytometer for FACS.
22. Flow Cytometric software: CellQuest™ (Becton Dickinson), FlowJo (Treestar Inc., Ashland, OR).

## 3. Methods

Carry out all procedures at room temperature unless otherwise indicated. Handling of human samples and disposal of biohazard waste should be performed according to the international guidelines on biosafety level 2 containment (or similar for each country, e.g. physical containment level 2 in Australia).

Allo-specific $CD8^+$ T cells can either be detected ex vivo by ELISPOT or tetramer staining, or after in vitro expansion in a mixed lymphocyte reaction (MLR), commonly utilised for $^{51}Cr$ release assays and ICS. For an MLR, responder (alloreactive) PBMC are stimulated with irradiated allogeneic PBMC at a 2:1 ratio. Antigen-specific $CD8^+$ T cells are generally used as positive controls and require stimulation of responder PBMC with irradiated, peptide-pulsed autologous PBMC at a 2:1 responder to stimulator ratio (see Note 5). Antigenic peptides derived from common viruses such as Influenza virus, EBV, or Cytomegalovirus (CMV) (59) with known HLA-restriction are utilised here. Selection of sterile cell culture plates depends on the seeding density of PBMC (see Table 1, adapted from Life Technologies (formerly Invitrogen) GIBCO cell culture system catalogue).

**Table 1**
**Selection of cell culture plates**

| Culture plates | Surface area ($cm^2$) | Seeding density (maximum) | Culture volume (mL) |
|---|---|---|---|
| 6-well | 9.6 | $30 \times 10^6$ | 10 |
| 12-well | 3.8 | $10 \times 10^6$ | 4 |
| 24-well | 2.0 | $5 \times 10^6$ | 2 |
| 48-well | 0.75 | $2.5 \times 10^6$ | 1 |

Adapted from GIBCO cell culture system catalogue

Following in vitro expansion in an MLR (see Subheading 3.1), alloreactive T cells can be detected directly by tetramer staining if the alloantigen and its HLA restriction are known (9) (see Subheading 3.2). Alternatively, the total alloresponse can be dissected following a short restimulation with B-lymphoblastoid cell lines (B-LCL) carrying the allogeneic HLA allotypes or restimulation with cell lines (such as the MHC class I reduced cell line, C1R) transfected with single HLA class I molecules similar to that of the allogeneic stimulators. These cell lines are referred to as "reporter cells" (see Note 6) and facilitate the determination of the contribution of each mismatched HLA alloantigen to the total alloresponse. Antigen-specific $CD8^+$ T cells expanded against known viral antigens (positive controls) are restimulated with peptide-pulsed reporter cells carrying the appropriate HLA. The restimulation of allo-specific T cells activates these cells, enabling functional characterisation via production or upregulation of both cell surface molecules and intracellular proteins/cytokines that can be analysed in an ELISPOT, $^{51}Cr$ release, or ICS assay.

### 3.1. Isolation of PBMC and In Vitro Expansion of Allo-Specific $CD8^+$ T Cells

1. Collect peripheral blood in appropriate blood collection tubes containing anti-coagulant (see Note 7).
2. To a 50 mL tube, add 5–20 mL of peripheral blood and an equal volume of RPMI to achieve a 1:2 dilution of the peripheral blood.
3. To another 50 mL tube, add 10 mL of Ficoll-Paque PLUS (see Note 8).
4. Using a 25 mL serological pipette gently overlay the diluted peripheral blood onto the Ficoll-Paque PLUS reagent using the slow setting on the pipette gun (see Note 9).
5. Centrifuge for 20 min at 931 ×*g*, room temperature with the brake setting = OFF (see Note 10).
6. Blood components will be fractionated and plasma can be collected using a 1 mL transfer pipette and stored at −80°C if required (see Fig. 2).
7. Using a sterile 1 mL transfer pipette, carefully collect lymphocyte/monocyte/platelet layer (interface) into a 30 mL V-bottom tube. Wash cells in a final volume of 20 mL of RPMI.
8. Centrifuge for 15 min at 524 ×*g*, room temperature.
9. A cell pellet should be visible at the bottom of the tube, discard supernatant by aspiration, leaving approximately 1 mL of residual volume and resuspend cell pellet.
10. Transfer the cell pellet to a 10 mL tube containing 8 mL of RPMI and centrifuge for 10 min at 524 ×*g*, room temperature. Repeat wash by resuspending the cell pellet in 8 mL of RPMI and centrifuging for 10 min at 524 ×*g*, room temperature.

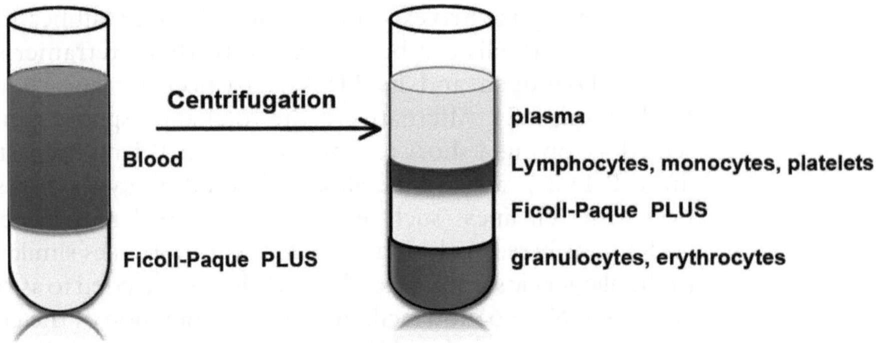


Fig. 2. Isolation of PBMCs. Peripheral blood is layered over the Ficoll-Paque and, following centrifugation (with brake OFF), the blood components are separated into (1) plasma, (2) lymphocytes, monocytes, platelets, and (3) granulocytes, erythrocytes. The lymphocytes, monocytes, and platelets layer can be extracted, centrifuged to remove platelets with the residual cells representing the peripheral blood mononuclear cell population.

11. Resuspend the cell pellet in 8 mL of RPMI and centrifuge for 2 min at 931 ×*g*, room temperature (see Note 11).
12. Discard supernatant by aspiration and resuspend the cell pellet in 1 mL of assay media or PBS.
13. Perform a cell count for viable cells, using 0.2% Trypan Blue.
14. PBMC can be used immediately or cryopreserved.
15. To set up an MLR: Resuspend the responder PBMC in an appropriate volume of assay media (RF10 + 20 U/mL IL-2) (see Note 12) to achieve a final concentration of $2 \times 10^6$ cells/mL. Add the right volume of responder cell suspension to a suitable cell culture plate (see Table 1) and incubate the plate at 37°C, 5% $CO_2$. For example, to achieve a 2:1 responder to stimulator ratio, one would add 1 mL of responders ($2 \times 10^6$ cells/mL) and 1 mL of stimulators ($1 \times 10^6$ cells/mL) to 1 well of a 24-well plate.
16. Allogeneic stimulator cells: Resuspend the allogeneic PBMC at a concentration of $3 \times 10^6$ cells/mL and gamma-irradiate at 3,000 Rad (30 cGy) (see Note 13). After irradiation, wash cells by resuspending in 10 mL of RPMI and centrifuging for 7 min at 524 ×*g*. Resuspend the cell pellet in assay media (RF10 + 20 U/mL IL-2) to achieve a final concentration of $1 \times 10^6$ cells/mL.
17. Preparation of peptide-pulsed autologous PBMC as positive control (for virus-specific T cells): Pellet autologous PBMCs and resuspend in plain RPMI to achieve $1 \times 10^6$ cells/100 μL at 10 μM final concentration of peptide (e.g. 5 μL of 200 μM peptide stock/100 μL of RPMI). Incubate at 37°C, 5% $CO_2$ for 1 h. Vortex every 15 min. Wash cells by resuspending in 10 mL of RPMI and centrifuging for 7 min at 524 ×*g*.

Resuspend the cell pellet in assay media (RF10 + 20 U/mL IL-2) to achieve a final concentration of $1 \times 10^6$ cells/mL.

18. Add the irradiated allogeneic PBMC and peptide-pulsed autologous PBMC to separate wells containing the responder PBMC, to achieve a 2:1 ratio of responder to stimulator. Mix cells gently and thoroughly and incubate the plate at 37°C, 5% $CO_2$ for 5–7 days.

19. The in vitro expansion of allo-specific or antigen-specific CD8⁺ T cells is dependent on the kinetics of the responder cell proliferation in response to the stimulus, and also on the cytokine/protein being measured (see Fig. 3, Note 14).

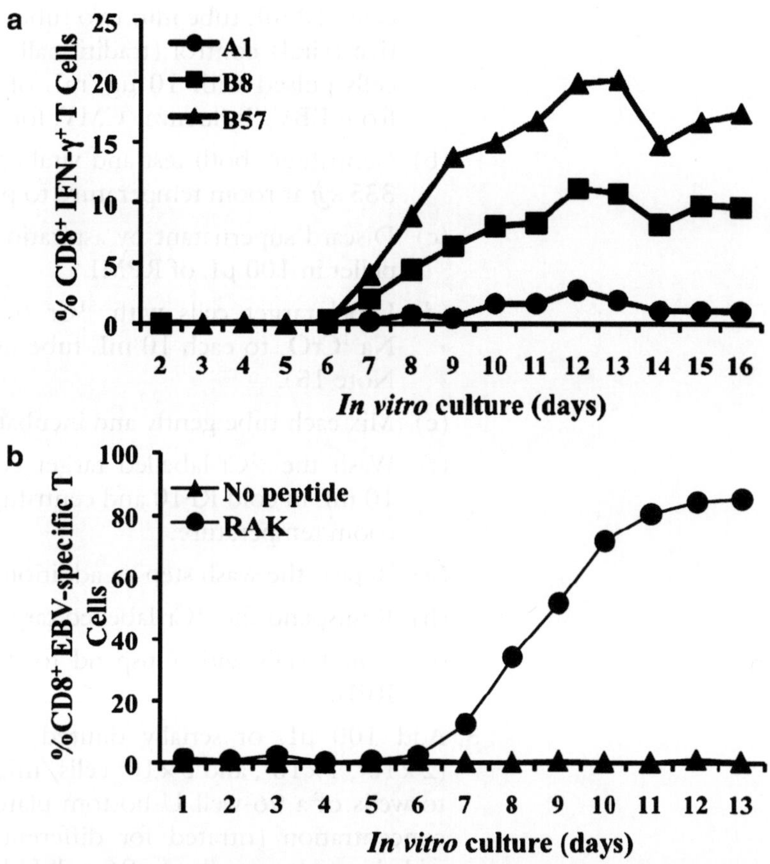


Fig. 3. In vitro expansion of allo-specific and antigen-specific CD8⁺ T cells. (**a**) PBMC from a healthy individual was stimulated for up to 16 days with allogeneic PBMC that enabled generation of allo-specific CD8⁺T cells against all three mismatched HLA-A1, -B8, and -B57 allotypes. The maximal CD8⁺ T cell response, measured by the production of IFN-γ, was observed at 12–13 days post-stimulation. (**b**) PBMC from a HLA-B8 healthy individual was stimulated with autologous PBMC pulsed with EBV peptide RAKFKQLL (RAK) for up to 13 days. The maximal response, measured in HLA-B8/RAK tetramer⁺CD8⁺ T cells by the production of IFN-γ, was observed at 12–13 days post-stimulation.

### 3.2. Dissection and Quantitation of the Alloreactive CD8+ T Cell Response

#### 3.2.1. $^{51}$Cr Release Assay

1. Preparation of responder (effector) cells: Count effector cells and serially dilute in 2 mL of RF10 in a series of 10 mL tubes to achieve a cell concentrations of $2 \times 10^6$, $1 \times 10^6$, and $5 \times 10^5$ cells/mL. The aim is to achieve multiple replicates of an effector:target (E:T) ratio of 100:1, 50:1, and 25:1 in the assay.
2. Preparation of reporter (target) cells—$^{51}$Cr labelling: Wear protective eyewear, gown, radiation badge, and double gloves. Scan the area in which you are planning to perform $^{51}$Cr labelling of target cells with a Geiger-Muller counter to assess if there is a pre-existing background level of radiation. Use the Geiger counter when using the isotope to monitor spills and exposure (see Note 15).
   (a) Count allogeneic reporter or target cells and aliquot $3 \times 10^6$ cells/10 mL tube into two tubes for test sample and positive (viral) control (traditionally viral controls are target cells pulsed with 10 μg/mL of peptide antigen derived from EBV/Influenza/CMV, for 1 h at 37°C).
   (b) Centrifuge, both test and viral control tubes for 7 min at $335 \times g$ at room temperature to pellet the cells.
   (c) Discard supernatant by aspiration and resuspend the cell pellet in 100 μL of RPMI.
   (d) Label target cells with $^{51}$Cr by adding 50–100 μL of $Na^{51}CrO_4$ to each 10 mL tube using a 1-mL syringe (see Note 15).
   (e) Mix each tube gently and incubate for 1 h at 37°C.
   (f) Wash the $^{51}$Cr-labelled target cells in a final volume of 10 mL in cold RF10 and centrifuge for 7 min at $800 \times g$ at room temperature.
   (g) Repeat the wash step an additional two times.
   (h) Resuspend the $^{51}$Cr-labelled target cells in 1 mL of RF10.
   (i) Count cells and resuspend to $2 \times 10^4$ target cells/mL in RF10.
3. Add 100 μL of serially diluted responder (effector) cells ($2 \times 10^6$, $1 \times 10^6$, and $5 \times 10^5$ cells/mL—as described in step 1) to wells of a 96-well U-bottom plate. Cells at each different concentration (titrated for different E:T ratios) should be added into three wells of a 96-well U-bottom plate (see Fig. 4).
4. Add 100 μL of $^{51}$Cr-labelled target cells ($2 \times 10^3$ target cells) as described in step 2 to each well of the 96-well U-bottom plate.
5. Negative controls (media only): 3–6 wells containing 100 μL of $2 \times 10^3$ target cells/well (without responders) plus an additional 100 μL RF10/well is used to calculate the spontaneous release of $^{51}$Cr from the target cells.

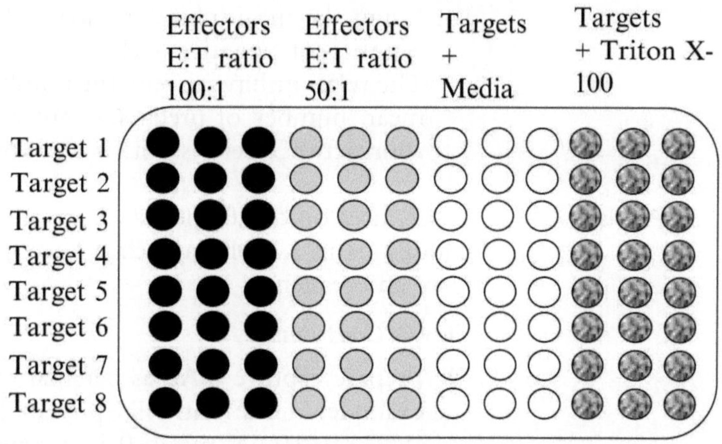


Fig. 4. Proposed plan for setting up the $^{51}$Cr release assay at an E:T ratio of 100:1 and 50:1. Other ratios may be tested similarly in different plates. Target 1–8 represent the different cell lines (BLCL or transfected C1R) that need to be tested for allogeneic reactivity to the responders (or effectors), the untransfected parent C1R cell line and a positive control (reporter cell line pulsed with a viral peptide). All targets are resuspended in the assay media at a set concentration (e.g. $2 \times 10^4$ target cells/mL) and the effectors or responder cells are serially diluted to achieve an E:T ratio of 100:1, 50:1, and 25:1 (and more if required).

6. Positive controls (1% of Triton X-100): 3–6 wells containing 100 μL of $2 \times 10^3$ target cells/well (without responders) plus 100 μL of 1% Triton X-100/well is used to calculate the maximal release of $^{51}$Cr from the target cells (see Note 16).
7. Ensure that each well contains $^{51}$Cr-labelled target cells with effector cells, media (RF10) only, or 1% of Triton X-100 (see Fig. 4).
8. Centrifuge the plate at $233 \times g$ for 3 min, to pellet cells.
9. Incubate at 37°C, 5% $CO_2$ for 4–5 h.
10. Centrifuge the plate at $233 \times g$ for 3 min, to ensure cells are at the bottom of the well.
11. Using a multichannel pipette, remove 25 μL of supernatant from each well and transfer directly to the same position on a LumaPlate, which already contains scintillant.
12. Leave LumaPlate at room temperature to dry overnight.
13. The $^{51}$Cr levels in assay supernatant samples collected on the LumaPlate are measured on a beta scintillation counter and the % Specific Lysis is calculated using the following formula (see Note 17):

$$\frac{(\text{Experimental release} - \text{Spontaneous release})}{(\text{Maximal release} - \text{Spontaneous release})} \times 100$$

14. Using the mean plus 3 standard deviations (SD) cut-off, the number of negative wells is determined for each dilution. The relationship between the number of negative wells and the mean number of precursors are plotted, and a frequency of alloreactive T cells is obtained (3, 60, 61).

#### 3.2.2. ELISPOT Assay

Procedures on day 0 and day 1 are to be performed under sterile conditions in a Biohazard class II cabinet to maintain sterility of plate and reagents.

*Day 0: Coat Plate*

1. Prepare capture mAb as per manufacturer's instructions. For example: dilute anti-IFN-γ mAb (1-DIK anti-IFN-γ mouse IgG1) to 10 μg/mL in 0.1 M sodium bicarbonate buffer pH 9.6 or 1× PBS and dispense 100 μL to each well of the ELISPOT plate (see Notes 18 and 19). Incubate plate with lid overnight (approximately 18 h) at 4°C (refrigerator) on a level surface.

*Day 1:*

2. *Plate blocking*: After overnight incubation, retrieve test plate from 4°C incubation and wash wells by flicking off coating mAb solution into discard tray. Then add 200 μL sterile PBS per well and flick off into discard tray. Repeat washing another five times. After the final wash add 200 μL per well of sterile PBS with 5% FCS (blocking solution) to test plate, incubate for 1 h at 37°C (or at room temperature if to be left longer).
3. *Prepare effectors*: PBMC (fresh or cryopreserved) or in vitro expanded alloreactive T cells can be used as effector cells for assessing the alloreactive response (see Note 20). Perform cell count and adjust cell concentration to $2 \times 10^6$ cells/mL to seed at a final concentration of $2 \times 10^5$ cells/well/100 μL in the ELISPOT plate (see Note 19). If using in vitro expanded alloreactive T cells, the cell concentration should be between $1 \times 10^3$–$5 \times 10^4$cells/well.
4. *Prepare targets*: Allogeneic PBMC depleted of $CD3^+$ T cells (B cell enriched) are utilised (see Note 21). Relevant B-LCLs or reporter cell lines (see Subheading 3 introduction) can also be used although they may give a high background. Seed target cells in limiting dilution ($5 \times 10^4$, $2.5 \times 10^4$, and $1 \times 10^4$ cells/well) in triplicate in a total volume of 100 μL to appropriate wells.
5. *Positive control*: A final concentration of 10 μg/mL of either phytohemagglutinin (PHA) or a known anti-viral peptide (EBV, CMV, or Influenza A) restricted to the same HLA molecules expressed by the effector cells, in a total volume of 5 μL serves as positive control.

6. *Negative control:* Replicate wells with effector cells only (without targets) and targets only (without effectors) serve as negative control.
7. The ELISPOT plate is incubated for 20–24 h at 37°C, 5% $CO_2$ (see Note 22).

*Day 2:*

8. After incubation remove cells by flicking plate over a discard tray in the biosafety cabinet. Wash wells with 200 μL/well of filtered 0.05% PBST (PBS containing 0.05% Tween 20; see Note 23) using a multichannel pipette (can use a wash bottle with a blunt nozzle positioned very close to the well). Wash an additional two times.
9. Change pipette tips and repeat three washes with 200 μL/well of filtered PBS (no Tween) (see Note 24). Dry the ELISPOT plate by gently blotting inverted plate on a stack of tissues or paper towels just before adding the next reagent.
10. Dilute biotinylated detection mAb (7-B6-1 anti-IFN-γ mouse IgG1) in filtered PBS to a final concentration of 1 μg/mL in a 10-mL tube.
11. Dispense 100 μL of detection mAb to each well of ELISPOT plate and incubate for 4 h at room temperature on a level surface, in darkness.
12. After 4 h incubation, wash ELISPOT plate six times, as described in steps 8 and 9. This step can be performed over the sink, rather than within the biosafety cabinet.
13. Dilute stock Streptavidin-alkaline phosphatase (SAP) (1 mg/mL) in filtered PBS to a final concentration of 10 μg/mL in a 10-mL tube.
14. Dispense 100 μL (1 μg) of SAP to each well of ELISPOT plate and incubate for 2 h at room temperature (see Note 25).
15. Prepare substrate for the SAP by dissolving one BCIP/NBT tablet in 10 mL of sterile $H_2O$, filter through syringe filter (0.2 μm ministart filter, Sartorius) (see Note 26). The substrate should be prepared no more than 15 min prior to use as the solution is light sensitive and, once prepared, it should be stored in the dark/wrapped in foil.
16. Wash ELISPOT plate (from step 14) six times as described in step 8 and dispense 100 μL/well of BCIP/NBT substrate solution. Wrap plate in aluminium foil and incubate at room temperature, on a flat surface. The plate is usually left for 10–60 min, although in some cases it may take longer for full development.
17. When the spots are visible (see Fig. 1), stop colour development by washing in tap water.

18. Tease away the bottom plastic covering gently and wash the bottom of the ELISPOT plate. Allow the plates to dry overnight in open air on bench top. Once dry, the plate is ready to be analysed using an ELISPOT reader.
19. Results are presented as mean values of spots detected in triplicate wells containing effectors plus stimulator cells or antigen, after subtracting the response of wells with responder cells or effector cells alone (normally less than 10 spots per 200,000 cells).

#### *3.2.3. Intracellular Cytokine Staining Assay*

Before an ICS is conducted, individual mAbs (to be used for phenotyping and functional analysis) should be titrated to determine amounts for optimal staining (see Table 2). Prior to the assay, alloreactive/responder T cells derived from an MLR are restimulated by specific reporter cells (i.e. transfected cell lines or B-LCLs), and the antigen-specific $CD8^+$ T cells are restimulated by appropriate reporter cells pulsed with the relevant peptide. Reporter cells for alloreactive T cells should carry HLA allotypes corresponding to the allogeneic stimulator (PBMC utilised for the initial stimulation). For example, for dissecting T cells from an MLR in which responder PBMC were expanded with an allogeneic stimulator carrying: HLA-A*0101, A*0201; HLA-B*0801, B*5701, the following reporter cell lines would be required:

Transfected cell line panel: C1R parental, C1R.A*0101, C1R.A*0201, C1R.B*0801, C1R.B*5701.

B-LCL panel: Cell lines expressing individual HLA allotypes-A*0101, A*0201, B*0801, or B*5701.

1. Calculate the total number of T cells and reporter cells required for the assay (for the test sample, negative controls, and compensation controls) considering that you will require $2 \times 10^5$ T cells/100 μL of assay media (RF10 + 20 U/mL of IL-2) per well and $1 \times 10^5$ reporter cells/100 μL of assay media

**Table 2**
**Selection of monoclonal antibodies used for characterising cell phenotype and function**

| Antibody | Flurochrome | Clone | Isotype | Dilution | Manufacturer |
|---|---|---|---|---|---|
| CD3 | APC | SK7 | IgG1 | 1:20 | Becton Dickinson |
| CD4 | PE | SK3 | IgG1 | 1:20 | Becton Dickinson |
| CD8 | PE-Cy5 | HIT8a | IgG1 | 1:20 | Becton Dickinson |
| CD107a | FITC | H4A3 | IgG1 | 1:20 | Becton Dickinson |
| IFN-γ | APC | B27 | IgG1 | 1:1,000 | Becton Dickinson |
| TNF-α | PE | MAb11 | IgG1 | 1:20 | Becton Dickinson |

(RF10+20 U/mL of IL-2) per well. Each test sample should be assessed in duplicate or triplicate. In a 96-well U-bottom plate:

(a) Test: Dispense $2 \times 10^5$ cells/100 μL/well of responder T cells and $1 \times 10^5$ cells/100 μL/well of transfected C1R cell line or B-LCL.

(b) Negative control: Dispense $2 \times 10^5$ cells/100 μL/well of responder T cells and add 100 μL of assay media.

(c) Negative control: Dispense $1 \times 10^5$ cells/100 μL/well of transfected C1R cell line or B-LCL and add 100 μL of assay media.

(d) FACS compensation control: Dispense $2 \times 10^5$ cells/100 μL/well of responder T cells and add 100 μL of assay media into multiple wells for FACS compensation. For example, for 4 fluorochromes you will require 5 wells: Unstained, FL1 (FITC), FL2 (PE), FL3 (PE-Cy5, PerCP), and FL4 (APC) (see Note 27).

2. Add 10 μL/well of CD107a FITC (see Note 28) and mix carefully to avoid excess bubbles.
3. After 1 h incubation at 37°C, 5% $CO_2$, add 1.46 μL/well of 500 μg/mL Monensin (5 μM final concentration, see Note 29).
4. After 2 h incubation at 37°C, 5% $CO_2$, add 23 μL/well of 100 μg/mL Brefeldin A (10 μg/mL final concentration, see Note 30).
5. Incubate for 4 h at 37°C, 5% $CO_2$.
6. Centrifuge plate for 5 min at 335 ×*g*, room temperature.
7. Discard supernatant by flicking off in a single, sharp motion.
8. Resuspend cells in 20 μL of antibody mix/well (antibody mix should contain all the desired antibodies for surface staining, e.g. anti-CD3, CD8, etc.). The following panels are included:

   (a) Allo-specific $CD8^+$ T cells are stained with antibody mix containing anti-CD8 (and other desired antibodies for surface staining of phenotypic markers) diluted in PBS (see Table 2).

   (b) Antigen-specific $CD8^+$ T cells are stained with tetramer (see Table 3) and antibody mix with anti-CD8 (and other antibodies, see Table 2) diluted in PBS.

   (c) Compensation controls: Responder T cells in PBS only (unstained) and T cells with individual FL1 to FL4 antibodies diluted in PBS (see Note 31).

9. Wrap plate in foil and incubate for 30 min at 4°C in the dark.
10. Wash cells with 150 μL/well of PBS.
11. Centrifuge plate for 5 min at 335 ×*g*, room temperature.
12. Discard supernatant by flicking off in a single, sharp motion.

**Table 3**
**Selection of pMHC tetramers used to quantify and dissect antigen-specific T cells**

| Tetramer | HLA restriction | Virus | Protein | Sequence | Dilution | Manufacturer |
|---|---|---|---|---|---|---|
| B8/RAK | B8 | EBV | BZLF1 | RAKFKQLL | 1:50 | The University of Melbourne |
| B8/FLR | B8 | EBV | EBNA3A | FLRGRAYGL | 1:50 | The University of Melbourne |
| A1/YSE | A1 | CMV | pp65 | YSEHPTFTSQY | 1:40 | Monash University |
| A2/NLV | A2 | CMV | pp65 | NLVPMVATV | 1:100 | Monash University |
| B7/TPR | B7 | CMV | pp65 | TPRVTGGGAM | 1:40 | Monash University |
| B8/DAN | B8 | CMV | pp65 | DANDIYRIF | 1:40 | Monash University |

13. Resuspend cells in 100 μL/well of 1% Paraformaldehyde (16% stock diluted in PBS, see Note 32).
14. Wrap plate in foil and incubate for 20 min on bench at room temperature.
15. Wash cells with 100 μL/well of PBS.
16. Centrifuge plate for 5 min at 335 ×*g*, room temperature.
17. Discard supernatant by flicking off in a single, sharp motion.
18. Resuspend cells in 50 μL/well of anti-IFN-γ (and/or mAb for other desirable cytokines) in 0.3% Saponin (1% stock diluted in PBS, see Note 33).
19. Wrap plate in foil and incubate for 1 h at room temperature in the dark or overnight at 4°C in the dark.
20. Wash cells with 100 μL/well of PBS.
21. Centrifuge plate for 5 min at 335 ×*g*, room temperature.
22. Discard supernatant by flicking off in a single, sharp motion.
23. Resuspend cells in 60–100 μL/well of PBS.
24. Transfer cells into 5 mL polystyrene FACS tube. (This step is unnecessary, if a flow cytometer with a 96-well plate reader is available; as samples can be acquired directly from the plate).
25. Acquire by FACS.
26. Analyse data using flow cytometric software package (e.g.: CellQuest™, FlowJo).
27. Gating strategies for allo-specific $CD8^+$ T cells and antigen-specific $CD8^+$ T cells are shown in Figs. 5 and 6 respectively.

*3.2.4. Tetramer Staining*

Following generation of in vitro expanded allo-specific or antigen-specific T cells (see Subheading 3.1), the use of pMHC tetrameric complexes in combination with mAb specific for cell surface markers

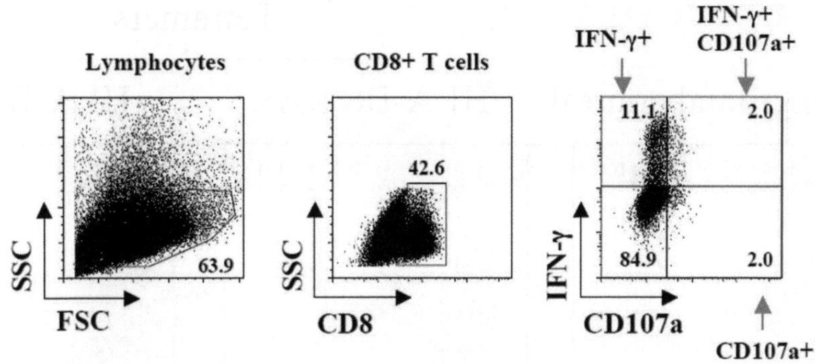


Fig. 5. Gating strategy for allo-specific CD8+ T cells. Identification of lymphocytes is achieved using a forward scatter (FSC) vs. side scatter (SSC) dot plots. From the lymphocyte population, the percentage of CD8+ T cells can be measured using a CD8 (FL3 channel) vs. SSC dot plot. Functional analysis of the CD8+ T cells can be quantitated using a CD107a (cytolytic potential; FL1 channel) vs. IFN-γ (cytokine production; FL4 channel).

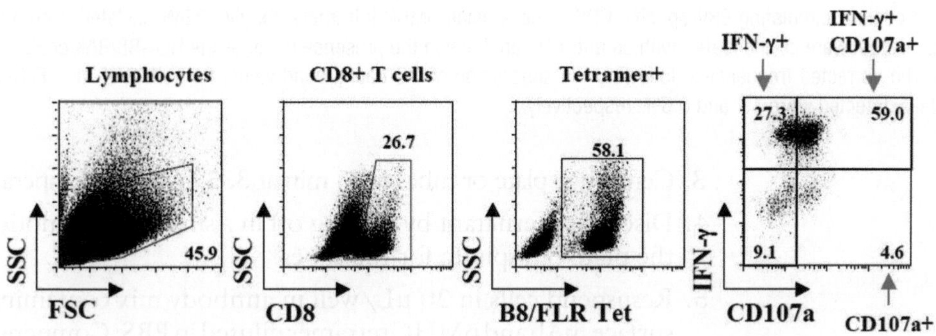


Fig. 6. Gating strategy for antigen-specific CD8+T cells. Identification of lymphocytes is achieved using a FSC vs. SSC dot plots. From the lymphocyte population, the percentage of CD8+ T cells can be measured using a CD8 (FL3 channel) vs. SSC dot plot. Antigen-specific CD8+T cells are identified using a HLA-B8/FLRGRAYGL (FLR) Tetramer (FL2 channel) vs. SSC. Functional analysis of the CD8+ T cells can be quantitated using a CD107a (cytolytic potential; FL1 channel) vs. IFN-γ (cytokine production; FL4 channel).

or intracellular proteins can be used for powerful quantitation and characterisation of T cell subsets. The number of T cells needed for the analysis depends on the frequency of T cell subsets being investigated. For example, low frequency cells (≈1%) require higher numbers of cells (≈$1 \times 10^6$ cells) to be stained, in order to generate sufficient data to analyse (minimum 10,000 events) using flow cytometry. Individual mAbs and/or pMHC tetramers should be titrated to determine optimal staining amounts prior to use in the assay.

1. To a 96-well U-bottom plate or 5 mL polystyrene FACS tube, add $2 \times 10^5$/well of T cells.
2. Add responder cells (PBMC or T cells) in separate wells or 5 mL polystyrene FACS tubes for FACS compensation. Example: Unstained FL1, FL2, FL3, and FL4.

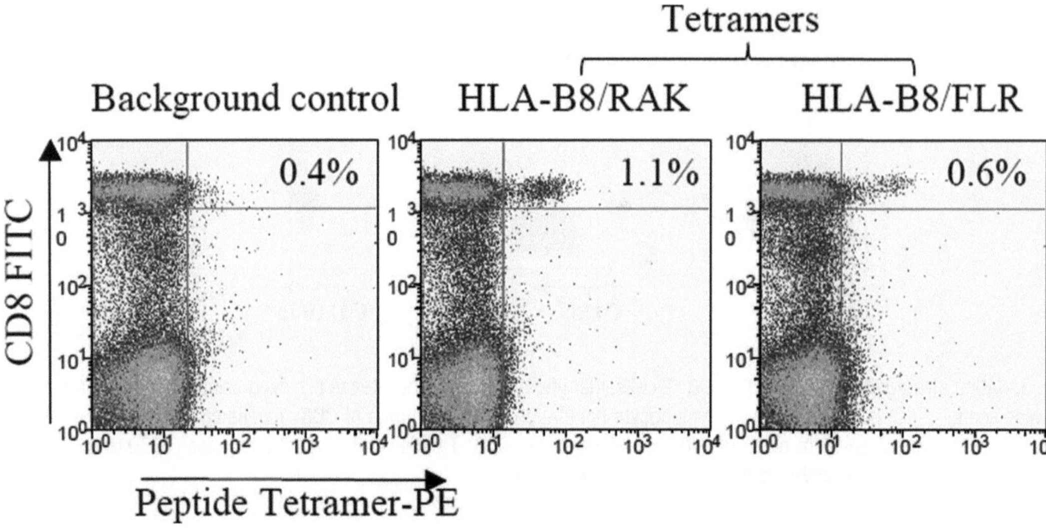


Fig. 7. Detection of circulating EBV-specific CD8+ T cells using pMHC tetramers. Ex vivo PBMC isolated from a HLA-B8 healthy individual were co-incubated with an anti-CD8 antibody in the presence of either the HLA-B8/RAK or HLA-B8/FLR tetramer. The corrected frequencies, following the subtraction of the background value, for both RAK- and FLR-specific CD8+ T cells detected were 1.1 and 0.6%, respectively.

3. Centrifuge plate or tubes for 5 min at 335 × *g*, room temperature.
4. Discard supernatant by flicking off in a single, sharp motion for the plate or aspirate for the tubes.
5. Resuspend cells in 20 μL/well in antibody mix containing cell surface mAb and pMHC tetramer diluted in PBS. Compensation controls: Unstained cells in PBS only and FL1 to FL4 (tetramer or antibody diluted in PBS, see Note 31).
6. Wrap plate/tubes in foil and incubate for 30 min at 4°C in the dark.
7. Wash cells with 150 μL/well or 1 mL/tube of PBS.
8. Centrifuge plate for 5 min at 335 × *g*, room temperature.
9. Discard supernatant by flicking off in a single, sharp motion for the plate or aspirate for the tubes.
10. If combining tetramer staining with intracellular detection of proteins, follow steps 13–25 of Subheading 3.2.3.
11. A gating strategy for antigen-specific CD8+ T cells is shown in Fig. 7.

## 4. Notes

1. *ELISPOT reagents*: The capture and secondary antibodies will vary depending on the cytokine that needs to be detected. Here we describe reagents obtained from (Mabtech, Sweden)

for an IFNγ ELISPOT. Detection kits and individual antibodies are available for an array of cytokines (TNFα, Granzyme B, Perforin, IL2, IL10, IL4, IL5, and others) from Mabtech and other manufacturers such as PharMingen, Endogen, Woburn, MA, USA; Cell Sciences, Norwood, MA, USA; R & D Systems etc. ELISPOT plates are also available from different manufacturers (Mabtech, Millipore), and come with different membranes custom made to increase specificity and/or sensitivity of the assay. Plates with polyvinylidene difluoride (PVDF) membranes such as the ELIIP and MSIP plates from Mabtech require pre-treatment with ethanol.

2. Monoclonal antibodies (mAb) can be purchased from an array of manufacturers. In our methodologies antibodies were purchased from Becton Dickinson Biosciences. Regardless of the manufacturer, each mAb should be titrated to determinate optimal dilution (range 1:10 to 1:1,000) for use in the assay, without compromising both specificity and sensitivity. A loss of detectable signal, or a high background staining are clear indicators that these dilutions are below or above the desired mAb amounts, respectively.
3. HLA class I tetramers can either be purchased from manufacturers including National Institutes of Health, Tetramer Core Facility, USA, or ProImmune, UK, or if you have the available technology and reagents can be produced "in-house" as were those used in our assays from either The University of Melbourne or Monash University. The optimal amount of tetramer used in an assay must also be evaluated using a similar titration range (1:10 to 1:500) as discussed in Note 2 for mAbs.
4. The method described uses CellQuest™ (Becton Dickinson) for acquisition of samples and FlowJo (Treestar Inc., Ashland, OR) for analysing the data. The softwares can vary depending on the Flow cytometer used for acquiring the samples. Generally, Cell Quest™ software is used on the FACSCalibur, and FACSDiva™ (Becton Dickinson) on a FACSCanto. The software for both Cell Quest™ and FACSDiva™ is suitable for data acquisition, as well as analysis.
5. Generation, expansion, and detection of allo-specific T cells requires prior knowledge of HLA mismatches between responder and stimulator and HLA-restricted molecule, whilst expansion and detection of antigen-specific T cells requires the knowledge of the viral epitope (minimal antigen and its HLA restriction).
6. Target cell lines (B-LCLs and transfected parental lines: C1R, 721.221, K562) are cultured in RF10. Depending on methodology utilised some transfected cell lines require additional antibiotic selection [Geneticin (G418) or Hygromycin B, Life Technologies] and the optimal antibiotic concentration varies

between cell lines. The type of antibiotic and its optimal concentration is determined at the time of transfection of the parental cell line.

7. Peripheral blood samples collected in the anticoagulant sodium or lithium heparin should be stored at room temperature and the blood should be processed within 24 h of collection.
8. Ficoll-Paque PLUS: Layering of anticoagulant-treated blood onto Ficoll-Paque PLUS followed by centrifugation enables differential migration of cell types and results in the formation of distinct layers (see Fig. 2). Ficoll-Paque Plus is stored at room temperature and protected from direct light.
9. When overlaying blood onto Ficoll-Paque PLUS reagent, it is very important to hold the end of the serological pipette towards the top of the 50 mL tube and, holding the tube at a 45° angle, trickle the very first 1–5 mL of diluted blood down the lower side of the tube. This will ensure that the layer of diluted blood will remain intact and undisturbed. Once the first 5 mL has been overlayed, the rate of loading can be increased. Do not let the samples stand for too long as cells will start to sediment through the interface between the blood and the Ficoll-Paque PLUS, which may affect your lymphocyte recovery.
10. It is very important that the brake setting is OFF, otherwise the Ficoll-Paque PLUS layer will be disturbed and separation of blood components will not be achieved. However, if this does occur, then mix the entire sample and repeat overlay step in a new 50 mL tube. The *g* values provided herewith are quoted for Beckman Coulter Allegra X-12-R centrifuge for which, 2,000 rpm = 931 × *g*, 1,500 rpm = 524 × *g*, 1,200 rpm = 335 × *g*, and 1,000 rpm = 233 × *g*.
11. Wash to remove residual platelets. This generally only requires one wash, but two washes may be needed for heavily contaminated preparations (i.e. if supernatant looks cloudy). Additionally, if heavy red blood cell (RBC) contamination is observed, the cells may require treatment with a commercial RBC lysis buffer as per the manufacturer's instructions.
12. Assay media: RF10 + 20 U/mL IL-2, media conditions have been optimised for expansion of either allo-specific or antigen-specific $CD8^+$ T cells. IL-2 cytokine mediates its effects by binding to IL-2 receptors, expressed by lymphocytes. In this in vitro culture system, the IL-2/IL-2R interaction then stimulates the growth, differentiation, and survival of allo-specific or antigen-specific $CD8^+$ T cells.
13. Gamma irradiation: Stimulator cells are gamma irradiated to ensure that either the MLR or auto-stimulation for antigen-specific T cells is uni-directional. Stimulator cells are unable to undergo proliferation due to DNA damage caused by effects of the ionising radiation.

14. Bulk T cell cultures should be observed every day. It is paramount that adequate cell density is maintained to promote cell–cell contact and interactions essential for T cell activation and expansion. Media colour changes is an indicator of proliferation. It is recommended that sub-culturing of bulk T cell cultures (split 1:2 only) is not performed until at least day 3 in order to maximise priming events. Replenish media every 3–4 days if not actively sub-culturing the T cells. The number of days for in vitro expansion of T cells may vary depending on (1) stimulator potency, (2) kinetics of cell proliferation, and (3) kinetics of protein to be measured.
15. Safety Precautions: $^{51}Cr$ is a strong gamma-emitter. A lead shield should be used at all times between the $^{51}Cr$ source and user when labelling the targets. Wear protective eyewear, radiation badge, gown, and double gloves. Make sure there is no spill. Record any spills and contain them according to institutional procedures prescribed for $^{51}Cr$ spill containment. Discard the syringe in a yellow syringe disposal bin reserved for radioactive waste. When using the isotope, use a Geiger counter to monitor spills and exposure. Dispose off high-level $^{51}Cr$ waste in a lead bucket surrounded by a lead shield in a designated area. $^{51}Cr$-labelled target cells should be transported in an esky lined with lead.
16. Take care not to splash 1% Triton X-100 into any of the surrounding wells as this will lyse all targets and confound results for target-specific lysis. It might be easier to leave 1% Triton X-100 addition until the very end of the assay just before incubating the plate.
17. The mean spontaneous lysis for target cells in culture medium should always be less than 10%, and the variation about the mean specific lysis, less than 5%.
18. ELISPOT plates may need to be pre-treated as per manufacturers instructions and buffer used for diluting the antibodies may also vary between suppliers.
19. Avoid touching the bottom of the wells of the ELISPOT plate with the pipette tips as this may disrupt the membrane or give the impression of artificial spots. Dispense down the side of the wells with the tips touching the walls.
20. To use cryopreserved PBMC, retrieve cell vials from liquid nitrogen storage. Pre-fill 10 mL yellow capped tubes with 8 mL RPMI or RF10. Thaw vials in warm tap water (37°C) in beaker and transfer cells to 10 mL tubes containing RPMI or RF10. Centrifuge 10 mL tubes immediately for 5 min at 1,026 × *g*. Remove supernatant and resuspend pellet in 2–5 mL RF10 and incubate for 2 h at 37°C, 5%$CO_2$ before use.
21. $CD3^+$ T cells can be separated from the whole blood using Rosette sep (StemCell Biotechnologies, CellSystems GmbH,

St Katherinen, Germany) as recommended by the manufacturer. Alternatively, Dynabeads® CD3 (Cat. no. 111.51D, Invitrogen) can be used to deplete $CD3^{+}$ T cells directly from whole blood, buffy coat, or PBMCs.

22. The incubation time for the responder cells with the antigen in the ELISPOT assay can vary depending on the cytokine to be detected. For example, for IL-2 or IFN-$\gamma$, the recommended incubation time is 20–24 h whilst for IL-10, a longer incubation period of up to 48 h may be required.
23. Caution! Tween 20 may be harmful and should be treated as hazardous. Avoid inhalation and contact with skin and eyes.
24. Between and after final wash steps (in steps 8, 9, 12, and 16 of ELISPOT assay), do not let the plate dry. Leave last wash solution (PBS) in the plate until the reagent for the next step has been prepared and ready to be used.
25. Caution! Streptavidin-alkaline phosphatase can be hazardous. Avoid inhalation and skin contact.
26. Caution! BCIP/NBT is an irritant causing irritation to eyes, respiratory system, and skin. Avoid contact to these areas of the body.
27. Number of fluorochromes (FL) would depend on the phenotypic and functional markers to be assessed and the tetramers utilised.
28. CD107a, also known as Lysosomal-associated membrane protein 1 (LAMP1), is a marker of degranulation on lymphocytes.
29. Monensin, isolated from *Streptomyces cinnamonensis*, blocks intracellular protein transport.
30. Brefeldin A is a lactone antibiotic produced by fungal organisms such as *Penicillium brefeldianum*. Brefeldin A interferes with protein transport from the endoplasmic reticulum (ER) to the Golgi apparatus by inhibiting transport in Golgi, which leads to proteins accumulating inside the endoplasmic reticulum.
31. Compensation controls are important to select markers of proteins that have relatively high density on surface of cells, not rare events.
32. Paraformaldehyde is used to fix the cells prior to permeabilisation to stabilise the integrity of the cell.
33. Saponin is a surfactant, extracted from the Quillaja Bark. It enhances penetration of proteins and other macromolecules through cell membranes. Saponin is diluted to 0.3% to ensure permeability but not potent haemolysis of the cells.

## Acknowledgements

The authors would like to thank Ms Patricia Therese Illing, The University of Melbourne, Australia, for her help in proofreading the manuscript.

## References

1. Burrows SR, Khanna R, Burrows JM, Moss DJ (1994) An alloresponse in humans is dominated by cytotoxic T lymphocytes (CTL) cross-reactive with a single Epstein–Barr virus CTL epitope: implications for graft-versus-host disease. J Exp Med 179(4):1155–1161
2. Brunner KT, Mauel J, Cerottini JC, Chapuis B (1968) Quantitative assay of the lytic action of immune lymphoid cells on 51-Cr-labelled allogeneic target cells in vitro; inhibition by isoantibody and by drugs. Immunology 14(2): 181–196
3. Lefkovits I (1972) Induction of antibody-forming cell clones in microcultures. Eur J Immunol 2(4):360–366
4. Lefkovits I, Waldmann H (1984) Limiting dilution analysis of cells of the immune system I. The clonal basis of the immune response. Immunol Today 5:265–268
5. Waldmann H, Lefkovits I (1984) Limiting dilution analysis of cells of the immune system II: what can be learnt? Immunol Today 5:295–298
6. Sharrock CE, Kaminski E, Man S (1990) Limiting dilution analysis of human T cells: a useful clinical tool. Immunol Today 11(8): 281–286
7. Hickling JK (1998) Measuring human T-lymphocyte function. Expert Rev Mol Med 1:1–20
8. Kaminski E, Hows J, Brookes P, Mackinnon S, Hughes T, Avakian O et al (1989) Alloreactive cytotoxic T-cell frequency analysis and HLA matching for bone marrow transplants from HLA matched unrelated donors. Transplant Proc 21(1 Pt 3):2976–2977
9. Macdonald WA, Chen Z, Gras S, Archbold JK, Tynan FE, Clements CS et al (2009) T cell allorecognition via molecular mimicry. Immunity 31(6):897–908
10. Bharadwaj M, Thammanichanond D, Aitken CK, Moneer S, Drummer HE, Tracy S et al (2009) TCD8 response in diverse outcomes of recurrent exposure to hepatitis C virus. Immunol Cell Biol 87(6):464–472
11. Bharadwaj M, Burrows SR, Burrows JM, Moss DJ, Catalina M, Khanna R (2001) Longitudinal dynamics of antigen-specific CD8+ cytotoxic T lymphocytes following primary Epstein–Barr virus infection. Blood 98(8):2588–2589
12. Kaminski E, Hows J, Man S, Brookes P, Mackinnon S, Hughes T et al (1989) Prediction of graft versus host disease by frequency analysis of cytotoxic T cells after unrelated donor bone marrow transplantation. Transplantation 48(4):608–613
13. Schwarer AP, Jiang YZ, Deacock S, Brookes PA, Barrett AJ, Goldman JM et al (1994) Comparison of helper and cytotoxic antirecipient T cell frequencies in unrelated bone marrow transplantation. Transplantation 58(11): 1198–1203
14. Roelen DL, Stobbe I, Young NT, van Bree SP, Doxiadis II, Oudshoorn M et al (2001) Permissible and immunogenic HLA-A mismatches: cytotoxic T-cell precursor frequencies reflect graft survival data. Hum Immunol 62(7):661–667
15. Dolezalova L, Vrana M, Dobrovolna M, Loudova M, Cukrova V, Vitek A et al (2002) Cytotoxic T lymphocyte precursor frequency analysis in the selection of HLA matched unrelated donors for hematopoietic stem cell transplantation: the correlation of CTLp frequency with HLA class I genotyping and aGVHD development. Neoplasma 49(1):26–32
16. Fussell ST, Donnellan M, Cooley MA, Farrell C (1994) Cytotoxic T lymphocyte precursor frequency does not correlate with either the incidence or severity of graft-versus-host disease after matched unrelated donor bone marrow transplantation. Transplantation 57(5):673–676
17. Eberspacher ML, Otto G, Herfarth C, Kabelitz D (1994) Frequency analysis of donor-reactive cytotoxic T lymphocyte precursors in in allograft recipients. Lack of correlation with clinical outcome. Transplantation 57(12): 1746–1752
18. Wang XN, Taylor PR, Skinner R, Jackson GH, Proctor SJ, Hedley D et al (2000) T-cell frequency analysis does not predict the incidence of graft-versus-host disease in HLA-matched

sibling bone marrow transplantation. Transplantation 70(3):488–493

19. Tan LC, Gudgeon N, Annels NE, Hansasuta P, O'Callaghan CA, Rowland-Jones S et al (1999) A re-evaluation of the frequency of CD8+ T cells specific for EBV in healthy virus carriers. J Immunol 162(3):1827–1835
20. Lalvani A, Brookes R, Hambleton S, Britton WJ, Hill AV, McMichael AJ (1997) Rapid effector function in CD8+ memory T cells. J Exp Med 186(6):859–865
21. Murali-Krishna K, Altman JD, Suresh M, Sourdive DJ, Zajac AJ, Miller JD et al (1998) Counting antigen-specific CD8 T cells: a reevaluation of bystander activation during viral infection. Immunity 8(2):177–187
22. Kuzushima K, Hoshino Y, Fujii K, Yokoyama N, Fujita M, Kiyono T et al (1999) Rapid determination of Epstein–Barr virus-specific CD8(+) T-cell frequencies by flow cytometry. Blood 94(9):3094–3100
23. Hernandez-Fuentes MP, Warrens AN, Lechler RI (2003) Immunologic monitoring. Immunol Rev 196:247–264
24. Miyahira Y, Murata K, Rodriguez D, Rodriguez JR, Esteban M, Rodrigues MM et al (1995) Quantification of antigen specific CD8+ T cells using an ELISPOT assay. J Immunol Methods 181(1):45–54
25. Czerkinsky C, Andersson G, Ekre HP, Nilsson LA, Klareskog L, Ouchterlony O (1988) Reverse ELISPOT assay for clonal analysis of cytokine production. I. Enumeration of gamma-interferon-secreting cells. J Immunol Methods 110(1):29–36
26. Elliott SL, Suhrbier A, Miles JJ, Lawrence G, Pye SJ, Le TT et al (2008) Phase I trial of a CD8+ T-cell peptide epitope-based vaccine for infectious mononucleosis. J Virol 82(3):1448–1457
27. Scheibenbogen C, Romero P, Rivoltini L, Herr W, Schmittel A, Cerottini JC et al (2000) Quantitation of antigen-reactive T cells in peripheral blood by IFNgamma-ELISPOT assay and chromium-release assay: a four-centre comparative trial. J Immunol Methods 244(1–2):81–89
28. Pelfrey CM, Rudick RA, Cotleur AC, Lee JC, Tary-Lehmann M, Lehmann PV (2000) Quantification of self-recognition in multiple sclerosis by single-cell analysis of cytokine production. J Immunol 165(3):1641–1651
29. Bestard O, Nickel P, Cruzado JM, Schoenemann C, Boenisch O, Sefrin A et al (2008) Circulating alloreactive T cells correlate with graft function in longstanding renal transplant recipients. J Am Soc Nephrol 19(7):1419–1429
30. Sherritt MA, Bharadwaj M, Burrows JM, Morrison LE, Elliott SL, Davis JE et al (2003) Reconstitution of the latent T-lymphocyte response to Epstein–Barr virus is coincident with long-term recovery from posttransplant lymphoma after adoptive immunotherapy. Transplantation 75(9):1556–1560
31. Gazagne A, Claret E, Wijdenes J, Yssel H, Bousquet F, Levy E et al (2003) A Fluorospot assay to detect single T lymphocytes simultaneously producing multiple cytokines. J Immunol Methods 283(1–2):91–98
32. Altman JD, Moss PA, Goulder PJ, Barouch DH, McHeyzer-Williams MG, Bell JI et al (1996) Phenotypic analysis of antigen-specific T lymphocytes. Science 274(5284):94–96
33. McMichael AJ, O'Callaghan CA (1998) A new look at T cells. J Exp Med 187(9):1367–1371
34. Ogg GS, McMichael AJ (1998) HLA-peptide tetrameric complexes. Curr Opin Immunol 10(4):393–396
35. Miles JJ, Thammanichanond D, Moneer S, Nivarthi UK, Kjer-Nielsen L, Tracy SL et al (2011) Antigen-driven patterns of TCR bias are shared across diverse outcomes of human hepatitis C virus infection. J Immunol 186(2):901–912
36. James EA, LaFond R, Durinovic-Bello I, Kwok W (2009) Visualizing antigen specific CD4+ T cells using MHC class II tetramers. J Vis Exp (25) pii:1167
37. Landais E, Romagnoli PA, Corper AL, Shires J, Altman JD, Wilson IA et al (2009) New design of MHC class II tetramers to accommodate fundamental principles of antigen presentation. J Immunol 183(12):7949–7957
38. Vollers SS, Stern LJ (2008) Class II major histocompatibility complex tetramer staining: progress, problems, and prospects. Immunology 123(3):305–313
39. Raddassi K, Kent SC, Yang J, Bourcier K, Bradshaw EM, Seyfert-Margolis V et al (2011) Increased frequencies of myelin oligodendrocyte glycoprotein/MHC class II-binding CD4 cells in patients with multiple sclerosis. J Immunol 187(2):1039–1046
40. Laughlin E, Burke G, Pugliese A, Falk B, Nepom G (2008) Recurrence of autoreactive antigen-specific CD4+ T cells in autoimmune diabetes after pancreas transplantation. Clin Immunol 128(1):23–30
41. Bonvalet M, Wambre E, Moussu H, Horiot S, Kwok WW, Louise A et al (2011) Comparison between major histocompatibility complex class II tetramer staining and surface expression of activation markers for the detection of allergen-specific CD4(+) T cells. Clin Exp Allergy 41(6):821–829

42. Ayyoub M, Dojcinovic D, Pignon P, Raimbaud I, Schmidt J, Luescher I et al (2010) Monitoring of NY-ESO-1 specific CD4+ T cells using molecularly defined MHC class II/His-tag-peptide tetramers. Proc Natl Acad Sci USA 107(16):7437–7442
43. Cusick MF, Yang M, Gill JC, Eckels DD (2011) Naturally occurring CD4+ T-cell epitope variants act as altered peptide ligands leading to impaired helper T-cell responses in hepatitis C virus infection. Hum Immunol 72(5):379–385
44. Sun Y, Iglesias E, Samri A, Kamkamidze G, Decoville T, Carcelain G et al (2003) A systematic comparison of methods to measure HIV-1 specific CD8 T cells. J Immunol Methods 272(1–2):23–34
45. McMichael AJ, Ogg G, Wilson J, Callan M, Hambleton S, Appay V et al (2000) Memory CD8+ T cells in HIV infection. Philos Trans R Soc Lond B Biol Sci 2355(1395):363–367
46. Ogg GS, Jin X, Bonhoeffer S, Dunbar PR, Nowak MA, Monard S et al (1998) Quantitation of HIV-1-specific cytotoxic T lymphocytes and plasma load of viral RNA. Science 279(5359):2103–2106
47. Callan MF, Tan L, Annels N, Ogg GS, Wilson JD, O'Callaghan CA et al (1998) Direct visualization of antigen-specific CD8+ T cells during the primary immune response to Epstein–Barr virus In vivo. J Exp Med 187(9):1395–1402
48. Mifsud NA, Nguyen TH, Tait BD, Kotsimbos TC (2010) Quantitative and functional diversity of cross-reactive EBV-specific CD8+ T cells in a longitudinal study cohort of lung transplant recipients. Transplantation 90(12):1439–1449
49. Nguyen TH, Sullivan LC, Kotsimbos TC, Schwarer AP, Mifsud NA (2010) Cross-presentation of HCMV chimeric protein enables generation and measurement of polyclonal T cells. Immunol Cell Biol 88(6):676–684
50. Pala P, Hussell T, Openshaw PJ (2000) Flow cytometric measurement of intracellular cytokines. J Immunol Methods 243(1–2):107–124
51. Prussin C, Metcalfe DD (1995) Detection of intracytoplasmic cytokine using flow cytometry and directly conjugated anti-cytokine antibodies. J Immunol Methods 188(1):117–128
52. Goulder PJ, Tang Y, Brander C, Betts MR, Altfeld M, Annamalai K et al (2000) Functionally inert HIV-specific cytotoxic T lymphocytes do not play a major role in chronically infected adults and children. J Exp Med 192(12):1819–1832
53. Asemissen AM, Nagorsen D, Keilholz U, Letsch A, Schmittel A, Thiel E et al (2001) Flow cytometric determination of intracellular or secreted IFNgamma for the quantification of antigen reactive T cells. J Immunol Methods 251(1–2):101–108
54. Whiteside TL, Zhao Y, Tsukishiro T, Elder EM, Gooding W, Baar J (2003) Enzyme-linked immunospot, cytokine flow cytometry, and tetramers in the detection of T-cell responses to a dendritic cell-based multipeptide vaccine in patients with melanoma. Clin Cancer Res 9(2):641–649
55. Koehne G, Smith KM, Ferguson TL, Williams RY, Heller G, Pamer EG et al (2002) Quantitation, selection, and functional characterization of Epstein–Barr virus-specific and alloreactive T cells detected by intracellular interferon-gamma production and growth of cytotoxic precursors. Blood 99(5):1730–1740
56. Waldrop SL, Pitcher CJ, Peterson DM, Maino VC, Picker LJ (1997) Determination of antigen-specific memory/effector CD4+ T cell frequencies by flow cytometry: evidence for a novel, antigen-specific homeostatic mechanism in HIV-associated immunodeficiency. J Clin Invest 99(7):1739–1750
57. Mifsud NA, Purcell AW, Chen W, Holdsworth R, Tait BD, McCluskey J (2008) Immunodominance hierarchies and gender bias in direct T(CD8)-cell alloreactivity. Am J Transplant 8(1):121–132
58. Allen KJ, Mifsud NA, Williamson R, Bertolino P, Hardikar W (2008) Cell-mediated rejection results in allograft loss after liver cell transplantation. Liver Transpl 14(5):688–694
59. Elkington R, Walker S, Crough T, Menzies M, Tellam J, Bharadwaj M et al (2003) Ex vivo profiling of CD8+-T-cell responses to human cytomegalovirus reveals broad and multispecific reactivities in healthy virus carriers. J Virol 77(9):5226–5240
60. Taswell C (1981) Limiting dilution assays for the determination of immunocompetent cell frequencies. I. Data analysis. J Immunol 126(4):1614–1619
61. Strijbosch LW, Buurman WA, Does RJ, Zinken PH, Groenewegen G (1987) Limiting dilution assays. Experimental design and statistical analysis. J Immunol Methods 97(1):133–140

# Chapter 19

# Detection of Allo-HLA Cross-Reactivity by Virus-specific Memory T-Cell Clones Using Single HLA-Transfected K562 Cells

**Lloyd J. D'Orsogna, Ellen M.W. van der Meer-Prins, Yvonne M. Zoet, Dave L. Roelen, Ilias I.N. Doxiadis, and Frans H.J. Claas**


## Abstract

The ability to directly measure virus-specific lymphocytes using fluorochrome-labeled tetrameric complexes has proven a great advancement for the transplantation field. Viral peptide/HLA tetrameric complexes allow the rapid generation of virus-specific clones using single cell sorting apparatus, permitting the determination of alloreactivity from a single TCR with known specificity. When combined with new target "detector" cells called single HLA antigen-transfected K562 cells (SALs), the human alloresponse can for the first time be examined specifically and reliably. Here we describe a method for detection of "heterologous immunity" from virus-specific memory T-cells using single HLA expressing cell lines as allogeneic targets.


**Key words:** Heterologous immunity, Memory T-cells, Viral immunity, Alloreactivity, SALs

## 1. Introduction

The mechanisms by which alloreactive memory T-cells are generated in nonsensitized individuals have begun to be elucidated. It is generally accepted that a very high level of cross-reactivity is an essential feature of the T-cell receptor, e.g., memory T-cells that have been generated as a result of a previous viral infection can subsequently respond to a second unrelated infection. However, it has only recently been shown that alloreactivity from virus-specific memory T-cells is far more common than predicted; 45% of virus-specific T-cell clones were found to be allo-HLA cross-reactive (1).

Detection of alloreactivity from virus-specific memory T-cells should first be performed by screening against a panel of cells expressing most common HLA molecules, such as a panel of EBV

Frank T. Christiansen and Brian D. Tait (eds.), *Immunogenetics: Methods and Applications in Clinical Practice*, Methods in Molecular Biology, vol. 882, DOI 10.1007/978-1-61779-842-9_19, © Springer Science+Business Media New York 2012

LCLs as described elsewhere (1). However, cross-reactivity should be confirmed using a single HLA-transfected cell type. This will not only confirm the individual HLA molecule recognized but also exclude the possibility of the clone recognizing viral peptides presented on allo-HLA.

Single HLA-transfected K562 cells (SALs) are a new sensitive and specific tool to detect alloresponses from virus-specific T-cells (2). SALs express only the transfected HLA class I molecule (3), unlike C1R cells that may have low expression of other HLA molecules. For example, the previously described alloreactivity of the EBV EBNA3A specific T-cell against HLA-B*4402 has been confirmed using SALs (2). Furthermore, the same T-cell clone was also found to recognize HLA-B*5501 expressing SALs (2), suggesting that SALs may be a more sensitive target than other cells expressing multiple HLA molecules. Therefore, detection of HLA-specific alloresponses from virus-specific T-cells in vitro is now feasible in the routine laboratory.

This technique to define cross-reactive T-cells may lead to important future improvements in donor selection and monitoring. The ability to define public TCR responses that give specific allo-HLA cross-reactivity may assist in the definition of (un) acceptable mismatches. If in vitro tools can more specifically predict which transplant recipients are at risk for rejection and which patients are predisposed to tolerance, the immunosuppressive regimen could be adjusted accordingly. We also hypothesize that antiviral therapy may decrease the proportion and activation status of these alloreactive T-cells.

## 2. Materials

### *2.1. Virus-specific T-Cell Cloning Using Single Cell Sorting*

1. Viral peptide/HLA tetrameric complex of interest (see Note 1).
2. PBMCs from donor known to have viral peptide/HLA tetramer complex binding T-cells in the peripheral blood (or at least known to be serologically positive for virus of interest) (see Notes 2–3).
3. Iscoves Modified Dulbecco Medium (IMDM) with 1% l-glutamine.
4. Fetal Calf Serum (FCS) made to 1 and 10% solutions in IMDM.
5. Human Serum (HS) made to 5% HS and 5% FCS in IMDM.
6. Phytohaemagglutinin (PHA) 800 ng/mL.
7. Interleukin-2 (IL-2).
8. Freshly collected human PBMCs to be used as feeder cells (see Note 4).

9. Sterile 96-well round bottom plates.
10. Sterile 24-well flat bottom plates.
11. FACS sorting apparatus, e.g., FACSAriaII.

#### 2.2. Generation of Single HLA-Transfected K562 Cells Lines (SALs)

1. K562 cell line.
2. Plasmid (pLNCX, pCDNA3.0, resistant to neomycin (G418), pEAK10 resistant to puromycin, with the HLA-cDNA construct of interest (10 μg of plasmid cDNA per transfection)) (obtained from 13th international histocompatibility working group) (3, 4).
3. IMDM supplemented with 1% l-glutamine.
4. 10% FCS in IMDM supplemented with penicillin/streptomycin.
5. G418 (200 μg/mL) (see Note 5).
6. Gene pulser (Biorad).
7. Dynabeads Sheep anti-Mouse Immunoglobulin—Dynal.
8. w6/32 (anti-MHC class I antibody), w6/32-PE, w6/32-FITC (Abcam, United Kingdom).
9. Anti-IgG antibody (Goat anti-Mouse-FITC) (BD, the Netherlands).
10. Puromycin (0.5 μg/mL) (Invitrogen).
11. Hygromycin (50 μg/mL) (Clontech).
12. Sterile Gen pulser 0.4-cm cuvettes (Biorad).
13. FACS calibur flow cytometer.
14. FACS tubes.
15. Solution of 0.1% bovine serum albumin (BSA) in phosphate buffered saline (PBS).
16. HLA-specific Monoclonal Antibodies (Leiden University Medical Centre (LUMC), Leiden, the Netherlands) (see Note 6).
17. Rabbit anti-Human IgG FITC.
18. Rabbit anti-Human IgM FITC.
19. Dimethyl sulfoxide (DMSO).
20. Incubator.
21. PBS/1% paraformaldehyde.
22. 15-mL falcon tubes (BD biosciences).
23. 75-cm$^2$ culture flask (Corning).
24. Dynal magnet.

#### 2.3. IFNγ ELISA

1. Virus-specific T-cell clone—see Subheading 3.1.
2. SALs transfected with the HLA molecule of interest—see Subheading 3.2.

3. Nontransfected K562 cells.
4. Viral peptide for which the clone is specific (positive control), and a control viral peptide (see Note 7).
5. IMDM supplemented with 1% l-glutamine.
6. Freshly prepared T-cell culture medium—see Subheading 3.1, step 9.
7. PHA 800 ng/mL.
8. Interleukin-2 (IL-2).
9. Sterile 96-well round bottom plates.
10. Human IFN-γ Elisa kit (U-Cytech, Netherlands).

### 2.4. Cytotoxicity Assay

1. Virus-specific T-cell clone—see Subheading 3.1.
2. SALs transfected with the HLA molecule of interest—see Subheading 3.2.
3. Nontransfected K562 cells.
4. Viral peptide for which the clone is specific (positive control), and a control viral peptide (see Note 7).
5. IMDM supplemented with 1% l-glutamine.
6. Freshly prepared T-cell culture medium—see Subheading 3.1, step 9.
7. PHA 800 ng/mL.
8. Interleukin-2 (IL-2).
9. Sodium Chromate (1 mCi/mL (370mBq)).
10. 1% Triton X-100.
11. 96-well round bottom plates.

## 3. Methods

### 3.1. Virus-specific CD8 T-Cell Cloning Using Single Cell Sorting

1. Perform all steps at 4°C (see Note 8).
2. Ensure cell donor for single cell sorting is serologically positive for the virus and has a population of the relevant tetramer binding T-cells (see Notes 2 and 9).
3. Count the ficoll hypaque separated PBMCs ensuring you have at least $1 \times 10^6$ cells. Wash twice in medium containing 1% FCS/IMDM by spinning down the cells at 700 G for 8 min.
4. After second wash, resuspend the pellet in the residual medium and transfer to a FACS tube (see Note 9).
5. Add 1 μL tetramer-PE to the FACS tube on ice (see Note 1).
6. Add markers CD45Ra/CD4/CD14-FITC (see Note 10).

7. Incubate on ice for 30 min.
8. Wash PBMCs twice in 1% FCS/IMDM medium as for step 3.
9. Place up to 5 million cells for sorting in 1 mL 10% FCS/ IMDM *without* phenol red.
10. Prepare T-cell Medium—5% FCS/5% Human serum in IMDM medium with 1% penicillin/streptomycin, 3 mg l-Glutamine and IL-2 100 IU/mL (see Note 11).
11. Prepare T-cell feeder mix for stimulation of sorted virus-specific T-cells in 96 well plate—To the T-cell medium add 0.5 million irradiated feeder cells, $0.05 \times 10^6$ EBV LCLs, and 2 μL PHA per mL of required feeder mix (approximately 10 mL per plate is required) (see Notes 11–13).
12. Add 100 μL feeder mix per well to 96-well round bottom plates(s).
13. Perform single cell sorting into preprepared 96-well round bottom plate (with feeder mix) based on tetramer positive gate using single cell sorting apparatus. After sorting place 96-well plates into incubator at 37°C (see Notes 14–16).
14. Add further 100 μL T-cell medium per well on day 7.
15. At day 14 check the plates for cell growth. Select the growing clones and transfer the contents to individual wells in a 24-well plate to which 1 mL feeder cell mix has already been added. Continue to culture at 37°C.
16. Check daily for growth and if wells are full split the culture into a separate well containing 1 mL of T-cell culture medium.
17. After day 6 confirm tetramer positivity of T-cell clones by resuspending and taking 100 μL aliquot for FACS analysis.
18. Determine Vβ IOtest TCR usage using Vβ kit (Beckman Coulter) and/or TCR PCR using primers designed to cover the complete TCR repertoire.
19. Continue to culture cells. Freeze interesting clones if required for later use (freeze before day 10 since last stimulation).
20. These T-cell clones are now ready for use in IFNγ ELISA assays (see Subheading 3.3) or cytotoxicity assays (see Subheading 3.4). However defrosted T-cell clones can also be used but must be restimulated prior to use. $1 \times 10^6$ defrosted T-cell clone should be restimulated in T-cell medium with 5 million feeder cells, $0.5 \times 10^6$ EBV LCLs and 2 μL/mL PHA in a T75 flask. IFNγ ELISA is usually performed 9–10 days after stimulation and cytotoxicity 7–8 days after stimulation.

### 3.2. Generation of Single HLA-Transfected K562 Cells Lines (SALs)

1. Culture K562 until you have $10 \times 10^6$ cells per transfection in IMDM supplemented with 10% FCS and penicillin/streptomycin.
2. Spin down the cells and wash two times in IMDM/10%FCS.
3. Count the cells and resuspend the cells in IMDM/10%FCS at a concentration of $10 \times 10^6$ cells per mL.
4. Mix 1 mL of the cells with 10 μg of the plasmid DNA containing the HLA-cDNA construct of the HLA specificity required.
5. Put 1 mL of the cell/DNA mixture in a 0.4-cm cuvette and store on ice for a minimum of 5 min.
6. Mix and pulse (960 μF, 230 V).
7. Store on ice for 15 min.
8. Add a few drops of IMDM/10%FCS/pen/strep medium to the cuvette and transfer the cells to a culture flask containing 9 mL of the same medium.
9. Culture the cells for 2 days at 37°C.
10. Add selection antibiotic at the correct final concentration (see manufacturers protocol) (see Note 5).
11. Culture for another week at 37°C. If culture flasks become full then split flasks and add new medium.
12. Perform a flow cytometry test to see whether there are HLA-positive cells (incubate $10^5$ cells with w6/32-PE for 30 min on ice, wash twice, take up in 100 μL PBS/1% paraformaldehyde, read in FACS calibur and analyze) (see Note 17).
13. If positive cells are present, separate positive cells from negative cells (described in steps 14–31) (see Notes 18 and 19).
14. Take 20–25 mL of your cultured cells (leave some in the flask and continue culturing them).
15. Spin down, remove supernatant, and resuspend the cell pellet.
16. Add 0.5 mL unlabeled-w6/32 antibody and vortex.
17. Incubate on ice for 30 min.
18. Wash three times with ice cold medium (IMDM/10%FCS) in a 15-mL tube.
19. Resuspend the cells and add 30 μL Sheep anti-Mouse dynabeads.
20. Incubate on a rollerbench in 4°C room for 30 min.
21. Put the tube in the magnet, add 10 mL ice cold medium.
22. Wait for 5 min.
23. Discard the medium with the nonbound cells.
24. Repeat from step 21 twice.
25. Add 10 mL ice cold medium and resuspend the cells bound to the beads, put them in a small culture flask, and culture at 37°C.

26. Wait for the cells to grow and expand. Check daily (see Notes 19 and 20).
27. When the cells have expanded, remove the beads as follows.
28. Put the cells in a 15-mL tube within the dynal magnet.
29. Wait for 5 min.
30. Collect the medium with the cells into a culture flask leaving the beads in the tube.
31. Add 10 mL of fresh medium (10%FCS/IMDM) to the tube.
32. Repeat twice from step 28 and on the last removal of beads transfer the cells to a culture flask, add 10% of fresh culture medium.
33. Culture at 37°C.
34. After a few days growth, test the class I expression of the cells using HLA-specific monoclonal antibodies and FACS analysis (step 12).
35. If there still are cells with no expression at all, repeat the bead sorting (repeat from step 14 onwards).
36. If the cells all have a good expression, they can be used in the IFNγ assay (see Subheading 3.3) or cytotoxicity assay (see Subheading 3.4). Alternatively the cells can be frozen in several aliquots for subsequent use in these assays.
37. Test the cells with a flow cytometry test against a panel of anti-HLA monoclonal antibodies to confirm the HLA expression of the K562 cell (see Note 17).

### 3.3. IFNγ ELISA Using Responder Virus-specific T-Cell Clones and SAL Stimulator Cells

1. Spin down the virus-specific T-cell clone (generated using method in Subheading 3.1), resuspend and count (see Notes 21 and 22).
2. Make a T-cell clone solution of $0.1 \times 10^6$ T-cells/mL in T-cell medium (see Subheading 3.1, step 10).
3. Dilute the SALs and the K562 line in T-cell medium to a concentration of $0.25 \times 10^6$ cells/mL.
4. Add 50 μL/well of the T-cell clone solution to a sterile 96-well plate.
5. Add 100 μL/well of the different SALs in duplicate to the T-cell clone. Include:
   (a) A SAL transfected with the restricting HLA molecule loaded with the viral peptide that is recognized by the clone as a positive control. To load peptides onto SALs first incubate harvested cell pellet with 100 μg/mL of peptide for 30 min at room temperature, then wash twice and resuspend to required concentration of $0.25 \times 10^6$ cells/mL.

(b) A SAL transfected with the restricting HLA molecule loaded with the control peptide that is not recognized by the clone as a negative control (see Notes 23–25).

(c) A nontransfected K562 as a negative control.

(d) As background control also add only T-cell medium to some of the wells without SALs.

6. Incubate for 24 h at 37°C.

7. Transfer 120 μL supernatant from each well by pipetting to a new 96-well plate and store the samples at −20°C till use in IFNγ ELISA (see Notes 26 and 27).

8. Thaw the supernatants and use in an IFN-γ ELISA according to the manufacturer's protocol.

### 3.4. Cytotoxicity Assay Using Effector Virus-specific T-Cell Clones and SAL Target Cells

1. Spin down the SALs and the nontransferred K562 cell line (see Subheading 3.2, step 36) direct from the culture medium or following thawing. Do not resuspend. The cell pellets must first be labeled with chromium (see Note 28). Include:

   (a) A SAL transfected with the restricting HLA molecule loaded with the viral peptide that is recognized by the clone as a positive control (see Notes 23–25).

   (b) A SAL transfected with the restricting HLA molecule loaded with the control peptide that is not recognized by the clone as a negative control.

   (c) A nontransfected K562 as a negative control.

2. Add the appropriate amount of sodium chromate to the cell pellets (see Note 29)

3. Incubate the cells in a 37°C water bath for 1 h.

4. Meanwhile spin down, resuspend, and count the T-cell clone and make the necessary dilutions of the clone (see Note 30). Add 100 μL/well to a 96-well plate.

5. Wash the chromium-labeled SAL and K562 cells three times with 4 mL IMDM + 1%FCS.

6. Add 100 μL of the labeled target cells (concentration of 5,000 cells/100 μL) to each of the wells already containing the T-cell clone.

7. Make a control plate for spontaneous and maximum release. For each target make 3 wells with 100 μL TCM and 3 wells 100 μL 1% Triton X-100. Add 100 μL target suspension per well.

8. Spin the plates for 1 min at 550×*g*.

9. Incubate the plates for 4 h at 37°C, 5%$CO_2$.

10. Spin the plates for 1 min at 550×*g*.

11. Harvest the supernatants.

12. Measure the chromium release and calculate the specific lysis (see Note 31).

## 4. Notes

1. We recommend using PE-labeled tetrameric complexes for brighter cell staining. However, other conjugates may be used. The tetramers used were produced in-house. However, a number of companies (e.g., ProImmune, United Kingdom) have a range of available tetramers.
2. Prior to attempting sorting we recommend screening first for the presence of viral peptide/HLA tetramer complex binding T-cells within the peripheral blood of the donor. Ensuring the donor has a high proportion of the virus-specific T-cells of interest in the peripheral blood increases the probability of successful sorting and cloning. Viral seropositivity does not guarantee the donor blood will contain T-cells with the viral specificity of interest.
3. PBMCs should be prepared by Ficoll hypaque gradient centrifugation. Freshly defrosted PBMCs are also suitable for single cell sorting.
4. Cells from a single random volunteer donor are suitable irrespective of HLA typing. $5 \times 10^6$ donor cells are required for every $1 \times 10^6$ virus-specific T-cells to be stimulated.
5. A G418 resistance gene has been added to some of the plasmid constructs. SALs generated with such constructs are also cultured with G418 added to the culture medium to provide a selection advantage and facilitate growth of the transfectant.
6. The antibodies were obtained in-house from the Department of Immunohematology and Blood Transfusion, LUMC, the Netherlands. They are available commercially on request at a.mulder@lumc.nl.
7. Peptides were produced in-house at LUMC, the Netherlands. These are available for purchase; however, a number of companies will synthesize peptides on request.
8. Perform all steps prior to sorting at 4°C. When tetramers are used at room temperature they are capable of activating the virus-specific T-cells for sorting.
9. Do not forgot positive and negative control tubes for set up of single cell sorting apparatus.
10. It is most convenient to use a pool of FITC-labeled conjugates which will mark the cells which are not of interest. For example, if CD8 memory T-cells are to be sorted then CD45Ra/CD4/

CD19-FITC will exclude naïve cells, CD4 T-cells, and B-cells. In this case the CD8 T-cells to be sorted would be PE positive (tetramer positive) and FITC negative.

11. We recommend using fresh T-cell medium for every T-cell sorting or stimulation (Maximum 2 weeks old).
12. Only freshly collected PBMCs are suitable as feeder cells. Previously frozen cells are not suitable.
13. EBV LCLs are used to provide additional nonspecific stimulation to the sorted T-cells. However, they are not definitely required for successful stimulation. The HLA expression of the EBV LCLs is not important.
14. Virus-specific T-cell clones are used to confirm that the alloreactivity and viral specificity are mediated by the same TCR. Virus-specific T-cell lines can also be generated by sorting multiple tetramer complex binding T-cells per well (e.g., 25 cells/well). T-cell lines are useful for screening purposes and may contain T-cells with the same viral specificity but different TVR Vb usage to that of the single cell sorted clones.
15. For single cell sorted wells expect growth at day 12–14.
16. The TCR will often be absent from the cell surface for the first 5 days after sorting/stimulation.
17. Flow cytometry tests for HLA should always be performed on ice to avoid capping.
18. When you have a low number of HLA-positive cells (before sorting) use PE-labeled w6/32, it is more sensitive than FITC-labeled w6/32.
19. If NO positive cells are present consider repeating procedure from Subheading 3.2, step 1. If repeatedly negative seek specialist advice.
20. Usually there is evidence of cell growth by day 3–4. SALs will continue to grow as long as they are split and supplied with fresh medium. You may wish to freeze aliquots for future use.
21. Virus-specific T-cell clones should be used in IFNγ ELISA assays at day 9–10 after stimulation. Earlier use of the T-cell clone may be associated with ongoing IFNγ production from the T-cells.
22. The cells survive better if the wash medium contains protein (e.g., 1% FCS). Instead of IMDM you can also use other media for harvesting and washing, e.g., RPMI.
23. Leaving SALs at 26°C for two nights increases HLA expression.
24. IFNγ stimulation probably does increase HLA expression.
25. K562 cells do not have functional CIITA gene product (5). Therefore, K562 cells will not express HLA class II molecules.

26. For easy transfer of your supernatants, make the layout of your culture plate the same as the layout of the ELISA plate and leave wells open for your standard dilutions and blank.
27. When the supernatants have to be stored for a longer period (>1 month), it is better to store them in small siliconized vials.
28. Cytotoxicity assays are best performed at day 7–8 after stimulation of the T-cell clone.
29. The half life off sodium chromate is short, be sure to use the correct amount according to the manufacturers instructions.
30. The effector target ratios commonly used are 30:1, 10:1, 1:1, and 0.1:1. Therefore, given that there are 5,000 target cells/well then the number of effector cells to be added are 150,000, 50,000, 5,000, and 500 (each in 100 μL), i.e., cell concentrations $1.5 \times 10^6$, $0.5 \times 10^6$, $0.05 \times 10^6$, and $0.005 \times 10^6$/mL respectively.
31. % specific lysis = ((test release–spontaneous release) (maximum release–spontaneous release)) × 100%. For more details on calculations of % specific lysis, see ref. (2).

## References


1. Amir A, D'Orsogna L, Roelen D, van Loenen M, Haagedoorn R, de Boer R et al (2010) Allo-HLA reactivity of viral specific memory T-cells is common. Blood 115:3146–3157
2. D'Orsogna LJA, Amir A, Zoet Y, van der Meer-Prins P, van der Slik A, Kester M et al (2009) New tools to monitor the impact of viral infection on the alloreactive T-cell repertoire. Tissue Antigens 74:290–297
3. Zoet Y, Eijsink C, Kardol M, Franke-van Dijk M, Wilson G, de Paus R et al (2005) The single antigen expressing lines (SALs) concept: an excellent tool for screening for HLA-specific antibodies. Hum Immunol 66: 519–525
4. Mulder A, Zoet Y, Eijsink C. Single MHC antigen expressing cell lines for the definition of monoclonal antibody specificities. In: Hansen JA(ed) Histocompatibility testing 2002, HLA 2002, Munksgaard, 2005
5. van der Stoep N, Biesta P, Quinten E, van den Elsen P (2002) Lack of IFNγ mediated induction of the class II transactivator (CIITA) through promoter methylation is predominantly found in developmental tumor cell Lines. Int J Cancer 97:501–507

# Chapter 20

# Separation and Cryopreservation of Lymphocytes from Spleen and Lymph Node

## Gabriella Tassone and Samantha J. Fidler

## Abstract

Spleen and lymph node retrieved post-mortem from deceased organ donors are a rich source of lymphocytes. Storage of lymphocytes separated from these sources can be valuable where post-transplant testing (crossmatching) is required. DNA extraction from stored lymphocytes also allows further genetic testing where required, for example additional HLA typing not performed at the time of transplant for donor-specific antibody monitoring. Methods for the isolation and freezing of such cells is described.

**Key words:** Lymphocytes, Spleen, Lymph node, Cryopreservation

## 1. Introduction

Peripheral blood is readily available as a source of lymphocytes for serological HLA typing and histocompatibility testing, however for some individuals such as deceased organ donors, high volumes of peripheral blood are not available and re-bleeds are not possible. Alternative sources, such as spleen and lymph node, can be utilised for bulk separation of lymphocytes for immediate use and or cryopreservation. The Ficoll-Hypaque density gradient separation technique used for peripheral blood lymphocyte separation can also be utilised for spleen and lymph node preparations (1). A cell suspension is layered over the density gradient. On centrifugation, the denser erythrocytes and granulocytes pass through the gradient and pellet at the bottom of the tube. Platelets remain in the supernatant, while lymphocytes remain at the plasma/gradient interface. The interface is removed and washed to remove any platelet contamination. The lymphocytes may then be used immediately or cryopreserved for future use (2, 3).

Frank T. Christiansen and Brian D. Tait (eds.), *Immunogenetics: Methods and Applications in Clinical Practice*, Methods in Molecular Biology, vol. 882, DOI 10.1007/978-1-61779-842-9_20, © Springer Science+Business Media New York 2012

## 2. Materials

### *2.1. Isolation of Spleen and Lymph Node Cells*

1. RPMI medium 1640 (Gibco Invitrogen) (see Note 1).
2. Sections of fresh lymph node or spleen (see Note 2).
3. Ficoll-Paque (GE Healthcare Bioscience) (see Note 1).
4. Sterile Petri dishes (Sarstedt) (see Note 1).
5. Disposable sterile scalpels (Swann- Morton).
6. 30-mL round bottom capped tubes (Sarstedt).
7. 30-mL syringes (Becton Dickinson).
8. Cannulae (Maerski Medical).
9. Size 7 and/or size 9 sterile plastic pasteur pipettes (Samco Scientific).
10. Centrifuge (Beckman TJ-6 or equivalent).
11. 50-mL Cellstar tubes (Greiner).
12. 20% Foetal calf serum (FCS)/RPMI (see Note 3).

### *2.2. Cryopreservation of Separated Lymphocytes*

1. Lymphocytes prepared in Subheading 3.1.
2. 20% FCS/RPMI (see Note 3).
3. 15% Dimethyl sulphoxide (DMSO)/RPMI (see Note 3).
4. Nunc cryo tube vials (Thermo Scientific).
5. Neubauer cell counting chamber (see Note 4).
6. Light microscope.

### *2.3. Thawing Frozen Lymphocytes for Histocompatibility Testing*

1. 10% FCS/RPMI (see Note 3).
2. FCS (Gibco).
3. 15-mL round bottomed tubes (Sarstedt).
4. 1.5-mL microtubes (Sarstedt).
5. Microfuge (Hetlich Mikro 22R or equivalent).
6. 37°C water bath (Thermoline Scientific or equivalent).
7. Citrated phosphate-buffered saline (PBSC) (see Note 5).

## 3. Methods

### *3.1. Isolation of Spleen and Lymph Node Cells*

1. Place an approximate 2 $cm^3$ section of spleen onto a sterile Petri dish and using a sterile scalpel, trim the capsule from the spleen and discard.
2. In a separate Petri dish, place the lymph nodes and remove any fatty tissue from around the nodes.

3. Using sterile forceps and scalpels, gently tease spleen or lymph node cells into approximately 5 mL of RPMI placed in the Petri dish (see Note 6).
4. Using a sterile pasteur pipette, place the cell suspension into 2 × 30-mL round bottom capped tubes. Wash the Petri dish out with RPMI to get all of the cell suspension. Avoid picking up pieces of tissue.
5. Spin the tubes at 1,800 × *g* for 30 s (see Note 7).
6. Transfer 15 mL aliquots of cell suspension (supernatant) into an appropriate number of 50-mL CellStar tubes.
7. Dilute the transferred supernatant 1:2 with RPMI, making up to a volume of 30 mL. Underlay 10 mL of sterile Ficoll-paque using a cannula attached to a 30-mL syringe (see Notes 8 and 9).
8. Centrifuge the cell suspension/gradient for 30 min at 4,000 × *g*.
9. Using a sterile pasteur pipette, carefully remove the cells at the gradient interface and transfer to clean 30-mL round bottomed capped tubes. Wash by filling the tube to 30 mL with RPMI and centrifuging at 1,500 × *g* for 10 min.
10. Carefully pour out and discard the RPMI and resuspend the remaining cell pellet in 5 mL of 20% FCS/RPMI.

### 3.2. Freezing of Isolated Lymphocytes for Storage

1. Determine the lymphocyte concentration using a Neubauer chamber (see Notes 4 and 10).
2. Adjust the cell concentration to $20 \times 10^6$/mL by the addition or removal of 20% FCS/RPMI as described in Note 11.
3. Place the tube of cell suspension onto wet ice to begin the cooling process. Leave to cool for a few minutes before proceeding to step 4.
4. Add an equal volume of 15% DMSO/RPMI to the cell suspension drop-wise with gentle constant mixing (see Note 12).
5. Transfer 1 mL aliquots of cell suspension into an appropriate number of Nunc tubes and freeze at −80°C overnight or for at least 1.5 h before transferring into liquid nitrogen (see Note 13).

### 3.3. Thawing Frozen Lymphocytes in Preparation for Dynabead Separation for Serological HLA Class I or II Typing

1. Place a 1 mL Nunc containing frozen cells prepared in Subheading 3.2 in 37°C water bath to thaw (see Note 14).
2. Immediately add 0.5 mL FCS drop-wise and transfer the cells to a 1.5-mL microtube (see Note 15).
3. Microfuge for 1 min at 1,000 × *g*.
4. Remove the supernatant by tipping off slowly taking care not to disturb the cell pellet and lose cells, and resuspend cells in 1 mL 10% FCS/RPMI.

5. Incubate at 37°C in a waterbath for 10 min, mix by gentle inversion after 5 min.
6. Centrifuge the cell suspension at 1,000 × *g* for 1 min, remove the supernatant by tipping off slowly.
7. Resuspend in 1 mL 10% FCS/RPMI, transfer to a 15-mL round bottomed tube and repeat step 6.
8. Slowly add 8 mL PBSC. Cells are ready for T- and B- cell separation—refer to Chapter 22 (see Note 16).

## 4. Notes

1. Use sterile equipment and reagents throughout this procedure. Perform in a Class II Biosafety cabinet.
2. Spleen and lymph node should be collected fresh and aseptically by the surgical retrieval team with appropriate donor consent. The material should be placed in RPMI at room temperature and expeditiously transported to the laboratory for processing. The specimens should be processed within 12 h of donor retrieval. After this time, cells may still be extracted but viability may not be sufficient for use in crossmatching or any assay requiring viable cells. However, these cells can still be used as a source of DNA.
3. 10% FCS/RPMI, 20% FCS/RPMI, and 15% DMSO/RPMI should be made in a sterile cabinet using aseptic techniques.
4. Coulter cell counter or equivalent may be used to determine cell numbers if available.
5. pH 7.4 PBS can be made easily in-house or bought commercially from suppliers, such as MP Biomedicals and Dako. PBSC is PBS pH7.4 + 0.6% Tri-sodium citrate, i.e. 12 g Tri-sodium citrate in 2 L filtered PBS.
6. To extract the cells hold the tissue firmly with the forceps. With the scalpel use minimal pressure to gently tease the cells into the RPMI. From time to time, wash the tissue with RPMI using a pasteur pipette. A cloud of cells should be seen coming into the media. Do not allow the media to become too overloaded with cells, add more RPMI as required so that the medium looks opaque.

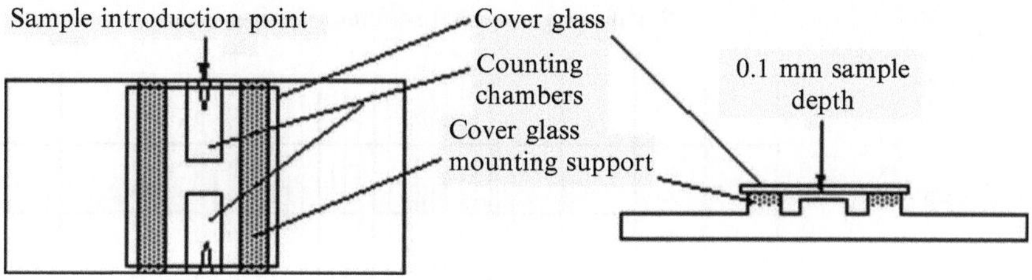


Fig. 1. The Neubauer chamber, indicating sample introduction point, and counting chamber.

7. This centrifugation will spin down any tissue debris but is short and gentle enough to leave the cells in suspension. This step can be repeated if necessary.
8. Remove the syringe plunger from the barrel and discard. Place a cannula on the end (where a hypodermic needle is usually placed) and carefully place the cannula into the cell suspension so the end sits on the bottom of the tube. Pour 10 mL of density gradient into the syringe barrel and lift the syringe slightly to allow flow of gradient.
9. If the tubes are accidently knocked or dropped resulting in mixing of the gradient/cell suspension interface, the samples can be recovered by underlaying the gradient/cell mix with a further 10 mL of density gradient.
10. Cell concentration determination using a Neubauer chamber (see Fig. 1):
    - Clean lens thoroughly prior to use.

    Ensure cover slip is also thoroughly cleaned.
    - Place cover slip over the counting surface. Add the cell suspension using a pipette. (The area under the cover slip fills by capillary action).
    - Place the counting chamber on the microscope stage and bring the counting grid into focus at low power (40×).
    - There are 9 large squares, each of which contains 16 medium squares, each of which contains 25 small squares. One large square has 0.1 μL volume (see Fig. 2).
    - Count the number of lymphocytes in 5 of the medium squares and multiply by 5 (=number of cells/0.1 μL).

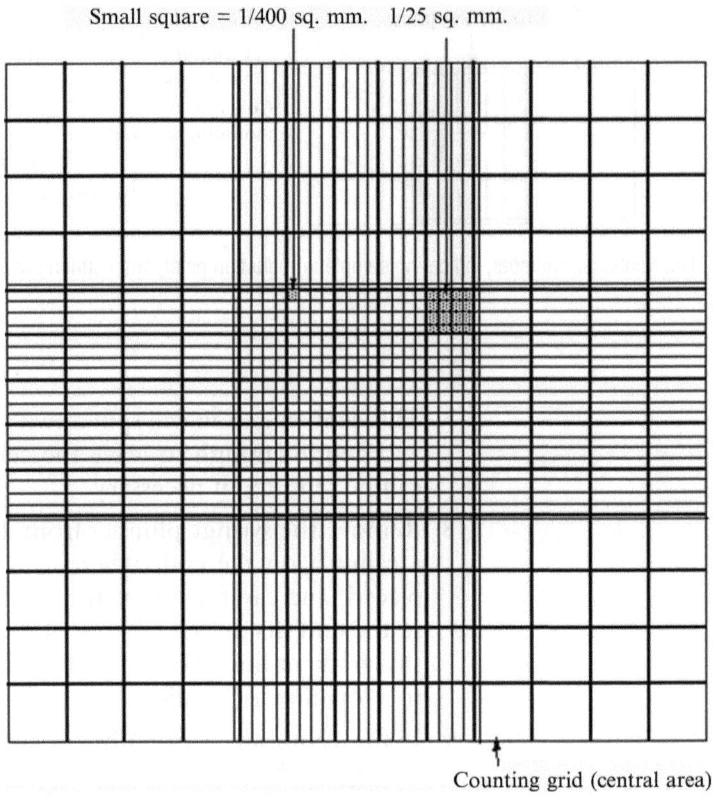


Fig. 2. Diagrammatic representation of the Neubauer counting chamber. One large square have 0.1 μL volume.

11. Remove FCS/RPMI by centrifuging the cell suspension at 1,500×*g* for 10 min. Resuspend the cell pellet in an appropriate volume of FCS/RPMI to adjust to the correct concentration.
12. DMSO minimises cell damage in the freezing process by gradually replacing water within the cells.
13. The cooling rate should be approximately −1°C per minute and can be assisted by first placing the Nunc tubes in a cryo container, such as "Mr Frosty" from Nalgene and placing the container in the −80°C freezer, or by using a controlled rate freezer.
14. Cells should be thawed as rapidly as possible as prolonged exposure to DMSO will compromise cell viability.
15. DMSO is toxic to lymphocytes at room temperature so rapid washing of the cells is essential.
16. You can at this stage check the cell count (see Note 9) and viability. This can be prudent if you are suspicious about the

storage conditions of the cryopreserved cells or the viability of the cells prior to freezing. However, if you have a limited number of cells stored, you may wish to proceed to T-and B-cell separation and check the viability and cell count following separation.

## References

1. Bøyum A (1968) Isolation of mononuclear cells and granulocytes from human blood. Scand J Clin Lab Invest Suppl 97:77–87
2. Strong DM (2000) Cryopreservation of lymphocytes in bulk. ASHI Laboratory Manual 4th Edition, vol 1
3. Lorentzen D (2000) Cell preservation. ASHI Laboratory Manual 4th Edition, vol 1

# Chapter 21

# Crossmatching by Complement-Dependent Lymphocytotoxicity


## Samantha J. Fidler



## Abstract

The presence of preformed donor-specific HLA antibodies detected by Complement-dependent cytotoxicity (CDC) crossmatch assay is associated with a high incidence of hyperacute or accelerated rejection and remains one of the gold standard tests pre-transplant. The standard CDC crossmatch detects IgG1, IgG3, and IgM antibody, i.e. complement fixing, bound to the native viable cell surface of lymphocytes. The crossmatch can be enhanced with the addition of anti-human-globulin to detect non-complement fixing antibodies (IgG2 and IgG4), and sensitivity can be improved with prolonged incubation times.



**Key words:** Crossmatch, Complement-dependent cytotoxicity, Alloantibody, Autoantibody, IgG, IgM


## 1. Introduction

Since the landmark paper by Patel and Terasaki (1) was published in the late 1960s, a positive (T cell) lymphocytotoxic crossmatch has been considered a contraindication to renal transplantation. The crossmatch assay detects high levels of recipient antibodies against donor HLA antigens, and a positive crossmatch is associated with hyperacute and accelerated acute rejection, and long-term graft failure. The complement-dependent lymphocytotoxicity (CDC) crossmatch remains to this day the gold standard as the final pre-transplant check for donor-specific anti-HLA antibodies. Since the 1960s a number of modifications, such as the AHG-CDC crossmatch and treatment of sera to remove IgM reactivity, have been made to improve sensitivity and specificity. The barrier of a positive crossmatch to transplantation has somewhat diminished in the current era of desensitisation protocols and effective treatment for rejection episodes. However, it is clear that the


Frank T. Christiansen and Brian D. Tait (eds.), *Immunogenetics: Methods and Applications in Clinical Practice*, Methods in Molecular Biology, vol. 882, DOI 10.1007/978-1-61779-842-9_21, © Springer Science+Business Media New York 2012

presence of class I anti-HLA antibodies pre-transplant is associated with poor graft survival and there is increasing evidence that class II anti-HLA antibodies are associated with an increase in rejection episodes and poor long-term survival, particularly in the presence of a positive B cell crossmatch (2, 3).

Serum samples from the recipient are incubated with separated T and B lymphocytes from a potential organ donor. If donor reactive antibodies are present, addition of complement results in cell death via activation of the complement cascade. A positive T cell crossmatch is usually due to antibodies against HLA class I and is a contraindication to transplantation. A positive B cell crossmatch in the absence of a positive T cell crossmatch may be due to antibodies against HLA class II or weak antibodies against HLA class I. A positive B cell crossmatch is not considered a contraindication to transplantation in all centres, but rather a risk factor for transplantation (4). Positive crossmatches due to IgM antibodies are not usually considered a contraindication to transplantation as many are due to the presence of harmless IgM autoantibody. IgM reactivity can be removed by dithiothreitol (DTT) treatment or heat treatment of sera.

## 2. Materials

### 2.1. Separation of T and B Lymphocytes

1. Anticoagulated blood samples (ACD) (see Note 1).
2. Human B cell whole blood (WB) positive selection EasySep beads—includes positive selection cocktail (StemCell Technologies Product Number 18184 HLA).
3. Human CD3 WB positive selection EasySep beads—includes positive selection cocktail (StemCell Technologies Product Number 18081HLA).
4. 15-mL round bottomed tubes.
5. Magnetic Separation Device-EasySep magnet.
6. Sterile phosphate buffered saline (PBS) pH 7.4-Filtered and stored at 4°C.
7. Carboxyfluorescein diacetate (CFDA) staining solution (stored at 4°C wrapped in aluminium foil) (see Notes 2 and 3).
8. McCoys 5A tissue culture medium + 5% heat-inactivated fFoetal calf serum (HIFCS).
9. Haemoglobin/ethidium bromide staining solution (stored at 4°C wrapped in aluminium foil) (see Notes 2 and 3).
10. 1× RBC lysis buffer (Made by diluting 10× RBS lysis buffer) (see Note 4).
11. Hamilton syringes—1 and 5-μL dispensing.

12. 10-, 20-, 100-, 200-, and 1,000-μL pipette—Gilson or equivalent.
13. Pipette tips (10, 20, 100, 200, 1,000 μL).
14. 60-Well Terasaki trays (containing 5 μL mineral oil per well).
15. RoboSep-automated cell separator (see Note 5).
16. 22°C incubator (see Note 6).
17. Inverted fluorescence microscope.

### 2.2. Standard CDC Crossmatch

1. 1 and 5-μL single dispense pipettes (e.g., Hamilton, Robbins).
2. 60- or 72-well microlymphocytotoxicity (Terasaki) trays (containing 5 μL mineral oil per well).
3. Recipient sera (see Notes 7 and 8).
4. Donor lymphocytes—refer to Subheading 2.1.
5. Fluorescent stain (Haemoglobin/ethidium bromide or alternative).
6. Pooled rabbit complement—refer to Subheading 3.5: Evaluation of complement—(PelFreeze) (see Note 9).
7. Citrated PBS pH 7.4.
8. PBS pH 7.4.
9. AB Negative serum (see Note 10)—negative control.
10. Anti-thymocyte globulin (ATG) (see Note 11)—positive control.
11. B cell positive control (see Note 12).
12. Inverted fluorescence microscope.
13. 37°C waterbath.
14. 22°C incubator (see Note 6).
15. 1- and 5-μL automatic dispensers (e.g. Greiner, OLI, Robbins).
16. 1% Kaolin (Sigma).

### 2.3. AHG-CDC Crossmatch

As Subheading 2.2 plus.

1. Anti-human globulin (AHG) (Biotest).
2. RPMI Media (Sigma).

### 2.4. Heat Treatment of Sera to Remove IgM Reactivity

As Subheading 2.2 plus.

1. 400-μL capped tubes (Beckman).
2. 60°C waterbath or thermal cycler.
3. Microfuge.
4. IgM control serum (see Note 13).
5. IgG control serum (see Note 14).

### 2.5. Complement Evaluation

As Subheading 2.2 plus.

1. Well-characterised antisera (see Note 15).

## 3. Methods

### 3.1. Separation of T and B Lymphocytes

1. Into a 15-mL round bottomed tube add 4 mL ACD blood and 4 mL of 1× RBC lysis buffer. Mix by gently inverting.
2. Add 200 μL of positive selection cocktail (Human B cell WB positive selection for B cells or Human CD3 WB positive selection for T cells) to the whole blood/lysis mixture. Incubate at room temperature for 15 min (see Note 6).
3. Mix the EasySep beads to ensure uniform suspension by pipetting up and down vigorously at least five times (DO NOT VORTEX).
4. Add 200 μL of the mixed EasySep beads to the respective tubes. Incubate for 10 min at room temperature.
5. Add 2 mL PBS pH 7.4 and mix gently by pipetting up and down.
6. Remove cap from tube and place on EasySep magnet. T cells require 5 min, B cells require 10 min on the magnet.
7. Pick up magnet and in one continuous motion pour contents out of the 15-mL tube, leave inverted for 2–3 s (DO NOT SHAKE OR BLOT ANY DROPS REMAINING ON THE MOUTH OF THE TUBE).
8. Remove tube from magnet and add 10 mL PBS pH 7.4. Place on magnet for another 5 min (both T and B cells).
9. Pick up magnet and in one continuous motion pour contents out leave inverted for 2–3 s as per step 7 (DO NOT SHAKE OR BLOT ANY DROPS REMAINING ON THE MOUTH OF THE TUBE).
10. Remove the 15-mL tube from magnet add 0.5 mL CFDA solution drop wise directly onto the cells in the 15-mL tube and incubate for 5 min at room temperature (mix the tube gently by hand from time to time during this period).
11. Place the 15-mL tube into the magnet and fill the tube to top of magnet with PBS pH 7.4. Incubate for 2 min.
12. Pick up magnet and in one continuous motion pour contents out leave inverted for 2–3 s (DO NOT SHAKE OR BLOT ANY DROPS REMAINING ON THE MOUTH OF THE TUBE).
13. Fill CTS tube to top of magnet with PBS pH 7.4 for 2 min.

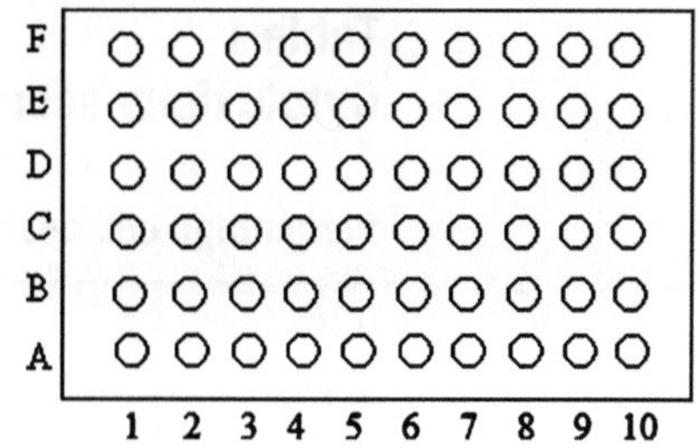


Fig. 1. Diagrammatic representation of the 60-well Terasaki tray.

14. Pick up magnet and in one continuous motion pour contents out of the 15-mL tube, leave inverted for 2–3 s (DO NOT SHAKE OR BLOT ANY DROPS REMAINING ON THE MOUTH OF THE TUBE).
15. Resuspend cells by adding fresh 5% HIFCS/McCoy's (1 mL for class I and 0.5 mL class II) to the 15-mL tube.
16. Using a Hamilton syringe spot 1 μL of cell suspension in triplicate onto an oiled Terasaki tray.
17. Add 5 μL Haemoglobin/ethidium bromide stain to each well (see Note 4). Allow cells to settle for approximately 20 min.
18. View the cells under the fluorescent microscope to determine cell concentration and viability. Concentration can be adjusted by addition or removal of 5% FCS/McCoys (see Note 16).
19. Hold the cells at room temperature for use in the crossmatch assay (see Note 17).

### 3.2. Standard CDC Crossmatch

#### 3.2.1. Tray Set-Up

1. Add 1 μL of ATG dilutions and AB negative sera to an oiled Terasaki tray using a Hamilton syringe (see Note 18, Fig. 1). 3A—ATG50, 3B—AB Neg, 3C—ATG500, 3D—ATG200, 3E—AB Neg, 3F—B Cell Pos, 4A—ATG400, 4B—ATG25, 4C—AB Neg, 4D—ATG100, 4E—ATG800, 4F—ATG1000.
2. Add 1 μL recipient serum to wells 1D, 1E, and 1F and 1 μL AB negative serum to wells 1A, 1B, and 1C using a Hamilton syringe. Historical peak sera can be added as appropriate in triplicate to wells 2A to 2F (see Note 8). Trays should be made at least in duplicate for both T and B cell crossmatch, i.e. at least four trays in total (see Note 19).

#### 3.2.2. Crossmatch Set-Up

1. Add 1 μL T or B cell suspension (refer to Subheading 3.1) using an automated cell dispenser to avoid cross-contamination. Ensure all wells are thoroughly mixed (see Note 20).
2. Incubate the trays for 45 min at 22°C (or room temperature—see Note 6) (see Note 21).

**Table 1**
**Cytotoxicity scores**

| Percentage cell death | Score | Conventional score |
|---|---|---|
| 0 | A | 1 |
| 1–2 | B | 1 |
| 3–5 | C | 1 |
| 6–10 | D | 1 |
| 11–15 | 1 | 1 |
| 15–25 | 2 | 1 |
| 25–35 | 3 | 2 |
| 35–45 | 4 | 2/4 |
| 45–55 | 5 | 4 |
| 55–65 | 6 | 4/6 |
| 65–75 | 7 | 6 |
| 75–85 | 8 | 8 |
| 85–100 | 9 | 8 |
| Empty well or unreadable | X | 0 |
| Insufficient cell numbers | 0 | 0 |

3. Following incubation, add 5 μL of previously screened pooled rabbit complement (see Subheading 3.5) to each well using an automated dispenser to avoid cross-contamination.
4. Incubate the trays for 45 min at 22°C (or room temperature—see Note 6) (see Note 21).
5. Following complement incubation, add 5 μL Haemoglobin/ethidium bromide stain to each well. Allow cells to settle for approximately 20 min.
6. Score the percentage cell death semi-quantitatively under the fluorescent microscope according to Table 1 (see Notes 22 and 23).

*3.2.3. Interpretation of Crossmatch Results*

1. A positive or negative crossmatch is determined by comparing the crossmatch score with the background reactivity, i.e. the AB negative control serum as shown in Fig. 2 (see Notes 24 and 25).
2. Results should be interpreted according to Table 2.

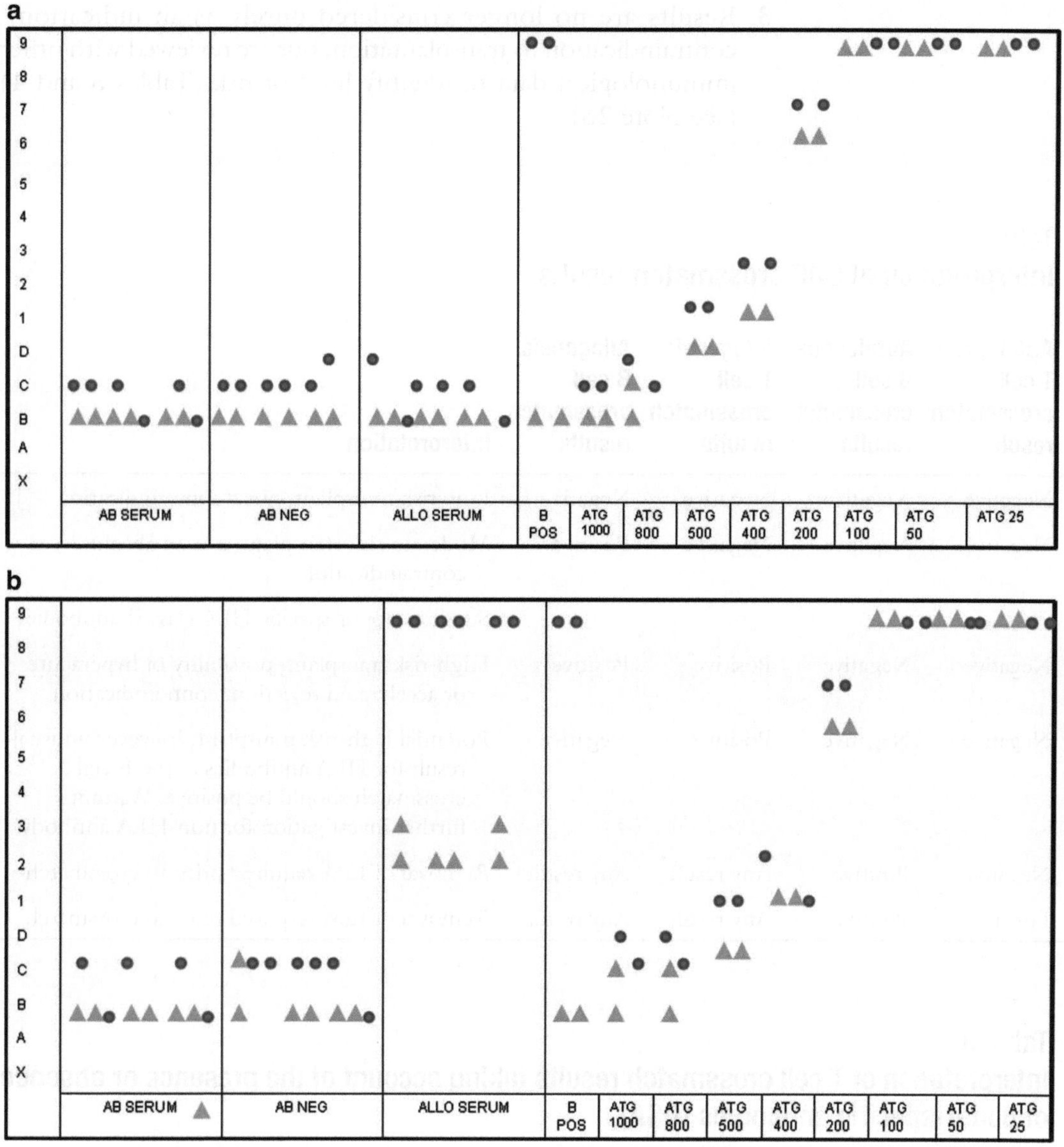


Fig. 2. (**a**) Autologous crossmatch (The *circle* denotes B cell crossmatch results, the *triangle* denotes T cell crossmatch results). Crossmatches are read according to Table 1. The AB serum is read as a background control, i.e. contains no HLA antibodies. The autologous crossmatch should be interpreted in relation to the crossmatch results of this control. The AB Neg is read as a carry-over control—this AB serum is located next to strongly positive ATG controls. The ATG controls can be used to monitor the sensitivity of the assay. The laboratory should determine its own QC criteria for example an assay might only pass QC if the ATG 400 dilution crossmatch result is >AB serum control. In this example, the autologous T and B cell crossmatches are negative. (**b**) Allogeneic crossmatch (the *circle* denotes B cell crossmatch results, the *triangle* denotes T cell crossmatch results). Crossmatches are read according to Table 2. The AB serum is read as a background control, i.e. contains no HLA antibodies. The allogeneic crossmatch should be interpreted in relation to the crossmatch results of this control. Other controls on this crossmatch tray follow the same criteria as those in the autologous crossmatch (**a**). In this example, both the T and B cell allogeneic crossmatches are positive.

3. Results are no longer considered purely as an indication/contraindication to transplantation; but are reviewed with other immunological data to identify level of risk (Tables 3 and 4) (see Note 26).

**Table 2**
**Interpretation of CDC crossmatch results**

| Autologous T cell crossmatch result | Autologous B cell crossmatch results | Allogeneic T cell crossmatch results | Allogeneic B cell crossmatch results | Interpretation |
|---|---|---|---|---|
| Negative | Negative | Negative | Negative | Low-risk transplant, not a contraindication |
| Negative | Negative | Negative | Positive | Moderate-risk transplant, not an absolute contraindication<br>Suggests donor-specific HLA class II antibodies |
| Negative | Negative | Positive | Positive | High-risk transplant, possibility of hyperacute or accelerated rejection, contraindication |
| Negative | Negative | Positive | Negative | Potential high-risk transplant, however unusual result for HLA antibodies as the B cell crossmatch should be positive. Warrants further investigation for non-HLA antibody |
| Negative | Positive | Any result | Any result | Removal of IgM required prior to crossmatch |
| Positive | Positive | Any result | Any result | Removal of IgM required prior to crossmatch |

**Table 3**
**Interpretation of T cell crossmatch results taking account of the presence or absence of donor-specific antibodies (DSA)**

| | Allogeneic T-cell crossmatch | | |
|---|---|---|---|
| DSA (MFI) | Negative | Positive—not reduced by heat or DTT | Positive—reduced by heat or DTT |
| >8,000 (strong) | These results are not an absolute contraindication to transplantation; however, the the presence of donor-specific HLA antibodies detected by Single Antigen Bead assay increases the risk of rejection episodes | These results are a contraindication to transplantation | These results are not an absolute contraindication to transplantation; however, the presence of donor-specific HLA antibodies detected by Single Antigen Bead assay increases the risk of rejection episodes |

(continued)

**Table 3**
**(continued)**

| DSA (MFI) | Allogeneic T-cell crossmatch | | |
|---|---|---|---|
| | Negative | Positive—not reduced by heat or DTT | Positive—reduced by heat or DTT |
| 2,000–8,000 (moderate) | These results are not an absolute contraindication to transplantation; however, the presence of donor-specific HLA antibodies detected by Single Antigen Bead assay may increase the risk of rejection episodes | These results are a contraindication to transplantation | These results are not an absolute contraindication to transplantation; however, the presence of donor-specific HLA antibodies detected by Single Antigen Bead assay may increase the risk of rejection episodes |
| 500–2,000 (weak) | These results are not a contraindication to transplantation. The clinical significance of weak donor-specific HLA antibodies detected by Single Antigen Bead assay is unknown | These results are a contraindication to transplantation | These results are not a contraindication to transplantation. The clinical significance of weak donor-specific HLA antibodies detected by Single Antigen Bead assay is unknown |
| <500 (negative) | These results are not a contraindication to transplantation | These results are a contraindication to transplantation | These results are not a contraindication to transplantation |

**Table 4**
**Interpretation of B cell crossmatch results taking account of the presence or absence of DSA**

| DSA (MFI) | Allogeneic B-cell crossmatch | | |
|---|---|---|---|
| | Negative | Positive—not reduced by heat or DTT | Positive—reduced by heat or DTT |
| >8,000 (strong) | These results are not an absolute contraindication to transplantation; however, the presence of donor-specific HLA antibodies detected by Single Antigen Bead assay increases the risk of rejection episodes | These results are a contraindication to transplantation | These results are not an absolute contraindication to transplantation; however, the presence of donor-specific HLA antibodies detected by Single Antigen Bead assay increases the risk of rejection episodes |

(continued)

**Table 4 (continued)**

| DSA (MFI) | Allogeneic B-cell crossmatch: Negative | Positive—not reduced by heat or DTT | Positive—reduced by heat or DTT |
|---|---|---|---|
| 2,000–8,000 (moderate) | These results are not an absolute contraindication to transplantation; however, the presence of donor-specific HLA antibodies detected by Single Antigen Bead assay may increase the risk of rejection episodes | These results are not an absolute contraindication to transplantation; however, the presence of donor-specific HLA antibodies detected by Single Antigen Bead assay in the presence of a positive B cell cross-match is associated with an increased risk of rejection episodes | These results are not an absolute contraindication to transplantation; however, the presence of donor-specific HLA antibodies detected by Single Antigen Bead assay may increase the risk of rejection episodes |
| 500–2,000 (weak) | These results are not a contraindication to transplantation. The clinical significance of weak donor-specific HLA antibodies detected by Single Antigen Bead assay is unknown | These results are not an absolute contraindication to transplantation; however, the risk of rejection episodes may be increased | These results are not a contraindication to transplantation. The clinical significance of weak donor-specific HLA antibodies detected by Single Antigen Bead assay is unknown |
| <500 (negative) | These results are not a contraindication to transplantation | These results are not an absolute contraindication to transplantation. The presence of a positive B cell crossmatch in the absence of DSA is uncertain but may increase the risk of rejection episodes | These results are not a contraindication to transplantation |

### 3.3. AHG-CDC Crossmatch

#### 3.3.1. Tray Set Up

Follow Subheading 3.2.1 for tray set up.

#### 3.3.2. Crossmatch Method

1. Follow Subheading 3.2.2 to step 3 (see Note 27).
2. Wash trays with RPMI. Add 10 μL RPMI to each well. Centrifuge for 1 min at 1,000 rpm. Quickly flick out the RPMI in one swift movement.
3. Repeat step 2 two more times, then add 1 μL AHG to each well. Leave for 1 min.
4. Follow Subheading 3.2.2 from step 4 until the end.

#### 3.3.3. Interpretation of Results

As per Subheading 3.2.3.

### 3.4. Heat Treatment of Sera to Remove IgM Reactivity

See Note 28.

#### 3.4.1. Preparation of Sera

1. Pre-warm the waterbath to 60°C (see Note 29).
2. Aliquot 200 μL of patient crossmatch sera and control sera (AB Neg, IgG, and IgM controls) into suitably labelled Beckman tubes.
3. Place the tubes into the waterbath ensuring that the sera are fully submerged (see Note 30).
4. Incubate the tubes for exactly 13 min (see Note 31).
5. Remove the samples from the waterbath and immediately microfuge at 10,000 rpm for 1 min.
6. Remove the supernatant into a clean Beckman tube, taking care not to disturb the gelatinous protein precipitate.

#### 3.4.2. Tray Set-Up

1. Add ATG dilutions as per step 1 of Subheading 3.2.1.
2. Add 1 μL AB Negative serum to wells 1A and 1B and 1 μL heat treated (HT) AB negative serum to wells 1C and 1D using a Hamilton syringe.
3. Add 1 μL IgG control serum to wells 1E and 1F and 1 μL HT IgG control serum to wells 2E and 2F.
4. Add 1 μL IgM control serum to wells 2C and 2D and 1 μL HT IgM control serum to wells 2A and 2B.
5. Add 1 μL patient serum to wells 5A and 5B and 1 μL HT patient serum to wells 5C and 5D. Historical peak sera can be added as appropriate in duplicate to wells 5E to 6F (see Note 8). Trays should be made in duplicate for both T and B cell crossmatch, i.e. four trays in total.

#### 3.4.3. Crossmatch Method

The standard CDC crossmatch as described in Subheading 3.2.2, or the AHG crossmatch as described in Subheading 3.3.2 may be performed.

#### 3.4.4. Interpretation of Results

1. A positive or negative crossmatch is determined by comparing the crossmatch score with the background reactivity, i.e. the AB negative control serum as shown in Fig. 3 (see Notes 24 and 25).
2. Results should be interpreted according to Tables 5 and 6.

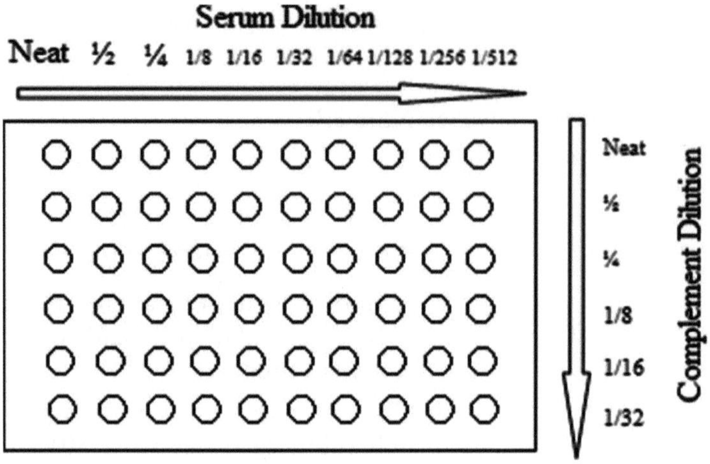


Fig. 3. Suggested layout for complement evaluation titration.

**Table 5**
**Interpretation of heat-treated T cell crossmatch results**

| Allogeneic T cell crossmatch result | | | |
|---|---|---|---|
| **Neat (non-heat treated)** | **Heat treated** | **Interpretation of crossmatch** | **Conclusion** |
| Positive | Positive | Positive | IgG alloantibodies detected. High risk, possibility of hyperacute or accelerated rejection, contraindication |
| Positive | Weak positive | Indeterminate | Possible IgG alloantibodies and IgM autoantibodies detected. Requires further investigation |
| Positive | Negative | Negative | IgM autoantibodies detected. Not a contraindication |

**Table 6**
**Interpretation of heat-treated T cell crossmatch results**

| Allogeneic T cell crossmatch result | | | |
|---|---|---|---|
| **Neat (non-heat treated)** | **Heat treated** | **Interpretation of crossmatch** | **Conclusion** |
| Positive | Positive | Positive | IgG alloantibodies detected. Moderate risk, not a contraindication |
| Positive | Weak positive | Indeterminate | Possible IgG alloantibodies and IgM autoantibodies detected. Requires further investigation |
| Positive | Negative | Negative | IgM autoantibodies detected. Not a contraindication |

3. Results are no longer considered purely as an indication/contraindication to transplantation; but are reviewed with other immunological data to identify level of risk (Tables 3 and 4) (see Note 26).

### 3.5. Complement Evaluation

Pooled rabbit serum is used as a source of complement (see Note 9).

#### 3.5.1. Tray Set-Up

1. Serially dilute the complement N/2 with McCoys medium (see Note 32).
2. Serially dilute antisera with well-characterised reactivity N/2 in AB negative serum (see Note 33).
3. Add 1 μL of serum to a Terasaki tray from Neat to 1/512 (see Fig. 3).

#### 3.5.2. Crossmatch Set-Up

1. Add 1 μL T or B cell suspension (refer to Subheading 3.1) using an automated cell dispenser to avoid cross-contamination (see Note 34). Ensure all wells are thoroughly mixed (see Note 20).
2. Add 5 μL of diluted complement according to the format in step 3. Incubate at room temperature for 45 min (see Note 21).
3. Add 5 μL ethidium bromide/haemoglobin stain and allow to rest for 20 min (see Note 3).
4. Score the percentage cell death under the fluorescent microscope according to Table 1 (see Notes 22 and 23).

#### 3.5.3. Interpretation of Results

1. A positive or negative crossmatch is determined by comparing the crossmatch score with the background reactivity, i.e. the AB negative control serum as shown in Fig. 4 (see Notes 24 and 25).

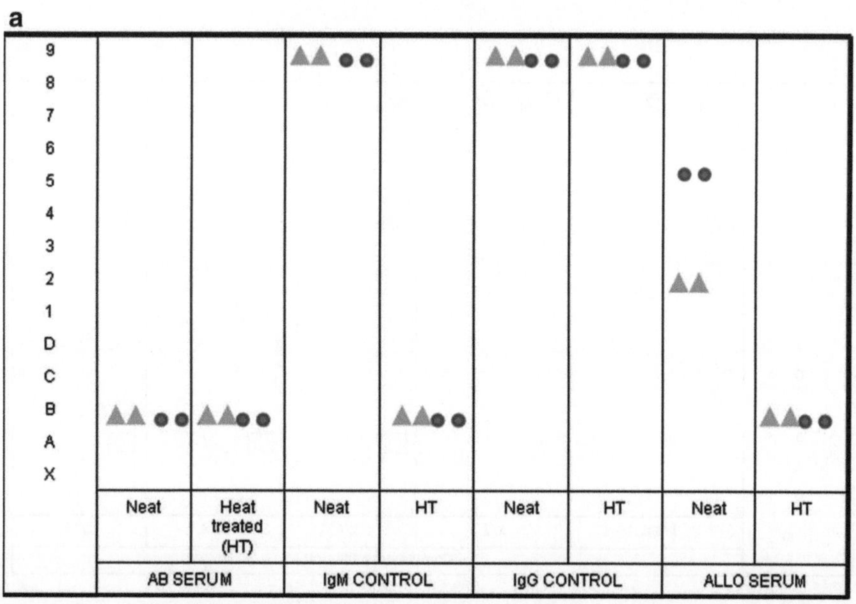


Fig. 4. (**a**) Autologous crossmatch (the *circle* denotes B cell crossmatch results, the *triangle* denotes T cell crossmatch results). Crossmatches are read according to Table 1. The AB serum is read as a background control, i.e. contains no

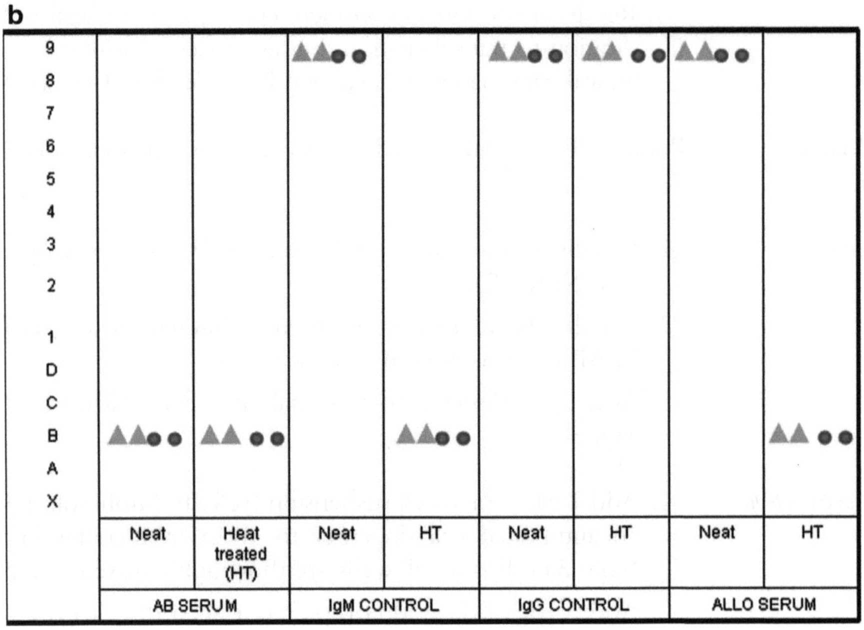


Fig. 4. (continued) HLA antibodies. The autologous crossmatch should be interpreted in relation to the crossmatch results of this control. The IgG control should not reduce with heat treatment (HT). Reduction may be due to over-incubation of serum or incubation at the incorrect temperature (>63°C) leading to denaturation of IgG antibody. The IgM control should reduce with HT. Failure to reduce may be due to under-incubation of serum or incubation at the incorrect temperature (<60°C). In this example, the autologous T and B cell crossmatches are positive, and reduce with HT indicating the presence of IgM autoantibody. (**b**) Allogeneic crossmatch (the *circle* denotes B cell crossmatch results, the *triangle* denotes T cell crossmatch results). Crossmatches are read according to Table 2. The AB serum is read as a background control, i.e. contains no HLA antibodies. The allogeneic crossmatch should be interpreted in relation to the crossmatch results of this control. The IgG control and IgM controls follow the same criteria as in the autologous crossmatch (**a**). In this example, the allogeneic T and B cell crossmatches are positive, and reduce with HT consistent the presence of IgM autoantibody.

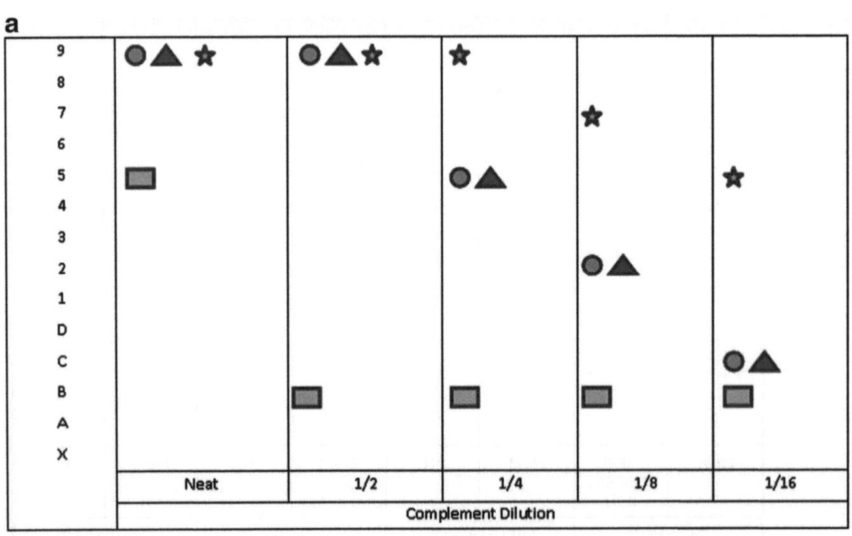


Fig. 5. (**a**) Example of crossmatch results of a homozygous cell against neat antiserum where the *circle* is the current complement, the *triangle* is evaluation complement 1, the *rectangle* is evaluation complement 2 and the *star* is evaluation complement

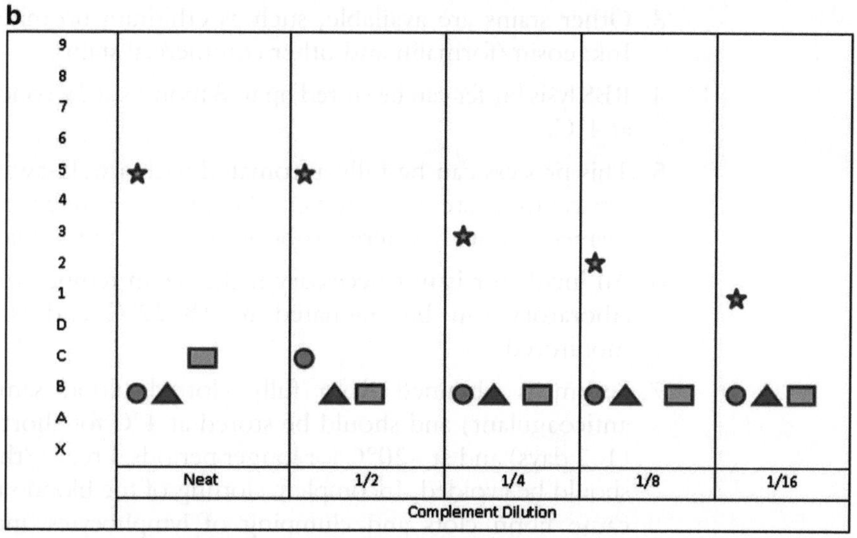


Fig. 5. (continued) 3. Evaluation complement 2 has low reactivity and should be discarded. Complement 1 appears to have reactivity similar to the current complement. Complement 3 has increased reactivity, this may be due to high background or stronger complement activity (see (**b**)). (**b**) Example of crossmatch results of a negative cell against neat antiserum where the *circle* is the current complement, the *triangle* is evaluation complement 1, the rectangle is evaluation complement 2 and the *star* is evaluation complement 3. Complement 5 has high reactivity and should be discarded. Complement 1 appears to have consistent reactivity with the current complement.

2. Crossmatch scores of the current and evaluation complement should be plotted to compare reactivity (see Fig. 5).
3. Evaluation complement can be immediately discarded if it consistently has high reactivity with cells which are negative for the antigen against which the antiserum is reactive, i.e. high background/non-specific reactivity.
4. Evaluation complement can be discarded if it consistently has low reactivity (compared to the current batch) with cells that are homozygous or heterozygous for the antigen against which the antiserum is reactive, i.e. low reactivity.
5. Complement should be re-tested at delivery to ensure shipment has not caused any reduction in reactivity.

## 4. Notes

1. Heparin blood is also suitable for cell extraction by this method; however, EDTA blood is unsuitable. The volume of blood required is determined by the number of crossmatch tests (trays), but as a guideline 2 × 10 mL of blood is sufficient for approximately 10 B cell crossmatch trays and 20 T cell crossmatch trays.
2. Solutions containing fluorescent dyes must be kept in the dark to prevent quenching.

3. Other stains are available, such as ethidium bromide/Indian Ink; eosin/formalin and other commercial stains.
4. RBS lysis buffer can be stored up to 3 months at 1× concentration at 4°C.
5. This process can be fully automated with a walk-away robotic separation system. However, the process can be easily performed manually where a robotic system is not available.
6. An incubator is not necessary if the room temperature of the laboratory can be regulated to 18–22°C and is carefully monitored.
7. Serum is obtained from fully clotted blood samples (no anticoagulant) and should be stored at 4°C for short intervals (1–2 days) and at −20°C for longer periods. Freeze/thaw cycles should be avoided. Incomplete clotting of the blood sample can cause fibrin clots and clumping of lymphocytes and can be rectified by incubation with 1% Kaolin at 37°C for 1 h. The serum is frozen and thawed to remove the clot. Approximately 5 μL of serum is required per crossmatch test (tray), i.e. 20 μL of serum is required for 2 × T cell and 2 × B cell crossmatches.
8. Historical peak sera should be selected according to laboratory protocol but in general should be the serum with the highest antibody reactivity (highest PRA). If the recipient has had a previous transplant, then two historical sera should be chosen: one with the highest PRA, and one immediately following the previous graft failure if available.
9. Alternative suppliers of Rabbit complement include CSix, GTI Diagnostics and BAG.
10. Blood group AB Negative serum from untransfused Male donors is used as a negative control. It is often pooled from three or more donations in order to increase volume and decrease QC frequency. The sera must be screened for the presence of lymphocyte antibodies prior to use by the most sensitive screening method available in the laboratory and at the very minimum by CDC crossmatch.
11. We use ATG serially diluted to determine assay sensitivity (1/25, 1/50, 1/100, 1/200, 1/400, 1/800, 1/1,000, 1/1,200). An alternative IgG control can be obtained commercially or by pooling sera positive for IgG HLA antibodies. However, this control must be carefully and thoroughly tested to ensure that a positive crossmatch will be consistently obtained against all cells tested.
12. A positive control specific for B cells should be sought. We find a 1/10,000 dilution of Rituximab to be a good quality control which shows no T cell reactivity.

13. An IgM control which is strongly reactive neat, but reduces completely with heat-treatment (or DTT treatment) should be sought. This can be obtained commercially, e.g. anti-lymphocyte serum IgM (ALSM) from OneLambda Inc. Alternatively pooled IgM antisera may used. The control must be carefully and thoroughly tested to ensure it reacts with all cells (T and B cells of any HLA type) and reduces completely and consistently with heat-treatment, i.e. it contains no IgG antibody.
14. An IgG control which is strongly reactive neat, but does not reduce with heat-treatment (or DTT treatment) should be sought. This can be obtained commercially e.g. anti-lymphocyte serum IgG (ALSG) from OneLambda Inc. Alternatively pooled IgG antisera may used. The control must be carefully and thoroughly tested to ensure it reacts with all cells (T and B cells of any HLA type) and does not reduce with heat-treatment.
15. Sera fully characterised by CDC crossmatch are used in evaluation and should be monospecific for a particular HLA antigen (class I or II) if possible. The corresponding cells used in the complement evaluation crossmatch should include (1) cells homozygous for the antigen against which the antiserum reacts; (2) cells heterozygous for the antigen against which the antiserum reacts; and (3) cells negative for the antigen against which the antiserum reacts.
16. With experience, cell numbers can be estimated manually under the fluorescent microscope. 100–150 cells per well equate to a cell concentration of $1 \times 10^5$/mL. Alternatively, a Neubauer chamber can be used to count the cells more accurately. The concentration can be adjusted to $1 \times 10^5$/mL by the addition/removal of cell medium.
17. Cells should be kept at room temperature for crossmatch. If a delay of over a few hours should occur cells may be stored at 4°C, however they should be brought back to room temperature before use. Cells extracted by this method are not suitable for freezing.
18. Trays can be pre-prepared up to 6 months in advance and stored at −20°C. Ensure the trays are fully enclosed and preferably vacuum packed in plastic bags prior to freezing to avoid ice crystal formation in the trays and subsequent diluting of controls on thawing. Trays must be thawed to room temperature before use.
19. If more than one donor is to be crossmatched (i.e. $n$ donors), the total number of trays required should be at least $4 \times n$.
20. Trays can be mixed using static by rubbing a latex gloved hand across the bottom of the tray. Alternatively, the trays may be centrifuged for a few seconds to bring the cell/serum mixture to the bottom of the tray well.

21. Incubation times can be increased/decreased according to the complement used (see Subheading 3.4) and the sensitivity required. B cells are more sensitive than T cells and therefore a shorter incubation time with complement is often required. However, use of a weaker complement for B cell crossmatching may compensate the difference in reactivity, and with careful selection the incubation times of T and B cell crossmatches can be synchronised.
22. Live cells are stained with CFDA and appear green under the fluorescent microscope, dead cells take up ethidium bromide and appear red. It is not necessary to count individual cells in each well but rather given an average 2,000 cells are added per well for lower cytotoxicity an approximation of dead cell numbers can be made and an estimate of proportion of total cells determined. For higher cytotoxicity, it is easier to estimate live cell numbers.
23. We find that by reading standard crossmatch trays in a sensitive manner, distinguishing between lower differences in cytotoxicity than the conventional scoring system, we can achieve crossmatch results with the same sensitivity as an AHG-enhanced crossmatch. We have found with experience cytotoxicity can be reliably scored by different readers to an average ±1 cytotoxicity score.
24. Some laboratories read the negative serum as background and visually subtract this from all other readings. We recommend that each of the wells are scored independently and according to the scale in Table 1, and the results interpreted in relation to the negative control as shown in Fig. 2.
25. Many laboratories categorise crossmatches according to crossmatch score in terms of strength of reactivity, i.e. weak positive, moderate positive, strong positive.
26. Crossmatch data should be interpreted in combination with donor-specific antibody data. We use the Luminex Single Antigen Bead Assay to derive our antibody results and therefore Table 3 may need to be tailored for your own requirements depending on local MFI cut-offs for positivity or the antibody detection method used.
27. The AHG crossmatch is usually only performed with T cells.
28. DTT is still widely used for the removal of IgM from sera but has the distinct disadvantage that dilution of the sera is required and weak IgG alloantibodies may become negative by dilution and not reduction. In addition, the assay is poorly standardised between laboratories so exchange of crossmatch trays for local or national exchange of organs is problematic.

29. The precise temperature is critical for this assay. We prefer to use a waterbath as the temperature can be constantly monitored and adjusted as necessary.
30. Place tubes in polystyrene floats so that the serum is fully submerged in the waterbath. These floats can be easily made by cutting the bottom from polystyrene cups and making small holes in which the tubes are held snugly.
31. The precise timing and incubation temperature should be validated in your laboratory to ensure IgM antibody is reduced and IgG reactivity is not affected.
32. Perform the evaluation in parallel with the current batch of complement. It is reasonable to request evaluation samples from several different commercial companies for comparison.
33. Well-characterised class I and class II antisera previously tested by CDC crossmatch should be selected. Monospecific sera, or sera against well-defined epitopes present in several antigens (e.g. Bw4 or Bw6) are ideal for this evaluation.
34. A number of cells should be chosen with the following characteristics: (1) homozygous for the antigen against which the antiserum is reactive; (2) heterozygous for the antigen against which the antiserum is reactive; and (3) negative for the antigen against which the antiserum is reactive.

## References


1. Patel R, Terasaki PI (1969) Significance of the positive crossmatch test in kidney transplantation. N Engl J Med 280:735–739
2. Nickerson P, Pochinco D, Karpinski M et al (2004) Class II donor specific antibodies are pathogenic in primary renal allografts. Am J Transplant 4:257
3. Eng HS, Bennett G, Humphreys I et al (2008) Anti-HLA donor-specific antibodies detected in positive B-cell crossmatches by Luminex predict late graft loss. Am J Transplant 8: 2335–2342
4. Gebel HM, Bray RA, Nickerson P (2003) Pretransplant assessment of donor-reactive. HLA specific antibodies in renal transplantation: contraindication vs risk. Am J Transplant 3: 1488–1500

# Chapter 22

# The Lymphocyte Crossmatch by Flow Cytometry for Kidney Transplantation

Jonathan Downing

## Abstract

The flow cytometric lymphocyte crossmatch is a standard technique for evaluating the compatibility of potential kidney transplant recipients and donors. Recipient serum is incubated with donor lymphocytes and the latter are analysed in a flow cytometer for the presence of bound IgG antibodies. An increase in the level of IgG binding compared to a negative control indicates the presence of donor-specific antibodies which may lead to deleterious graft function. Described here is a method to perform T and B lymphocyte crossmatching in the same tube to detect IgG donor-reactive antibodies.

**Key words:** Flow cytometry, Lymphocyte crossmatch, Kidney transplantation, Human leukocyte antigen, Pronase treatment

## 1. Introduction

The flow cytometric lymphocyte crossmatch (FCXM) was first described by Garovoy et al. (1), and has since become a standard test performed prior to kidney transplantation. The FCXM examines potential donor lymphocytes for recipient antibody binding by passing the cells one at a time through a laser and measuring the amount of a fluorescently labelled secondary anti-Ig antibody. With the use of labelled monoclonal antibodies differentiation can be made between IgG and IgM antibodies and between reactivity towards T and B lymphocytes (2).

A positive complement-dependent cytotoxicity (CDC) crossmatch in the presence of CDC detectable donor-specific HLA antibodies is a contraindication to transplant, and its link to hyperacute rejection is well established (3). However, it was recognised that a proportion of transplant recipients experienced early graft loss despite a negative CDC crossmatch test. The FCXM is able to

Frank T. Christiansen and Brian D. Tait (eds.), *Immunogenetics: Methods and Applications in Clinical Practice*, Methods in Molecular Biology, vol. 882, DOI 10.1007/978-1-61779-842-9_22, © Springer Science+Business Media New York 2012

detect HLA antibodies of low titre or of a non-complement binding nature that may be responsible for this early graft loss. Numerous studies have since described a link between positive T and B lymphocyte FCXM and graft rejection and, or loss in both primary and re-graft recipients and in highly sensitised patients (4–12). Despite these studies, controversy has persisted as to the clinical relevance of a pre-transplant T or B cell positive FCXM test.

During the interpretation of the crossmatch result, it is essential to determine the nature of the antibody causing the reactivity. The most clinically relevant antibodies are donor reactive, HLA-specific, IgG antibodies (10, 12). Irrelevant positive reactions can be caused by antibodies reacting with self epitopes shared by the donor cells; Fc receptors that bind antibodies in a non-specific manner; or antibodies against non-HLA antigens. Thus, extensive characterization of patient HLA antibody must always occur alongside the crossmatch test.

The era of fluorescent bead solid phase HLA antibody detection has led to a rethink of FCXM relevance. It is now reasonable to consider the strength of positivity of FCXM in relation to quantitative, precise detection of donor-specific antibody (DSA) and assess a degree of risk of rejection for each individual patient and donor pair (12–14). Thus, a positive FCXM result even in the presence of DSA may not be considered as a contraindication to transplant. Rather it allows the clinician to stratify risk for each patient.

## 2. Materials

1. 2 × 10 mL anti-coagulated peripheral blood sample on donor and patient (see Note 1).
2. 1 × 10 mL clotted peripheral blood sample on patient.
3. Phosphate buffered saline (Invitrogen, Carlsbad, CA, USA) (see Note 2).
4. Ficoll-Paque™ Plus (GE Healthcare Biosciences, Uppsala, Sweden).
5. 50-mL plastic centrifuge tubes (Thermo-Fisher, Waltham, MA, USA).
6. 15-mL plastic centrifuge tubes (Greiner-Bio-one, Monroe, NC, USA).
7. RPMI 1640 (Invitrogen) with 20% v/v foetal bovine serum (Invitrogen).
8. Pronase/Protease XIV (Sigma, St. Louis, MO, USA).
9. 3-mL flow cytometry tubes (Becton Dickinson Labware, Franklin Lakes, NJ, USA).

10. Negative control serum—male blood group AB blood donor serum tested for the absence of HLA antibodies (see Note 3).
11. Positive control serum—human serum known to contain broad specificity IgG HLA antibodies (see Note 4).
12. PBS-Azide: 1 L PBS containing 10% sodium azide (Scharlau Chemicals, Sentmenant, Spain).
13. Anti-human IgG conjugated to fluorescein isothiocyanate (FITC) (Jackson Immunoresearch, West Grove, PA, USA) (see Note 5).
14. Anti-CD3 conjugated to peridinin chlorophyll protein (PERCP) (Becton Dickinson, San Jose, CA, USA).
15. Anti-CD19 conjugated to phycoerythrin (PE) (Becton Dickinson).
16. Three colour flow cytometer (Becton Dickinson FACSCalibur).

## 3. Methods

### *3.1. Isolation of Peripheral Blood Mononuclear Cells*

Peripheral blood lymphocytes (PBL) are the main target of the crossmatch test. Anti-coagulated blood samples should be stored at room temperature and should be no older than 48 h before isolating the lymphocytes, where possible.

1. Transfer 10 mL of anti-coagulated peripheral blood into two labelled 50-mL centrifuge tubes.
2. Dilute with PBS to a total volume of 30 mL.
3. Underlay diluted blood with Ficoll-Paque™ Plus taking care not mix the blood-Ficoll interface.
4. Centrifuge for 10 min at 1,600 × *g*.
5. Carefully aspirate the mononuclear cell layer at the Ficoll—plasma interface from each 50-mL centrifuge tube into clean labelled 15-mL centrifuge tubes and top up to 15 mL with PBS.
6. Centrifuge for 3 min at 650 × *g*.
7. Decant the supernatant and re-suspend the cell button in 15 mL of PBS.
8. Centrifuge for 3 min at 650 × *g*.
9. Decant the supernatant.
10. Pool and re-suspend the cell buttons from the two 15-mL centrifuge tubes into 1 mL of RPMI cell medium (see Note 6).
11. Adjust the mononuclear cell count to $8 \times 10^6$ cells/mL (see Note 7).

### 3.2. Cleavage of Fc Receptors Using Pronase

T and B lymphocyte cell surface Fc receptors can bind IgG molecules non-specifically and lead to a high anti-IgG FITC measurement on the cell. This can lead to difficulty in discriminating between negative and positive crossmatch results. Cleavage of Fc receptors using Pronase at can lead to a reduction in the incidence of false negative crossmatch due to the presence of excess irrelevant IgG bound to Fc receptors (15) (see Note 8).

1. Add 0.5 mL of 1 mg/mL Pronase to 1 mL of donor or recipient cells.
2. Incubate for 30 min at 37°C.
3. After incubation top up to 15 mL with RPMI.
4. Centrifuge for 3 min at 650 × *g*.
5. Decant the supernatant and re-suspend the cell button in 0.5 mL RPMI.
6. Re-adjust the mononuclear cell count to $8 \times 10^6$ cells/mL.

### 3.3. Crossmatch Procedure

PBLs should be prepared from the donor sample for the allo-crossmatch and from the patient sample where an auto-crossmatch test is required (see Note 9).

1. Label 7× 3-mL flow cytometry tubes in the following sequence: 3 negative control serum vs. donor cells; 3 patient serum vs. donor cells; 1 positive control serum vs. donor cells. Additionally, if required, label a series of flow tubes for an auto control crossmatch to include a negative control serum vs. patient cells and at least two replicates of patient serum vs. patient cells (see Note 10).
2. In each tube, add 50 μL of appropriate serum to 50 μL of appropriate cells, mix by gentle vortexing and incubate at room temperature for 30 min.
3. After incubation, wash each tube by adding approximately 2 mL of cold PBS-azide (see Note 11) and centrifuging for 2 min at 1,800 × *g*. Decant the supernatant and gently re-suspend the cell button. Alternatively an automated cell washer can be employed.
4. Repeat the wash process twice. After the third wash remove as much supernatant as possible and gently re-suspend the cell button (see Note 12).
5. Add 50 μL of diluted anti-human-IgG FITC to each tube, mix by gentle vortexing, and incubate for 15 min in the dark at 5°C (see Note 13).
6. Wash once as described in step 3 above.
7. To each tube add 2 μL each of anti-CD3 and anti-CD19 reagents (see Note 14). Mix by gentle vortexing and incubate for 15 min in the dark at 5°C.

8. Wash once as described in step 3 above. Re-suspend the cells in 200 μL of PBS-azide. The tubes are ready for flow analysis (see Note 15).

### 3.4. Flow Cytometric Analysis

The flow cytometer instrument must be set up correctly before use. The manufacturer's daily start-up and shut-down procedures must be followed and a daily calibration using commercial standard reagents performed. In addition, optimisation (see Note 16) and colour compensation must be performed (see Note 17).

1. Collect data on 1,200 B lymphocyte events as follows, see Fig. 1 (see Note 18).
2. Use the cytometer acquisition and analysis software to create a 1,024 channel 4-decade log plot of forward scatter (FSC) vs. side scatter (SSC) (Fig. 1a).
3. Draw a polygon gate around the lymphocyte population and use this gate to create a dot plot to show FL2 (PE) vs. FL3 (PerCP) to discriminate the B and T lymphocytes, respectively (Fig. 1b) (see Note 19).
4. Draw a rectangular gate around each of the lymphocyte populations, and use these to plot an FL1 (FITC) vs. cell count histogram for each population (Fig. 1c, d). Draw a histogram

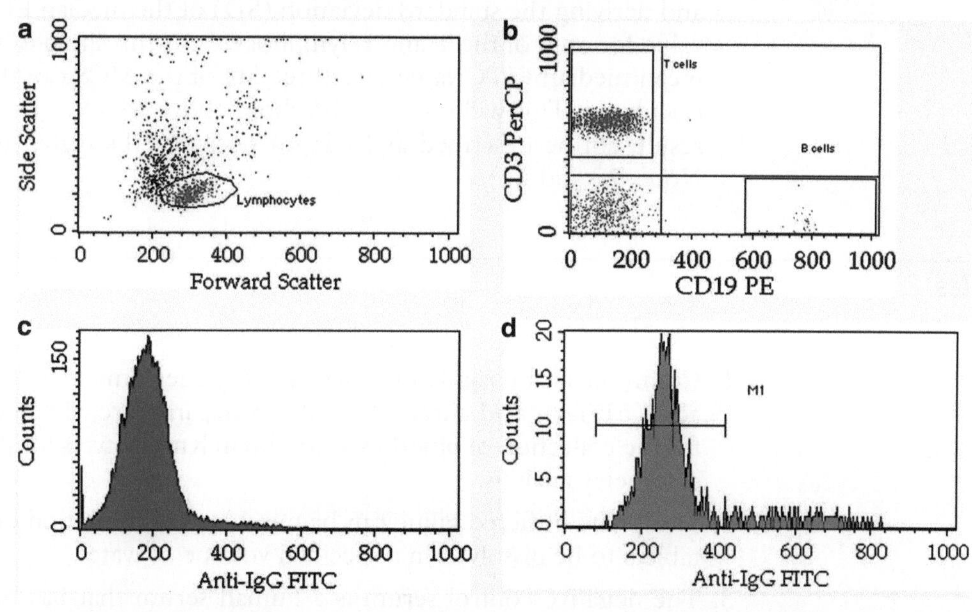


Fig. 1. Flow cytometer analysis histograms. Flow analysis histograms created using Becton Dickinson Cell Quest Pro analysis software. Lymphocytes are displayed by plotting forward scatter (FSC) against side scatter light on a 1,024 channel log-scale plot (**a**). A gate is drawn around the lymphocytes and gated data used to populate a CD19-PE against CD3-PERCP plot to distinguish the B and T population, respectively (**b**). Rectangular gates are drawn around each lymphocyte population and gated data used to plot anti-IgG FITC on a log scale against count on a linear scale for T lymphocytes (**c**) and B lymphocytes (**d**).

marker around the main peak of the B lymphocyte FITC histogram (see Note 20).

5. Obtain the median FITC channel value from each histogram, in the case of the B lymphocytes this will be the M1 median value (see Note 21).

### 3.5. Interpretation

To determine whether a crossmatch result is negative or positive, the median FITC channel in the patient serum—donor lymphocyte reactions is compared to that of the negative control serum—donorlymphocyte reactions. The following method is recommended as it uses median FITC values simply obtained from the analysis software of the cytometer and applies a statistical method to determine whether the result is in the normal range expected if no donor-reactive antibody is present. It must be made clear, however, that there are a number of alternative methods (see Note 22).

1. For each lymphocyte population, subtract the mean of the median FITC channel values of the negative serum vs. donor lymphocyte replicates from the mean of the median FITC channel values of the patient serum vs. donor lymphocyte replicates to give the median channel shift (MCS).
2. An absolute MCS value can be established as a positive threshold by testing the negative control serum used in the assay against a panel of lymphocytes from 30 healthy individuals and deriving the standard deviation (SD) of the median FITC value for each of the T and B lymphocytes. A threshold of the mean median FITC value plus three SD of the MCS can then calculated. This will give the threshold above which a patient result can be described as having a positive crossmatch (see Notes 23 and 24).

## 4. Notes

1. Common anti-coagulants, such as ethylenediaminetetracetic acid (EDTA), acid citrate dextrose or heparin, are all suitable for the collection of blood used to obtain lymphocytes for flow cytometry analysis.
2. Phosphate buffered saline can be purchased as a solution or as tablets to be dissolved in a specified volume of water.
3. The negative control serum is a human serum that has been shown to contain no reactivity to T or B lymphocytes. This serum can be sourced locally from male blood group AB blood donors or can be obtained commercially from suppliers, such as Invitrogen or One Lambda (Canoga Park, CA, USA). The negative control serum should be evaluated for lack of reactivity

before used routinely. This should consist of testing to confirm lack of HLA antibodies using a solid phase method, and by testing by flow cytometry using the above FCXM method with lymphocytes from a number of individuals to show lack of reactivity.

4. The positive control serum is required to establish that correct binding of the anti-IgG FITC secondary antibody has occurred during the assay. A pool of locally available highly sensitised transplant patients is a common source for this positive control. Pools of up to ten individuals known to possess strong IgG HLA antibodies can be made and aliquots stored at –30°C for continued used. Each pool should be evaluated for reactivity before use, by testing by flow cytometry using the above FCXM assay. Alternatively, a commercial source of a monoclonal antibody, such as w6/32 (Abcam, Cambridge, MA, USA) could be used.
5. The fluorophore-labelled antibodies, anti-human-IgG-FITC, anti-CD19-PE, and anti-CD3-PERCP fluoresce at particular light wavelengths so that they can be detected by the flow cytometer fluorescence (FL) detectors, FL1, FL2, and FL3, respectively. These detectors collect signals at 530, 585, and >670 nm, respectively, in a BD FACSCalibur instrument. The fluorophores emit at 519, 578, and 675 nm for FITC, PE and PERCP, respectively. Thus, if a particular labelled antibody is not available, any replacement needs to emit in the correct range for it to be collected by a specific FL detector. The anti-CD19 and anti-CD3 antibodies are required to discriminate between B and T lymphocytes and this can give valuable information as to the nature of the specificity and strength of patient antibody binding. It is possible to perform the crossmatch without these, but no B and T lymphocyte discrimination will be possible.
6. If the cell buttons are quite large, increase the re-suspension volume. This will ease the process for adjusting the cell count to the optimum.
7. It is important to adjust the cells to the correct optimum concentration. Too few cells will make interpretation of the results difficult. With too many cells, there is a risk of diluting any allo-antibody to levels below detection. In addition, an exceedingly high cell event rate can lead to inaccurate data capture.
8. The pronase cleavage of FC receptors could be considered as an optional step and is not performed by all laboratories. Pronase can potentially reduce the incidence of false negative results by reducing background fluorescence caused by irrelevant binding of IgG to Fc receptors (15). The requirement for pronase treatment is difficult to predict as the incidence of

background can vary depending on patient serum and donor lymphocytes and it is recommended that this step be carried out with all crossmatch tests. In addition, for patients undergoing treatment with Rituximab, the anti-CD20 monoclonal antibody, binding of Rituximab will lead to high levels of binding of FITC. Using pronase will cleave the anti-CD20 and hence remove Rituximab binding.

9. An auto crossmatch result will aid interpretation where the allo crossmatch result is positive for either T or B lymphocyte, but no donor-specific HLA antibody can be detected in the patient. If the auto crossmatch is also positive and of a similar magnitude, this can indicate non-HLA auto-reactive antibodies that are also able to bind to donor lymphocytes. It must be stressed though, that this interpretation can only be made in the presence of precise determination of patient HLA antibody using sensitive solid phase methodology.
10. Each laboratory will have its own requirements for the number of replicate reactions performed during the crossmatch. Flexibility may be required in the event of low serum or cell preparation volumes.
11. Sodium azide is typically included in the wash buffer to prevent the modulation and internalisation of surface antigens which can produce a loss of fluorescence intensity.
12. Careful removal of most of the wash supernatant is important at this stage to ensure that the volume of FITC that the cells are incubated in the following stage is optimum and consistent.
13. The optimum dilution of anti-IgG FITC should be determined in each laboratory by testing a range of dilutions against known positive and negative serum/cell combinations. An optimum dilution will give the best differentiation between the negative and positive reactions.
14. The anti-CD3 and anti-CD19 can be combined in equal volumes before addition to the cells. This reduces the number of low volume reagent dispensing steps required. Thus, 4 μL of the combined reagent can be added to each crossmatch tube.
15. At this stage, the cells should be kept in the dark until ready for analysis. This should be performed within an hour of the end of the assay. Alternatively, a cell fixing reagent such as paraformaldehyde can be used to preserve the cells for a number of days.
16. The flow cytometer must be set up before analysis of the crossmatch assay in order to optimally record the amount of patient IgG antibody binding to cells. Using lymphocytes prepared in the same manner as the crossmatch assay, adjust the FSC amp gain and SSC voltage to display the lymphocytes appropriately on the scale of a log-scale FSC vs. SSC plot. When prepared in

the manner described above, lymphocytes should represent the densest population recorded and thus be easily identifiable. Adjust the FSC threshold in order to exclude the collection of data on unwanted small particles and debris.

17. At some stage prior to analysis, colour compensation should be performed in order to optimise the instrument settings for use with the lymphocyte crossmatch assay. Compensation is required where the emission spectra of fluorophores used in an assay overlap, as is the case for example with FITC and PE and with PE and PERCP. Compensation ensures that fluorescence emitted by FITC is not detected by the FL2 photomultiplier as a PE signal. Compensation is performed by individually preparing lymphocytes with the fluorophores to be used in the assay and then using the flow cytometer acquisition software compensation controls to ensure there is minimal overlap between the FL detectors. It is recommended that compensation be performed using lymphocytes in addition to any manufacturer's calibration reagents. This is because lymphocytes have different optical properties to these reagents. Once compensation is performed, the saved instrument settings should be used when subsequently analysing lymphocytes from the crossmatch test. Compensation does not need to be performed before each analysis, but should be carried approximately 6 monthly to monitor wear of the cytometer optics or in the event that changes are made to the optics.

18. As B lymphocytes are usually less numerous than T lymphocytes, setting a minimum number of B lymphocyte events is important to ensure enough data is collected to be able to make an accurate interpretation. Generally, enough T cell events will be collected under these conditions. In the case of samples with low B lymphocyte counts, where 1,200 events cannot be obtained, a time limit should be placed on each acquisition such that all 200 μL of the sample is acquired at a high flow rate. It is useful to have a minimum T and B lymphocyte count, for example, 2,000 T and 350 B, so that accurate interpretation can be made. If the counts obtained fall below this the crossmatch should be repeated. With very low cell counts, natural variation in FITC level can introduce inaccuracy that may lead to false interpretation of the test result.

19. The T and B lymphocyte population should show as clearly defined clusters of events segregated to high on the PERCP axis for T lymphocytes and high on the PE axis for B lymphocytes. Quadrant markers are placed on the plot to indicate the areas of negative and positive cell populations (see Fig. 1b). If either of these populations or the negative population (which should appear low on both axis) appear outside of the expected areas, this may indicate poor compensation set up of the cytometer

or contamination from other sources of fluorescence that emit at the same wavelength, e.g. ethidium bromide. Failure to recognise this problem could lead to a false positive result. Note also that the count scale for B lymphocytes is lower than that of T lymphocytes in Fig. 1c, d, so that the peak is appropriately sized.

20. B lymphocyte preparations may display low numbers of events with high levels of bound FITC that manifest as very small peaks towards the right of the *x* axis of an FITC vs. cell count histogram derived from the B lymphocyte gate. This is due to non-specific IgG binding that can be disregarded from the analysis by placing a histogram marker (M1 in Fig. 1d) symmetrically around the main peak and deriving the median FITC value from this marker. FITC values outside of the marker will not be included in the median value, and this has the effect of lowering the overall median value but potentially lowering the signal-to-noise ratio.

21. The FITC histograms should show roughly symmetrical peaks with a clearly defined population based around a single maximum FITC level. Poorly defined peaks will lead to less accurate definition of the median FITC level and may be caused by low cell counts, inadequate mixing of cells, serum or fluorescent labels during the assay, or by the labelling of abnormal donor or patient lymphocyte subpopulations.

22. Each laboratory must establish its own criteria for a threshold for a positive crossmatch and there are a variety of methods available to do this. The method described above utilises an absolute cut-off of MCS calculated by testing the negative control serum against a panel of healthy cells to determine the normal range of background FITC binding. An alternative is to calculate the SD of the FITC channel values of the negative control replicates derived from the crossmatch. If the patient FITC channel value exceeds the negative value plus three SD this can be described as a positive crossmatch. Another way of comparing the patient and negative channel values is to calculate the relative fluorescence by dividing the mean of patient median FITC channel value by that of the negative control, and a cut-off value of 1.5 or 2 used to indicate a positive result. A further method for comparing the patient and negative values is to employ calibration beads to convert the arbitrary FITC channel values into molecules of equivalent soluble fluorochrome (MESF). In this process, fluorescence from commercially available combinations of precisely quantitated solutions and microbead suspensions is measured in the cytometer. The results are used to create a standard curve which can be used to convert any cytometer reading into an MESF value.

Thus, median FITC values can be converted into MESF values and the shift of patient MESF from negative MESF applied to a threshold level in a similar way as MCS described above. MESF methods are particularly useful when comparing data from crossmatch tests performed at different times or in different centres.

23. The use of a fixed threshold, however it is determined, is problematic when trying to interpret a result that is close to this threshold. Whether or not a particular result relates to the presence of donor-specific HLA antibody is not always well reflected by a fixed threshold. It might be useful to have a second threshold to indicate weak positive reactions, for example, the MCS of the negative plus two SD. A threshold of the negative median plus two SD relates to the fact that 95% of "normal" negative reactions, i.e. those reactions that do not show increased specific FITC binding will fall within this threshold. Only 5% of reactions that exceed the threshold will be due to "normal" negative reactions, all others being defined as true positive due to increased FITC binding. Using three SD assumes that only 0.3% of negative reactions will exceed this level and that 99.7% of reactions above this level are of a true positive nature and hence is a more stringent definition of a positive result.

24. By testing the negative control serum against a range of different lymphocyte samples it is possible to establish ranges of reactivity that can be used as acceptance criteria for the assay. For example, it is desirable to have a minimum and maximum acceptable median FITC value for the negative serum against any particular donor lymphocyte. If the negative serum median FITC is too high, this can lead to a false negative interpretation as a large amount of "background" is subtracted from the patient FITC value during calculation of the MCS. When the negative serum is tested against 30 healthy individuals, the lowest and highest FITC value obtained for each lymphocyte population can be used as the lower and upper range. If, during a crossmatch test, these ranges are exceeded, then the crossmatch may be repeated or the interpretation questioned.

## References

1. Garovoy MR et al (1983) Flow cytometry analysis: a high technology crossmatch technique facilitating transplantation. Transplant Proc 15:1939–1944
2. Bray RA, Lebeck LK, Gebel HM (1989) The flow cytometric crossmatch: dual-colour analysis of T and B cell reactivities. Transplantation 48:834–840
3. Patel R, Terasaki PI (1969) Significance of the positive crossmatch test in kidney transplantation. N Engl J Med 280:735–739
4. Chapman JR et al (1985) Analysis of flow cytometry and cytotoxic crossmatches in renal transplantation. Transplant Proc 17:2480–2481
5. Ogura K et al (1993) The significance of a positive flow cytometry crossmatch test in primary

kidney transplantation. Transplantation 56: 294–298

6. Sridhar NR et al (1992) Evaluation of flowcytometric crossmatching in renal allograft recipients. Nephron 62:262–266
7. Lazda VA (1994) Identification of patients at risk for inferior renal allograft outcome by a strongly positive B cell flow cytometry crossmatch. Transplantation 57:964–969
8. Talbot D et al (1995) Flow cytometric crossmatching in renal transplantation—the long term outcome. Transpl Immunol 3:352–355
9. Graff RJ et al (2009) The role of positive flow cytometry crossmatch in late renal allograft loss. Hum Immunol 70:502–505
10. Lefaucher C et al (2008) Clinical relevance of preformed HLA donor-specific antibodies in kidney transplantation. Am J Transplant 8:324–331
11. Delgado JC, Eckels DD (2008) Positive B-cell only flow cytometric crossmatch: implications for renal transplantation. Exp Mol Pathol 85: 59–63
12. Gebel HM, Bray RA, Nickerson P (2003) Pretransplant assessment of donor-reactive. HLA-specific antibodies in renal transplantation: contraindication vs. risk. Am J Transplant 3:1488–1500
13. Taylor CJ et al (2009) Back to the future: application of contemporary technology to longstanding questions about the clinical relevance of human leukocyte antigen-specific alloantibodies in renal transplantation. Hum Immunol 70:563–568
14. Riethmuller S et al (2010) Donor-specific antibody levels and three generations of crossmatches to predict antibody mediated rejection in kidney transplantation. Transplantation 90:160–167
15. Vaida S et al (2001) Improved flow cytometric detection of HLA alloantibodies using pronase. Transplantation 71:422–428

# Chapter 23

# Overview of the Killer Cell Immunoglobulin-Like Receptor System

**Raja Rajalingam**

## Abstract

Natural killer (NK) cells are more than simple killers and have been implicated in control and clearance of malignant and virally infected cells, regulation of adaptive immune responses, rejection of bone marrow transplants, and autoimmunity and the maintenance of pregnancy. Human NK cells largely use a family of germ-line encoded killer cell immunoglobulin-like receptors (KIR) to respond to the perturbations from self-HLA class I molecules present on infected, malignant, or HLA-disparate fetal or allogenic transplants. Genes encoding KIR receptors and HLA class I ligands are located on different chromosomes, and both feature extraordinary diversity in the number and type of genes. The independent segregation of KIR and HLA gene families produce diversity in the number and type of KIR-HLA gene combinations inherited in individuals, which may determine their immunity and susceptibility to diseases. This chapter provides an overview of NK cells and their unprecedented phenotypic and functional diversity within and between individuals.

**Key words:** NK cells, Innate immunity, HLA, KIR, Polymorphism, Immune genes

## 1. Natural Killer Cells

Natural killer (NK) cells are the third population of lymphocytes defined by $CD3^-$, $CD56^+$ cell surface phenotype, and they represent 5–25% of the mononuclear cell fraction of normal human peripheral blood (1, 2). NK cells share several features with $CD8^+$ cytolytic T lymphocytes (CTL) in their development, morphology, cell-surface phenotypes, killing mechanism, and cytokine production (3). Compared to T and B lymphocytes, NK cells are larger and contain preformed cytolytic granules (granzymes and perforin) as well as an exponential amount of constitutively expressed transcripts for interferon-γ (IFN-γ) and certain cytokines that activate other immune cell types. The fundamental function of NK cells is

Frank T. Christiansen and Brian D. Tait (eds.), *Immunogenetics: Methods and Applications in Clinical Practice*, Methods in Molecular Biology, vol. 882, DOI 10.1007/978-1-61779-842-9_23, © Springer Science+Business Media New York 2012

to provide the first line of defense by inherently responding to infection and tumor transformation without any prior sensitization, and therefore NK cells are considered to be the integral component of innate immunity (4, 5). Recent reports suggest that similar to B and T cells, NK cells exhibit many features normally associated with adaptive immunity. These include the expansion of pathogen-specific cells, the generation of long-lasting "memory" cells that persist after cognate antigen encounter, and the ability to mount an enhanced secondary recall response to rechallenge (6).

On the basis of adhesion molecule CD56 expression level, two subsets of NK cells have been distinguished in human peripheral blood (7). Over 90% belong to the $CD56^{dim}$ subset that expresses high levels of CD16 and KIR receptors, and represent the most differentiated and mature NK cell type, and have superior cytotoxicity capacity (1, 8). The remaining 10% are the $CD56^{bright}$ phenotype ($CD16^{-}$, $KIR^{+/-}$) representing the precursors of $CD56^{dim}$ subset, and have greater ability to produce proinflammatory cytokines (9). In contrast to blood, the $CD56^{bright}$ cells are the dominant NK cell subset in human lymph nodes and they interact with dendritic cells (10, 11). During pregnancy, the placenta houses unique subsets of NK cells that contribute to successful implant and function of the placenta by secreting angiogenetic factors, such as vascular endothelial growth factor (VEGF) (12). Gut-associated lymphoid tissues harbor a unique NK cell subset that specializes in production of interleukin (IL)-22, a proinflammatory cytokine that mediates host defense against extracellular pathogens (13). NK cells are therefore an unexpectedly heterogeneous population involving both innate and adoptive immune responses and successful pregnancies, which altogether promote human health and survival.

## 2. Natural Killer Cell Receptors

NK cells have a highly specific and complex target cell recognition receptor system arbitrated by the integration of signals triggered by a multitude of inhibitory and activating receptors, which trigger cytotoxicity and the secretion of chemokines and cytokines (14, 15). Unlike T and B lymphocytes, NK cells do not express receptors that require somatic gene rearrangements to generate receptor diversity and specificity. Instead, NK cells express a wide array of conventional germline-encoded receptor families with inhibitory or activating functions, including (i) killer cell immunoglobulin-like receptors (KIR), (ii) killer cell lectin-like receptors (KLR) such as CD94/NKG2, (iii) leukocyte immunoglobulin-like receptors (LILR), and (iv) natural cytotoxicity receptors (NCR), such as NKp46, NKp44, and NKp30, and 2B4 (2, 16–18). Most of these receptors are expressed in stochastic, variegated combinations of activating and inhibitory receptors, resulting in many subsets of functionally distinct

NK cells (19, 20). In addition to the receptor–ligand-mediated regulation, the lytic potential of NK cells and their ability to produce IFN-γ is enhanced by type I IFNs (IFN-α and IFN-β), IL-2, IL-18, and IL-15 that are secreted by dendritic cells, macrophages as well as pathogen-infected tissue (21).

Because NK cells circulate in a state that can spontaneously deliver effector function, it is critical that they do not attack surrounding healthy cells. To prevent such detrimental autoreactivity, NK cells express an array of inhibitory receptors recognizing self-HLA class I molecules (Fig. 1). Abundant expression of four

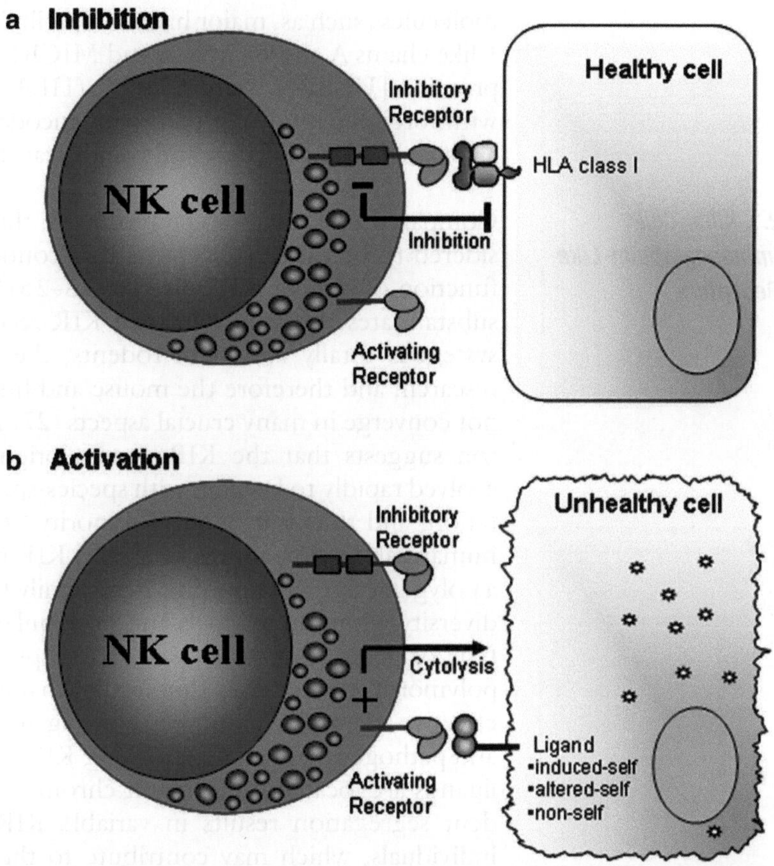


Fig. 1. Natural killer (NK) cell response against healthy and unhealthy cells. NK cells express both inhibitory and activating receptors. Inhibitory receptors recognize self HLA class I molecules and trigger signals that stop the natural lytic function of NK cells. By expressing normal levels of multiple HLA class I molecules, the healthy cells are resistant to NK cell attack (**a**). Downregulation of HLA class I expression due to tumor transformation or viral infection relieves the inhibitory influence on NK cells (**b**), permitting NK cells to lyse these unhealthy target cells, a phenomenon first described as the "missing-self" hypothesis. Upon transformation or infection, the unhealthy cells express ligands for activating receptors, which could be either "induced-self" (MICA, MICB, ULBP), "altered-self" (HLA-class I loaded with foreign peptide), and/or "non-self" (pathogen-encoded molecules). Upon recognizing these ligands, the activating receptors trigger signals that augment NK cell lysis of unhealthy targets.

distinct HLA class I molecules (HLA-A, -B, -C, and -E) on normal healthy cells provide ligands for a variety of inhibitory receptors of NK cells, and consequently are resistant to NK cell attack. Downregulation of HLA class I expression due to certain viral infections, neoplastic transformations or other forms of stress, relieves the inhibitory influence on NK cells, permitting NK cells to eliminate these unhealthy target cells, a phenomenon originally described as the "missing-self" hypothesis (22). In addition to the "missing-self" mechanism, the expression of ligands for activating receptors on target cell surface might also contribute to NK cell attack (Fig. 1). The ligands identified for activating receptors are either "induced-self" that are structurally related to HLA class I molecules (such as, major histocompatibility complex [MHC] class I-like chains A and B [MICA and MICB] and unique long binding proteins [ULBP]), "altered-self" (HLA class I molecule loaded with foreign peptide) or pathogen encoded "non-self" (molecules associated with infection and tumor transformation).

### 2.1. Killer Cell Immunoglobulin-Like Receptors

Compared to other NK cell receptors, the KIR receptors are considered to be the key receptors that control the development and function of human NK cells (16, 23–26). The following rationale substantiates the importance of KIR receptors: (i) KIR receptor system is totally absent in rodents, the basic model for clinical research, and therefore the mouse and human NK cell biology do not converge in many crucial aspects (27, 28); (ii) species comparison suggests that the KIR system originated in mammals, and evolved rapidly to keep up with species-specific evolution and adaptation, and thus only a small minority of KIR genes is shared by humans and chimpanzees (29); (iii) KIR receptors are encoded by a polygenic and polymorphic gene family that produces remarkable diversity within individuals and in populations in the number and type of genes (30, 31); (iv) KIR receptors recognize an array of polymorphic HLA class I molecules that evolved rapidly to mount effective adaptive immune response against rapidly evolving viruses and pathogens; (v) genes encoding KIR receptors and HLA class I ligands are located on different chromosomes, and their independent segregation results in variable KIR-HLA combinations in individuals, which may contribute to the individual's health and disease. Consistent with this theory, combinations of certain KIR-HLA genes have been associated with diseases as diverse as autoimmunity, infection, cancer, and reproductive failure (32, 33).

Fourteen KIR receptors triggering either inhibition (3DL1-3, 2DL1-3, 2DL5) or activation (3DS1, 2DS1-5), or both (2DL4) have been identified in humans (Fig. 2) (34–36). KIR receptors possess two or three extracellular Ig-like domains involved in ligand binding and either a long or short cytoplasmic tail involved in signaling. KIRs are named on the basis of their number of Ig domains and type of cytoplasmic tail (37). The first digit following the

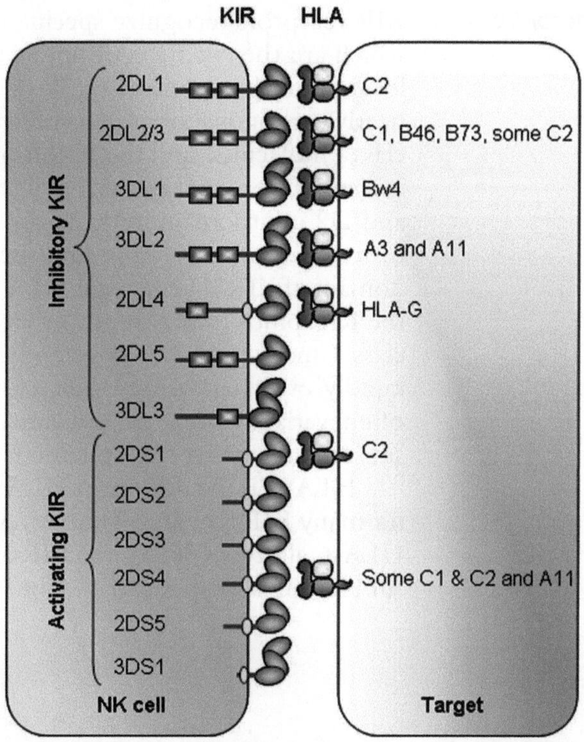


Fig. 2. Killer cell immunoglobulin-like receptors (KIR). Fourteen distinct KIR receptors have been characterized in humans that comprise either two (2D) or three (3D) extracellular Ig-like domains and either a long (L) or short (S) cytoplasmic tail. Six KIR receptors are activating types and the remaining KIR are inhibitory types. The ITIM motifs in the cytoplasmic tails of inhibitory KIRs are shown as *boxes*, and positively charged residues in the transmembrane regions of activating KIRs are shown as *circles*. The inhibitory KIR receptors bind to distinct HLA class I allotypes and the ligands for most activating KIR receptors are unknown.

KIR acronym corresponds to the number of Ig-like domains in the molecule and the "D" denotes "domain." The "D" is followed by either an "L" indicating a "Long" cytoplasmic tail, an "S" indicating a "Short" cytoplasmic tail or a "P" for pseudogenes (2DP1 and 3DP1). The final digit indicates the number of the gene encoding a protein with this structure. Thus, KIR2DL1, KIR2DL2, and KIR2DL3 all encode receptors having two extracellular Ig-like domains and long cytoplasmic tails, while KIR3DS1 encodes a receptor having three extracellular Ig-like domains and a short cytoplasmic tail. The long tails contain immune-receptor tyrosine-based inhibitory motifs (ITIMs) that trigger inhibitory signals. The short cytoplasmic tails lack ITIM but possess a positively charged residue in the transmembrane domain that interacts with the signaling adaptor DAP12 (38). DAP12 contains immune-receptor tyrosine-based activation motifs (ITAM), which trigger activating signals upon the short-tailed KIR receptor recognizing a ligand.

### 2.2. Ligands for KIR Receptors

KIR receptors recognize specific motifs of HLA class I molecules, which are the products of highly polymorphic genes of the MHC located on chromosome 6 (39–41) (Figs. 2 and 3). KIR binds in a nearly orthogonal orientation across the α1 and α2 helices of HLA class I molecules, and the KIR footprint on HLA overlaps with but is distinct from that of the T cell receptor (42). The six loops of D1 and D2 interdomain hinge region of KIR2DL as well as KIR3DL form the HLA class I binding site, while the membrane-distal D0 domain of KIR3D enhances HLA class I ligand binding (43). Since the KIR binds to the polymorphic peptide binding groove of HLA class I molecules, it is constantly subjected to changes driven by rapidly evolving viruses. Therefore, the KIR binding motifs are often variable between individuals and their distribution differs substantially between populations (39, 44, 45).

HLA-C is the dominant HLA class I locus that provides ligands for many KIR receptors (Fig. 2). Amino acid residues 76 and 80 on HLA-C allotypes determine KIR binding epitopes (46–48) (Fig. 3). All HLA-C allotypes carry valine (V) at position 76, while position

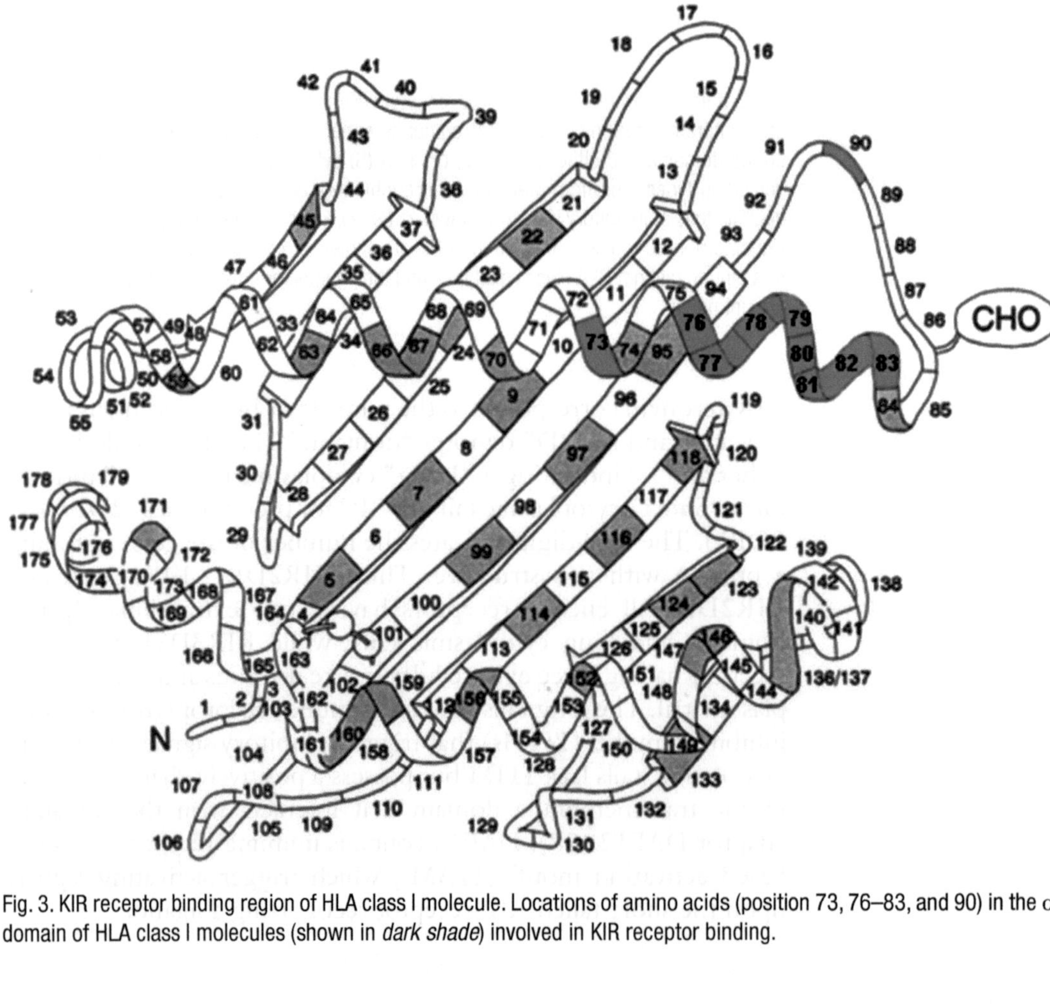


Fig. 3. KIR receptor binding region of HLA class I molecule. Locations of amino acids (position 73, 76–83, and 90) in the α1 domain of HLA class I molecules (shown in *dark shade*) involved in KIR receptor binding.

80 displays a dimorphism of either asparagine (N) or lysine (K). Nearly half of the HLA-C allotypes (Cw2, Cw4, Cw5, Cw6, and Cw15) carry a K80 (conventionally termed C2 epitope) that binds inhibitory receptor KIR2DL1 (49–51). The remaining HLA-C allotypes (Cw1, Cw3, Cw7, and Cw8) carry N80 (termed C1 epitope) and bind inhibitory receptors KIR2DL2 and 2DL3. Two exceptionally diverse HLA-B allotypes, B46 and B73 that both have V76 and N80 motifs are good ligands for KIR2DL2/3 (52). In addition to C1 binding, the KIR2DL2/3 can also interact with several C2 allotypes, notably C*0501 and C*0202 (52). The inhibitory signals triggered by the 2DL2/3-C1 interaction is relatively weaker as compared to those triggered by the 2DL1-C2 interaction (52, 53). The activating KIR receptor KIR2DS1 has similar Ig-like domains to inhibitory KIR2DL1 and also binds HLA-C2, but with reduced avidity (54). KIR2DS2 is an activating receptor that has similar Ig-like domains to inhibitory KIR2DL2 but has no detectable avidity for HLA-C1 (53). KIR2DS4 is the oldest and most prevalent activating receptor and has unique ligand specificity for subsets of HLA-C allotypes carrying C1 or C2 epitopes and HLA-A11 (55).

Since the C1 and C2 are nonoverlapping subsets of HLA-C allotypes, individuals can be either C1 homozygous, C2 homozygous or C1/C2 heterozygous. Contrarily, only a subset of HLA-A (HLA-A23, 24, 25, and 32) and HLA-B (40% of the known B allotypes) molecules that carry a Bw4 epitope in a similar region (residues 77–83) function as ligands for the KIR3DL1 receptor (56–58) (Fig. 3). KIR3DL2 binds to only HLA-A3 and A11 allotypes and the strength of this interaction is highly sensitive to the bound peptide sequence (59–61). The KIR2DL4 receptor binds to the extravillous trophoblast-specific HLA-G molecule and induces rapid IFN-γ production that promotes vascularization of the maternal decidua, which provides the placenta with blood and the growing fetus with gases and nutrients (62–65). In addition to its activation function, the KIR2DL4 receptor carries a single ITIM motif in its cytoplasmic tail and exhibits an inhibitory function (66, 67). The ligand specificities for KIR2DS2, 2DS3, 2DS5, 3DS1, and 2DL5 remain elusive. Epidemiological studies implicate HLA-Bw4 specificity for KIR3DS1 (68).

## 3. Extraordinary Diversity of KIR Receptor System

The unique feature of the KIR system that distinguishes it from other types of NK cell receptors is its substantial diversity, which is contributed by various factors such as individual-specific KIR gene content, nucleotide sequence polymorphism of each KIR gene, and stochastic and variegated expression of KIR receptor repertoires on individual NK cell clones.

### *3.1. Gene Content Diversity of KIR Gene Complex*

KIR receptors are encoded by a family of tightly clustered genes on the leukocyte receptor complex (LRC) that spans a region of about 150 kb on chromosome 19q13.4 (34, 35). The number and type of KIR genes vary substantially between haplotypes (Fig. 4). Over 30 distinct KIR haplotypes with distinct gene content have been characterized to date by sequencing genomic clones and haplotype segregation analysis in families (34, 69–74). The most commonly occurring haplotype in most human populations is conventionally called the "group-A haplotype," which carries a fixed gene content comprising KIR3DL3-2DL3-2DP1-2DL1-3DP1-2DL4-3DL1-2DS4-3DL2 (Fig. 4; haplotype 1) (31, 34). Remaining KIR haplotypes are collectively referred to as "group-B haplotypes," which have variable gene content comprising several genes that are not part of the A haplotype (Fig. 4; haplotypes 2–22). Particularly, KIR2DS1, 2DS2, 2DS3, 2DS5, 2DL2, 2DL5, and 3DS1 are associated only with group-B haplotypes, and thus B haplotypes generally encode more activating KIR receptors than the A haplotype that encodes a single activating receptor, KIR2DS4 (34, 69, 73, 74). Despite such extraordinary gene-content diversity, four KIR genes, 2DL4, 3DL2, 3DL3, and 3DP1, are present on virtually all KIR

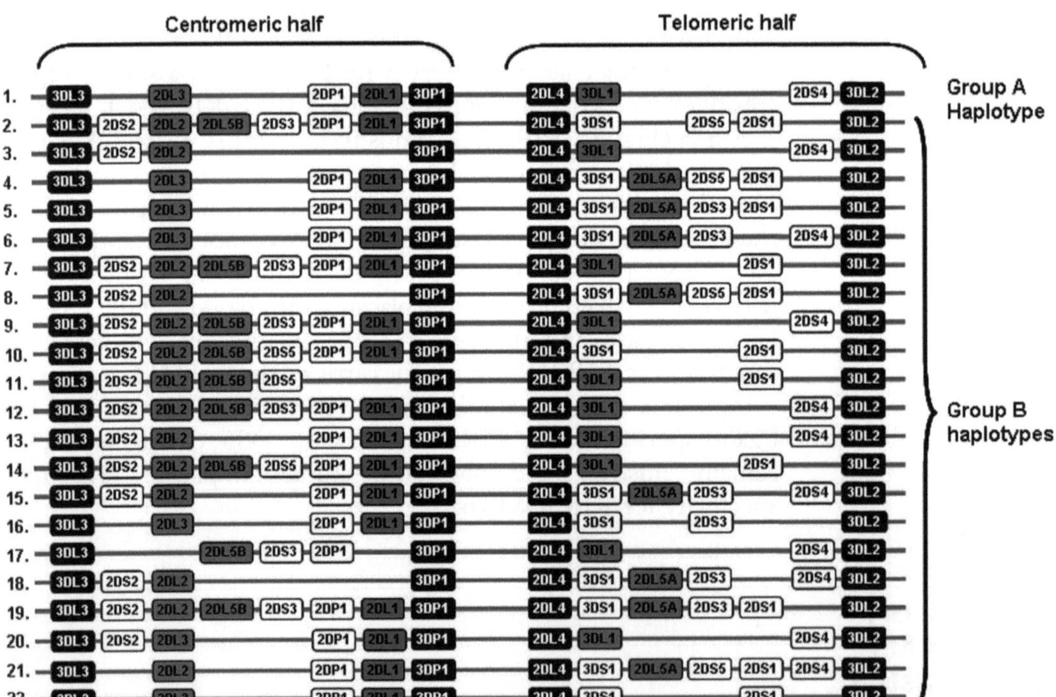


Fig. 4. KIR haplotypes differ by gene content. Map of KIR haplotypes as determined by family segregation analysis. Haplotype 1 represents group-A KIR haplotype and the remainder group-B haplotypes. The framework genes, present in all haplotypes are shown in *dark boxes*; genes encoding activating KIR are in *white boxes*; and those for inhibitory receptors are in *gray boxes*. The KIR2DP1 and 3DP1 are pseudogenes that do not express a receptor. Maps are not drawn to scale.

haplotypes and therefore have been referred to as "framework" genes (34). Inheritance of paternal and maternal haplotypes comprising different KIR gene content haplotypes (A+A, A+B, or B+B) generates extraordinary diversity between humans. For example, homozygotes for group-A haplotypes have only seven functional KIR genes (Fig. 5; sibling-1), while heterozygotes for group-A and group-B haplotypes may have all 14 functional KIR genes (Fig. 5; sibling-2). Data from various populations revealed over 240 genotypes that differ in their KIR gene content, of which only a single genotype, suggestive of the homozygote for group-A haplotype, occurs in all 51 studied populations (75, 76) (http://www.allelefrequencies.net/). The gene content for the ten KIR genotypes that occur most frequently in populations are listed in Fig. 6.

A stretch of 14 kb enriched with L1 repeats upstream of KIR2DL4 divides the KIR haplotype into two halves (34) (Figs. 4 and 7). The centromeric half is delimited by 3DL3 at the 5′-end and 3DP1 at the 3′-end, while the telomeric half is delimited by 2DL4 at the 5′-end and 3DL2 at the 3′-end. These four framework genes

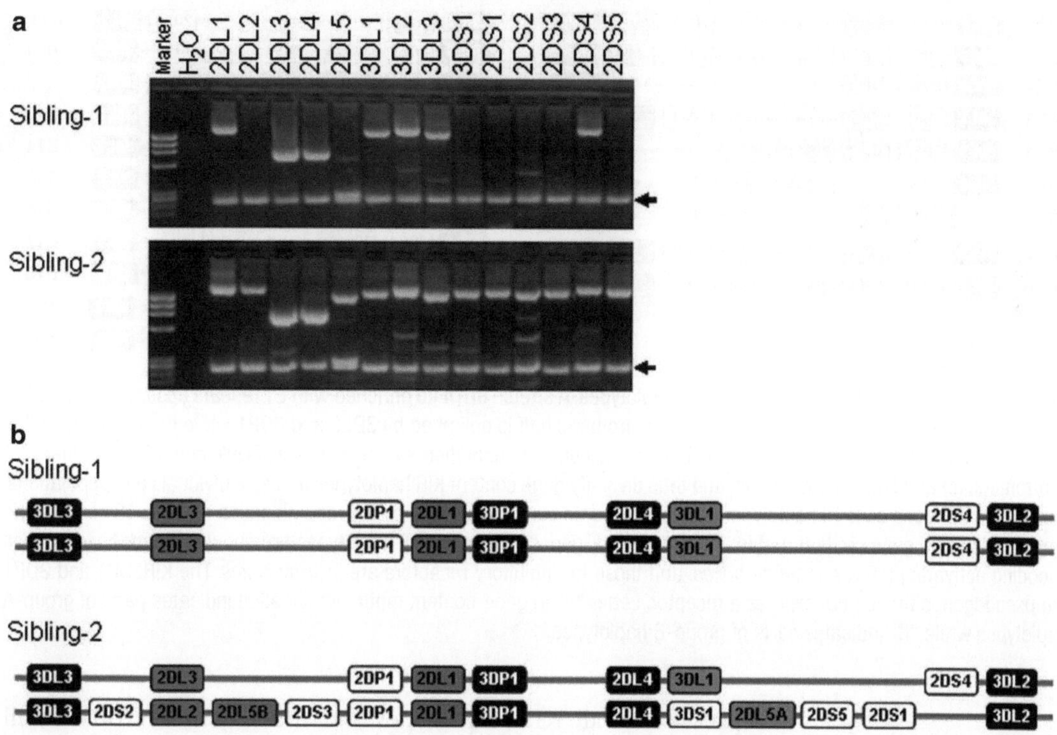


Fig. 5. KIR gene content differs between individuals. The number and type of KIR genes can be substantially variable between individuals, even within a family. (**a**) Is the gel picture indicating the extreme difference in the KIR gene content of two siblings. Sibling-1 has fewer genes and sibling-2 has all known genes. *Arrows* indicate internal positive control bands specific to an invariant gene. The pseudogenes KIR2DP1 and 3DP1 are not typed. (**b**) Shows the possible KIR haplotype composition of each sibling.

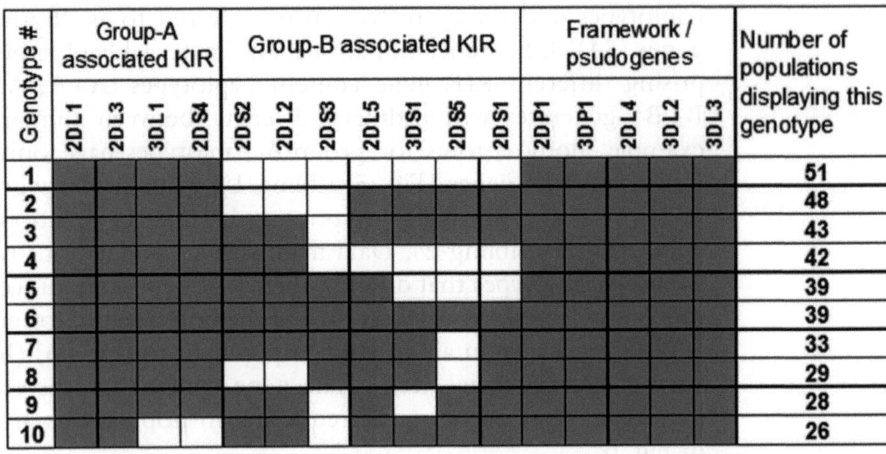


Fig. 6. Ten most commonly occurring KIR genotypes in populations. Genotyping studies revealed a significant ethnic difference in the distribution of KIR genotypes. Listed are the ten most frequently occurring KIR genotypes in 51 distinct human populations. The presence of a gene is indicated by a *shaded box* while the absence of a gene is indicated by a *white box*.

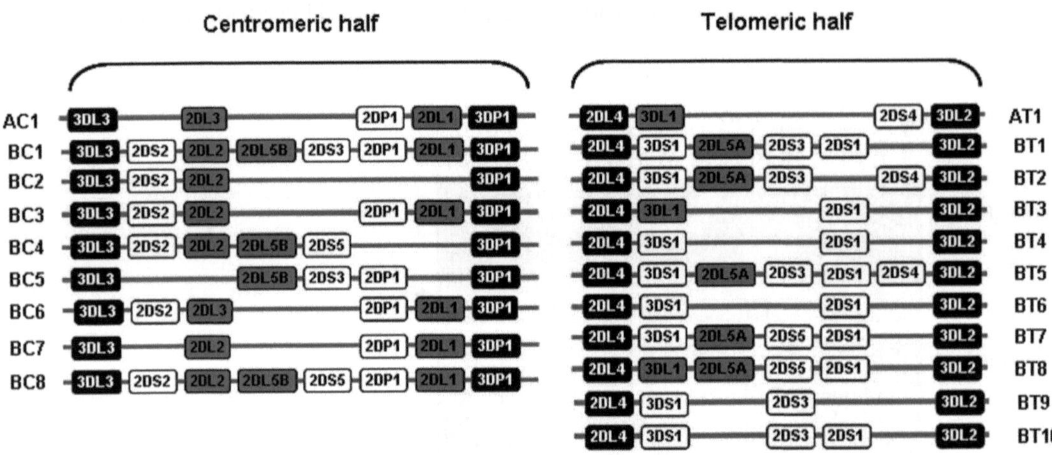


Fig. 7. Cetromeric and telomeric halves of KIR haplotypes. A stretch of 14 kb enriched with L1 repeats upstream of KIR2DL4 divides the KIR haplotype into two halves. The centromeric half is delimited by 3DL3 and 3DP1 while the telomeric half is delimited by 2DL4 and 3DL2. Multiple reciprocal meiotic recombination events between 3DP1 and 2DL4 shuffled the centromeric (c) and telomeric (t) motifs, and thus diversify gene content KIR haplotypes across individuals and populations. Most of the KIR gene content haplotypes published to date can be explained by the recombination of these 10 centromeric and 10 telomeric gene content motifs. The framework genes, present in all haplotypes are shown in *dark boxes*; genes encoding activating KIR are in *white boxes*; and those for inhibitory receptors are in *gray boxes*. The KIR2DP1 and 3DP1 are pseudogenes that do not express a receptor. Letter "A" in gene-content motif identification indicates parts of group-A haplotypes while "B" indicates parts of group-B haplotypes.

are present on all KIR haplotypes and thus occur in 100% of all populations (75). In contrast, the existence of the other 12 KIR genes is considerably variable. The inhibitory receptors KIR2DL2 and 2DL3 segregate as alleles of a single locus at the centromeric half. Similarly, the inhibitory KIR3DL1 and activating KIR3DS1 behave as alleles of the same locus at the telomeric half. Almost all haplotypes contain these two loci, such that virtually every one has either 2DL2 or 2DL3, and 3DL1 or 3DS1 within their KIR genome. KIR2DL1, 2DL2, 2DL3, and 2DS2 are specific to the centromeric half while KIR3DL1, 3DS1, 2DS1, and 2DS4 are specific to the telomeric half. Three KIR genes, 2DL5, 2DS3, and 2DS5, are found in both centromeric and telomeric locations (70, 74). For genes within each half, there is significant linkage disequilibrium, but much less for genes in the two different halves (73, 77).

Multiple reciprocal recombination events at the center of the KIR complex, between 3DP1 and 2DL4, presumably diversify gene content for KIR haplotypes across individuals and populations (75, 78). Most of the KIR gene content haplotypes published to date can be explained by the recombination of 10 centromeric and 10 telomeric gene content motifs (Figs. 4 and 7). For example, haplotype 1 listed in Fig. 4 is a recombinant of the centromeric half cA01 and telomeric half tA01; similarly, haplotype 8 is a recombinant of the centromeric half cB02 and telomeric half tB02. The reciprocal recombination also results haplotypes carrying both group-A and group-B haplotype-specific motifs. For instance, haplotype 6 listed in Fig. 4 is a recombinant of the centromeric half cA01 and telomeric half tB04, and haplotype 9 is a recombinant of the centromeric half cB01 and telomeric tA01. Recombination events also are reported outside the region between 3DP1 and 2DL4. These are generally nonallelic crossovers generating several unusual haplotypes, including truncated haplotypes that are missing some framework genes (70, 77) or elongated haplotypes that contain duplicated genes (79–81). It is important to remark here that the current genotyping methods used to detect the presence and absence of individual KIR gene will not identify the copy number of each KIR gene within a given individual. Therefore, more precise typing methods, such as a yet to be developed quantitative real-time PCR assay are necessary to investigate the KIR gene copy number and their impact on human disease.

All human populations have both group-A and B haplotypes, but their distribution varies considerably across distinct populations. Individuals carrying both A and B haplotypes are more common in Caucasians and Africans, and therefore A and B haplotypes are approximately equally distributed in these populations (31, 75). In contrast, the prevalence of inhibitory haplotypes (group-A) dominates over the activating haplotypes (group-B) in one population and vice versa in others. Individuals carrying homozygous group-A KIR haplotypes (AA genotypes) are common in Northeast Asians (Chinese, Japanese, and Koreans) (72, 82, 83). Conversely, individuals carrying AB or BB genotypes are common in the natives of America (84, 85), Australia (86), and India (87–89). The NK cells from AA homozygous individuals can express a maximum of four inhibitory KIRs (2DL1, 2DL3, 3DL1, and 3DL2) and one activating KIR (2DS4). In contrast, individuals carrying AB or BB genotypes can express a maximum of six inhibitory KIRs (2DL1-3, 2DL5, 3DL1, and 3DL2) and 2–6 activating KIRs (3DS1, 2DS1-5). NK cells of group-B haplotype carriers express more activating KIR receptors and respond more vigorously to pathogens. These data suggest that the aboriginal populations of India, Australia, and America acquired activating KIR genes to survive the environmental challenges during their extensive prehistoric migrations from Africa (87).

### 3.2. Nucleotide Polymorphism of KIR Genes

In addition to gene content diversity, each KIR gene itself exhibits considerable nucleotide sequence polymorphism (37, 73, 77, 90, 91). Allelic sequence variants of KIR genes are named in a fashion analogous to that used for HLA alleles (37) (Fig. 8). After the gene name, an asterisk is used as a separator before a numerical allele designation. The first three digits of the numerical designation indicate alleles that differ in the sequences of their encoded proteins. The next two digits distinguish alleles that differ only by synonymous (noncoding) differences within the coding sequence. The final two digits distinguish alleles that only differ by substitutions in an intron, promoter, or other noncoding region of the sequence.

To date, 614 KIR nucleotide sequences encoding 321 distinct KIR proteins have been deposited in IPD-KIR database (Release 2.4.0, 15 April 2011), the database that provides a centralized repository for human KIR sequences (http://www.ebi.ac.uk/ipd/kir/). Inhibitory KIR receptors are more polymorphic than the activating KIR receptors. The highest allelic polymorphisms are reported for 3DL1, 3DL2, and 3DL3 loci, which is probably due to the subjective sequencing analyses of large cohorts by certain laboratories that focus on these loci (92–95).

The functional consequence of sequence polymorphism has been studied in great detail for the KIR3DL1 locus. The amino

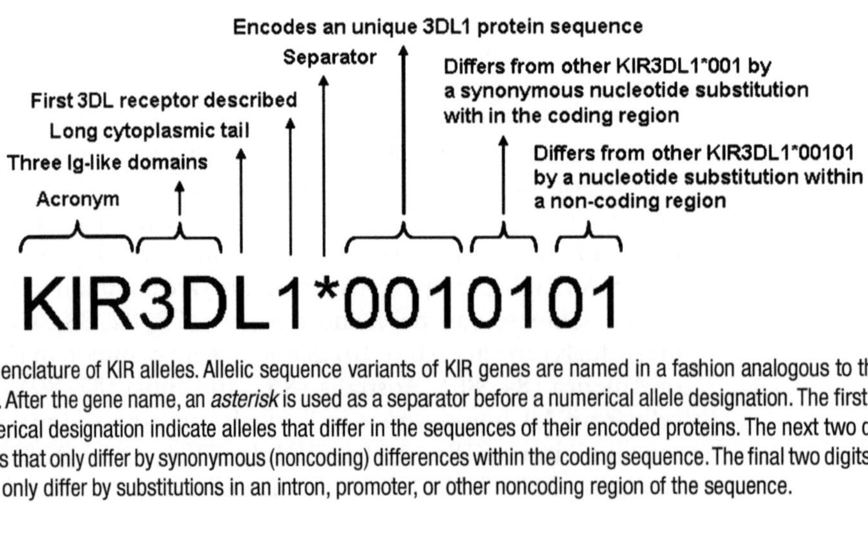


Fig. 8. Nomenclature of KIR alleles. Allelic sequence variants of KIR genes are named in a fashion analogous to that used for HLA alleles. After the gene name, an *asterisk* is used as a separator before a numerical allele designation. The first three digits of the numerical designation indicate alleles that differ in the sequences of their encoded proteins. The next two digits distinguish alleles that only differ by synonymous (noncoding) differences within the coding sequence. The final two digits distinguish alleles that only differ by substitutions in an intron, promoter, or other noncoding region of the sequence.

acid substitutions that distinguish allelic diversity of 3DL1 are enriched in polymorphic HLA-Bw4 ligand-binding Ig-like domains compared to the cytoplasmic tail region, and such diversity appears to be the result of natural selection (92). The sequence polymorphism of 3DL1 is known to influence their expression, ligand binding and cytolytic and cytokine secretion functions (53, 71, 93, 96, 97). Some KIR sequences are null alleles that carry either a premature stop codon or one or more nucleotide substitution/deletion/insertion(s) that alter the reading frame of protein synthesis, which affect their cell surface expression. The most frequently encountered unexpressed alleles belong to KIR2DS4 locus, which is the most polymorphic among the activating KIR gene exhibiting 13 distinct protein variants. Nine (2DS4*003, *004, *006, *007, *008, *009, *010, *012, and *013) have a 22 bp deletion in exon-5, which shifts the reading-frame and results in a premature stop codon causing this receptor to be unexpressed at the cell surface (70, 98). Individuals homozygous for group-A haplotypes carrying 2DS4-deletion alleles will not express any activating KIR receptors as they carry only 2DS4 as an activating KIR gene. Frequencies of individuals with zero activating KIR genotypes vary between ethnic populations (17% of Caucasians, 9% of Hispanics, 10% of Africans, and 11% of Asians) (70, 98, 99).

The other frequently occurring unexpressed alleles belong to KIR2DL4 locus. Based on the presence of a sequence of 9 or 10 adenine residues at the end of exon 6, all 46 alleles of 2DL4 can be divided into two groups, 9A and 10A (100). The deletion of one adenine in group 9A alleles results in a frame-shift and the production of either a protein with a truncated cytoplasmic tail or one lacking the transmembrane region, both of which are not expressed at the cell surface. In contrast, the 10A alleles, which can be further divided into the 10A-A and 10A-B subgroups, encode receptors that may be expressed at the cell surface (101). Sequence variation in the promoter region is implicated with the lack of 2DL5B expression (102). Certain amino acid residues that distinguish allelic polymorphism are known to be largely responsible for the intracellular retention of 3DL1*004 (103) and 2DL2*004 (104). The synergistic combination of allelic polymorphism and variable gene content individualize KIR genotypes to an extent where unrelated individuals almost always have different KIR genotypes (77). This level of diversity likely reflects a strong pressure from pathogens on the human NK cell response.

### 3.3. KIR Receptor Repertoire Diversity of NK Cell Clones

In addition to the gene content variation and sequence polymorphism, the level of mRNA expression varies among KIR genes and alleles. For instance, the KIR3DL3 transcripts are detected at low levels in peripheral blood when compared to other KIR genes (24, 105). Further, alternatively spliced mRNA are reported for most KIR genes, and such isoforms can hinder the cell surface

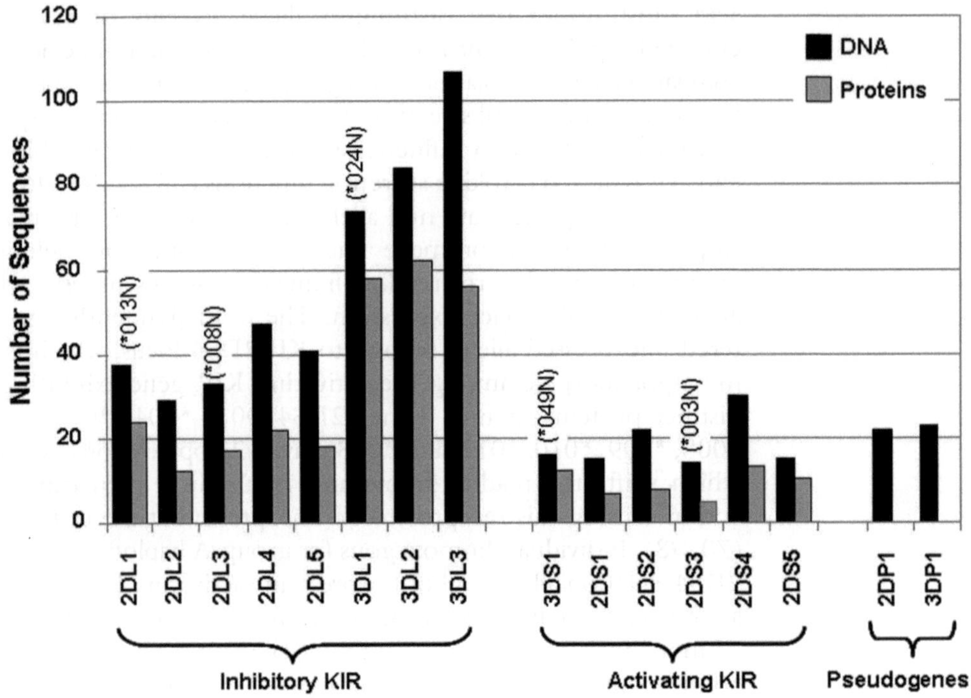


Fig. 9. Sequence polymorphism of KIR receptors. The number of nucleotide sequences (*black bars*) and their predicted protein variants (*gray bars*) characterized to date for each KIR locus are shown. This data was extracted from IPD-KIR database (http://www.ebi.ac.uk/ipd/kir/stats.html; Release 2.4.0; April 2011) that provides a centralized repository for human KIR sequences. Null alleles identified for each locus are given in the parenthesis.

receptor expression (106). Although mRNA expressions have been detected for all KIR genes (except for pseudogenes KIR2DP1 and 3DP1), due to the lack of specific antibodies, the cell surface expression of KIR3DL3, 2DS3, and 2DS5 proteins is not confirmed (Fig. 9).

The KIR receptors are clonally expressed on mature NK cells in a stochastic manner such that each NK cell clone within a given individual does not express the entire set of KIR genes present in that individual's genome, but rather only a portion of the genes in a apparently random combination (20, 107). Combinatorial diversity of KIR expression yields a broad range of functionally distinct NK cell clones, which presumably are critical for a rapid and sensitive detection of reduced HLA class I expression on target cells. The NK cell clone stably maintains its acquired KIR receptor repertoire throughout subsequent cell divisions. Although the KIR repertoire is largely determined by genetically defined factors (108), there is increasing evidence that epigenetic mechanisms modulate KIR receptor expression patterns. The methylation state of cytosines within CpG islands at the promoter regions of KIR loci is implicated in perpetual expression of KIR receptors on NK cell clones (105, 109, 110). Furthermore, the presence of the cognate

HLA class I ligand is shown to increase the frequency of NK cells expressing the specific inhibitory KIR receptor (71), but these findings are challenged by another study (111). Finally, a recent study indicates an unexpected and strong epistatic influence on the expression of one KIR receptor (KIR2DL1) by other KIRs (2DL2 and 2DS2) (112).

The majority of NK cells in peripheral blood express at least one inhibitory receptor for self-MHC class I and are functionally competent to recognize and eliminate target cells that have down-regulated their respective MHC class I ligands (20, 107). Additionally, a subpopulation of developmentally immature NK cells exists that lacks inhibitory receptors for self-MHC class I and is generally hyporesponsive to target cells that are deficient in MHC class I expression (113–115). Developmental interactions of the KIRs with HLA class I trigger the acquisition of functional competence in a process called "licensing" (114, 116), "arming" (117), or "education" (113). Therefore, individuals carry a minimum of one inhibitory KIR-HLA gene pair, crucial for the development of functional NK cells (99). Consistent with this, the NK cells from MHC-deficient mice and humans are shown to be defective in target killing (118, 119). Expression of progressively higher numbers of inhibitory KIRs for self-HLA-B and HLA-Cw molecules has been correlated with an increased effector capacity (120). In summary, interactions of KIR to HLA class I ligands set the threshold of NK cell capacity as well as control the NK cell response.

Unlike T and B cells, NK cells use a multiple receptor recognition strategy, whereby an individual NK cell can be triggered through various receptors independently or in combination, depending on the ligands presented by the target cell in a given encounter (20, 25, 107). If a given NK cell uses both inhibitory and activating receptors to recognize the target, the balance between these disparate signals determines the action of that NK cell (18). In addition to NK cells, KIR receptors are expressed on a subset of T lymphocytes, in particular on γδ T cells and memory/effector $CD8^+$ T cells indicating that the KIRs can regulate the antigen-specific T cell immune response (121, 122).

## 4. Diversity of KIR-HLA Compound Genotypes and Relavance in Disease

KIR and HLA loci are both highly polymorphic and they map to distinct human chromosomes (Chromosomes 19 and 6, respectively). KIR and HLA gene families segregate independently, yielding many individuals who express KIR receptors for which they lack HLA class I ligands, and vice versa, thus creating human diversity in the number and type of KIR-HLA inherited gene pairs (99). Nevertheless, at the population level there is compelling evidence for coevolution of interacting KIR-HLA pairs (123, 124). Although most individuals have all four well-defined inhibitory KIR receptors (3DL1, 3DL2, 2DL1, and 2DL2/3), we found only a subset that expresses all relevant HLA class I ligands, HLA-Bw4 (3DL1), HLA-A3/11 (3DL2), HLA-C2 (2DL1), and HLA-C1 (2DL2/3) (99). The majority of Caucasians, Hispanics, and African Americans carry either two or three inhibitory KIR-HLA combinations. Interestingly, one out of five individuals in these populations carries only a single receptor–ligand pair, KIR2DL3 + HLA-C1. Environmental invectives, such as viral infections, affecting HLA-C expression in individuals carrying this single KIR-HLA combination can break self-tolerance and may endorse autoimmunity. Furthermore, all 759 individuals tested in our study had at least one of the four inhibitory KIR-HLA class I ligand gene pairs (99). Similar studies of KIR-HLA gene combinations are warranted in populations enriched with either group-A or group-B KIR haplotypes, such as Chinese, Japanese, and natives of Australia, America, and India, which will enlighten how the epistatic interactions between KIR and HLA involved in the survival of modern human populations.

The interaction between KIR2DL3 and HLA-C1 is weak and signals triggered by this low affinity combination are shown to be overridden by activating signals compared to those triggered through the stronger inhibitory interactions of KIR2DL1 + HLA-C2 (53). The clinical implication of such strength variation in KIR-HLA-mediated inhibitions is evidenced from two lines of research. Firstly, the poorly inhibiting KIR2DL3 + HLA-C1 gene combination more readily resolves infection with hepatitis C virus than infected individuals of other genotypes (125). Secondly, the stronger inhibitory interaction of KIR2DL1 + HLA-C2 was shown to affect placental development causing many common reproductive disorders, such as preeclampsia, recurrent miscarriage, and fetal growth restriction (63, 126, 127). Moreover, these pregnancy disorders were found to be less frequent in mothers that possessed the telomeric end of the group-B KIR haplotype, which contains KIR3DS1, 2DL5A, 2DS1, and 2DS5 (127) (Fig. 7, telomeric half tB02).

Although the cell surface expression and ligands for activating KIR receptors have not been clearly defined, a series of genetic epidemiological data have revealed the association of distinct activating KIR in antiviral immunity, autoimmune diseases, and cancer progression (32, 33, 128). In these models, the activation signals were proposed to prevail over HLA-dependent inhibition that presumably exacerbates NK cell response (18). KIR2DS2 or 2DS1 were found to be strongly associated with most of the autoimmune conditions. A recent study with Japanese, a highly homogeneous population appropriate for studying genetic associations, found a strong association between the telomeric KIR3DS1-2DL5A-

2DS1-2DS5 gene content motif and patients with Vogt-Koyanagi-Harada (VKH) disease (129).

In contrast to the autoimmune conditions, the presence of activating receptor KIR3DS1 slowed down the AIDS progression in HIV-1 infected patients, compared to patients lacking KIR3DS1, thus indicating a potential anti-HIV effect of KIR3DS1 (68). The KIR3DS1 receptor was also shown to be protective to hepatitis-C virus (HCV) infection (125, 130). Furthermore, KIR3DS1 and KIR2DS1 genes protect from developing a severe form of recurrent respiratory papillomatosis (RRP), a rare disease of the larynx and upper airway caused by human papilloma viruses (HPV)-6/11 (131). Nonetheless, the presence of KIR3DS1 was shown to be associated with cervical neoplasia progression to cervical cancer, a tumor that is strongly associated with another HPV strain, HPV-16/18 (132). The difference in clinical disease expression induced by different HPV strains in 3DS1 carriers could be interaction of 3DS1 with putative HPV strain-specific ligands leading to either killing of HPV-6/11-infected cells keeping the host from developing RRP, or leading to inappropriate tissue-specific hyperresponsiveness promoting growth of cervical cancer, vs. benign respiratory papillomas.

Taken together, the genotypes encoding a dominant inhibitory KIR receptor repertoire is likely protective against autoimmunity but susceptible for infection and reproductive disorders, while the genotypes encoding a dominant activating KIR receptor repertoire are presumably detrimental to autoimmunity and cancer growth but instrumental against viral infection. Greater understanding of KIR-HLA diversity and functional distinctions between NK cell subsets are needed to strengthen the ability to harness the power of NK cells for therapeutic aims.

## 5. Alloreactive NK Cells in Hematopoietic Stem Cell Transplantation

HLA-matched allogeneic hematopoietic stem cell transplantation (HSCT) is an effective treatment for hematologic malignancies, including leukemia, lymphoma, and inherited hematopoietic stem cell diseases (133). Donor T cells in the allograft are critical for promoting engraftment and eradicating malignant cells. Unfortunately, alloreactive T cells also cause graft-versus-host disease (GVHD), which is an attack on recipient tissues, primarily the gastrointestinal tract, liver, and skin. T cell depletion prevents GVHD but increases the risk of graft rejection and leukemic relapse.

Following allogeneic HSCT, the progeny of the donor stem cells repopulate the entire hematopoietic system of the recipient. NK cells are the first lymphocyte population to appear in peripheral blood shortly after HSCT. KIR receptor repertoires of NK cells reconstituted from the donor hematopoietic precursors are consistently of donor type (108). The donor-derived NK cells can be alloreactive if their inhibitory KIRs do not see a relevant HLA class I ligand that was present in the donor. Such alloreactive NK cells greatly contribute many potential benefits, including decreased rates of GVHD, decreased rates of graft rejection mediated by NK lysis of host T cells, decreased relapse, improved engraftment mediated by NK-cell release of hematopoietic cytokines, and enhanced immune reconstitution and decreased infectious complications mediated by NK-cell antiviral activity. Such beneficial NK cell alloreactivity, which can be predicted from the differences in KIR-binding HLA class I ligands between donor and recipient based on their HLA class I type, was first described for HLA haploidentical transplantation by the use of an extensively T cell-depleted graft in acute myeloid leukemia (AML) patients (134) and later investigated in other transplantation settings (135, 136).

The patients with myeloid malignancies were more responsive to treatment than those with lymphoid malignancies. Several studies have suggested that adult acute lymphoid leukemia (ALL) is not as susceptible to KIR ligand-mismatched haploidentical allogeneic HSCT (134, 137–139). However, alloreactive NK cell-mediated effects can impact childhood ALL (140). Beneficial effects from KIR-ligand mismatch have not been seen in the T cell-replete setting (141, 142).

In addition to the recipient lacking HLA class I ligands for the donor-derived NK cells, expression of activating KIR receptors on donor NK cells is also shown to influence HSCT outcome. Compared to donors with AA genotypes (express one or no activating KIR), the Bx genotype (express 1–6 activating KIRs) donors were shown to contribute significantly superior relapse protection and improved disease-free survival for AML patients (143). Gene content motif analyses further reveal that the centromeric and telomeric B haplotype-specific motifs both contribute to relapse protection and improved survival, but centromeric B homozygosity (Cen-B/B) has the strongest independent effect (143). Further studies are required to determine if the clinical benefit conferred by Cen-B/B is caused by a single KIR gene (such as 2DS2, 2DS3, or KIR2DL2) or by the combination of specific KIR genes.

Recent studies reveal the strongest clinical impact of telomeric B haplotype-specific activating KIR genes (144, 145). Compared with KIR3DS1-negative donors, a donor with KIR3DS1 was shown to be associated with lower-grade II–IV acute GVHD, but not with relapse (144). Furthermore, grade II–IV acute GVHD, overall mortality, and transplantation-related mortality all decreased as the number of copies of donor KIR3DS1 increased, with the lowest failure rate occurring among patients homozygous for donor KIR3DS1 (144). Functional experiments reveal that the activating

KIR2DS1 plays a substantial role in mediating alloreactivity and confers an advantage in the ability of NK cell alloreactivity to kill dendritic cells and T cell blasts (145). In summary, knowing the KIR genotype of the donor, and HLA types of both the donor and recipient, it is possible to predict the degree of KIR-HLA interactions that may determine an enhanced ability to limit GVHD and improve engraftment for certain leukemias.

## Acknowledgment

This work was supported by start-up funds from the UCLA Department of Pathology and Laboratory Medicine.

## References


1. Caligiuri MA (2008) Human natural killer cells. Blood 112:461–469
2. Vivier E et al (2011) Innate or adaptive immunity? The example of natural killer cells. Science 331:44–49
3. Colucci F et al (2003) What does it take to make a natural killer? Nat Rev Immunol 3:413–425
4. Lee SH et al (2007) Keeping NK cells in highly regulated antiviral warfare. Trends Immunol 28:252–259
5. Smyth MJ et al (2002) New aspects of natural-killer-cell surveillance and therapy of cancer. Nat Rev Cancer 2:850–861
6. Sun JC et al (2010) Immune memory redefined: characterizing the longevity of natural killer cells. Immunol Rev 236:83–94
7. Cooper MA et al (2001) Human natural killer cells: a unique innate immunoregulatory role for the CD56 (bright) subset. Blood 97:3146–3151
8. Freud AG, Caligiuri MA (2006) Human natural killer cell development. Immunol Rev 214:56–72
9. Jacobs R et al (2001) CD56bright cells differ in their KIR repertoire and cytotoxic features from CD56dim NK cells. Eur J Immunol 31:3121–3127
10. Fehniger TA et al (2003) CD56bright natural killer cells are present in human lymph nodes and are activated by T cell-derived IL-2: a potential new link between adaptive and innate immunity. Blood 101:3052–3057
11. Cooper MA et al (2004) NK cell and DC interactions. Trends Immunol 25:47–52
12. Manaster I, Mandelboim O (2008) The unique properties of human NK cells in the uterine mucosa. Placenta 29(suppl A):S60–S66
13. Colonna M (2009) Interleukin-22-producing natural killer cells and lymphoid tissue inducer-like cells in mucosal immunity. Immunity 31:15–23
14. Bryceson YT, Long EO (2008) Line of attack: NK cell specificity and integration of signals. Curr Opin Immunol 20:344–352
15. Lanier LL (2003) Natural killer cell receptor signaling. Curr Opin Immunol 15:308–314
16. McQueen KL, Parham P (2002) Variable receptors controlling activation and inhibition of NK cells. Curr Opin Immunol 14: 615–621
17. Moretta L et al (2000) Human NK-cell receptors. Immunol Today 21:420–422
18. Lanier LL (2005) NK cell recognition. Annu Rev Immunol 23:225–274
19. Lanier LL (2008) Up on the tightrope: natural killer cell activation and inhibition. Nat Immunol 9:495–502
20. Valiante NM et al (1997) Functionally and structurally distinct NK cell receptor repertoires in the peripheral blood of two human donors. Immunity 7:739–751
21. Biron CA (2001) Interferons alpha and beta as immune regulators—a new look. Immunity 14:661–664
22. Ljunggren HG, Karre K (1990) In search of the 'missing self': MHC molecules and NK cell recognition. Immunol Today 11:237–244
23. Lanier LL (1998) NK cell receptors. Annu Rev Immunol 16:359–393

24. Long EO et al (2001) Inhibition of natural killer cell activation signals by killer cell immunoglobulin-like receptors (CD158). Immunol Rev 181:223–233
25. Moretta A et al (2001) Activating receptors and coreceptors involved in human natural killer cell-mediated cytolysis. Annu Rev Immunol 19:197–223
26. Vilches C, Parham P (2002) KIR: diverse, rapidly evolving receptors of innate and adaptive immunity. Annu Rev Immunol 20:217–251
27. Lanier LL (2008) Evolutionary struggles between NK cells and viruses. Nat Rev Immunol 8:259–268
28. Parham P (2003) Immunogenetics of killer-cell immunoglobulin-like receptors. Tissue Antigens 62:194–200
29. Abi-Rached L et al (2010) Human-specific evolution and adaptation led to major qualitative differences in the variable receptors of human and chimpanzee natural killer cells. PLoS Genet 6:e1001192
30. Parham P (2005) MHC class I molecules and KIRs in human history, health and survival. Nat Rev Immunol 5:201–214
31. Uhrberg M et al (1997) Human diversity in killer cell inhibitory receptor genes. Immunity 7:753–763
32. Khakoo SI, Carrington M (2006) KIR and disease: a model system or system of models? Immunol Rev 214:186–201
33. Bashirova AA et al (2006) The killer immunoglobulin-like receptor gene cluster: tuning the genome for defense. Annu Rev Genomics Hum Genet 7:277–300
34. Wilson MJ et al (2000) Plasticity in the organization and sequences of human KIR/ILT gene families. Proc Natl Acad Sci USA 97: 4778–4783
35. Trowsdale J (2001) Genetic and functional relationships between MHC and NK receptor genes. Immunity 15:363–374
36. Steffens U et al (1998) Nucleotide and amino acid sequence alignment for human killer cell inhibitory receptors (KIR), 1998. Tissue Antigens 51:398–413
37. Marsh SG et al (2003) Killer-cell immunoglobulin-like receptor (KIR) nomenclature report, 2002. Tissue Antigens 62:79–86
38. Lanier LL (2009) DAP10- and DAP12-associated receptors in innate immunity. Immunol Rev 227:150–160
39. Marsh SG et al (2011) Nomenclature for factors of the HLA system, 2010. Tissue Antigens 75:291–455
40. Klein J, Sato A (2000) The HLA system. Second of two parts. N Engl J Med 343:782–786
41. Klein J, Sato A (2000) The HLA system. First of two parts. N Engl J Med 343:702–709
42. Boyington JC et al (2000) Crystal structure of an NK cell immunoglobulin-like receptor in complex with its class I MHC ligand. Nature 405:537–543
43. Khakoo SI et al (2002) The D0 domain of KIR3D acts as a major histocompatibility complex class I binding enhancer. J Exp Med 196:911–921
44. Prugnolle F et al (2005) Pathogen-driven selection and worldwide HLA class I diversity. Curr Biol 15:1022–1027
45. Parham P, Ohta T (1996) Population biology of antigen presentation by MHC class I molecules. Science 272:67–74
46. Colonna M et al (1992) Alloantigen recognition by two human natural killer cell clones is associated with HLA-C or a closely linked gene. Proc Natl Acad Sci USA 89: 7983–7985
47. Mandelboim O et al (1996) Protection from lysis by natural killer cells of group 1 and 2 specificity is mediated by residue 80 in human histocompatibility leukocyte antigen C alleles and also occurs with empty major histocompatibility complex molecules. J Exp Med 184:913–922
48. Mandelboim O et al (1997) The binding site of NK receptors on HLA-C molecules. Immunity 6:341–350
49. Colonna M et al (1993) HLA-C is the inhibitory ligand that determines dominant resistance to lysis by NK1- and NK2-specific natural killer cells. Proc Natl Acad Sci USA 90:12000–12004
50. Wagtmann N et al (1995) Molecular clones of the p58 NK cell receptor reveal immunoglobulin-related molecules with diversity in both the extra- and intracellular domains. Immunity 2:439–449
51. Winter CC, Long EO (1997) A single amino acid in the p58 killer cell inhibitory receptor controls the ability of natural killer cells to discriminate between the two groups of HLA-C allotypes. J Immunol 158:4026–4028
52. Moesta AK et al (2008) Synergistic polymorphism at two positions distal to the ligand-binding site makes KIR2DL2 a stronger receptor for HLA-C than KIR2DL3. J Immunol 180:3969–3979
53. Winter CC et al (1998) Direct binding and functional transfer of NK cell inhibitory receptors reveal novel patterns of HLA-C allotype recognition. J Immunol 161:571–577
54. Stewart CA et al (2005) Recognition of peptide-MHC class I complexes by activating

killer immunoglobulin-like receptors. Proc Natl Acad Sci USA 102:13224–13229

55. Graef T et al (2009) KIR2DS4 is a product of gene conversion with KIR3DL2 that introduced specificity for HLA-A*11 while diminishing avidity for HLA-C. J Exp Med 206:2557–2572
56. Gumperz JE et al (1995) The Bw4 public epitope of HLA-B molecules confers reactivity with natural killer cell clones that express NKB1, a putative HLA receptor. J Exp Med 181:1133–1144
57. Cella M et al (1994) NK3-specific natural killer cells are selectively inhibited by Bw4-positive HLA alleles with isoleucine 80. J Exp Med 180:1235–1242
58. Thananchai H et al (2007) Cutting edge: allele-specific and peptide-dependent interactions between KIR3DL1 and HLA-A and HLA-B. J Immunol 178:33–37
59. Pende D et al (1996) The natural killer cell receptor specific for HLA-A allotypes: a novel member of the p58/p70 family of inhibitory receptors that is characterized by three immunoglobulin-like domains and is expressed as a 140-kD disulphide-linked dimer. J Exp Med 184:505–518
60. Dohring C et al (1996) A human killer inhibitory receptor specific for HLA-A1,2. J Immunol 156:3098–3101
61. Hansasuta P et al (2004) Recognition of HLA-A3 and HLA-A11 by KIR3DL2 is peptide-specific. Eur J Immunol 34:1673–1679
62. Rajagopalan S, Long EO (1999) A human histocompatibility leukocyte antigen (HLA)-G-specific receptor expressed on all natural killer cells. J Exp Med 189:1093–1100
63. Moffett-King A (2002) Natural killer cells and pregnancy. Nat Rev Immunol 2:656–663
64. Rajagopalan S et al (2006) Activation of NK cells by an endocytosed receptor for soluble HLA-G. PLoS Biol 4:e9
65. Kikuchi-Maki A et al (2003) KIR2DL4 Is an IL-2-regulated NK cell receptor that exhibits limited expression in humans but triggers strong IFN-gamma production. J Immunol 171:3415–3425
66. Faure M, Long EO (2002) KIR2DL4 (CD158d), an NK cell-activating receptor with inhibitory potential. J Immunol 168: 6208–6214
67. Ponte M et al (1999) Inhibitory receptors sensing HLA-G1 molecules in pregnancy: decidua-associated natural killer cells express LIR-1 and CD94/NKG2A and acquire p49, an HLA-G1-specific receptor. Proc Natl Acad Sci USA 96:5674–5679
68. Martin MP et al (2002) Epistatic interaction between KIR3DS1 and HLA-B delays the progression to AIDS. Nat Genet 31:429–434
69. Uhrberg M et al (2002) Definition of gene content for nine common group B haplotypes of the Caucasoid population: KIR haplotypes contain between seven and eleven KIR genes. Immunogenetics 54:221–229
70. Hsu KC et al (2002) Killer Ig-like receptor haplotype analysis by gene content: evidence for genomic diversity with a minimum of six basic framework haplotypes, each with multiple subsets. J Immunol 169:5118–5129
71. Yawata M et al (2006) Roles for HLA and KIR polymorphisms in natural killer cell repertoire selection and modulation of effector function. J Exp Med 203:633–645
72. Whang DH et al (2005) Haplotype analysis of killer cell immunoglobulin-like receptor genes in 77 Korean families. Hum Immunol 66:146–154
73. Middleton D et al (2007) KIR haplotype content at the allele level in 77 Northern Irish families. Immunogenetics 59:145–158
74. Pyo C et al (2010) Different patterns of evolution in the centromeric and telomeric regions of group A and B haplotypes of the human killer cell Ig-like receptor locus. PLoS One 5:e15115
75. Yawata M et al (2002) Variation within the human killer cell immunoglobulin-like receptor (KIR) gene family. Crit Rev Immunol 22:463–482
76. Ashouri E et al (2009) KIR gene content diversity in four Iranian populations. Immunogenetics 61:483–492
77. Shilling HG et al (2002) Allelic polymorphism synergizes with variable gene content to individualize human KIR genotype. J Immunol 168:2307–2315
78. Norman PJ et al (2009) Meiotic recombination generates rich diversity in NK cell receptor genes, alleles, and haplotypes. Genome Res 19:757–769
79. Martin AM et al (2000) The genomic organization and evolution of the natural killer immunoglobulin-like receptor (KIR) gene cluster. Immunogenetics 51:268–280
80. Williams F et al (2003) Multiple copies of KIR 3DL/S1 and KIR 2DL4 genes identified in a number of individuals. Hum Immunol 64:729–732
81. Ordonez D et al (2008) Duplication, mutation and recombination of the human orphan gene KIR2DS3 contribute to the diversity of KIR haplotypes. Genes Immun 9: 431–437

82. Jiang K et al (2005) Distribution of killer cell immunoglobulin-like receptor genes in the Chinese Han population. Tissue Antigens 65:556–563
83. Yawata M et al (2002) Predominance of group A KIR haplotypes in Japanese associated with diverse NK cell repertoires of KIR expression. Immunogenetics 54:543–550
84. Gendzekhadze K et al (2006) High KIR diversity in Amerindians is maintained using few gene-content haplotypes. Immunogenetics 58:474–480
85. Ewerton PD et al (2007) Amazonian Amerindians exhibit high variability of KIR profiles. Immunogenetics 59:625–630
86. Toneva M et al (2001) Genomic diversity of natural killer cell receptor genes in three populations. Tissue Antigens 57:358–362
87. Rajalingam R et al (2008) Distinct diversity of KIR genes in three southern Indian populations: comparison with world populations revealed a link between KIR gene content and pre-historic human migrations. Immunogenetics 60:207–217
88. Rajalingam R et al (2002) Distinctive KIR and HLA diversity in a panel of north Indian Hindus. Immunogenetics 53:1009–1019
89. Kulkarni S et al (2008) Comparison of the rapidly evolving KIR locus in Parsis and natives of India. Immunogenetics 60:121–129
90. Garcia CA et al (2003) Human KIR sequences 2003. Immunogenetics 55:227–239
91. Rajalingam R et al (2001) Identification of seventeen novel KIR variants: fourteen of them from two non-Caucasian donors. Tissue Antigens 57:22–31
92. Norman PJ et al (2007) Unusual selection on the KIR3DL1/S1 natural killer cell receptor in Africans. Nat Genet 39:1092–1099
93. Gardiner CM et al (2001) Different NK cell surface phenotypes defined by the DX9 antibody are due to KIR3DL1 gene polymorphism. J Immunol 166:2992–3001
94. Jones DC et al (2006) Nature of allelic sequence polymorphism at the KIR3DL3 locus. Immunogenetics 58:614–627
95. Hou L et al (2007) Seventeen novel alleles add to the already extensive KIR3DL3 diversity. Tissue Antigens 70:449–454
96. O'Connor GM et al (2007) Functional polymorphism of the KIR3DL1/S1 receptor on human NK cells. J Immunol 178:235–241
97. Carr WH et al (2005) KIR3DL1 polymorphisms that affect NK cell inhibition by HLA-Bw4 ligand. J Immunol 175:5222–5229
98. Maxwell LD et al (2002) A common KIR2DS4 deletion variant in the human that predicts a soluble KIR molecule analogous to the KIR1D molecule observed in the rhesus monkey. Tissue Antigens 60:254–258
99. Du Z et al (2007) Receptor-ligand analyses define minimal killer cell Ig-like receptor (KIR) in humans. Immunogenetics 59:1–15
100. Witt CS et al (2000) Detection of KIR2DL4 alleles by sequencing and SSCP reveals a common allele with a shortened cytoplasmic tail. Tissue Antigens 56:248–257
101. Goodridge JP et al (2003) KIR2DL4 (CD158d) genotype influences expression and function in NK cells. J Immunol 171: 1768–1774
102. Vilches C et al (2000) Gene structure and promoter variation of expressed and nonexpressed variants of the KIR2DL5 gene. J Immunol 165:6416–6421
103. Pando MJ et al (2003) The protein made from a common allele of KIR3DL1 (3DL1*004) is poorly expressed at cell surfaces due to substitution at positions 86 in Ig domain 0 and 182 in Ig domain 1. J Immunol 171:6640–6649
104. VandenBussche CJ et al (2006) A single polymorphism disrupts the killer Ig-like receptor 2DL2/2DL3 D1 domain. J Immunol 177: 5347–5357
105. Trompeter HI et al (2005) Three structurally and functionally divergent kinds of promoters regulate expression of clonally distributed killer cell Ig-like receptors (KIR), of KIR2DL4, and of KIR3DL3. J Immunol 174:4135–4143
106. Dohring C et al (1996) Alternatively spliced forms of human killer inhibitory receptors. Immunogenetics 44:227–230
107. Raulet DH et al (2001) Regulation of the natural killer cell receptor repertoire. Annu Rev Immunol 19:291–330
108. Shilling HG et al (2002) Genetic control of human NK cell repertoire. J Immunol 169:239–247
109. Santourlidis S et al (2002) Crucial role of DNA methylation in determination of clonally distributed killer cell Ig-like receptor expression patterns in NK cells. J Immunol 169:4253–4261
110. Chan HW et al (2003) DNA methylation maintains allele-specific KIR gene expression in human natural killer cells. J Exp Med 197:245–255
111. Andersson S et al (2009) KIR acquisition probabilities are independent of self-HLA class I ligands and increase with cellular KIR expression. Blood 114:95–104
112. Schonberg K et al (2011) Analyses of HLA-C-specific KIR repertoires in donors with

group A and B haplotypes suggest a ligand-instructed model of NK cell receptor aquisition. Blood 117:98–107
113. Anfossi N et al (2006) Human NK cell education by inhibitory receptors for MHC class I. Immunity 25:331–342
114. Kim S et al (2005) Licensing of natural killer cells by host major histocompatibility complex class I molecules. Nature 436:709–713
115. Cooley S et al (2007) A subpopulation of human peripheral blood NK cells that lacks inhibitory receptors for self MHC is developmentally immature. Blood 110:578–586
116. Yokoyama WM, Kim S (2006) How do natural killer cells find self to achieve tolerance? Immunity 24:249–257
117. Raulet DH, Vance RE (2006) Self-tolerance of natural killer cells. Nat Rev Immunol 6:520–531
118. Bix M et al (1991) Rejection of class I MHC-deficient haemopoietic cells by irradiated MHC-matched mice. Nature 349:329–331
119. Furukawa H et al (1999) Tolerance of NK and LAK activity for HLA class I-deficient targets in a TAP1-deficient patient (bare lymphocyte syndrome type I). Hum Immunol 60:32–40
120. Yu J et al (2007) Hierarchy of the human natural killer cell response is determined by class and quantity of inhibitory receptors for self-HLA-B and HLA-C ligands. J Immunol 179:5977–5989
121. Chang C et al (1995) Molecular characterization of human CD94: a type II membrane glycoprotein related to the C-type lectin superfamily. Eur J Immunol 25:2433–2437
122. Uhrberg M et al (2001) The repertoire of killer cell Ig-like receptor and CD94:NKG2A receptors in T cells: clones sharing identical alpha beta TCR rearrangement express highly diverse killer cell Ig-like receptor patterns. J Immunol 166:3923–3932
123. Single RM et al (2007) Global diversity and evidence for coevolution of KIR and HLA. Nat Genet 39:1114–1119
124. Gendzekhadze K et al (2009) Co-evolution of KIR2DL3 with HLA-C in a human population retaining minimal essential diversity of KIR and HLA class I ligands. Proc Natl Acad Sci USA 106:18692–18697
125. Khakoo SI et al (2004) HLA and NK cell inhibitory receptor genes in resolving hepatitis C virus infection. Science 305:872–874
126. Hiby SE et al (2004) Combinations of maternal KIR and fetal HLA-C genes influence the risk of preeclampsia and reproductive success. J Exp Med 200:957–965
127. Hiby SE et al (2011) Maternal activating KIRs protect against human reproductive failure mediated by fetal HLA-C2. J Clin Invest 120:4102–4110
128. Terme M et al (2008) Natural killer cell-directed therapies: moving from unexpected results to successful strategies. Nat Immunol 9:486–494
129. Levinson RD et al (2010) Killer cell immunoglobulin-like receptor gene-cluster 3DS1-2DL5-2DS1-2DS5 predisposes susceptibility to Vogt-Koyanagi-Harada syndrome in Japanese individuals. Hum Immunol 71:192–194
130. Lopez-Vazquez A et al (2005) Protective effect of the HLA-Bw4I80 epitope and the killer cell immunoglobulin-like receptor 3DS1 gene against the development of hepatocellular carcinoma in patients with hepatitis C virus infection. J Infect Dis 192:162–165
131. Bonagura VR et al (2010) Activating killer cell immunoglobulin-like receptors 3DS1 and 2DS1 protect against developing the severe form of recurrent respiratory papillomatosis. Hum Immunol 71:212–219
132. Carrington M et al (2005) Hierarchy of resistance to cervical neoplasia mediated by combinations of killer immunoglobulin-like receptor and human leukocyte antigen loci. J Exp Med 201:1069–1075
133. Appelbaum FR (2003) The current status of hematopoietic cell transplantation. Annu Rev Med 54:491–512
134. Ruggeri L et al (2002) Effectiveness of donor natural killer cell alloreactivity in mismatched hematopoietic transplants. Science 295: 2097–2100
135. Giebel S et al (2003) Survival advantage with KIR ligand incompatibility in hematopoietic stem cell transplantation from unrelated donors. Blood 102:814–819
136. Davies SM et al (2002) Evaluation of KIR ligand incompatibility in mismatched unrelated donor hematopoietic transplants. Killer immunoglobulin-like receptor. Blood 100: 3825–3827
137. Kawase T et al (2009) HLA mismatch combinations associated with decreased risk of relapse: implications for the molecular mechanism. Blood 113:2851–2858
138. Clausen J et al (2007) Impact of natural killer cell dose and donor killer-cell immunoglobulin-like receptor (KIR) genotype on outcome following human leucocyte antigen-identical haematopoietic stem cell transplantation. Clin Exp Immunol 148:520–528
139. Willemze R et al (2009) KIR-ligand incompatibility in the graft-versus-host direction improves outcomes after umbilical cord blood transplantation for acute leukemia. Leukemia 23:492–500

140. Pende D et al (2009) Anti-leukemia activity of alloreactive NK cells in KIR ligand-mismatched haploidentical HSCT for pediatric patients: evaluation of the functional role of activating KIR and redefinition of inhibitory KIR specificity. Blood 113:3119–3129
141. Lowe EJ et al (2003) T-cell alloreactivity dominates natural killer cell alloreactivity in minimally T-cell–depleted HLA-non-identical paediatric bone marrow transplantation. Br J Haematol 123:23–326
142. Farag SS et al (2006) The effect of KIR ligand incompatibility on the outcome of unrelated donor transplantation: a report from the center for international blood and marrow transplant research, the European blood and marrow transplant registry, and the Dutch registry. Biol Blood Marrow Transplant 12: 876–884
143. Cooley S et al (2010) Donor selection for natural killer cell receptor genes leads to superior survival after unrelated transplantation for acute myelogenous leukemia. Blood 116: 2411–2419
144. Venstrom JM et al (2010) Donor activating KIR3DS1 is associated with decreased acute GVHD in unrelated allogeneic hematopoietic stem cell transplantation. Blood 115: 3162–3165
145. Sivori S et al (2011) Natural killer cells expressing the KIR2DS1-activating receptor efficiently kill T-cell blasts and dendritic cells: implications in haploidentical HSCT. Blood 117:4284–4292

# Chapter 24

# KIR Typing by Non-Sequencing Methods: Polymerase-Chain Reaction with Sequence-Specific Primers

**David Ordóñez, Manuela Moraru, Natalia Gómez-Lozano, Elisa Cisneros, and Carlos Vilches**

## Abstract

The killer-cell immunoglobulin-like receptors (KIR), which enable NK cells to detect allogeneic target cells and abnormalities in the expression of self-HLA molecules, are encoded by genes that display extensive copy number variation. These variations in the *KIR* genotype are relevant for multiple aspects of human health, including therapy of cancer. PCR with sequence-specific primers (SSP) is simplest and most widely used among techniques for studying *KIR* genotypes. Here, we present a protocol that details the critical steps of a method for *KIR* genotyping by PCR-SSP.

**Key words:** Alloreactivity, Copy number variation, Electrophoresis, Genotyping, Killer-cell immunoglobulin-like receptors, Hemopoietic transplant, HLA, Natural killer cells, PCR, Quality assurance

## 1. Introduction

### 1.1. Background

Killer-cell immunoglobulin-like receptors (KIR) provide NK cells with the capacity of surveying normal expression of MHC class I molecules, frequently altered in intracellular infection and tumours (1). Human KIR are encoded in chromosome 19 by a gene complex that displays extensive copy number variation—most commonly, an individual lacks one or more *KIR* genes, and, conversely, some chromosomes carry *KIR*-gene duplications (2–4). Certain arrangements of *KIR* genes, or haplotypes, are more common than others, their frequencies varying in different populations and ethnic groups. Variability of *KIR* genotypes influences human health in several ways, and is consistent with selective pressures having favoured functional diversification of KIR in manners and degrees that resemble those of their HLA ligands.

Frank T. Christiansen and Brian D. Tait (eds.), *Immunogenetics: Methods and Applications in Clinical Practice*, Methods in Molecular Biology, vol. 882, DOI 10.1007/978-1-61779-842-9_24, © Springer Science+Business Media New York 2012

### 1.2. Role of KIR Genotyping in the Clinical Context

#### 1.2.1. Exploiting NK-Cell Alloreactivity Against Cancer

NK cells kill target cells that lack HLA ligands for the inhibitory receptors of the NK cell, as it often happens in tumours and infected cells. Killing can also occur when an NK cell meets an allogeneic target that lacks one or more of the polymorphic HLA epitopes that "educated" or "licensed" the NK cell. This phenomenon has been proposed to mediate beneficial effects on patient survival, and on graft vs. host and leukaemia-relapse rates after hemopoietic transplant from non-HLA identical donors (5). Similarly, adoptive transfer of allogeneic NK cells is a promising form of immunotherapy against cancer. In both clinical settings, selection of the appropriate donors requires identification of the HLA epitopes recognised by the inhibitory KIR 2DL1, 2DL2/2DL3, 3DL1, and 3DL2 (lysine-80 of HLA-C; asparagine-80 of HLA-C; the Bw4 motif of HLA-B and HLA-A; and alleles HLA-A*03 and -A*11, respectively). Furthermore, because NK-cell alloreactivity is based on the presence in the allogeneic NK cells of certain inhibitory KIR, optimal donor selection for transplant or adoptive NK-cell therapy should include KIR genotyping (and, if possible, surface KIR phenotyping by flow cytometry) to ensure that the necessary receptors are included in the donor KIR repertoire.

Independently of the predictable NK-cell alloreactivity determined by mismatch between the HLA epitopes of donors and recipients, some transplant centres have observed that patients transplanted from donors carrying certain combinations of *KIR* genes have better outcomes than patients who received hemopoietic transplants from donors that lacked those genes (6). According to this, *KIR* genotyping should be part of the protocol for donor selection.

#### 1.2.2. Other Clinical Conditions

KIR polymorphisms can influence multiple aspects of human health, including at least: (a) reproduction and its complications; (b) chronic infection; (c) inflammatory disease and autoimmunity; (d) solid organ transplant; and (e) tumours. In none of these clinical settings is *KIR* genotyping yet unanimously accepted as a part of decision making for patient care. Further research is needed to understand how KIR participate in the physiopathology of those processes, which should allow for predictive models of clinical outcomes based on the patient *KIR* genotype, and also for therapies based on a more comprehensive knowledge of NK-cell physiology. In addition, subsequent studies will likely identify new diseases in which risk or clinical course is influenced by the diversity of *KIR* genotypes.

### 1.3. KIR Typing Using a PCR-SSP Method

The diversity of *KIR* genotypes was discovered by means of a polymerase-chain reaction with sequence-specific primers (PCR-SSP) technique that detected distinctive motifs of each *KIR* gene (7). Different PCR-SSP methods are still most widely used for exploring the genetic diversity of KIR. Here, we provide a detailed protocol for performing a PCR-SSP method for *KIR* genotyping that amplifies short DNA fragments (8). The method comprises 16 reactions, one of them multiplexed, that enable quick and simple detection of all *KIR* genes and pseudogenes.

## 2. Materials

### 2.1. Special Equipment

1. Electronic repetitive pipettors (e.g. EDP-1 or -3 from Rainin) can be programmed to dispense multiple aliquots of the desired volume after a single aspiration step. They are of extraordinary help for dispensing primer mixes and liquid wax into typing sets; DNA:buffer:Taq mixes for PCR setup; and the loading dye to processed reactions before electrophoresis.
2. Thermal cycler with a 96-well block. We have used models PTC-100 and PTC-200 from MJR, and models 2720 and Veriti 96-Well from Applied Biosystems.
3. Electrophoresis system. A horizontal electrophoresis chamber with a tray that accommodates six 17- or 18-well combs enables genotyping six DNAs (96 reactions) in a single run (16 reactions and 1 or 2 size markers per row). Moreover, multichannel pipette-compatible combs greatly speed up the loading of a full gel (see Notes 1 and 2).
4. A multichannel pipettor in the 0.5–10.0 μL range (e.g. CAPP) for gel loading (see Note 3).

### 2.2. Consumables and Reagents

1. Strips of eight attached 0.2-mL PCR microtubes are the most convenient format. The primer set for typing one DNA will comprise two such strips (16 reactions).
2. The oligonucleotides primers used in this method have been described previously (8). Standard quality (desalted) oligonucleotides are sufficient.
3. Polymerases: regular Taq polymerase is fine; hot start is not necessary (see Note 4). Proof-reading polymerases with 3′–5′ exonuclease activity must not be used for PCR-SSP.
4. Other speciality reagents: Chill-out red Liquid Wax (Bio-Rad) for storage of aliquoted primer mixes; store at room temperature or 4°C.

## 3. Methods

### 3.1. Prepare Primer Mixes

1. These primer sets (Tables 1 and 2), designed in 2007 (8), detected all 168 KIR alleles of the KIR-IPD database release 1.4.0 (http://www.ebi.ac.uk/ipd/kir/). Current release of the database (2.3.0) includes 614 alleles: 608 are still detected

**Table 1**
**Chart for preparing primer mixes for *KIR* genotyping**

| | | | | Forward primer, 100 μM | | Reverse primer, 100 μM | |
|---|---|---|---|---|---|---|---|
| **Mix** | **Gene** | **Water (μL)** | **IPC283 (μL)** | **Name** | **Volume (μL)** | **Name** | **Volume (μL)** |
| 1 | *KIR2DL1* | 925.0 | 50 | Fa517[a] | 12.5 | Rc621 | 12.5 |
| 2 | *KIR2DL2* | 825.0 | 50 | Fcon750 | 62.5 | Rt854 | 62.5 |
| 3 | *KIR2DL3* | 825.0 | 50 | Fcon1254 | 62.5 | Rt1375 | 62.5 |
| 4 | *KIR3DL1* | 762.5 | 50 | Ft624<br>Ftt624 | 62.5<br>62.5 | Rt697 | 62.5 |
| 5 | *KIR3DL2* | 932.5 | 50 | Fg864 | 12.5 | Rc962 | 5.0 |
| 6 | *KIR2DS1* | 762.5 | 50 | Fg621<br>Fa621b | 62.5<br>62.5 | Rcon682 | 62.5 |
| 7 | *KIR2DS2* | 825.0 | 50 | Fa546 | 62.5 | Rcon621 | 62.5 |
| 8 | *KIR2DS3* | 887.5 | 50 | Ft803[a] | 31.25 | Ra925 | 31.25 |
| 9 | *KIR2DS4* | 825.0 | 50 | Fat781 | 62.5 | Rca877 | 62.5 |
| 10 | *KIR2DS5* | 825.0 | 50 | Fc551 | 62.5 | Rcon662 | 62.5 |
| 11 | *KIR3DS1* | 762.5 | 50 | Fg624<br>Fg624b | 62.5<br>62.5 | Rt697 | 62.5 |
| 12 | *KIR2DP1* | 918.8 | 50 | Fc567 | 15.62 | Rdel674 | 15.62 |
| 13 | *KIR3DL3*<br>*KIR3DX1* | 700.0 | 50 | Fg510<br>Fma920 | 62.5<br>62.5 | Rta669b<br>Rdel967b | 62.5<br>62.5 |
| 14 | *KIR2DL4* | 825.0 | 50 | Ftgc157b | 62.5 | Rga250b | 62.5 |
| 15 | *KIR2DL5* | 887.5 | 50 | Fag843 | 31.25 | Rc953 | 31.25 |
| 16 | *KIR3DP1* | 856.3 | IPC608: 50 μL | Fi2–89<br>Fa–97b | 31.25<br>31.25 | Rg287 | 31.25 |

[a]See Note 5

by the correct primer mix; none is predicted to cross-react with a wrong mix; and six new alleles are missed—*2DL1*013N*, *2DL2*009*, *2DL3*010* and **017*, *2DS3*004*, and *3DL1*054* (see Note 5).

2. Dissolve all your lyophilised primers at 100 μM in 10 mM Tris–HCl pH 8.0 (e.g. if you receive 78.6 nmol of a given primer, add 786 μL solvent) (primers will be more stable at pH 8 than dissolved in $H_2O$).
3. Prepare a primer mix for the 283-bp internal positive control (IPC) by combining 720 μL $H_2O$, 40 μL 100 μM FDRA360,

**Table 2**
**Oligonucleotide primers for *KIR* typing by PCR-SSP (8) (primers sequences reproduced with permission from John Wiley and Sons)**

| Primer name | Sequence |
|---|---|
| Fa–97b | gtacgtcaccctcccatgatgta |
| Fi2–89 | gtgtggtaggagccttag |
| Ftgc157b | tcaggacaagcccttctgc |
| Fg510 | aatgttggtcagatgtcag |
| Fa517 | gttggtcagatgtcatgtttgaa |
| Fa546 | tgcacagagaggggaagta |
| Fc551 | agagaggggacgtttaacc |
| Fc567 | cgacactttgcacctcac |
| Fg621 | tctccatcagtcgcatgag |
| Fa621b | tctccatcagtcgcatgaa |
| Fg624 | catcggttccatgatgcg |
| Fg624b | catcagttccatgatgcg |
| Ft624 | ccatyggtcccatgatgct |
| Ftt624 | tccatcggtcccatgatgtt |
| Fcon750 | aaaccttctctctcagccca |
| Fat781 | ggttcaggcaggagagaat |
| Ft803 | cttgtcctgcagctcct |
| Fag843 | atctatccagggaggggag |
| Fg864 | catgaacgtaggctccg |
| Fma920 | tttctgtgggccgtgcaa |
| Fcon1254 | agaccctcaggaggtga |
| Rga250b | ggacagggaccccatcttc |
| Rg287 | gaaaacggtgtttcggaatac |
| Rc621 | cctgccaggtcttgcg |
| Rcon621 | ccctgcaaggtcttgca |
| Rcon662 | ctgatagggggagtgagt |
| Rta669b | gcygacaactcatagggta |
| Rdel674 | gggagctgacaactgatg |
| Rcon682 | ggtcactgggagctgac |

(continued)

**Table 2 (continued)**

| Primer name | Sequence |
|---|---|
| Rt697 | ccacgatgtccagggga |
| Rt854 | gccctgcagagaacctaca |
| Rca877 | ctggaatgttccgtkgatg |
| Ra925 | gcatctgtaggttcctcct |
| Rc953 | catagggtgagtcatggag |
| Rc962 | gaccacacgcagggcag |
| Rdel967b | gtcactgggggcttatag |
| Rt1375 | caggagacaactttggatca |
| FDRA360 | gaggtaactgtgctcacgaacagc |
| RDRA595 | ggtccataccccagtgcttgagaag |
| RDRA633 | cacgttctctgtagtctctggg |

and 40 μL 100 μM RDRA595 (each primer will be at 5 μM). This volume will be enough for preparing all primer mixes 1–15 described in Table 1. Label it IPC283.

4. For primer mix 16, you will use 50 μL of an oligonucleotide pair for a 608 bp IPC. You can prepare it in advance (e.g. 45 μL $H_2O$, 2.5 μL 100 μM FDRA360, and 2.5 μL 100 μM RDRA633, or scaled-up volumes), and label it IPC608; or add its components directly when you prepare primer mix 16.
5. Prepare primer mixes 1–16 according to Table 1. Store all primer mixes and stocks at −20°C or below.

### 3.2. Prepare Sets of Ready-to-Use PCR Primers in Strips

A stock of ready-to-use primer mixes, pre-aliquoted into two 8-tube strips, will allow you to determine quickly the *KIR* genotypes of any number DNA samples as soon as you receive them.

1. Prepare an appropriate number of 0.2 mL, 8-tube strips (e.g. 24–48, see Note 6) and set them in 96-well trays (empty tip cases are handy). Mark the left side of each strip with *one* dot or line—this tube will hold reaction 1. Mark an identical number of strips with *two* dots or lines—the labelled tube will be reaction 9.
2. Thaw primer mixes 1–8, and homogenise them by inversion.
3. Using an electronic repetitive pipettor, dispense 4 μL primer mix 1 in tube 1 of all strips. Follow with reactions 2–8.
4. Using an electronic repetitive pipettor, overlay the mixes with 5–7 μL Chill-out red Liquid Wax (see Note 7 and Fig. 1).

5. Cap one of every eight strips, stack groups of eight strips, and lay them into one or more boxes (again, empty cases of 1,000-μL tip racks are handy) (Fig. 2 and video in http://www.yotube.com/watch?v=8wU55yu-BgA). You can hold the strips

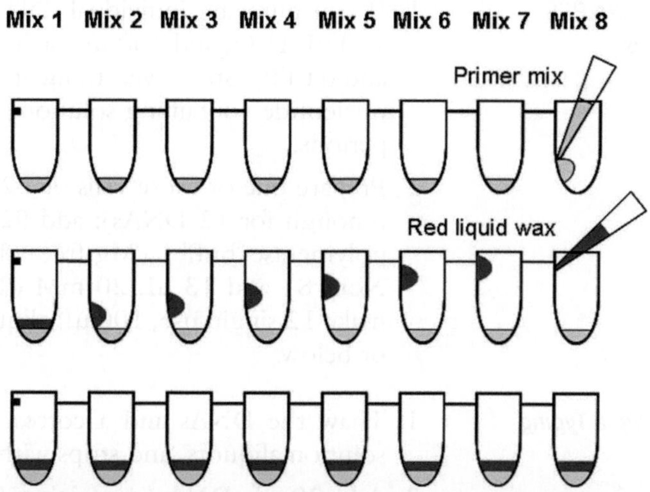


Fig. 1. A few microliters of liquid wax laid over the aliquoted primer mixes avoid their evaporation during long-term storage in the freezer.

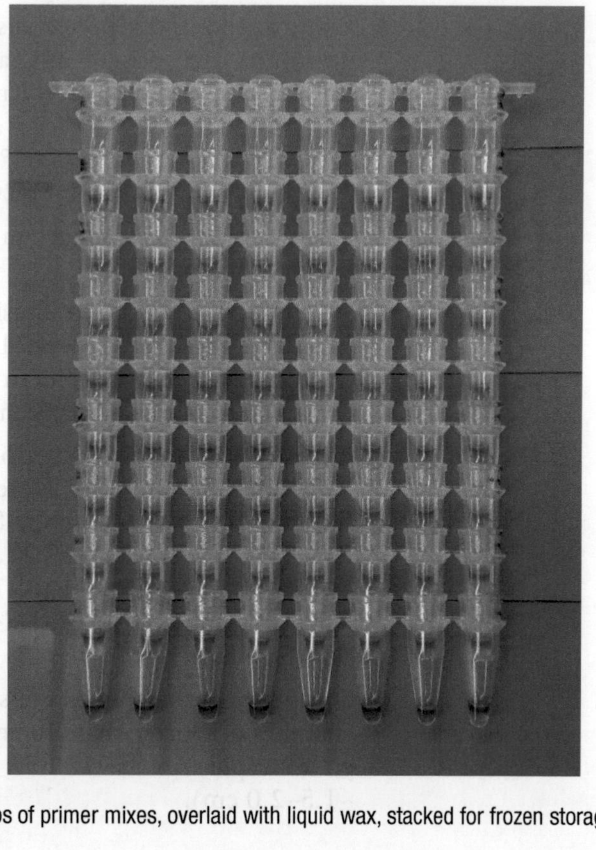

Fig. 2. Strips of primer mixes, overlaid with liquid wax, stacked for frozen storage.

together with small rubber bands, which will avoid accidental loss of their frozen content during storage and manipulation. Label the boxes "KIR typing, strip 1", and store them frozen.

6. Repeat steps 2–5 for primer mixes 9–16.

### 3.3. Prepare PCR Solutions

1. If you purchase individual dNTPs, make a 20 mM mix (e.g. 100 μL $H_2O$, and 100 μL each 100 mM dATP, dCTP, dGTP, and dTTP). Store everything at –20°C or below. Do not leave nucleotide-containing solutions at room temperature for long periods.
2. Prepare one or more vials of a 2×-concentrated PCR solution (enough for 12 DNAs): add 923 μL $H_2O$, 260 μL 10× Taq polymerase buffer (Mg-free), 104 μL 50 mM $MgCl_2$ (see Note 8), and 13 μL 20 mM dNTPs. Mix well by inversion, make 12 single-use, 100 μL aliquots, and store them at –20°C or below.

### 3.4. Setup a Typing Assay

1. Thaw the DNAs and a corresponding number of 2× PCR-solution aliquots, and strips with pre-dispensed primer mixes.
2. Add 20 μL DNA (containing 0.2–3.0 μg, see Note 9) and 1.2 μL Taq (5 U/μL) to a 100 μL aliquot of 2× PCR solution, and mix thoroughly. Prepare as many similar mixes as DNAs you have to analyse (six is a convenient number).
3. Using a repetitive pipettor, dispense 6 μL aliquots of this solution onto each primer mix, and cap the strips tightly. Make sure that reagents have fallen to the tube bottoms, transfer the strips to the thermocycler, and start cycling (denaturation at 95°C, 2 min; 10 cycles of 94°C, 10 s, and 65°C, 40 s; and 20 cycles of 94°C, 20 s, 61°C, 20 s, and 72°C, 30 s).
4. Prepare a 2% agarose gel in your preferred electrophoresis buffer.
5. When thermocycling has finished, add 10 μL of a 2×-concentrated loading dye (see Note 10) to the wall of each tube using an electronic repetitive pipettor, and let the dye fall to the bottom. The same pipette tip can be used for all reactions.
6. Load 10 μL of each reaction in the agarose gel, using an 8-channel pipettor (see Notes 11–13 and video in http://www.youtube.com/watch?v=8wU55yu-BgA). Leave an empty well between strips 1 and 2, and load in it ~300 ng of a size marker that covers the range 100–600 bp. Save the remaining reaction volume for *KIR2DS4* subtyping (see Note 14) or for possible reanalysis.
7. Set the power supply to constant 200 V (or 9 V/cm if your chamber is shorter than 20 cm) with no current limit, and let your samples run 10–15 min (bromophenol blue will migrate ~1.5–2.0 cm).

8. Stain the gel 15–20 min in ethidium bromide, or, preferably, a non-toxic alternative (e.g. GelRed from Biotium or SYBR Safe from Invitrogen), reveal by UV exposure, and photograph.

### 3.5. Quality Control

1. Contamination tests. Before you use your 2× PCR solution and *KIR*-typing sets, you should verify that they are not contaminated with DNA. To that end, run one typing assay in which you substitute 20 μL $H_2O$ for the DNA, and make sure that you see no amplification bands (other than possible primer multimers). If you prepare single-use aliquots of all reagents (namely, the 2× PCR solution, and the primer-mix strips), you only have to test periodically that your Taq polymerase is not contaminated. To that end, you can perform a single-tube PCR using the 283 bp IPC primers: these will detect contamination with genomic DNA or with any product derived from the 16 reactions of the *KIR* typing set.
2. Reference samples. It is advisable to control that the method is working properly on reference DNAs with known KIR genotypes (9). You can obtain reference DNAs from another lab, or purchase them from a repository of well-characterised cell lines (e.g. http://www.hpacultures.org.uk/collections/ecacc.jsp). In addition, you can test your proficiency by participating in a DNA exchange, such as those organised by UCLA (http://www.hla.ucla.edu/cellDna.htm).

### 3.6. Interpretation Hints, Potential Errors

1. Acceptability of results.
   (a) *IPC.* Each reaction should yield one or more PCR products. If one or more mixes yield no amplification product of the correct size, those particular reactions must not be interpreted (i.e. they are neither negative nor positive). An IPC band will appear in most or all reactions: in mixes 1–15, it will migrate just below 300 bp (or above if you prefer to see your gels with the wells in the bottom); and at approximately 600 bp in mix 16. In the presence of a strong specific band, the IPC band may disappear, which shall not be considered a reaction failure, but a positive result.
   (b) *KIR-gene-specific bands: size.* All specific bands will have smaller sizes than their IPCs in this method, which helps avoid falsely negative results in partially degraded DNA (8). A reaction will be considered positive when you see a neat band of the correct size, which varies according to the primer mix (see Table 3 and Note 15). If no bands other than the IPC are seen, or if any other bands have the wrong size (an indication that the PCR conditions need optimization), the reaction is negative. Small-size specific amplicons (e.g. those derived from *KIR2DS1*, 96 bp, and

**Table 3**
**Amplicon sizes (8)**

| Mix | Gene | Amplicon length (bp) |
|---|---|---|
| 1 | *KIR2DL1* | 142 |
| 2 | *KIR2DL2* | 142 |
| 3 | *KIR2DL3* | 156 |
| 4 | *KIR3DL1* | 108/109 |
| 5 | *KIR3DL2* | 131 |
| 6 | *KIR2DS1* | 96 |
| 7 | *KIR2DS2* | 110 |
| 8 | *KIR2DS3* | 158 |
| 9 | *KIR2DS4* (canonical)<br>*KIR2DS4* (exon 5-deleted) | 133<br>111 |
| 10 | *KIR2DS5* | 147 |
| 11 | *KIR3DS1* | 107 |
| 12 | *KIR2DP1* | 141 |
| 13 | *KIR3DL3*<br>*KIR3DX1* | 196<br>88 |
| 14 | *KIR2DL4* | 131 |
| 15 | *KIR2DL5* | 147 |
| 16 | *KIR3DP1* (canonical)<br>*KIR3DP1* (exon 2-deleted) | 279<br>398 |
| 1–15 | Internal positive control | 283 |
| 16 | Internal positive control | 608 |

*KIR3DX1*, 88 bp) must not be confused with primer multimers that migrate with just faster mobility.

(c) *KIR-gene-specific bands: intensity.* Specific amplicons should be of greater or similar intensity than the IPC band; weak amplicons of the correct size should not be seen. Should such weak reactivities appear, they must not be considered definitely positive or negative, and they are an indication to repeat that test, and, in case they occur frequently, to adjust the amplification conditions (reagents stability and concentration, polymerase performance, thermalcycler calibration, etc.).

2. Knowledge on the organisation of *KIR* genes will also help troubleshoot your results (see Note 16):
   (a) The genes *KIR3DL3* and *KIR3DX1* are seemingly present in all humans.
   (b) *KIR3DL2*, in the telomeric end of the *KIR* complex, and two genes in its middle, *KIR3DP1* and *KIR2DL4*, are also very well conserved. Exceptions are: deletions of the *KIR*-complex central region, and haplotypes carrying chimeras of *KIR3DL1* and *KIR3DL2*, which will lack the latter gene. Both traits are more common in Black populations.
   (c) Some pairs of genes are normally inherited as alleles of the same conserved locus: *KIR3DL1* and *KIR3DS1*; *KIR2DL3* and *KIR2DL2*; *KIR2DS1* and *KIR2DS4*. Therefore, the vast majority of haplotypes contain one or both members of those pairs. However, the aforementioned deletions of the central *KIR* genes often affect *KIR3DL1/KIR3DS1*; and haplotypes that contain a *KIR3DL1/KIR3DL2* chimera could lack the intervening *KIR2DS1/KIR2DS4* locus.
   (d) Some genes are infrequently seen in the absence of certain others: *KIR2DS2* and *KIR2DL2*; *KIR2DL1* and *KIR2DP1*; *KIR2DL3* and the latter two genes (which, in turn, are not uncommon in the absence of *KIR2DL3*); *KIR3DL1* and *KIR2DS4*; *KIR2DL5* and either *KIR2DS3* or *KIR2DS5*; *KIR3DS1* and the *KIR2DL5-KIR2DS3/S5-KIR2DS1* cluster. Again, exceptions to these associations, derived from recombinant haplotypes created by unequal crossing-over events, are not rare in some populations.

### 3.7. Other KIR Typing Methods

1. Variations of PCR-SSP.
   (a) The PCR-SSP technique can discriminate between sequences that differ by a single nucleotide substitution; therefore, it can be used, not only for detecting presence or absence of a *KIR* gene, but also for allelic typing (9).
   (b) PCR-SSP typing comprises multiple amplification reactions, and uses more DNA than methods based on a single PCR. To minimise the use of DNA, whole genome amplification can be performed before *KIR* typing by PCR-SSP (10).
   (c) Multiplexing (i.e. including multiple primer pairs that will produce distinguishable amplicons from two or more *KIR* genes in the same reaction) also helps reduce reagent and DNA expense by limiting the number of reactions, but it needs extra optimisation to avoid preferential amplification of certain genes. Our method includes one multiplexed reaction (number 13, for *KIR3DL3* and *KIR3DX1*), and

complete *KIR* typing methods based on this principle have been reported (11–13).

(d) PCR-SSP can be adapted to real-time technology in order to eliminate post-PCR processing and reduce DNA expense (14).

(e) The PCR-SSP principle can also be applied to cDNA to determine the *KIR* genes expressed by an NK- or T-cell clone or subpopulation (7, 15). Lack of IPC bands in RT-PCR-SSP techniques makes more difficult (in comparison with assays on genomic DNA) to detect possible failure of individual reactions within an assay.

2. Probe hybridization of *KIR* amplicons has also been used to determine *KIR* geno- and allotypes. Both the classical PCR-SSOP (hybridization of labelled probes to immobilised PCR products) and the fluorescent bead-attached probe formats have been reported (16–18), and they facilitate the analysis of high numbers of samples.

3. Other non-sequencing methods for analysis of *KIR* polymorphism.

(a) High resolution melting analysis after real-time PCR can discriminate between amplicons differing at a single nucleotide and has been used to type for *KIR2DS4*, *KIR2DL4*, and *KIR3DL2* alleles (19).

(b) Differences in the spatial conformation (thus, the electrophoretic mobility) of slightly different sequences are the basis for sequence-specific conformational polymorphism analysis (SSCP). This technique, in combination with capillary electrophoresis in an automated DNA sequencer has been applied to allelic typing of *KIR2DL4* alleles (20).

(c) MALDI-TOF mass spectrometry is a powerful, high-throughput technique that exploits small differences in the molecular mass to discriminate between similar DNA sequences. Mass spectrometry has been used for both generic and allelic typing of *KIR* genes, and for identifying novel *KIR* alleles (21).

## 4. Notes

1. Appropriate electrophoresis systems can be obtained from a few providers (e.g. 96Q High Throughput PCR Sub System, from Denville Scientific; horizontal systems from CBS Scientific; SUB25C from Hoefer; and Sub-Cell Model 192 from Bio-Rad). A power supply should provide constant voltage of 200 V and support 100–200 mA (current varies with the electrophoresis

chamber; you will need twice as much current—not voltage—if you plan to run two chambers in parallel).

2. Make sure that the gel will fit in your UV-transilluminator screen.
3. Do not use higher volume multichannel pipettors (e.g. 5.0–50.0 μL), they will spill your PCR products.
4. We use BioTaq from Bioline (UK), or Ecotaq from a local provider, both with an $NH_4$-based buffer (10×: 160 mM $(NH_4)_2SO_4$, 670 mM Tris–HCl (pH 8.8 at 25°C), 0.1% Tween-20). For other brands and 10× buffers you may need to adjust the amount of Taq and $MgCl_2$ concentration (see Note 3). With some KCl-buffer formulations, the IPC band may be amplified preferentially over the specific bands (which, in extreme situations, will result in false negatives).
5. Substitution of a new primer (Fy803, cttgtcctgmagctccy) for Ft803 in mix 8 would suffice for detecting all *KIR2DS3* alleles. Adding a new primer (Fa517b, gttggtcagatgtcatgttttaa) to mix 1 (besides Fa517 and Rc621) should ensure detection of *2DL1*013N* (you may not want to detect a null *KIR2DL1* allele in certain cases, though). Detecting the four new other alleles would require substantial modifications to the method design.
6. Primer-strips preparation is a tedious task; once you set to it, you may want to prepare a generous amount of strips. We strongly discourage preparing a primer set for just one or a few DNAs: in the long term, you will waste an enormous amount of time and pipette tips, and your primer stocks will suffer an unnecessarily high number of freeze-thaw cycles, favouring both degradation and contamination. Preparing 48 typing sets from primer mixes will take ~30–40 min.
7. You need not change the tip if you dispense the wax on the tube wall. The wax (liquid at room temperature and solid below 10°C) forms a red meniscus on top of the primer mixes (Fig. 1), and minimises evaporation during long-term storage in the freezer. If you plan to use all your strips in less than 2–4 weeks, you need not use wax.
8. The 2× concentrated PCR solution serves several purposes: (a) it avoids repeated reagent thawing and freezing, (b) reduces contaminations, and (c) increases reproducibility by minimising pipetting steps and errors. If your 10× Taq polymerase buffer contains 15 mM $MgCl_2$, add only 26 μL 50 mM $MgCl_2$ (instead of 104 μL) and increase water to 1,001 μL. Volumes can be scaled up using devices appropriate for the volumes to be pipetted.
9. We adjust DNA concentration at ~50–150 ng/μL, but the method can work with good quality DNA as diluted as 10 ng/μL.

Within that DNA concentration range (10–150 ng/μL) you need not adjust the 20 μL DNA volume in the mix. We have analysed DNAs isolated from peripheral blood, spleen and lymph node lymphocytes, paraffin-embedded tissue, and mouth wash, using salting-out methods, DNAzol (MRC), and a Maxwell-16 machine (Promega).

10. Prepare a 2×-concentrated loading dye by diluting a 6×- or 10×-concentrated loading dye with an appropriate volume of $H_2O$ or electrophoresis buffer (e.g. 0.67 mL of a 6× loading dye, and 1.33 mL $H_2O$; 160 μL of this solution are needed for each *KIR* typing). Increasing the reaction volume right before electrophoresis facilitates aspiration of the sample with the multichannel pipettor, and loading it into the gel wells. If you did not use wax, just add 1.0–1.5 μL of the 6×- or 10×-concentrated loading dye to each tube, and load 5 μL into each well.
11. You need not remove the red wax, just aspirate the reaction underneath. The electrophoresis buffer will get somewhat oleaginous, and you will have to change it periodically, but it does not affect migration. Should you feel uncomfortable in the beginning with pipetting below the wax meniscus, reduce the amount of wax to 3 μL in Subheading 3.2, step 4, harden the wax by putting the strips on ice, and poke the pipette tips through the thin hardened wax film.
12. Make sure that the ends of the tips inserted in the multichannel pipettor are well aligned—any misaligned tip will add difficulty to the loading process.
13. You need not change the pipette tips after each loading step. Instead, wash them by pipetting two or three times in the electrophoresis buffer before aspirating the next strip. The degree of contamination between samples with this procedure is undetectable (unless you want to re-amplify a PCR product for any reason), and you will save a considerable amount of time (and pipette tips).
14. Canonical and exon-5-deletion carrying *KIR2DS4* alleles can be distinguished from each other by their different amplicon sizes (133 bp vs. 111 bp, respectively). This is easiest if you run in parallel reaction 9 of multiple DNAs, which facilitates comparing amplicon sizes. To this end, load the remaining 5 μL of reaction 9 in a 2.0–2.5% agarose gel and allow a longer run (e.g. 25 min at 200 V) before staining and photographing. This can also be done in a smaller electrophoresis chamber at lower voltage.
15. Amplicon sizes in reactions 9 and 16 allow for discrimination between major structural allotypes of *KIR2DS4* and *KIR3DP1*, respectively (6).

16. None of the following indications on *KIR*-gene organisation is an absolute rule, and you will probably meet occasional exceptions when you type multiple individuals. However, you should pay attention to any exceptions because they may indicate either that you have found some interesting genotypes, or that there is a typing error. In either case, some extra work is warranted before accepting unusual genotypes (e.g. revising the results, repeating the test with the same or an alternative method, checking reagents integrity, optimising the typing procedure, et cetera). Our initial approach to deal with unusual *KIR* genotypes is, first, to repeat the test, and, second, to use a previously published PCR-SSP method that uses different primer combinations (7).

## Acknowledgements

This work was supported by grant SAF2010-22153-C03-03 from the Spanish *Ministerio de Ciencia e Innovación*. DO was supported by a grant from "Fundación LAIR". NGL is supported by a grant from Instituto de Salud Carlos III (CP09/182). The authors have no conflicts of interest.

### References

1. Wagtmann N et al (1995) Molecular clones of the p58 NK cell receptor reveal immunoglobulin-related molecules with diversity in both the extra- and intracellular domains. Immunity 2:439–449
2. Vilches C, Parham P (2002) KIR: diverse, rapidly evolving receptors of innate and adaptive immunity. Annu Rev Immunol 20:217–251
3. Gómez-Lozano N et al (2005) The silent KIR3DP1 gene (CD158c) is transcribed and might encode a secreted receptor in a minority of humans, in whom the KIR3DP1, KIR2DL4 and KIR3DL1/KIR3DS1 genes are duplicated. Eur J Immunol 35:16–24
4. Ordonez D et al (2008) Duplication, mutation and recombination of the human orphan gene KIR2DS3 contribute to the diversity of KIR haplotypes. Genes Immun 9:431–437
5. Velardi A et al (2009) Natural killer cell allorecognition of missing self in allogeneic hematopoietic transplantation: a tool for immunotherapy of leukemia. Curr Opin Immunol 21: 525–530
6. Cooley S et al (2010) Donor selection for natural killer cell receptor genes leads to superior survival after unrelated transplantation for acute myelogenous leukemia. Blood 116:2411–2419
7. Uhrberg M et al (1997) Human diversity in killer cell inhibitory receptor genes. Immunity 7:753–763
8. Vilches C et al (2007) Facilitation of KIR genotyping by a PCR-SSP method that amplifies short DNA fragments. Tissue Antigens 70:415–422
9. Gómez-Lozano N, Vilches C (2002) Genotyping of human killer-cell immunoglobulin-like receptor genes by polymerase chain reaction with sequence-specific primers: an update. Tissue Antigens 59:184–193
10. Chainonthee W et al (2010) Improved KIR gene and HLA-C KIR ligand sequence-specific primer polymerase chain reaction genotyping using whole genome amplification. Tissue Antigens 76:135–143
11. Sun JY et al (2004) Development of a multiplex PCR-SSP method for Killer-cell immunoglobulin-like receptor genotyping. Tissue Antigens 64:462–468
12. Ashouri E et al (2009) A novel duplex SSP-PCR typing method for KIR gene profiling. Tissue Antigens 74:62–67
13. Kulkarni S, Martin MP, Carrington M (2010) KIR genotyping by multiplex PCR-SSP. Methods 612:365–375

14. Alves LG, Rajalingam R, Canavez F (2009) A novel real-time PCR method for KIR genotyping. Tissue Antigens 73:188–191
15. Thompson A et al (2006) An improved RT-PCR method for the detection of killer-cell immunoglobulin-like receptor (KIR) transcripts. Immunogenetics 58:865–872
16. Crum KA et al (2000) Development of a PCR-SSOP approach capable of defining the natural killer cell inhibitory receptor (KIR) gene sequence repertoires. Tissue Antigens 56: 313–326
17. Halfpenny IA et al (2004) Investigation of killer cell immunoglobulin-like receptor gene diversity: IV. KIR3DL1/S1. Hum Immunol 65:602–612
18. Nong T et al (2007) KIR genotyping by reverse sequence-specific oligonucleotide methodology. Tissue Antigens 69(suppl 1):92–95
19. Gonzalez A et al (2009) Killer cell immunoglobulin-like receptor allele discrimination by high-resolution melting. Hum Immunol 70: 858–863
20. Witt CS, Martin A, Christiansen FT (2000) Detection of KIR2DL4 alleles by sequencing and SSCP reveals a common allele with a shortened cytoplasmic tail. Tissue Antigens 56:248–257
21. Houtchens KA et al (2007) High-throughput killer cell immunoglobulin-like receptor genotyping by MALDI-TOF mass spectrometry with discovery of novel alleles. Immunogenetics 59:525–537

# Chapter 25

# Killer Cell Immunoglobulin-Like Receptors (*KIR*) Typing by DNA Sequencing

**Lihua Hou, Minghua Chen, Noriko Steiner, Kanthi Kariyawasam, Jennifer Ng, and Carolyn K. Hurley**

## Abstract

DNA sequencing is a powerful technique for identifying allelic variation within the natural killer cell immunoglobulin-like receptor genes. Because of the relatively large size of the *KIR* genes, each locus is amplified in two or more overlapping segments. Sanger sequencing of each gene from a preparation containing one or two alleles yields a sequence that is used to identify the alleles by comparison with a reference database.

**Key words:** Natural killer cell, Killer immunoglobulin-like receptor, DNA sequencing, Alleles

## 1. Introduction

The human killer cell immunoglobulin-like receptors (KIR) are encoded by 14 genes: *KIR2DL1*, *KIR2DL2*, *KIR2DL3*, *KIR2DL4*, *KIR2DL5*, *KIR2DS1*, *KIR2DS2*, *KIR2DS3*, *KIR2DS4*, *KIR2DS5*, *KIR3DL1*, *KIR3DL2*, *KIR3DL3*, *KIR3DS1* (1). These genes likely arose from gene duplications and unequal crossing over since they share extensive sequence homology. Each gene is divided into 8–9 exons that encode the signal peptide, two or three extracellular domains, stem, transmembrane region, and cytoplasmic tail. The genes are about 9–16 kb in length. The number of *KIR* loci present varies among individuals. For example, some individuals might carry only seven of the 14 *KIR* genes while other individuals might carry 12 of the 14 *KIR* genes. A clear understanding of the *KIR* gene system will be important to understand the basis for the strategies described in this chapter and to correctly interpret the sequencing results.

Frank T. Christiansen and Brian D. Tait (eds.), *Immunogenetics: Methods and Applications in Clinical Practice*, Methods in Molecular Biology, vol. 882, DOI 10.1007/978-1-61779-842-9_25, © Springer Science+Business Media New York 2012

### 1.1. Overview of Methods

This protocol describes the amplification and sequencing of each *KIR* gene from genomic DNA. The polymerase chain reaction is used to obtain two or more overlapping amplicons covering all or most of each gene (Fig. 1). The nucleotide sequences of the exons carried by each amplicon are determined using Sanger sequencing (2) with primers that anneal in the introns and flank each exon. Both alleles of a locus, if present, are sequenced concurrently and the allele assignments made by comparison to a *KIR* reference database. Some loci (*KIR2DL1*, *KIR2DL2*, *KIR2DL3*, *KIR2DL5*, *KIR2DS4*) require special steps in order to obtain unambiguous sequences as described in Table 1. An initial survey of the *KIR* genes present or absent in the sample using sequence-specific priming will provide the information necessary to determine the additional steps required to obtain allele assignments.

### 1.2. Use of Methods in Clinical Practice

The impact of genetic variation in the *KIR* gene complex on the functional activity of NK cells is yet to be fully understood. The presence of specific *KIR* genes has been associated with susceptibility or resistance to infectious and autoimmune diseases and to malignancy (1, 3). In hematopoietic progenitor cell transplantation for acute myelogenous leukemia, a decreased frequency of relapse and infection has been noted in transplants with donors carrying haplotypes with increased numbers of activating *KIR*

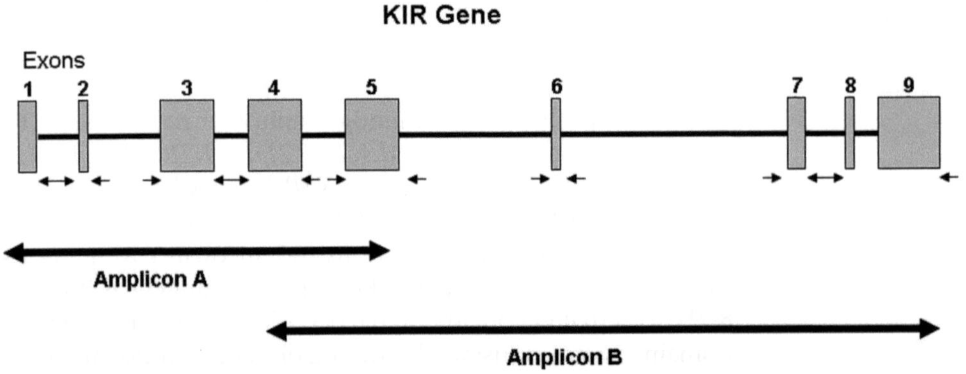


Fig. 1. Amplification of overlapping amplicons covering the *KIR2DL1* coding region sequence. *KIR* genes have eight to nine exons. PCR amplification primers are designed to generate two or more overlapping amplicons. The figure shows the three amplicons, A, B, and A2, that cover the coding sequence of the *KIR2DL1* gene. If the sample does not contain *KIR2DS1*, the laboratory needs only to generate the A and B amplicons for sequencing as described in Table 1. Amplicon A will allow the sequence determination from nucleotide 11 of exon 1 through nucleotide 632 of exon 5; amplicon B will cover nucleotide 332 in exon 4 through the last nucleotide of exon 9. If the sample contains the *KIR2DS1* gene, the laboratory will perform instead three amplifications generating amplicons A, B, and A2. The A2 amplicon will contain only *KIR2DL1* and will provide the sequence covering nucleotide 1 in exon 1 through nucleotide 330 of exon 4. The A amplicon which contains DNA from both *KIR2DL1* and *KIR2DS1* genes will provide sequence information covering the region where the A2 antisense and the B sense primers anneal, i.e., around nucleotide 331 in exon 4. The small arrows under the exons denote the positions of sequencing primers that anneal in the introns and that provide the sequence of both sense and antisense DNA strands for each exon. Tables 2 and 3 list the amplification and sequencing primers for all the *KIR* loci and describe their annealing sites.

**Table 1**
**Summary of amplification protocols for 15 *KIR* Loci[a]**

| Locus | Specific amplification or allele isolation protocol required |
|---|---|
| *KIR2DL1* | Amplicon A—General PCR in Subheading 3.2 with genomic DNA. If *KIR2DS1* is present, it will coamplify with this amplicon. When *KIR2DS1* is present, amplicon A should be characterized to obtain DNA sequence in the area where the antisense A2 and sense B primers anneal (i.e., in region of nucleotide 331)<br>Amplicon A2—General PCR in Subheading 3.2 with genomic DNA. In cells carrying *KIR2DS1*, coamplification of *KIR2DS1* is eliminated in this additional reaction. This amplification is not required if the cell does not carry *KIR2DS1*<br>Amplicon B—General PCR in Subheading 3.2 with genomic DNA |
| *KIR2DL2* | Amplicon A—General PCR in Subheading 3.2 with genomic DNA<br>Amplicon B—General PCR in Subheading 3.2 with genomic DNA with the following exception. For those cells shown to carry *KIR2DL1* or *KIR2DS2* or both *KIR2DL2* and *KIR2DL3*, use haplotype-specific extraction with probe *KIR2DL2*-999T as described in Subheading 3.4 prior to general PCR in Subheading 3.2 to isolate *KIR2DL2*<br>Amplicon C— General PCR in Subheading 3.2 with genomic DNA with the following exception. For those cells shown to carry *KIR2DL1* or *KIR2DS2* or both *KIR2DL2* and *KIR2DL3*, use haplotype-specific extraction with probe *KIR2DL2*-999T as described in Subheading 3.4 prior to general PCR in Subheading 3.2<br>Amplicon D—If *KIR2DL2* and *KIR2DL3* are both present in the cell, perform nested PCR with these primers using the amplicon B template to eliminate the highly homologous *KIR2DL3* gene as described in Subheading 3.3 |
| *KIR2DL3* | Amplicon A—If the cell is *KIR2DL2* negative, follow the general PCR protocol in Subheading 3.2 beginning with *Bc1I* digested genomic DNA as described in Subheading 3.5. Cleavage of *KIR2DP1* with the restriction enzyme *BclI* eliminates its coamplification. If the cell is *KIR2DL2* positive, follow the general PCR protocol in Subheading 3.2 beginning with haplotype-specific extraction with the *KIR2DL3*-1316T probe as described in Subheading 3.4<br>Amplicon B1—If the cell is *KIR2DL2* negative, follow the general PCR protocol in Subheading 3.2 beginning with the *Bc1I* digested genomic DNA as described in Subheading 3.5. Cleavage of *KIR2DP1* with the restriction enzyme *BclI* eliminates its coamplification. If the cell is *KIR2DL2* positive, do not prepare the B1 amplicon but instead use the amplicon B2 primers described below<br>Amplicon B2—If the cell is *KIR2DL2* positive, use this primer pair and follow the general PCR protocol in Subheading 3.2 beginning with haplotype-specific extraction with the *KIR2DL3*-1316T probe as described in Subheading 3.4. If the cell is *KIR2DL2* negative, do not prepare the B2 amplicon but instead use the amplicon B1 primers described above<br>Amplicon C1—General PCR in Subheading 3.2 with genomic DNA<br>Amplicon C2—General PCR in Subheading 3.2 with genomic DNA. Together, the information provided by the C1 and C2 amplicons produces more robust sequence results<br>Amplicon D—This is a nested PCR of amplicon A required to clarify the sequence in this region |
| *KIR2DL4* | Amplicon A—General PCR in Subheading 3.2 with genomic DNA<br>Amplicon A2—General PCR in Subheading 3.2 with genomic DNA. This amplicon will allow characterization of exon 1<br>Amplicon B—General PCR in Subheading 3.2 with genomic DNA |

(continued)

**Table 1**
**(continued)**

| Locus | Specific amplification or allele isolation protocol required |
|---|---|
| *KIR2DL5* | Amplicon A—General PCR in Subheading 3.2 with genomic DNA. The A amplicon includes 254 bp of the 5′ upstream region<br>Amplicon B—General PCR in Subheading 3.2 with genomic DNA<br>Amplicon A*001+—Use this primer pair with genomic DNA to clarify results for cells that carry more than two alleles of *KIR2DL5*<br>Amplicon B*002+—Use this primer pair with genomic DNA to clarify results for cells that carry more than two alleles of *KIR2DL5* |
| *KIR2DS1* | Amplicon A—General PCR in Subheading 3.2 with genomic DNA<br>Amplicon B—General PCR in Subheading 3.2 with genomic DNA |
| *KIR2DS2* | Amplicon A—General PCR in Subheading 3.2 with genomic DNA<br>Amplicon B—General PCR in Subheading 3.2 with genomic DNA |
| *KIR2DS3* | Amplicon A—General PCR in Subheading 3.2 with genomic DNA<br>Amplicon B—General PCR in Subheading 3.2 with genomic DNA |
| *KIR2DS4* | Amplicon A—General PCR in Subheading 3.2 with genomic DNA<br>Amplicon B—General PCR in Subheading 3.2 with genomic DNA<br>Amplicon C—In those cells with both full and deletion alleles, an exon 5 nested PCR is performed using amplicon B as a template (see Subheading 3.3). Cloning as described in Subheading 3.6 is used to separate alleles for sequencing in these samples |
| *KIR2DS5* | Amplicon A—General PCR in Subheading 3.2 with genomic DNA<br>Amplicon B—General PCR in Subheading 3.2 with genomic DNA |
| *KIR3DL1* | Amplicon A—General PCR in Subheading 3.2 with genomic DNA<br>Amplicon B—Perform the long template PCR protocol described in Subheading 3.7 with genomic DNA<br>Amplicon M—General PCR in Subheading 3.2 with genomic DNA. This amplicon overlaps the sequences of Amplicon A and Amplicon B |
| *KIR3DL2* | Amplicon A—General PCR in Subheading 3.2 with genomic DNA<br>Amplicon A2— General PCR in Subheading 3.2 with genomic DNA. This amplicon will allow characterization of exon 1<br>Amplicon B—General PCR in Subheading 3.2 with genomic DNA |
| *KIR3DL3* | Amplicon A—General PCR in Subheading 3.2 with genomic DNA<br>Amplicon A2—General PCR in Subheading 3.2 with genomic DNA. This amplicon will allow characterization of exon 1<br>Amplicon B—General PCR in Subheading 3.2 with genomic DNA |
| *KIR3DS1* | Amplicon A—General PCR in Subheading 3.2 with genomic DNA<br>Amplicon B—Perform the long template PCR protocol described in Subheading 3.7 with genomic DNA |

[a]Samples will differ in their requirement for the strategies listed in this table depending on the *KIR* genes present in each sample. Once the *KIR* genes present and absent are evaluated by an initial assay (as described in Chap. 24), the laboratory should use this table to select the methods required to obtain DNA for sequencing. For example, to obtain the allele assignments of *KIR2DL1*: If a cell carries *KIR2DL1* and not *KIR2DS1*, two PCR amplifications are performed to yield *KIR2DL1* amplicon A (yielding the sequence of nucleotide 10 through nucleotide 632) and *KIR2DL1* amplicon B (nucleotide 332 through the last nucleotide of exon 9). These two overlapping amplicons are subsequently sequenced to identify the *KIR2DL1* alleles. However, if the cell carries both *KIR2DL1* and *KIR2DS1*, amplicon A will include both *KIR2DL1* and *KIR2DS1* which makes it difficult to interpret the sequence data. In this case, it is necessary to perform an additional amplification of *KIR2DL1* generating amplicon A2 (nucleotide 1 through nucleotide 330) which does not include *KIR2DS1*. Because the antisense primer generating amplicon A2 anneals at nucleotide 331 which is the annealing site of the sense primer for amplicon B, the A2 amplicon does not provide a clear assessment of the sequence in the region of nucleotide 331. This information is provided by amplicon A

genes (4, 5). Less is known about the impact of *KIR* allelic polymorphism on the immune response. Allelic variation alters the level of protein expression and the affinity of ligand binding as demonstrated for KIR2DL2/KIR2DL3 (6) and KIR3DL1 (7, 8). For example, in HIV infection, allotypic variation of KIR3DL1 influences disease progression and levels of the pathogen in plasma (9). Thus, as we learn more about their impact, identification of *KIR* alleles may be used to predict the response of an individual to a disease or to therapy and to select optimal stem cell donors for patients with some malignancies.

## 2. Materials

Use reagent grade water (e.g., UltraPure™ distilled water, Invitrogen, Carlsbad, CA, USA) unless noted. Storage conditions of commercial reagents are indicated by the vendor.

### 2.1. DNA Preparation

1. Whole blood drawn into a standard blood tube containing the anti-coagulant acid citrate dextrose (ACD) (see Note 1).
2. QIAamp® DNA Blood Mini Kit (QIAGEN, Valencia, CA, USA): The kit contains buffers AL, AW1, AW2, protease and solvent for protease, spin columns, collection tubes, and instruction manual. The buffers in the kit, AW1 and AW2, are provided as concentrates. When opening a new bottle, add the appropriate amount of 96–100% ethanol (as written on the label). To reconstitute the protease, add the supplied solvent to the protease powder and invert the bottle several times to mix. Store for 2 months at 4°C after preparation.
3. 96–100% ethanol.
4. Phosphate buffered saline (PBS).
5. 1.5 mL microcentrifuge tubes.
6. Pipettor (5–200 μL) and tips.
7. Heat block or water bath at 56°C.
8. Vortex mixer.
9. Centrifuge capable of holding 1.5 mL tubes with a maximum speed of 20,000 ×*g* (14,000 rpm).

### 2.2. Polymerase Chain Reaction

1. Genomic DNA prepared as described in Subheading 3.1.
2. Positive and negative control genomic DNA (National Marrow Donor Program Cell Repository, Minneapolis, MN, USA; http://www.cibmtr.org/samples/) (see Note 2).
3. Taq polymerase and buffer: Platinum *Taq* DNA Polymerase High Fidelity 5 units/μL with 10× High Fidelity PCR Buffer (Invitrogen, Carlsbad, CA, USA).

4. 50 mM $MgSO_4$ (Invitrogen) according to Table 2.
5. 10 mM dNTP mixture (Roche, Mannheim, Germany).
6. *KIR* locus PCR primers: 10 μM of each oligonucleotide primer in water, store at −20°C. Table 1 describes the primer sets needed based on the presence or absence of specific *KIR* genes in the sample. Primers are listed in Table 2 (see Note 3).
7. Dimethyl sulfoxide (DMSO) (Sigma-Aldrich, St.Louis, MO).
8. 5 M betaine solution (Sigma-Aldrich).
9. Reagent grade water.
10. 1-kb DNA ladder (e.g., Tracklt™1Kb Plus DNA ladder, Invitrogen) (see Note 4).
11. Agarose (e.g., UltraPure™ Agarose, Invitrogen).
12. 10× TBE buffer (e.g., UltraPure™ 10× TBE buffer, Invitrogen) diluted with deionized water at an operational resistivity of 18.2 MΩ $cm^{-1}$ at 25°C to 1×.
13. Ethidium bromide solution (10 mg/mL) (Invitrogen) (see Note 5).
14. 5× sucrose cresol (0.04% cresol red in 30% sucrose) gel loading solution.
15. Agencourt AMPure kit (Beckman Coulter, Beverly, MA, USA).
16. 70% ethanol in water (e.g., Warner-Graham Company, Cockeysville, MD, USA).
17. 1.5-mL sterile disposable tubes (Fisher Scientific, Dallas, TX, USA).
18. Semi-skirted PCR tray (Fisher Scientific, Dallas, TX, USA).
19. Tape seals (One Lambda, Canoga Park, CA, USA).
20. Single channel and multichannel (8 or 12 channel) pipettors (0.5–200 μL) and tips.
21. Thermal cycler (e.g., model 2720, Applied Biosytems, Foster City, CA, USA).
22. Vortex mixer.
23. Flat bed slab gel unit (tray 11.9 cm (length) × 11.5 cm (width)) and power supply (e.g., RunOne™ Electrophoresis Unit, Embi Tec, San Diego, CA, USA).
24. UV transilluminator.
25. Gel photography system.
26. Agencourt SPRIPlate 96R magnet plate (Beckman Coulter).
27. Centrifuge capable of holding 1.5 mL tubes and plates with a maximum speed of 20,000 × *g* (14,000 rpm) (e.g., model 5424 (for tubes) and model 5804 (for plates with A-2-deep well plate rotor), Eppendorf, Hauppauge, NY, USA).

**Table 2**
***KIR* locus-specific polymerase chain reaction amplification primers[a] and conditions**

| | | | | Annealing sites: sense/ antisense[b] | Amplicon size (bp) | PCR reaction conditions | | PCR reaction components (50 μL) | | |
|---|---|---|---|---|---|---|---|---|---|---|
| *KIR* locus | Amplicon | Sense primer | Antisense primer | | | Annealing temp (°C)—initial/ secondary cycles | Extension time (min) | MgSO4 (μL) | DMSO/ Betaine (μL) | Taq |
| *KIR2DL1* | A | TGTAAAACGACGGC CAGTGGCAGCAC CATGTCGCTCT | CAAGCAGTGGG TCACTTGAC | 10T/633G | 5,605 | 64/61 | 5 | 2.0 | 2.5/– | High Fidelity |
| | A2 | ATAACATCCTG TGCGCTGCT | GGGTCACTGGG AGCTGACAC | 5UTR/331G | 3,825 | 66/64 | 5 | 1.5 | 3.0/– | High Fidelity |
| | B | ACTCACTCCC CCTATCAGG | TGTTGACTCCC TAGAAGACG | 331G/3UTR | 10,282 | 62/59 | 10 | 2.0 | –/– | High Fidelity |
| *KIR2DL2* | A | TCTCAGCACA GACAGCACC | GCCCTGCAGA GAACCTACA | 5UTR/505T | 5,382 | 62/58 | 7 | 2.0 | 2.0/– | High Fidelity |
| | B | CCATGATGGG GTCTCCAAA | TCAATGCCTGCATCG AAGGTTTCT | 246A/IN6 | 5,348 | 60/57 | 5 | 3.5 | –/10 | High Fidelity |
| | C | TCACCCACTGA ACCAAGCTCT | TGTTGACTCCC TAGAAGACG | 708T/3UTR | 5,228 | 62/58 | 7 | 2.0 | 2.0/– | High Fidelity |
| | D | AATGCCTCTTCT CCTCCAGGTCTA | CTCTCCTCTGGGTC TCTCCTGACCG | 375A/IN5 Nested Ex5 | 568 | 62/57 | 1.5 | - | –/10 | Taq/10× PCR buffer with MgCl2 |

(continued)

**Table 2 (continued)**

| | | | | Annealing sites: sense/antisense[b] | Amplicon size (bp) | PCR reaction conditions | | PCR reaction components (50 μL) | | |
|---|---|---|---|---|---|---|---|---|---|---|
| *KIR* locus | Amplicon | Sense primer | Antisense primer | | | Annealing temp (°C)—initial/secondary cycles | Extension time (min) | MgSO4 (μL) | DMSO/Betaine (μL) | Taq |
| *KIR2DL3* | A | TGTAAAACGACGGCCAGTGGCAGCACCATGTCGCTCA | GCCCTGCAGAGAACCTACG | 10A/505C | 5,385 | 62/58 | 5 | 3.0 | –/10 | High Fidelity |
| | B1 | GTTCTGTTACTCACTCCCCCT | CTCTCCTCTGGGTCTCTCCTGACCG | 325T/IN5 | 2,131 | 62/58 | 5 | 3.0 | –/10 | High Fidelity |
| | B2 | CGTTCTGCACAGAGAAGGGAA[c] | | 194A/IN5 | 2,262 | 62/58 | 5 | 3.0 | –/10 | High Fidelity |
| | C1 | TCAAGACAGTGGGCGTCACATACA | CTTCGTGAGACTTACTTT TTTTGTTGC | IN6/809G | 3,344 | 62/58 | 5 | 3.0 | –/10 | High Fidelity |
| | C2 | ACACCTGCATGTTCTGATTGG | GCAGGAGACAACTTTGGATCA | 746G/1024T | 879 | 62/58 | 5 | 3.0 | –/10 | High Fidelity |
| | D | AGCAAGGGGAAGCCTCACTCATTC | CCAATGACAATGAGAATG | IN2/IN4<br>Nested Ex4 | 419 | 62/57 | 1.5 | - | –/10 | Taq/10× PCR buffer with MgCl2 |

| | | | | | | | | | | |
|---|---|---|---|---|---|---|---|---|---|---|
| *KIR2DL4* | A | CACCCACGGTC ATCATCC | CCCTTTCSCTG TTGGAGTGT | 28C/IN6 | 5,378 | 64/57 | 6 | 2.0 | 2.0/– | High Fidelity |
| | A2 | TCCTGGCAGCAG AAGCTGCACC | GGAAAGAGCC GAAGCATC | 5UTR/581G | 2,564 | 64/57 | 5 | 2.0 | 2.0/– | High Fidelity |
| | B | CATGTTCTAGG AAACCCTTCT | TGGGCTAAGCA AAGGAGTGT | 666T/3UTR | 5,420 | 64/57 | 6 | 2.0 | 2.0/– | High Fidelity |
| *KIR2DL5* | A | ATCTTGTGTTC GGGAGGTTG | TCATAGGGTGA GTCATGGAG | 5UTR/589C | 3,274 | 64/62 | 5 | 2.0 | 2.0/– | High Fidelity |
| | B | GAGGGGAGGG CCCATGAACC | GGAAGAGCGAT CCCCTAAGA | 491C/3UTR | 6,193 | 64/62 | 7 | 2.0 | 2.0/– | High Fidelity |
| | A*001+ | CTCCCGTGATGTGG TCAACATGTAAA | TCATAGGGTG AGTCATGGAG | 5UTR/589C | 3,109 | 64/62 | 5 | 2.0 | 2.0/– | High Fidelity |
| | B*002+ | CTCCCATGATGTA GTCAACATGTAAG | TCATAGGGTG AGTCATGGAG | 5UTR/589C | 3,109 | 64/62 | 5 | 2.0 | 2.0/– | High Fidelity |
| *KIR2DS1* | A | GGCAGCACCAT GTCGCTCA | GCATCTGTAGG TCCCTCCA | 10A/576T | 5,540 | 64/60 | 7 | 1.5 | 1.0/– | High Fidelity |
| | B | TCTCCATCAGT CGCATGAR | GGGTGTCTTG GGCCTCTC | 272R/3UTR | 10,227 | 64/60 | 10 | 2.0 | 1.0/– | High Fidelity |
| *KIR2DS2* | A | ATCCTGTGCGCTG CTGAGCTGAG | CACGCTCTCT CCTGCCAA | 5UTR/418T | 5,239 | 62/58 | 7 | 1.5 | 2.0/– | High Fidelity |
| | B | CTTCTGCACAGAGA GGGGAAGTA | TTATGCGTATGACA CCTCCTGAT | 197A/893A | 10,253 | 62/58 | 10 | 1.5 | 2.0/– | High Fidelity |

(continued)

**Table 2 (continued)**

| *KIR* locus | Amplicon | Sense primer | Antisense primer | Annealing sites: sense/antisense[b] | Amplicon size (bp) | PCR reaction conditions: Annealing temp (°C)—initial/secondary cycles | PCR reaction conditions: Extension time (min) | PCR reaction components (50 μL): MgSO4 (μL) | PCR reaction components (50 μL): DMSO/Betaine (μL) | PCR reaction components (50 μL): Taq |
|---|---|---|---|---|---|---|---|---|---|---|
| *KIR2DS3* | A | ATCCTGTGCGCTGC TGAGCTGAG | GCATCTGTAG GTTCCTCCT | 5UTR/576A | 5,919 | 64/61 | 7 | 2.0 | –/– | High Fidelity |
| | B | GACATGTAC CATCTATCCAC | TTATGCGTATGAC ACCTCCTGA TGGTCC | 485C/888G | 8,427 | 60/57 | 10 | 2.0 | –/– | High Fidelity |
| *KIR2DS4* | A | CATGTCGCTCA TGGTCATCAT | ACACTCTCACCT ATGATCACC | 20T/360G | 5,122 | 64/58 | 7 | 2.0 | –/– | High Fidelity |
| | B | ATCCTGCAA TGTTGGTCG | TTATGCGTATGACAC CTCCTGAT | 153G/893A | 10,299 | 64/58 | 10 | 1.5 | –/– | High Fidelity |
| | C | CGCAGTGACCC TCTGGACATG[c] | GTGACGGAAACAA GCAGTGGA | 360G/642T Nested Ex 5 | 1,875 | 62/57 | 1.5 | - | –/10 | Taq/10× PCR buffer with MgCl2 |
| *KIR2DS5* | A | CCATCATGATCTT TCTTTCCAGC | CCTCCGTGGGTG GCAGGGT | 35C/563A | 4,541 | 62/58 | 5 | 2.0 | –/– | High Fidelity |
| | B | CATTGATGGGGT CTCCAAGGG | TTATGCGTATGACACC TCCTGATGGTCC | 248G/888G | 10,188 | 62/58 | 10 | 2.0 | –/– | High Fidelity |

| | | | | | | | | | | |
|---|---|---|---|---|---|---|---|---|---|---|
| *KIR3DL1* | A | TGTCKRCACC GGCAGCACC | TAGGTCCCTGC AAGGGCAA | 5UTR/560T | 3,454 | 60/57 | 5 | 1.5 | 2.0/– | High Fidelity |
| | B | CCATCGGTCC CATGATGCT | GACAACTTTGGA TCTGGGCTY | 560T/1303Y | 10,365 | 60/57 | 11 | - | –/– | Expand Long/ Buffer 3 |
| | M | CAARCCCTTCCT GTCTGCCT | GAGAGAGAAG GTTTCTCATATG | 100T/659C | 3,265 | 60/57 | 5 | 1.5 | 2.0/– | High Fidelity |
| *KIR3DL2* | A | GTCGTCAGCA TGGCGTGC | TGCATCCAAGG CTTCCACC | 30C/IN6 | 8,706 | 60/57 | 8 | 1.5 | 2.0/– | High Fidelity |
| | A2 | TGTCTGCACCG GCAGCACC | GACCACACG CAGGGCAG | 5UTR/898C | 5,421 | 60/57 | 5 | 2.0 | –/10 | High Fidelity |
| | B | TCACATCTC TCCTGTCCCG | GGCTGTTGTC TCCCTAGAAA | IN5/1362T | 7,693 | 60/57 | 8 | 1.5 | 2.0/– | High Fidelity |
| *KIR3DL3* | A | TTTCCAGGGTTCT TCTTGCTGG | TGACCCTCAG CACYGCAGT | 49G/799A | 4,415 | 62/60 | 5 | 3.0 | 2.0/– | High Fidelity |
| | A2 | TGTCTGCACCG GCAGCACC | CCGACAACTC ATAGGGTA | 5UTR/605T | 3,361 | 62/60 | 5 | 3.0 | –/10 | High Fidelity |
| | B | CCCGGAGCTTG TTTGACATT | AGAAGACAAC TTTGGATCTGC | 756T/3UTR | 6,569 | 58/54 | 7 | 3.0 | –/– | High Fidelity |
| *KIR3DS1* | A | TGTCKRCACCG GCAGCACC | CTGTGACCAT GATCACCAT | 5UTR/A337 | 2,116 | 60/57 | 3 | 1.0 | 1.5/– | High Fidelity |
| | B | GGCAGAATAT TCCAGGAGG | AGAGCGATGCC CTAAGATGA | 235G/3UTR | 12,324 | 60/57 | 11 | - | –/– | Expand Long/ Buffer 3 |

[a]Some of the primers have been previously described (19–23)

[b]UTR, untranslated region and/or other 5′ or 3′ noncoding sequences; IN, intron. The designations such as 10T/633G indicate the nucleotide at the annealing site of the 3′ end of the sense/antisense primers. Position 1 is defined as the first nucleotide of the ATG codon in exon 1 according to the IPD/*KIR* database (http://www.ebi.ac.uk/ipd/kir/). The numbering of *KIR2DS4* is based on an allele that does not contain the deletion

[c]Primer sequence is not identical to *KIR* gene sequence; a substitution was added to avoid the primer from self-annealing

#### 2.3. Nested PCR for KIR2DL2 Amplicon B, KIR2DL3 Amplicon A, and KIR2DS4 Amplicon B

1. AMPure-purified amplicons: *KIR2DL2* amplicon B, *KIR2DL3* amplicon A, and *KIR2DS4* amplicon B. Table 1 describes the use of nested PCR to either isolate the product of a specific gene or to clarify the sequence in a specific area.
2. *Taq* DNA Polymerase 5 units/μL (Roche, Mannheim, Germany) with 10× PCR Buffer with $MgCl_2$ (Roche).
3. 10 mM dNTP mixture (Roche).
4. *KIR* locus PCR primer solutions for nested PCR: 10 μM of each oligonucleotide primer in water. Primers are listed in Table 2.
5. Reagent grade water.
6. 5 M betaine solution (Sigma-Aldrich).
7. Supplies and equipment described in Subheading 2.2.

#### 2.4. Isolation of KIR2DL2 and KIR2DL3 by HaploPrep

1. Genomic DNA carrying *KIR2DL2* or *KIR2DL3*. Table 1 describes the use of HaploPrep to isolate a specific gene segment for sequencing in those samples containing a second gene sharing extensive sequence homology with the gene being characterized.
2. HaploPrep™ Kit (QIAGEN, Valencia, CA, USA) with hybridization buffer H.
3. *KIR* locus HaploPrep probes 2DL2-999T and 2DL3-1316T, 100 μM of each probe in 1× Tris–EDTA (TE) buffer (Invitrogen), stored at −20°C.
4. Reagent grade water.
5. Heating block with heated lid at 95°C (e.g., TruTemp DNA Microheating System, Robbins Scientific, Sunnyvale, CA, USA) (see Note 6).
6. BioRobot EZ1 (QIAGEN) with HaploPrep card and manual.

#### 2.5. Restriction Enzyme Digestion for the KIR2DL3 Locus

1. Genomic DNA from cells carrying *KIR2DL3*. Table 1 describes the use of restriction enzyme digestion to eliminate a highly homologous gene when present in the sample.
2. Restriction endonuclease *BclI* (15 U/μL) and 10× NE Buffer 3 (New England BioLabs, Ipswich, MA, USA).
3. Reagent grade water.
4. Phenol:chloroform:isoamyl alcohol 25:24:1,V/V/V (e.g., UltraPure™ phenol:chloroform:isoamyl alcohol, Invitrogen) (see Note 7).
5. 3M sodium acetate (Sigma-Aldrich).
6. 70% ethanol in water (Warner-Graham Company) at −20°C.
7. Heating block at 50°C.

8. –20°C freezer.
9. Supplies and equipment described in Subheading 2.2.

#### 2.6. *KIR2DS4* Allele Isolation by Cloning

1. Nested PCR amplicon of *KIR2DS4* from Subheading 2.3. Table 1 describes the use of cloning to separate alleles in specific *KIR2DS4* heterozygous samples.
2. TOPO TA Cloning Kit (Invitrogen) including SOC medium and instruction manual.
3. LB agar plates containing 50 μg/mL ampicillin.
4. 40 mg/mL X-gal (5-bromo-4-chloro-3-indolyl-b-D-galacto-pyranoside) in dimethylformamide.
5. 100 mM isopropyl β-D-1-thiogalactopyranoside (IPTG) in water.
6. Reagent grade water.
7. Sterile toothpicks.
8. 1.5 mL sterile disposable tubes (Fisher Scientific, Dallas, TX, USA).
9. 37°C Shaking and non-shaking bacterial incubators.
10. Centrifuge capable of holding 1.5 mL tubes with a maximum speed of 20,000×*g* (14,000 rpm) (e.g., model 5424 (for tubes), Eppendorf, Hauppauge, NY, USA).
11. Heating block at 42°C and 94°C.

#### 2.7. Long Template PCR for *KIR3DL1*/*KIR3DS1* Amplicon B

1. Genomic DNA from samples carrying *KIR3DL1* or *KIR3DS1*. Table 1 summarizes the strategies used to obtain amplicons for specific *KIR* genes.
2. Expand Long Template PCR System with *Taq* DNA polymerase and 10× Expand Long Template buffer 3 (Roche, Mannheim, Germany).
3. 10 mM dNTP mixture (Roche, Mannheim, Germany).
4. *KIR* locus PCR primer solutions for *KIR3DL1* and *KIR3DS1* B amplicons: 10 μM of each oligonucleotide primer in water. Primers are listed in Table 2.
5. Reagent grade water.
6. Supplies and equipment described in Subheading 2.2.

#### 2.8. DNA Sequencing

1. Amplified DNA purified with AMPure from Subheading 3.2.
2. BigDye Terminator v1.1 diluted 1:1 with 5× sequencing buffer (Applied Biosystems, Foster City, CA, USA).
3. *KIR* locus sequencing primers: 1.5 μM of each oligonucleotide primer in water. Store at –20°C (see Table 3) (see Note 8).
4. DMSO.
5. Agencourt CleanSEQ kit (Beckman Coulter, Beverly, MA, USA).

**Table 3**
**DNA sequencing primers for *KIR* loci**

| *KIR* locus | Primer | Sequence (5′–3′) | Strand | Nucleotide position[a] | Sequence covers exon[b] | Use with amplicon |
|---|---|---|---|---|---|---|
| 2DL1 | 2DL1-SEQ-E1R | GGCCCATCACTCCATCTCT | Antisense | 167–185 | Exon 1 | A/A2 |
| | 2DL1-SEQ-E2F | CAAGACTCACAGCCCAGTG | Sense | 917–935 | Exon 2 | A/A2 |
| | 2DL1-SEQ-E2R | GGAGGCAAGGTCAGAAATGT | Antisense | 1161–1180 | Exon 2 | A/A2 |
| | 2DL1-SEQ-E4F | GAYGCCTTCTRAACTCACAAC | Sense | 3450–3470 | Exon 4 | A/A2 |
| | 2DL1-SEQ-E4R | AAGTCCTRGATCATTCACTC | Antisense | 3825–3844 | Exon 4 | A |
| | 2DL1-SEQ-E5F | AAGATCCTCCCTGAGGAAAC | Sense | 5277–5296 | Exon 5 | A/B |
| | 2DL1-SEQ-E5R | AGGCTCTAGGATCATAGGACA | Antisense | 5634–5654 | Exon 5 | B |
| | 2DL1-SEQ-E6F | GCCTTTCTTTATGCCAATGT | Sense | 8488–8507 | Exon 6 | B |
| | 2DL1-SEQ-E6R | TGTCAGAGCTGTGAGATGCT | Antisense | 8887–8906 | Exon 6 | B |
| | 2DL1-SEQ-E7F | ATCTGGGTGCTTGTCCTAA | Sense | 12951–12969 | Exon 7 | B |
| | 2DL1-SEQ-E7R | AGGGACCATCCTGTTTGTGA | Antisense | 13252–13271 | Exon 7 | B |
| | 2DL1-SEQ-E89F | AAATGAGGACCCAGAAGTGC | Sense | 13580–13599 | Exons 8, 9 | B |
| | 2DL1-SEQ-E89R | TGTTGACTCCCTAGAAGACG | Antisense | 13987–14006 | Exons 8, 9 | B |
| 2DL2 | 2DL2-SEQ-E1R | GGCCCATCACTCCATCTCT | Antisense | 129–147 | Exon 1 | A |
| | 2DL2-SEQ-E2F | CAAGACTCACAGCCCAGTG | Sense | 861–879 | Exon 2 | A |
| | 2DL2-SEQ-E2R | TTGAGCACCCCAGTCTAACC | Antisense | 1170–1189 | Exon 2 | A |
| | 2DL2-SEQ-E4F | GACACCTTCTAAACTCACAAC | Sense | 3382–3402 | Exon 4 | A |
| | 2DL2-SEQ-E4R | AAGTCGTGGATCATTCACTC | Antisense | 3754–3773 | Exon 4 | A |
| | 2DL2-SEQ-E5F1 | GGTCATAGAGCAGGGGAGTG | Sense | 5136–5155 | Exon 5 | A |
| | 2DL2-SEQ-E5F2 | AATGCCTCTTCTCCTCCAGGTCTA | Sense | 5209–5233 | Exon 5 | D |
| | 2DL2-SEQ-E5R | TCTCTGCATCTGTCCATGCT | Antisense | 5602–5621 | Exon 5 | A/B/D |
| | 2DL2-SEQ-E6F | CCCAGGGCCCAATATTAGAT | Sense | 8681–8700 | Exon 6 | B |
| | 2DL2-SEQ-E6R | TCAATGCCTGCATCGAAGGTTTCT | Antisense | 9193–9217 | Exon 6 | B/C |
| | 2DL2-SEQ-E7F | ATCTGGGTGCTTGTCCTAA | Sense | 12993–13011 | Exon 7 | C |
| | 2DL2-SEQ-E7R | AGGGACCATCCTGTTTGTGA | Antisense | 13294–13313 | Exon 7 | C |
| | 2DL2-SEQ-E89F | AAATGAGGACCCAGAAGTGC | Sense | 13622–13641 | Exons 8, 9 | C |
| | 2DL2-SEQ-E89R | GGAGACAACTTTGGATCTGGA | Antisense | 13976–13996 | Exons 8, 9 | C |

| | | | | | | |
|---|---|---|---|---|---|---|
| 2DL3 | 2DL3-SEQ-E1R | GGCCCATCACTCCATCTCT | Antisense | 129–147 | Exon 1 | A |
| | 2DL3-SEQ-E2F | CAAGACTCACAGCCCAGTG | Sense | 861–879 | Exon 2 | A |
| | 2DL3-SEQ-E2R | TTGAGCACCCCAGTCTAACC | Antisense | 1170–1189 | Exon 2 | A |
| | 2DL3-SEQ-E4F | GACACCTTCTAAACTCACAAC | Sense | 3382–3402 | Exon 4 | A/D |
| | 2DL3-SEQ-E4R | CCAATGACAATGAGAATG | Antisense | 3731–3748 | Exon 4 | A/D |
| | 2DL3-SEQ-E4F-218T | TTAAGGACACTTTGCACCTCAT | Sense | 3542–3563 | Exon 4 | A/D |
| | 2DL3-SEQ-E4R-282T | TAGCATCTGTAGGTCCCTGCA | Antisense | 3627–3647 | Exon 4 | A/D |
| | 2DL3-SEQ-E4F-166C | TGGTCAGATGTCAGGTTT C | Sense | 3493–3511 | Exon 4 | A/D |
| | 2DL3-SEQ-E5F1 | GGTCATAGAGCAGGGGAGTG | Sense | 5136–5155 | Exon 5 | A/B1/B2 |
| | 2DL3-SEQ-E5F2 | AATGCCTCTTCTCCTCCAGGTCTA | Sense | 5209–5233 | Exon 5 | A/B1/B2 |
| | 2DL3-SEQ-E5R | TTCTCTCTGCATCTGTCCATG | Antisense | 5608–5628 | Exon 5 | B1/B2 |
| | 2DL3-SEQ-E5R-618A | AGTTTGACCACTCGTAT | Antisense | 5480–5496 | Exon 5 | B1/B2 |
| | 2DL3-SEQ-E6F | TGAACCAACCTCAAAGATTTCC | Sense | 8698–8719 | Exon 6 | C1 |
| | 2DL3-SEQ-E6R | TTCTACCTCCCCAGGTTT C | Antisense | 8860–8878 | Exon 6 | C1 |
| | 2DL2/3-SEQ-E7F | ATCTGGGTGCTTGTCCTAA | Sense | 12993–13011 | Exon 7 | C1/C2 |
| | 2DL3-SEQ-E7R | CCCACATGGCCCTGAGC | Antisense | 11966–11982 | Exon 7 | C2 |
| | 2DL3-SEQ-E89F | TGCTTATGAAATGAGGGCCC | Sense | 12336–12355 | Exons 8, 9 | C2 |
| | 2DL3-SEQ-E89R | AGGGCTCAGCATTTGGAAG | Antisense | 12683–12701 | Exons 8, 9 | C2 |
| 2DL4 | 2DL4-SEQ-E1R | CATCCTCACCACTCACTTGC | Antisense | 126–145 | Exon 1 | A2 |
| | 2DL4-SEQ-E2F | GGCTCAGGAGGAAAGGGTAG | Sense | 177–196 | Exon 2 | A/A2 |
| | 2DL4-SEQ-E2R | CAGGCCTTCCCATGGTCAG | Antisense | 374–392 | Exon 2 | A/A2 |
| | 2DL4-SEQ-E3F | GGGGAGAATCTTCTGAGCAC | Sense | 1063–1082 | Exon 3 | A/A2 |
| | 2DL4-SEQ-E3R | CACCAGAAGCTCTGGGACTC | Antisense | 1469–1488 | Exon 3 | A/A2 |
| | 2DL4-SEQ-E5F | AGAGCAGGGCAGTGAGTTCT | Sense | 2217–2236 | Exon 5 | A/A2 |
| | 2DL4-SEQ-E5R | TCCACATCTGTCCATGCTTC | Antisense | 2677–2696 | Exon 5 | A |
| | 2DL4-SEQ-E6F | CCAGGGCCCAACATTAGATA | Sense | 5074–5093 | Exon 6 | A |
| | 2DL4-SEQ-E6R | ATCACAGAGCTGGCAGGTG | Antisense | 5316–5334 | Exon 6 | A/B |
| | 2DL4-SEQ-E7F | CCTGGCAACCAAGAAATGAG | Sense | 9400–9419 | Exon 7 | B |
| | 2DL4-SEQ-E7R | AGACTTTCCTGCCAGTGAGG | Antisense | 9663–9682 | Exon 7 | B |
| | 2DL4-SEQ-E89F | CCCCCTGTGTGTTGGTATCT | Sense | 9965–9984 | Exons 8, 9 | B |
| | 2DL4-SEQ-E89R | TAAGCAAGAGACAGGCACCA | Antisense | 10519–10538 | Exons 8, 9 | B |

(continued)

**Table 3 (continued)**

| *KIR* locus | Primer | Sequence (5′–3′) | Strand | Nucleotide position[a] | Sequence covers exon[b] | Use with amplicon |
|---|---|---|---|---|---|---|
| 2DL5 | 2DL5-SEQ-E1F | ATCTTGTGTTCGGGAGGTTG | Sense | 5UTR (−274)–(−256) | 5′ noncoding region | A |
| | 2DL5-SEQ-E1R | AACTCCACCTCCAGGCCTAT | Antisense | 101–120 | Exon 1 | A |
| | 2DL5-SEQ-E2F | ACCAAGACTCACAGCCCAGT | Sense | 706–725 | Exon 2 | A |
| | 2DL5-SEQ-E2R | TCCCTCCTGTTTCAGGAAAAT | Antisense | 873–893 | Exon 2 | A |
| | 2DL5-SEQ-E3F | GGGGAGAATCTTCTGAGCACT | Sense | 1510–1529 | Exon 3 | A |
| | 2DL5-SEQ-E3R | TGCTCTGGGATTCAGGAAGT | Antisense | 1908–1927 | Exon 3 | A |
| | 2DL5-SEQ-E5F | GGGAGCTGTGACAAGGAAGA | Sense | 2697–2716 | Exon 5 | A/B |
| | 2DL5-SEQ-E5R | AGCAGGAAGCTCCTCAGCTA | Antisense | 3088–3107 | Exon 5 | B |
| | 2DL5-SEQ-E6F | GCCATGAACCAACCTCAAAG | Sense | 5131–5150 | Exon 6 | B |
| | 2DL5-SEQ-E6R | CTGAGCCAATGCTTGAATCC | Antisense | 5321–5340 | Exon 6 | B |
| | 2DL5-SEQ-E7F | GCTGGCAACCAAGAAATGAG | Sense | 7950–7969 | Exon 7 | B |
| | 2DL5-SEQ-E7R | ACCAGTGTGCTCCCATCCT | Antisense | 8187–8205 | Exon 7 | B |
| | 2DL5-SEQ-E89F | CCCTTCCAGCTGTTTTGATG | Sense | 8562–8581 | Exons 8, 9 | B |
| | 2DL5-SEQ-E89R | TGATGCCTTCAGATTCCAGC | Antisense | 9010–9029 | Exons 8, 9 | B |
| 2DS1 | 2DS1-SEQ-E1R | GGCCCATCACTCCATCTCT | Antisense | 470–488 | Exon 1 | A |
| | 2DS1-SEQ-E2F | CAAGACTCACAGCCCAGTG | Sense | 1220–1238 | Exon 2 | A |
| | 2DS1-SEQ-E2R | GGAGGCAAGGTCAGAAATGT | Antisense | 1464–1483 | Exon 2 | A |
| | 2DS1-SEQ-E4F | GAYGCCTTCTRAACTCACAAC | Sense | 3753–3773 | Exon 4 | A |
| | 2DS1-SEQ-E4R | AATTCCTGGATCATTCACTC | Antisense | 4128–4147 | Exon 4 | A/B |
| | 2DS1-SEQ-E5F | AAGGGAGCTGTGACAAGGAA | Sense | 5581–5600 | Exon 5 | A/B |
| | 2DS1-SEQ-E5R | TCTGCATCTGTCCATGCTTC | Antisense | 6008–6027 | Exon 5 | B |
| | 2DS1-SEQ-E6F | GCCTTTCTTTATGCCAGTGTC | Sense | 8785–8805 | Exon 6 | B |
| | 2DS1-SEQ-E6R | CTGAGTCAACGCCTGAATCC | Antisense | 9166–9185 | Exon 6 | B |
| | 2DS1-SEQ-E7F | CCAATCAAGAAATGCGAGACA | Sense | 13295–13315 | Exon 7 | B |
| | 2DS1-SEQ-E7R | CAGGGGAAGGGAATCTGGT | Antisense | 13609–13620 | Exon 7 | B |
| | 2DS1-SEQ-E89F | TCCCCCTGTTTGTTGGTATC | Sense | 13882–13901 | Exons 8, 9 | B |
| | 2DS1-SEQ-E89R | AAGGGCGAGTGATTTTTCTCT | Antisense | 14155–14175 | Exons 8, 9 | B |

| | | | | | | |
|---|---|---|---|---|---|---|
| 2DS2 | 2DS2-SEQ-E1R | GGCCCATCACTCCATCTCT | Antisense | 129–147 | Exon 1 | A |
| | 2DS2-SEQ-E2F | CAAGACTCACAGCCCAGTG | Sense | 745–763 | Exon 2 | A |
| | 2DS2-SEQ-E2R | GGAGGCAAGGTCAGAAATGT | Antisense | 989–1008 | Exon 2 | A |
| | 2DS2-SEQ-E4F | AAGGGGAAGCCTCACTCATT | Sense | 3216–3235 | Exon 4 | A |
| | 2DS2-SEQ-E4R | GCCCAATGACAATGAGAATG | Antisense | 3614–3633 | Exon 4 | A/B |
| | 2DS2-SEQ-E5F | TGAAGAGAGATGGGGTGGAG | Sense | 4977–4996 | Exon 5 | A/B |
| | 2DS2-SEQ-E5R | CTCTCTGCATCTGTCCATGC | Antisense | 5491–5510 | Exon 5 | B |
| | 2DS2-SEQ-E6F | CAGAGTGTTGGCCATGAACC | Sense | 8486–8505 | Exon 6 | B |
| | 2DS2-SEQ-E6R | CTGAGTCAACGCCTGAATCC | Antisense | 8686–8705 | Exon 6 | B |
| | 2DS2-SEQ-E7F | CCAATCAAGAAATGCGAGACA | Sense | 12818–12838 | Exon 7 | B |
| | 2DS2-SEQ-E7R | CAGGGGAAGGGAATCTGGT | Antisense | 13143–13161 | Exon 7 | B |
| | 2DS2-SEQ-E89F | CCTCCGAGCTCTTTTGTTGA | Sense | 13427–13446 | Exons 8, 9 | B |
| | 2DS2-SEQ-E89R | TTATGCGTATGACACCTCCTGAT | Antisense | 13633–13655 | Exons 8, 9 | B |
| 2DS3 | 2DS3-SEQ-E1R | AGGCCTATATCTCCACCTCTG | Antisense | 88–108 | Exon 1 | A |
| | 2DS3-SEQ-E2F | GCCTGGCTACCAAGACTCAC | Sense | 1247–1266 | Exon 2 | A |
| | 2DS3-SEQ-E2R | AGAGACTCCCCGACAGGACT | Antisense | 1443–1462 | Exon 2 | A |
| | 2DS3-SEQ-E4F | GGAAGCCTCACTCAATCCAG | Sense | 3739–3758 | Exon 4 | A |
| | 2DS3-SEQ-E4R | CCTCCAAGTCCTGGATCATT | Antisense | 4165–4184 | Exon 4 | A |
| | 2DS3-SEQ-E5F | AAGGGAGCTGTGACAAGGAA | Sense | 5581–5600 | Exon 5 | A |
| | 2DS3-SEQ-E5R | TCTGCATCTGTCCATGCTTC | Antisense | 6008–6027 | Exon 5 | A/B |
| | 2DS3-SEQ-E6F | CCCAGGGCCCAATATTAGAT | Sense | 8969–8988 | Exon 6 | B |
| | 2DS3-SEQ-E6R | GGTGGAAGACAGGGGTACAA | Antisense | 9229–9248 | Exon 6 | B |
| | 2DS3-SEQ-E7F | TCAATCAAGAAATGCGAGACA | Sense | 13321–13341 | Exon 7 | B |
| | 2DS3-SEQ-E7R | CACACCCACGTGCTAACATC | Antisense | 13556–13575 | Exon 7 | B |
| | 2DS3-SEQ-E89F | TCCCCCTGTTTGTTGGTATC | Sense | 13882–13901 | Exons 8, 9 | B |
| | 2DS3-SEQ-E89R | TTATGCGTATGACACCTC | Antisense | 14141–14158 | Exons 8, 9 | B |

(continued)

**Table 3 (continued)**

| *KIR* locus | Primer | Sequence (5′–3′) | Strand | Nucleotide position[a] | Sequence covers exon[b] | Use with amplicon |
|---|---|---|---|---|---|---|
| 2DS4 | 2DS4-SEQ-E1R | CAGGCCCATATCTCCACCT | Antisense | 91–109 | Exon 1 | A |
| | 2DS4-SEQ-E2F | GGGCTGGCTATCAAGACTCA | Sense | 2222–2241 | Exon 2 | A |
| | 2DS4-SEQ-E2R | TCCCGTTTCAGGAAAATCC | Antisense | 2396–2414 | Exon 2 | A |
| | 2DS4-SEQ-E4F | AGGCTCACTCATTCCAGGTG | Sense | 4736–4755 | Exon 4 | A |
| | 2DS4-SEQ-E4R | TTACAACCACCTGGGTCTCC | Antisense | 5174–5193 | Exon 4 | A/B |
| | 2DS4-SEQ-E5F | GGGAGCTGTGACAAGGAAGA | Sense | 6610–6630 | Exon 5 | B/C |
| | 2DS4-SEQ-E5R | CATGCTGCGTCTTCTCTCTG | Antisense | 7025–7044 | Exon 5 | B |
| | 2DS4-SEQ-E6F | GGCCATGAACCAAACTCAAA | Sense | 10016–10035 | Exon 6 | B |
| | 2DS4-SEQ-E6R | CAGGCGTACAATGTCAGAGC | Antisense | 10236–10256 | Exon 6 | B |
| | 2DS4-SEQ-E7F | GTGGTTACCTGCCAATCAAGA | Sense | 14327–14347 | Exon 7 | B |
| | 2DS4-SEQ-E7R | ATCCTGCTGGTGAGGAACAC | Antisense | 14592–14611 | Exon 7 | B |
| | 2DS4-SEQ-E89F | AAATGAGGACCCAGAAGTGC | Sense | 14927–14946 | Exons 8, 9 | B |
| | 2DS4-SEQ-E89R | TTATGCGTATGACACCTCCTGAT | Antisense | 15153–15175 | Exons 8, 9 | B |
| 2DS5 | 2DS5-SEQ-E2R | AGACTCCCTGACAGGACTTC | Antisense | 1613–1632 | Exon 2 | A |
| | 2DS5-SEQ-E4F | AGCCTCACTCAATCCAGGTG | Sense | 3915–3934 | Exon 4 | A |
| | 2DS5-SEQ-E4R | ACCTGTGATCACGATGTCCA | Antisense | 4273–4292 | Exon 4 | A/B |
| | 2DS5-SEQ-E5F | CAGAGCAGGGGAGTGAGTTC | Sense | 5731–5750 | Exon 5 | A/B |
| | 2DS5-SEQ-E5R | AGCAGGAAGCTCCTCAGCTA | Antisense | 6159–6178 | Exon 5 | B |
| | 2DS5-SEQ-E6F | CCCAGGGCCCAATATTAGAT | Sense | 9145–9164 | Exon 6 | B |
| | 2DS5-SEQ-E6R | GGTGGAAGACAGGGGTACAA | Antisense | 9405–9424 | Exon 6 | B |
| | 2DS5-SEQ-E7F | GCTAGGTCTCCCACCATTTG | Sense | 13440–13459 | Exon 7 | B |
| | 2DS5-SEQ-E7R | ATCCTGCCTGTGAGGAACAC | Antisense | 13752–13771 | Exon 7 | B |
| | 2DS5-SEQ-E89F | TCCCCCTGTTTGTTGGTATC | Sense | 14059–14079 | Exons 8, 9 | B |
| | 2DS5-SEQ-E89R | TTATGCGTATGACACCTC | Antisense | 14318–14335 | Exons 8, 9 | B |

| | | | | | | |
|---|---|---|---|---|---|---|
| 3DL1 | 3DL1-SEQ-E1R | CTCCACTTCAGGCCCATAAC | Antisense | 138–157 | Exon 1 | A |
| | 3DL1-SEQ-E2F | CAAGACKCACAGCCCAGTG | Sense | 953–971 | Exon 2 | A |
| | 3DL1-SEQ-E2R | TGGAGCACCCTAGTCTCACC | Antisense | 1262–1281 | Exon 2 | A |
| | 3DL1-SEQ-E3F | GAGAATCTTCTGGGCACTGG | Sense | 1739–1758 | Exon 3 | A |
| | 3DL1-SEQ-E3R | ATTCAGGAGGTGGGACAGTG | Antisense | 2126–2145 | Exon 3 | A/M |
| | 3DL1-SEQ-E4F | ACCCTCACTCATTCCAGGTG | Sense | 3136–3155 | Exon 4 | A/M |
| | 3DL1-SEQ-E4R | AAGTCCTRGATCATTCACTC | Antisense | 3555–3574 | Exon 4 | A/B/M |
| | 3DL1-SEQ-E5F1 | GGTCATAGAGCAGGGGAGTG | Sense | 4970–4989 | Exon 5 | B |
| | 3DL1/2-SEQ-E5F2 | CTTCTCTCTCAGCCCAGC | Sense | 5080–5097 | Exon 5 | B |
| | 3DL1-SEQ-E5R | TGCATCTGTCCATGCTTTTC | Antisense | 5434–5453 | Exon 5 | B |
| | 3DL1-SEQ-E6F | GCCTTTCTTTATGCCAATGT | Sense | 8254–8273 | Exon 6 | B |
| | 3DL1-SEQ-E6R | CCCTTTCACTGTTGGAGTGT | Antisense | 8708–8727 | Exon 6 | B |
| | 3DL1-SEQ-E7F | AGGGGTCAAACATCTCAACT | Sense | 12638–12657 | Exon 7 | B |
| | 3DL1-SEQ-E7R | AGCTGTGTGCTCCCATCCT | Antisense | 13016–13034 | Exon 7 | B |
| | 3DL1-SEQ-E89F | AAATGAGGACCCAGAAGTGC | Sense | 13372–13391 | Exons 8, 9 | B |
| | 3DL1-SEQ-E89R | GCCTCTGAGAAGGGCGA | Antisense | 13676–13692 | Exons 8, 9 | B |
| | 3DL1/2-SEQ-E89F | GGAGACAGAATCAATGGGAT | Sense | 15619–15638 | Exons 8, 9 | B |
| | 3DL1/2-SEQ-E89R | GGCTGTTGTCTCCCTAGAAA | Antisense | 16178–16197 | Exons 8, 9 | B |
| 3DL2 | 3DL2-SEQ-E1R | CGAGATCTCCATCCCCACT | Antisense | 66–84 | Exon 1 | A2 |
| | 3DL2-SEQ-E2F | AGTTTACCTTCAGCCCAGCA | Sense | 631–650 | Exon 2 | A/A2 |
| | 3DL2-SEQ-E2R | GAGACTCCCCGACAGGACTT | Antisense | 848–867 | Exon 2 | A/A2 |
| | 3DL2-SEQ-E3F | AGCGGAAATGGGAGAATCTT | Sense | 1436–1455 | Exon 3 | A/A2 |
| | 3DL2-SEQ-E3R | CAGAAGCTCTGGGATTCAGG | Antisense | 1847–1866 | Exon 3 | A/A2 |
| | 3DL2-SEQ-E4F | ACCCTCACTCATTCCAGGTG | Sense | 3196–3215 | Exon 4 | A/A2 |
| | 3DL2-SEQ-E4R | TCTGTGTCCCAATGACAATGA | Antisense | 3595–3615 | Exon 4 | A/A2 |
| | 3DL2-SEQ-E5F | CTCAGGTATGAGGGGAGCTG | Sense | 5078–5097 | Exon 5 | A/A2 |
| | 3DL2-SEQ-E5R | TCTGCATCTGTCCATGCTTC | Antisense | 5515–5534 | Exon 5 | A |
| | 3DL2-SEQ-E6F | AGGGTCCAACATTAGATAACA | Sense | 8492–8512 | Exon 6 | A/B |
| | 3DL2-SEQ-E6R | CCAGGTTTCCAAAAGCAGAG | Antisense | 8677–8696 | Exon 6 | B |
| | 3DL2-SEQ-E7F | GTCAATCAAGAAATGAGACAA | Sense | 15253–15273 | Exon 7 | B |
| | 3DL2-SEQ-E7R | GCAATGGTCTGTGAGCTGAA | Antisense | 15598–15617 | Exon 7 | B |
| | 3DL2-SEQ-E89F | TGAAATGAGGACCCAGAAGG | Sense | 15837–15856 | Exons 8, 9 | B |
| | 3DL2-SEQ-E89R | AACCCCCTCAAGACCTGACT | Antisense | 16231–16250 | Exons 8, 9 | B |

(continued)

**Table 3 (continued)**

| *KIR* locus | Primer | Sequence (5′–3′) | Strand | Nucleotide position[a] | Sequence covers exon[b] | Use with amplicon |
|---|---|---|---|---|---|---|
| 3DL3 | 3DL3-SEQ-E1R | CTCGATTCCCTTCCAGGACT | Antisense | 38–57 | Exon 1 | A2 |
| | 3DL3-SEQ-E2F | GAGATGTTGGCTTGGAGTGC | Sense | 442–461 | Exon 2 | A2 |
| | 3DL3-SEQ-E2R | ATCAGTCAACCCCCTGTGTC | Antisense | 820–839 | Exon 2 | A/A2 |
| | 3DL3-SEQ-E3F | AGAAACGTGGAAATGGGAGA | Sense | 1426–1445 | Exon 3 | A/A2 |
| | 3DL3-SEQ-E3R | GAGGTGGGACAGTGAGAAGC | Antisense | 1823–1842 | Exon 3 | A/A2 |
| | 3DL3-SEQ-E4F | TAGACACCATGGAGGGGAAG | Sense | 2982–3001 | Exon 4 | A/A2 |
| | 3DL3-SEQ-E4R | AAGTCCTRGATCATTCACTC | Antisense | 3418–3437 | Exon 4 | A |
| | 3DL3-SEQ-E5F | AGCTCAGGTGTGAGGAGAGC | Sense | 4890–4909 | Exon 5 | A |
| | 3DL3-SEQ-E5R | TGAGCCTAAGTTCACCGGC | Antisense | 5083–5101 | Exon 5 | A |
| | 3DL3-SEQ-E5F2 | ATCTATCCAGGGAGGCAGAG | Sense | 5063–5082 | Exon 5 | B |
| | 3DL3-SEQ-E5R2 | TGGCTCTAGGATCACAAGACA | Antisense | 5277–5297 | Exon 5 | A/B |
| | 3DL3-SEQ-E7F | CTCCTTGGGACAGCATTGAT | Sense | 10395–10414 | Exon 7 | B |
| | 3DL3-SEQ-E7R | AGAAAGTCCTGCCTCTGTGG | Antisense | 10938–10957 | Exon 7 | B |
| | 3DL3-SEQ-E89F | AAATGAGGACCCAGAAGTGC | Sense | 11231–11250 | Exons 8, 9 | B |
| | 3DL3-SEQ-E89R | CAGCATTTGGAAGTTCCGTGTT | Antisense | 11562–11583 | Exons 8, 9 | B |

| | | | | | | |
|---|---|---|---|---|---|---|
| 3DS1 | 3DS1-SEQ-E1R | AGGCCCATAACTCCACCTCT | Antisense | 109–128 | Exon 1 | A |
| | 3DS1-SEQ-E2F | AGTTTACCTTCAGCCCAGCA | Sense | 920–939 | Exon 2 | A |
| | 3DS1-SEQ-E2R | ACAGGACTTCCCTCCCATTT | Antisense | 1126–1145 | Exon 2 | A |
| | 3DS1-SEQ-E3F1 | TCTATGCAGGATGGGTCCTT | Sense | 1664–1683 | Exon 3 | A |
| | 3DS1-SEQ-E3F2 | CAACATGAGCCCTGTGACCA | Sense | 1982–2001 | Exon 3 | B |
| | 3DS1-SEQ-E3R1 | CAGAAGCTCTGGGATTCAGG | Antisense | 2137–2157 | Exon 3 | B |
| | 3DS1-SEQ-E3R2 | GGTGTGAACCCCGACATG | Antisense | 2023–2040 | Exon 3 | A |
| | 3DS1-SEQ-E4F | ACCCTCACTCATTCCAGGTG | Sense | 3509–3528 | Exon 4 | B |
| | 3DS1-SEQ-E4R | TCCAAGTCCTGGATCATTCAC | Antisense | 3929–3949 | Exon 4 | B |
| | 3DS1-SEQ-E5F | GGTCATAGAGCAGGGGAGTG | Sense | 5370–5389 | Exon 5 | B |
| | 3DS1-SEQ-E5R | ATGAAGGAGGGTTTGGAGGT | Antisense | 5911–5930 | Exon 5 | B |
| | 3DS1-SEQ-E6F | ACTCCCAGGGTCCAACATTA | Sense | 8811–8830 | Exon 6 | B |
| | 3DS1-SEQ-E6R | TTCACAGAGCTGGGAGGTTT | Antisense | 9055–9074 | Exon 6 | B |
| | 3DS1-SEQ-E7F | CATCTGGGTGCTTGTCCTAAA | Sense | 13138–13158 | Exon 7 | B |
| | 3DS1-SEQ-E7R | ATCCTGCTTCCCCACATGG | Antisense | 13402–13420 | Exon 7 | B |
| | 3DS1-SEQ-E89F | TCCCCCTGTTTGTTGGTATC | Sense | 13744–13763 | Exons 8, 9 | B |
| | 3DS1-SEQ-E89R | CTCTGAGAAGGGCGAGTG | Antisense | 14051–14068 | Exons 8, 9 | B |

[a]Numbering is based on the genomic sequences in the LRC database (http://www.ncbi.nlm.nih.gov/gv/lrc/). Nucleotide 1 is the first base of exon 1

[b]Exon numbering is based on nine total exons for each locus. Some of the *KIR* loci are missing an exon or have a pseudo exon that is not analyzed. *KIR2DL1*-3 and *KIR2DS1*-5 have a pseudo-exon 3 while *KIR2DL4* and *KIR2DL5* lack exon 4 (24)

6. Ethanol: 73% solution in water.
7. Reagent grade water.
8. Thermal cycler (e.g., model 2720, Applied Biosytems, Foster City, CA, USA).
9. 3730xl DNA Analyzer with POP7, 1× running buffer with EDTA, and manual (Applied Biosytems).
10. Centrifuge capable of holding plates with a maximum speed of 20,000 × *g* (14,000 rpm) (e.g., model 5804 (for plates), Eppendorf, Hauppauge, NY, USA).
11. Single channel and multichannel pipettors (0.5–200 μL) and tips.
12. Semi-skirted PCR tray (Fisher Scientific, Dallas, TX, USA).
13. Tape seals (One Lambda, Canoga Park, CA, USA).
14. Agencourt SPRIPlate 96R magnet plate (Beckman Coulter).

### 2.9. Sequence Analysis Including Preparation of Locus-Specific KIR Libraries

1. Analysis software: Assign SBT 3.2.7 (Conexio Genomics, Applecross, Western Australia), HLA Librarian (Conexio Genomics), Sequencher 4.6 (Ann Arbor, MI, USA) with manuals (see Note 9).
2. *KIR* nucleotide sequence databases: IPD-*KIR* curated coding region sequence database at http://www.ebi.ac.uk/ipd/kir/index.htmL; leukocyte receptor complex (LRC) database alignment viewer for genomic sequences at http://www.ncbi.nlm.nih.gov/gv/lrc/.

## 3. Methods

### 3.1. DNA Preparation

1. Label the appropriate number of 1.5 mL microcentrifuge tubes and QIAamp spin columns with sample identifier (see Note 10 on laboratory).
2. Add 200 μL whole blood sample to the tube (see Note 11). If the sample volume is less than 200 μL, add PBS to bring sample to volume.
3. Pipet 20 μL protease into the blood sample in the tube.
4. Add 200 μL buffer AL to the sample (see Note 12). Immediately mix by vortexing for 15 s.
5. Incubate at 56°C for 10 min.
6. Briefly centrifuge the microcentrifuge tube to remove condensation drops from the inside of the lid (see Note 13).
7. Add 200 μL 96–100% ethanol to the sample and mix again by vortexing for 15 s. Again briefly centrifuge the microcentrifuge tube.

8. Carefully apply the sample to the QIAamp spin column in a collection tube without wetting the rim of the spin column. Centrifuge at 6,000 × *g* (8,000 rpm) for 1 min. Place the QIAamp spin column into a clean 2-mL collection tube and discard the tube containing the filtrate.
9. After placing the spin column into a clean collection tube, carefully add 500 μL Buffer AW1 without wetting the rim of the spin column. Centrifuge at 6,000 × *g* (8,000 rpm) for 1 min.
10. Place the spin column into a clean 2-mL collection tube and discard tube with the filtrate. Carefully add 500 μL Buffer AW2 without wetting the rim. Centrifuge at 20,000 × *g* (14,000 rpm) for 3 min.
11. Place the QIAamp spin column in a clean 1.5 mL microcentrifuge tube and discard the tube with the filtrate. Add 200 μL water and incubate at room temperature for 1–5 min.
12. Centrifuge at 6,000 × *g* (8,000 rpm) for 1 min. The isolated DNA is in the liquid fraction.
13. Discard the spin column. Make sure the sample tube is labeled correctly. Store at 4°C for short term, or −20 to −80°C for long-term storage (see Note 14). See Note 15 for a discussion of potential problems.

### 3.2. Polymerase Chain Reaction Amplification of Individual KIR Loci: General

1. See Table 1 for a listing of those *KIR* loci that should be amplified following this protocol (see Note 16).
2. Thaw 10× High Fidelity PCR buffer, 50 mM $MgSO_4$, dNTP mix, primer solutions, and DMSO or 5M betaine solution (see Note 17). Mix the solutions thoroughly before use.
3. Prepare the reaction mix in a 1.5-mL tube as described in Table 4.
4. Vortex the reaction mix and dispense 45 μL volumes into each well of a semi-skirted PCR tray.
5. Add 5 μL of genomic DNA (50–200 ng), purified as described in Subheading 3.1, to each well containing reaction mix (see Note 18).
6. Set up positive and negative amplification control wells. The positive control for each primer pair is 5 μL DNA (50–200 ng) from a cell carrying that *KIR* locus. The negative control for each primer pair is 5 μL DNA (50–200 ng) from a cell lacking that *KIR* gene. For primers amplifying framework genes (*KIR2DL4*, *KIR3DL2*, and *KIR3DL3*), use 5 μL water as a negative control instead of DNA.
7. Place tape seal over entire tray and quick spin the plate in the centrifuge to ensure all the liquid is at the bottom of the wells. Place in the thermal cycler.

**Table 4**
**Composition of reaction master mix for Platinum Taq DNA Polymerase High Fidelity**

| Component | Volume in each reaction[a] |
|---|---|
| 10× High Fidelity PCR buffer | 5 μL |
| $MgSO_4$ (50 mM) | Variable (see Table 2) |
| dNTP (10 mM each) | 1 μL |
| Sense primer (10 μM) (see Table 2) | 2 μL |
| Antisense primer (10 μM) (see Table 2) | 2 μL |
| DMSO or 5 M betaine solution | Variable (see Table 2) |
| Platinum Taq DNA Polymerase High Fidelity (5 U/μL) | 0.5 μL |
| Template DNA | 5 μL (added in later step in protocol) |
| Water | Bring final volume excluding DNA to 45 μL |

[a]The volume for a single reaction is 50 μL including the DNA so multiply the number of amplification reactions desired by 50 to determine how much reaction master mix to make. Always make more than you need to account for losses during pipetting

8. Polymerase chain reaction (PCR) conditions are described in Table 5 (see Note 19).
9. Prepare a 1.5% agarose gel in 1× TBE. Ethidium bromide (2 μL) should be added to the gel solution.
10. After the amplification cycles are complete, confirm amplification by electrophoresis. Mix 5 μL of each amplification reaction with 2 μL of 5× sucrose cresol solution and load the entire sample into one well of the polymerized agarose gel. Electrophorese the DNA ladder as a molecular weight marker. Electrophorese at 100 V for 20 min until the cresol red dye has reached the bottom of the gel.
11. Visualize the bands by placing the gel on a UV translluminator. Photograph the gel. Using the molecular weight markers, determine the approximate molecular weight of the amplicons by comparison. The expected sizes of the amplicons for each locus are listed in Table 2. The presence of additional bands indicates a potential problem (see Note 20).
12. Add the AMPure solution directly to each PCR reaction in the PCR plate. The volume of AMPure to add is 1.8× the reaction volume (see Note 21).
13. Mix thoroughly by pipetting and place the PCR plate onto a magnetic plate to separate the AMPure beads from the solution. Incubate at room temperature for approximately 5–10 min.

**Table 5**
**Polymerase chain reaction amplification conditions**

| | General PCR conditions (see Subheading 3.2) | Nested PCR (see Subheading 3.3) | Long Template PCR (see Subheading 3.7) |
|---|---|---|---|
| Denaturation | 95°C for 5 min | 92°C for 4 min | 92°C for 2 min |
| Initial cycles | 10 cycles<br>95°C for 20 s<br>58–66°C for 30 s (see Table 2)<br>68°C for 3–10 min (see Table 2) | 10 cycles:<br>92°C for 45 s<br>62°C for 45 s<br>72°C for 1.5 min | 10 cycles<br>92°C for 10 s<br>60°C for 30 s<br>68°C for 11 min |
| Secondary cycles | 30 cycles<br>95°C for 20 s<br>52–64°C for 30 s (see Table 2)<br>68°C for 3–10 min (see Table 2) | 30 cycles<br>92°C for 45 s<br>57°C for 45 s<br>72°C for 1.5 min | 30 cycles<br>92°C for 15 s<br>57°C for 30 s<br>68°C for 11 min |
| Final extension | 68°C for 10 min | 72°C for 10 min | 68°C for 10 min |
| Final hold | 4°C | 4°C | 4°C |

14. With the PCR plate on the magnet, aspirate the cleared solution with a pipet and discard.
15. Keeping the PCR plate on the magnet, dispense 200 μL of 70% ethanol to each well. Allow to sit at least 30 s at room temperature. Aspirate the wash solution with a pipet, discard and repeat. Be sure to remove as much ethanol as possible to shorten the drying time. Dry at room temperature for 10 min.
16. To elute the purified DNA, add 30–50 μL (see Note 22) of reagent grade water to each well and mix well by pipetting up and down. Place the plate back on the magnet.
17. Remove the eluate containing the amplified DNA to a clean 96-well plate to begin the DNA sequencing reactions (see Subheading 3.8).

### *3.3. Nested PCR for KIR2DL2 Amplicon B, KIR2DL3 Amplicon A, and KIR2DS4 Amplicon B*

1. See Table 1 for a listing of those *KIR* loci that should be amplified following this protocol.
2. Thaw *Taq* DNA Polymerase, 10× PCR buffer with $MgCl_2$, dNTP mix, 5M betaine solution, and appropriate primer solutions (see Table 2). Mix the solutions thoroughly before use (see Note 23).
3. Prepare the nested PCR reaction master mix as shown in Table 6.
4. Aliquot 45 μL of master mix into each well of a semi-skirted PCR tray.

**Table 6**
**Composition of reaction master mix for nested polymerase chain reaction amplification**

| Components | Volume in each reaction[a] |
|---|---|
| 10× PCR Buffer with $MgCl_2$ | 5 μL |
| dNTP (10 mM each) | 1 μL |
| Sense primer (10 μM) (see Table 2) | 2 μL |
| Antisense primer (10 μM) (see Table 2) | 2 μL |
| 5 M betaine solution | 10 μL |
| Taq DNA Polymerase | 0.25 μL |
| Template DNA | 5 μL (added at later step) |
| Water | Bring final volume excluding DNA to 45 μL |

[a]The volume for a single reaction is 50 μL so multiple the number of amplification reactions desired by 50 to determine how much reaction master mix to make. Always make more than you need to account for losses during pipetting. If you need to add more or less volume of DNA to the reaction mix, adjust volume of water so that the final volume for each sample is 50 μL

5. Add 5 μL of each purified PCR product (i.e., *KIR2DL2* amplicon B, *KIR2DL3* amplicon A, and *KIR2DS4* amplicon B) (50–200 ng) to each well containing reaction mix.
6. Place in the thermal cycler and perform PCR using the protocol in Table 5.
7. Purify the nested PCR product of *KIR2DL2* and *KIR2DL3* for DNA sequencing with AMPure as described in Subheading 3.2, step 12. Purify the nested PCR product of *KIR2DS4* with AMPure as described in Subheading 3.2, step 12. If required, clone the *KIR2DS4* alleles as described in Subheading 3.6.

### 3.4. Isolation of *KIR2DL2* and *KIR2DL3* Using HaploPrep

1. Haplotype-specific extraction is performed using genomic DNA from some cells shown to carry *KIR2DL2* and *KIR2DL3* as described in Table 1.
2. Thaw HaploPrep *KIR2DL2* and *KIR2DL3* locus probes and hybridization buffer on ice (see Notes 24 and 25).
3. Prepare HaploPrep reaction mix as described in Table 7.
4. Pipet up and down to mix the reaction mix thoroughly and dispense the volume listed in Table 7 into 1.5 mL tubes.
5. Add 5 μL genomic DNA (30–150 ng) to each tube containing reaction mix (see Note 26).

**Table 7**
**HaploPrep reaction master mix**

| Components | Volume in each reaction[a] |
|---|---|
| Hybridization buffer H | 15 μL |
| HaploPrep Extraction Probe | 2 μL |
| 2DL2-999T or 2DL3-1316T | |
| Water | 8 μL |
| Genomic DNA | 5 μL (added at a later step) |

[a]The volume for a single reaction is 25 μL without the DNA added so multiply the number of reactions desired by 25 to determine how much reaction master mix to make. Always make more than you need to account for losses during pipetting

6. Cap the tubes, mix well by vortexing, and centrifuge briefly. Place the tubes in a heating block with a heated lid at 95°C and incubate for 15 min to denature the DNA.
7. Insert the EZ1 HaploPrep card into the BioRobot EZ1 following instructions from the instrument manual.
8. Switch on the EZ1 instrument and prepare the instrument as described in the instrument manual.
9. Allow the internal heating block of the EZ1 instrument to heat up to 64°C. After the 15-min incubation in step 6 is complete, remove the tubes from external heating block. Remove the caps, and place opened sample tube containing denatured samples immediately into the EZ1 instrument heating block (see Note 27).
10. Close the instrument door and continue to follow the instruction manual.
11. Once the HaploPrep-isolated DNA has been prepared, perform PCR amplification as described in Subheading 3.2 and proceed with DNA sequencing in Subheading 3.8.

### 3.5. Isolation of *KIR2DL3* Locus: Restriction Enzyme Digestion

1. This protocol is performed for some cells carrying *KIR2DL3* as described in Table 1.
2. Prepare the restriction enzyme reaction mix according to Table 8.
3. Mix the reaction thoroughly and dispense indicated volume from Table 8 into a 1.5-mL tube.
4. Add 20 μL genomic DNA (approximately 2 μg) to each tube containing reaction mix. Incubate at 50°C for 1 h.

**Table 8**
**Restriction enzyme reaction master mix**

| Components | Volume in each reaction[a] |
|---|---|
| 10× NE Buffer 3 | 20 μL |
| *BclI* | 3 μL |
| Genomic DNA | 20 μL (added at a later step) |
| Water | Bring final volume excluding DNA to 180 μL |

[a]The volume for a single reaction is 200 μL so multiple the number of digestion reactions desired by 200 to determine how much reaction master mix to make. Always make more than you need to account for losses during pipetting. If you need to add more or less volume of DNA to the reaction mix, adjust volume of water so that the final volume for each sample is 200 μL

5. Isolate DNA by adding 200 μL phenol:chloroform:isoamyl alcohol to each tube and vortexing (see Note 7).
6. Centrifuge briefly (1–2 min) and transfer the aqueous (top) phase to a clean tube.
7. Add 100 μL reagent grade water to the aqueous phase and vortex. Briefly centrifuge and transfer the aqueous phase (approximately 300 μL) to a clean tube.
8. Add 30 μL 3M sodium acetate to the aqueous phase and place the solution at −20°C for at least 30 min.
9. Centrifuge at 14,000 rpm for 20–30 min at room temperature. Remove the liquid with a pipettor.
10. Wash pellet by adding 200 μL cold 70% ethanol (see Note 28).
11. Centrifuge for 10 min, remove the liquid with a pipettor, and air dry the pellet for approximately 20 min at room temperature.
12. Redissolve the pellet in 20 μL reagent grade water.
13. Perform PCR amplification as performed as described in Subheading 3.2 and proceed with DNA sequencing in Subheading 3.8.

### 3.6. *KIR2DS4* Allele Isolation by Cloning

1. Cloning is required only for PCR amplicons containing both a full-length allele and an allele with a deletion (see Note 29). Prepare a nested *KIR2DS4* amplicon by PCR as described in Subheading 3.3.
2. Verify amplified products on a 1.5% agarose gel with 1Kb DNA ladder as described in Subheading 3.2, step 9.

3. Purify the PCR products using AMPure as described in Subheading 3.2, step 12.
4. Using the TOPO TA cloning kit, clone the PCR product into the pCR 2.1-TOPO vector following the manufacturer's instructions (see Note 30).
5. Add 2μl of the TOPO cloning reaction to a vial of One Shot Chemical *E. coli* and mix gently. Incubate on ice for 5–30 min.
6. Heat-shock the cells for 30 s at 42°C.
7. Add 250 μL of SOC at room temperature to the tube.
8. Incubate in a 37°C shaker (250 rpm) for 1 h before plating on LB agar.
9. Apply 40 μL Xgal (40 mg/mL) and 40 μL 100 mM IPTG to the surface of an LB agar plate containing ampicillin and let dry.
10. To optimize distinct colonies, plate 50 and 100 μL of each transformation onto two separate agar plates. Incubate at 37°C overnight.
11. Pick several isolated white colonies from the agar plate using a sterile toothpick. Transfer each colony of bacteria into a 0.5 mL tube containing 50 μL sterile water (see Note 31).
12. Place the tubes in a heating block at 94°C for 5 min to lyse the bacteria and to inactivate nucleases. Centrifuge at 2,000 rpm for 5 min.
13. Use 5 μL of the supernatant in a 50-μL PCR reaction with the same 2DS4 nested primers and protocol as described in Subheading 3.3.
14. Verify amplification on a 1% agarose gel as described in Subheading 3.2, step 9.
15. Purify the PCR fragments using AMPure as described in Subheading 3.2, step 12 and proceed with DNA sequencing in Subheading 3.8.

### 3.7. Long Template PCR for *KIR3DL1* B and *KIR3DS1* B Amplicons

1. Amplification of long segments of DNA from *KIR3DL1* and *KIR3DL2* will require this protocol (see Table 1). Thaw 10× Expand Long Template buffer 3, dNTP mix, and primer solutions for *KIR3DL1* B and *KIR3S1* B amplicons (see Table 2). Vortex the solutions thoroughly before use (see Note 32).
2. Assemble the reaction mix for the Expand Long Template PCR System as described in Table 9.
3. Vortex the reaction mix thoroughly and dispense 45 μL volumes into each well of semi-skirted PCR tray.
4. Add 5 μL template DNA (100–200 ng) to each well containing reaction mix (see Note 33).

**Table 9**
**Composition of reaction master mix for Expand Long Template PCR reaction**

| Components | Volume in each reaction[a] |
|---|---|
| 10× Expand Long Template buffer 3 | 5 μL |
| dNTP (10 mM) | 2.5 μL |
| Forward primer (10 μM) (see Table 2) | 1.5 μL |
| Reverse primer (10 μM) (see Table 2) | 1.5 μL |
| Expand Long Template Enzyme mix | 0.75 μL |
| Template DNA | 5 μL (added at later step) |
| Water | Bring final volume excluding DNA to 45 μL |

[a]The volume for a single reaction is 50 μL so multiply the number of amplification reactions desired by 50 to determine how much reaction master mix to make. Always make more than you need to account for losses during pipetting. If you need to add more or less volume of DNA to the reaction mix, adjust volume of water so that the final volume for each sample is 50 μL

5. Set up positive and negative control wells as described in Subheading 3.2, step 6.
6. Place in the thermal cycler and perform PCR using the protocol in Table 5.
7. Check for amplification of a band of appropriate size by electrophoresis on a 1.0% agarose gel stained with ethidium bromide as described in Subheading 3.2, step 9.
8. Purify and elute the PCR product with AMPure as described in 3.2, step 12 and proceed with DNA sequencing in Subheading 3.8.

### 3.8. DNA Sequencing

1. Sequence the amplicons using *KIR* loci sequencing primers (see Table 3). For each locus, both sense and antisense primers are used to cover the complete sequence of the exons (Fig. 1) (see Note 34).
2. To each well, add 2 μL of diluted Big Dye Terminator, 1 μL of the appropriate primer (see Table 3), and 3 μL of the purified PCR product. For exon 1 sequences for all *KIR* loci, add 0.3 μL DMSO to the reaction (see Note 35).
3. Place tape seal over entire tray and quick spin the plate in the centrifuge to ensure all liquid is at the bottom of the wells. Place in the thermal cycler.

**Table 10**
**DNA sequencing reaction conditions**

| Conditions for all exons except exon 1 | Conditions for exon 1 |
|---|---|
| 30 cycles | 30 cycles |
| 96°C for 10 s | 96°C for 10 s |
| 50°C for 5 s | 60°C for 1 min |
| 60°C for 4 min | Hold at 4°C |
| Hold at 4°C | |

4. Perform the DNA sequencing reaction using the protocol in Table 10.
5. Use the Agencourt CleanSEQ kit to remove excess dye terminators from the sequence reaction by adding 10 μL of CleanSEQ magnetic beads solution to each well of the sequencing plate.
6. For a 10 μL sequencing reaction, add approximately 75 μL 73% ethanol to each well and mix thoroughly.
7. Place the sequencing plate onto the magnet to separate the beads from the solution. Incubate approximately 3 min at room temperature.
8. With the sequencing plate on the magnet, aspirate the cleared solution with a pipet and discard.
9. Keeping the plate on the magnet, dispense 100 μL 73% ethanol to each well and allow it to sit for at least 30 s at room temperature. Aspirate the solution and discard.
10. Add 30 μL of water to each well. The reactions are now ready to electrophorese on the DNA analyzer.
11. Follow the instructions for operation of the DNA analyzer. The samples are electrophoresed using ABI RunModule "Rapidseq 36_POP7" with the default values. Longer electrophoresis times may be required for some sequences.
12. Sample files are analyzed as described in Subheading 3.9.

### 3.9. Sequence Analysis Including Preparation of Locus-Specific *KIR* Libraries

1. Locus-specific *KIR* libraries must be created prior to analysis of *KIR* sequencing data. Go to the IPD-*KIR* database downloads and open up the FTP directory. Obtain the nucleotide coding region sequences of all known alleles at each *KIR* locus as nuc. fasta files (e.g., *KIR2DL1*_nuc.fasta; one file for each locus). Create two separate libraries for *KIR2DS4*, one library with the full-length allele sequences and a second library with the

sequences of the alleles exhibiting the 22 base pair (bp) deletion.

2. Manually add the intron 8 genomic sequence from one representative allele from each locus to the nucleotide sequence of every allele at the locus. Use the database of the LRC to obtain the intron sequence from the genomic DNA (see Note 36).
3. Manually add the 247 bp genomic sequence found 5′ of exon 1 to each *KIR2DL5* locus allele sequence (see Note 37).
4. Use HLA Librarian to create a sequence library and reference file for each locus following the Library Builder user's guide.
5. Import each nuc.fasta file containing the intron 8 sequence into HLA Librarian assigning a name for the library and reference files (e.g., 2DL1). Enter information into the reference file as indicated including the position of nucleotides at the 5′ and 3′ ends of each exon.
6. Output the files to the Assign directory following instructions in the Assign user's guide.
7. The library should be validated by interpreting the sequences of multiple known *KIR* alleles obtained by sequencing both homozygous and heterozygous reference cell DNA.
8. Once the library has been created, use Assign SBT 3.2.7 software to interpret sequencing results and assign alleles (see Notes 38 and 39).
9. The library should be updated with newer versions of the IPD-*KIR* database as required (see Note 40).

## 4. Notes

1. Blood (8.5 mL) is collected by venipuncture into a yellow top ACD-A tube. ACD is the preferred anticoagulant. Other anticoagulants (e.g., heparin) may inhibit DNA amplification during the polymerase chain reaction. Blood can be aliquoted into 2 mL tubes and stored at -20°C until use. An alternative sample source is a buccal swab, but it is likely that the yield of DNA will be low and insufficient for sequencing of all *KIR* loci. Blood should be treated as a biohazard and handled with caution.
2. The panel of reference cells should include cells that lack specific *KIR* genes as well as cells that carry specific *KIR* genes. It is helpful to know the *KIR* alleles carried by the cells so that they can serve as controls for the assignment of *KIR* alleles.
3. Aliquot diluted primers. Repeated freezing and thawing of diluted oligonucleotide primers should be avoided.

4. The DNA ladder should range in size between 400 and 13,000 bp. It is helpful to have markers every 500–1,000 bp. A high DNA mass ladder (Invitrogen) is also helpful when judging the approximate quantity of amplicon present.
5. Handle carefully; ethidium bromide is a carcinogen.
6. It is critical to have a heated lid for the Haploprep protocol.
7. Handle phenol:chloroform:isoamyl alcohol carefully and work in a fume hood. Alternatives to phenol:chloroform:isoamyl alcohol extraction might be use of the Agencourt AMPure kit (Beckman Coulter, Beverly, MA, USA) or Amicon Ultra centrifugal filters (Millipore, Billerica, MA, USA), but the authors have not tested these products in this protocol.
8. Aliquot diluted primers. Repeated freezing and thawing of diluted oligonucleotide primers should be avoided.
9. Assign is used to obtain *KIR* allele assignments from the DNA sequences obtained. HLA Librarian is used to create the locus-specific *KIR* libraries. Sequencher with its library of full-length genomic sequences and coding region sequences is used to confirm the annealing site of PCR and sequencing primers, to design new primers, and to aid in assigning alleles in unusual sequences.
10. Amplicons generated in previous PCR reactions are a source of sample contamination. By separating the source of the amplicons (i.e., post-PCR activities as defined by thermal cycling and subsequent steps) from the pre-PCR activities (as defined by all steps up to and including assembly of the PCR reaction just prior to placing in the thermal cycler), the potential for contamination is greatly reduced. Ideally, the pre-PCR and post-PCR procedures should be performed in two different rooms, but, if not available, different areas of the laboratory should be set aside. If all activities are to be performed in a single room, pre-PCR activities should occur inside a laminar flow hood, preferably equipped with a UV light. The walls of the hood should be wiped with a freshly made 10% bleach solution (1 part regular bleach:9 parts tap water) before processing samples or preparing PCR samples. Dedicated equipment (e.g., pipettors, test tube racks) and lab coats should be set aside for pre-PCR procedures.
11. Typically, 200 μL of whole blood from a healthy individual will yield 3–12 μg of DNA. Sequencing of each *KIR* locus requires approximately 500 ng DNA. To sequence all the *KIR* loci, 5–10 μg of genomic DNA is required.
12. Never add Buffer AL directly to the protease. To obtain complete lysis, the sample and the Buffer AL must be mixed immediately and thoroughly.

13. The speed of the quick spin should be above 1,000 rpm. Set the speed to 8,000 rpm; press the button for 5 s and release to achieve this speed.

14. DNA should be stored in a neutral to slightly basic buffered solution to prevent degradation. Tris–EDTA (TE) buffer can be used for storage. TE contains EDTA which has a high affinity towards divalent ions like $Ca^{+2}$ and $Mg^{+2}$. These ions are cofactors for many enzymes including nucleases that digest DNA molecules. Since repeated access to a tube of genomic DNA may introduce nucleases, TE buffer will protect DNA from degradation during long-term storage. However, since EDTA can bind divalent ions, it can inhibit Taq polymerase in the PCR reaction. If DNA is stored in deionized water which is often at an acidic pH, DNA degradation can occur by acid hydrolysis.

15. Refer to the QIAamp® DNA Mini Kit handbook for trouble-shooting problems.

16. It is helpful to initially assay for the presence or absence of *KIR* genes using a sequence-specific priming assay as described in Chap. 24. This will facilitate the selection of protocols to use to isolate *KIR* genes for sequencing as described in Table 1. Methods described in this chapter have been published (10–13) (Hou, in preparation).
    Some *KIR* haplotypes include fusion genes. For example, *KIR3DL1/KIR3DL2* hybrid alleles have been found in populations of recent African origin (13, 14). These alleles carry the first five exons of *KIR3DL1* and exons 6–9 of *KIR3DL2*. The *KIR3DL1* primer pairs in this protocol will amplify this chimeric gene. When sequencing amplicon B of *KIR2DL4*, be alert for a single nucleotide deletion that removes the last nucleotide (811) of exon 7 in some alleles (e.g., *KIR2DL4**008). When sequencing *KIR2DL5*, it is possible that a cell may carry three or four alleles, i.e., two alleles of *KIR2DL5A* and two alleles of *KIR2DL5B* are potentially possible. An additional two primer pairs listed in Table 1 will assist in clarifying the allele calls in this situation. These pairs are each specific for a subset of *KIR2DL5* alleles. Sequencing primers used with *KIR2DL5* amplicon A will anneal to these two amplicons.

17. The polymerase and buffer used in the PCR reaction vary for different loci and are described in Table 2. DMSO or 5M betaine solution can improve and enhance the specificity of the polymerase chain reaction. The volumes in each reaction of $MgSO_4$, DMSO, and 5M betaine solution are provided in Table 2.

18. It is critical to have high-quality DNA for the PCR reaction. To quantify the DNA and to determine its purity, read its optical

density (OD) using a spectrophotometer. The NanoDrop spectrophotometer (e.g., NanoDrop ND-1000, NanoDrop Technologies, Inc. Wilmington, DE, USA) uses very small quantities of the solution so it or a similar instrument is recommended. The DNA concentration at OD 260 nm should be >10 ng/μL (OD260 × dilution factor × 50 = ng/μL). The purity as measured by the ratio of the absorbance at 260 nm/absorbance at 280 nm (measuring protein contamination) should be in the 1.65–1.9 range.

19. The thermal cycler should be calibrated at regular intervals to ensure that the temperatures required for PCR are achieved in all of the wells of the thermal cycler. This should be done at least every 6 months or more frequently depending on the usage. The Driftcon Temperature Verification System (CYCLERtest, Landgraaf, Netherlands) is one instrument that might be used if this calibration is performed in-house.
20. The molecular weight markers should be present as single sharp bands. The cresol red dye runs at approximately 125 bp. Each PCR reaction should yield a single bright band of the expected size (see Table 2). (The deletion present in some *KIR2DS4* alleles does not make a visible difference in the mobility of the band compared to alleles without the deletion.) The presence of additional bands suggests that the amplification conditions were less stringent than required and the primer annealing temperature should be raised until a single band is produced. The absence of a band may indicate that the gene is absent (see Note 16) or that the amplification conditions are too stringent. To reduce stingency, lower the annealing temperature until a single strong band is produced. Amplification of a locus or of one of two alleles at a locus may fail if the allele carries a nucleotide sequence variation in a primer annealing site.
21. The AMPure kit will remove unincorporated primers, dNTPs, and salts following the PCR.
22. Comparison of the intensity of staining of a reference mass ladder (see Note 4) to the staining intensity of an amplicon following gel electrophoresis can be used to estimate the amount of amplified DNA in the reaction. In turn, this information can be used to determine the amount of water used to elute purified DNA from the AMPure beads. If the concentration of DNA is low, elute with 30 μL instead of 50 μL of water.
23. Perform the protocol in the post-PCR laboratory since nested PCR uses amplified DNA as a template. Use aliquots of PCR reagents and do not return them to the pre-PCR room.
24. Probe 2DL2-999T targets nucleotide position 708 in exon 6 shared by all known *KIR2DL2* alleles except *KIR2DL2**004.

Probe 2DL3-1316T targets nucleotide position 1024T in exon 9 shared by all known *KIR2DL3* alleles. If *KIR2DL2**004 is present, the allele can be assigned based on amplicon A but cloning or allele-specific nested PCR of the B and C amplicons must be used to obtain the complete allele sequence. The strategies used will depend on the other *KIR* genes found in the sample and co-amplifying with *KIR2DL2**004.

25. It is critical that the buffer be thawed on ice. HaploPrep reagents must be always kept on ice when working with them on the bench.
26. It is critical that the DNA is not sheared so avoid excessive pipetting or vortexing.
27. It is critical that the solution be maintained at a high temperature to prevent renaturation of the DNA prior to exposure to the HaploPrep reagents.
28. Be careful not to lose the pellet.
29. A known 22 bp deletion in some alleles of *KIR2DS4* will make sequencing difficult if such an allele is found together with an allele lacking the deletion. The reading frame will be shifted resulting in uninterpretable sequences in the region of the deletion. In these cases, it is necessary to separate the two alleles by cloning in order to obtain a clear sequence of each allele in this region.
30. The amplified DNA should be obtained by PCR just prior to cloning.
31. The efficiency at which inserts are obtained should be at least 70–80%. The white colonies contain inserted DNA (e.g., *KIR2DS4*); the blue colonies do not contain an insert.
32. It is essential to vortex buffer 3 until the salt is in solution.
33. Ensure that template DNA is of sufficiently high quality and is not degraded. Avoid vigorous mixing or pipetting of the solution to prevent DNA from shearing.
34. The *KIR* sequencing primers flank each exon with the exception of exon 1 and the last two exons (exons 8 and 9). The sequences of exon 1 for all loci except *KIR2DL5* are obtained using only an antisense primer. Since the PCR amplification primers anneal just 5′ of exon 1, it is not possible to obtain a complete "read" of exon 1 sequence using either internal forward primers or the forward PCR primers as sense strand sequencing primers. The *KIR2DL5* A amplicon includes 274 bp of the 5′ upstream region so that transcription factor binding sites impacting gene expression (15) can be evaluated. For exons 8 and 9, one sequencing primer anneals 5′ of exon 8 and the second anneals 3′ of exon 9 so that the resultant sequence includes intron 8.

35. All exon 1 sequence reactions require 5% DMSO. The thermal cycler profile for the sequencing reaction for exon 1 is shown in Table 10 and does not include a primer annealing step. The sequence of exon 1 is very short and the antisense primer site has repeated sequences so that higher denaturation and annealing temperatures are required.

36. It is recommended that locus-specific libraries be created to facilitate the interpretation of *KIR* nucleotide sequences. The intron 8 data are not analyzed so it doesn't matter that the intron 8 sequence in the library comes from a single allele. It is also helpful to have the same length of nucleotides in the intron 8 library sequence so don't insert the intron 8 sequences from multiple alleles.

37. The 5′ sequence for each *KIR2DL5* allele can be found in the IPD-*KIR* database, in GenBank and in publications.

38. The primarily heterozygous sequences are compared to a database of known *KIR* sequences created in this section to identify alleles. The library does not need to be created each time DNA sequencing is performed. Manual inspection of the chromatograph should be performed to confirm assigned sequences and to exclude closely related sequences. Be alert to the presence of novel alleles.

    The allele assignments for multiple loci should be consistent with known telomere and centromere haplotype structures (summarized in ref. (5)). For example, essentially all *KIR* haplotypes carry the framework genes, *KIR3DL3*, *KIR2DL4*, and *KIR3DL2*. Since *KIR2DL2* and *KIR2DL3* are alleles at a single locus, the cell should not carry more than a total of 2 alleles (e.g., two alleles of *KIR2DL2* with *KIR2DL3* absent, not two alleles at *KIR2DL2* and one allele at *KIR2DL3*). The same is true for *KIR3DL1* and *KIR3DS1*. The *KIR2DL5* locus has been duplicated; the two genes are termed *KIR2DL5A* and *KIR2DL5B*. *KIR2DL5A* and *KIR2DL5B* should be associated with either *KIR2DS3* or *KIR2DS5* and specific combinations of alleles at these loci have been observed (11, 16). It should be noted that other *KIR* haplotypes have been described at lower frequencies, for example, a haplotype with a duplication so that an individual carries two *KIR3DL1* alleles and a *KIR3DS1* allele (14, 17, 18).

39. Poor quality sequences should not be interpreted and sequencing of those samples should be repeated.

40. The known *KIR* allele database, IPD-*KIR*, is updated at least annually with new, modified or deleted alleles.

## References


1. Bashirova AA et al (2006) The killer immunoglobulin-like receptor gene cluster: tuning the genome for Defense. Annu Rev Genomics Hum Genet 7:277–300
2. Sanger F, Nicklen S, Coulson AR (1977) DNA sequencing with chain-terminating inhibitors. Proc Natl Acad Sci USA 74:5463–5467
3. Khakoo SI, Carrington M (2006) KIR and disease: a model system or system of models? Immunol Rev 214:186–201
4. Tomblyn M et al (2010) Decreased infections in recipients of unrelated donor hematopoietic cell transplantation from donors with an activating KIR genotype. Biol Blood Marrow Transplant 16:1155–1161
5. Cooley S et al (2010) Donor selection for natural killer cell receptor genes leads to superior survival after unrelated transplantation for acute myelogenous leukemia. Blood 116:2411–2419
6. Moesta AK et al (2008) Synergistic polymorphism at two positions distal to the ligand-binding site makes KIR2DL2 a stronger receptor for HLA-C than KIR2DL3. J Immunol 180:3969–3979
7. Yawata M et al (2008) MHC class I-specific inhibitory receptors and their ligands structure diverse human NK-cell repertoires toward a balance of missing self-response. Blood 112:2369–2380
8. Sharma D et al (2009) Dimorphic motifs in D0 and D1 + D2 domains of killer cell Ig-like receptor 3DL1 combine to form receptors with high, moderate, and no avidity for the complex of a peptide derived from HIV and HLA-A*2402. J Immunol 183:4569–4582
9. Martin MP et al (2007) Innate partnership of HLA-B and KIR3DL1 subtypes against HIV-1. Nat Genet 39:733–740
10. Hou L et al (2010) African Americans exhibit a predominant allele in the midst of extensive KIR2DL1 allelic diversity. Tissue Antigens 76:31–34
11. Hou L et al (2010) Thirty allele-level haplotypes centered around KIR2DL5 define the diversity in an African American population. Immunogenetics 62:491–498
12. Hou L et al (2009) In contrast to other stimulatory natural killer cell immunoglobulin-like receptor loci, several KIR2DS5 alleles predominate in African Americans. Hum Immunol 70:733–737
13. Jiang B et al (2010) The profile of KIR3DL1 and KIR3DS1 alleles in an African American population resembles that found in African populations. Tissue Antigens 76:64–66
14. Norman PJ et al (2009) Meiotic recombination generates rich diversity in NK cell receptor genes, alleles, and haplotypes. Genome Res 19:757–769
15. Vilches C, Gardiner CM, Parham P (2000) Gene structure and promoter variation of expressed and nonexpressed variants of the KIR2DL5 gene. J Immunol 165:6416–6421
16. Ordonez D et al (2008) Duplication, mutation and recombination of the human orphan gene KIR2DS3 contribute to the diversity of KIR haplotypes. Genes Immun 9:431–437
17. Gomez-Lozano N et al (2005) The silent KIR3DP1 gene (CD158c) is transcribed and might encode a secreted receptor in a minority of humans, in whom the KIR3DP1, KIR2DL4 and KIR3DL1/KIR3DS1 genes are duplicated. Eur J Immunol 35:16–24
18. Martin MP et al (2003) Cutting edge: expansion of the KIR locus by unequal crossing over. J Immunol 171:2192–2195
19. Uhrberg M et al (1997) Human diversity in killer cell inhibitory receptor genes. Immunity 7:753–763
20. Vilches C et al (2007) Facilitation of KIR genotyping by a PCR-SSP method that amplifies short DNA fragments. Tissue Antigens 70:415–422
21. Gomez-Lozano N, Vilches C (2002) Genotyping of human killer-cell immunoglobulin-like receptor genes by polymerase chain reaction with sequence-specific primers: an update. Tissue Antigens 59:184–193
22. Murdoch S et al (2006) Detailed gene and allele content analysis of three homozygous KIR haplotypes. Tissue Antigens 68:72–77
23. Sun JY, Oki A, Senitzer D (2008) Alleles and intron polymorphism of KIR3DL1 shown by combination of allele group-specific primers and sequencing. Tissue Antigens 72: 578–580
24. Vilches C, Pando MJ, Parham P (2000) Genes encoding human killer-cell Ig-like receptors with D1 and D2 extracellular domains all contain untranslated pseudoexons encoding a third Ig-like domain. Immunogenetics 51:639–646

# Chapter 26

# An Overview of Methods Required to Evaluate Donor NK Cell Alloreactivity for Haploidentical Haemopoietic Stem Cell Transplantation

**Andrea Velardi**


## Abstract

Donor-vs.-recipient NK cell alloreactivity has been established as a key therapeutic element in HLA haplotypemismatched hematopoietic transplants in acute myeloid leukemia. NK cell allotherapy for leukemia is deployed through stem cell transplantation and ensuing NK cell reconstitution across KIR ligand mismatches. It is effected by functional NK cells which express inhibitory killer cell immunoglobulin-like receptor(s) (KIRs) for self-class I ligand(s), sense missing expression of donor KIR ligand(s) in the recipient, and mediate alloreactions. Donor-vs.-recipient NK cell alloreactivity is evaluated by integrating genetic, phenotypic, and functional features.


**Key words:** HLA, KIR, Alloreactivity, Cytotoxicity, Acute leukemia, Haploidentical hematopoietic transplantation

## 1. Introduction

Donor-vs.-recipient NK cell alloreactivity is a key therapeutic element in the success of HLA haplotype-mismatched ("haploidentical") hematopoietic stem cell transplants (HSCT) for acute leukemia. Milestones along the way towards this breakthrough discovery were observations that: (1) extensive ex-vivo T-cell depletion of the graft prevented graft-vs.-host disease (GvHD), in haploidentical transplants for patients with severe combined immunodeficiency (1); (2) a "megadose" of T-cell-depleted stem cells ensured engraftment across MHC barriers in mice (2), and across HLA barriers in clinical transplantation (3, 4); (3) human NK cells exerted alloreactivity (5, 6); (4) transplantation from haploidentical donors that were able to mount donor-vs.-recipient

Frank T. Christiansen and Brian D. Tait (eds.), *Immunogenetics: Methods and Applications in Clinical Practice*, Methods in Molecular Biology, vol. 882, DOI 10.1007/978-1-61779-842-9_26, © Springer Science+Business Media New York 2012

NK cell alloreactions eradicated acute myeloid leukemia (AML), favored engraftment, protected from GvHD and greatly improved survival, as demonstrated by integrating clinical and preclinical data ((7, 8) reviewed in refs. (9–13)).

Human NK cells possess clonally distributed inhibitory receptors termed "killer cell immunoglobulin-like receptors" (KIRs) that recognize allotypic determinants ("KIR ligands") shared by certain groups of HLA class I alleles. KIR2DL1 recognizes HLA-C alleles with a $Lys^{80}$ residue (HLA-Cw4 and related, "Group 2" alleles), KIR2DL2 and KIR2DL3 recognize HLA-C with an $Asn^{80}$ residue (HLA-Cw3 and related, "Group 1" alleles), KIR3DL1 is the receptor for HLA-B alleles sharing the Bw4 specificity.

All KIR genes are randomly expressed and KIR distribution varies on NK cells. Only NK cells which express inhibitory KIRs for self-HLA ligands are functionally active as they become "licensed/educated" upon interaction with self-HLA molecules and thus enabled to exert alloreactivity against mismatched allogeneic targets which do not express self-HLA inhibitory KIR ligands. NK cells which express, as their only inhibitory receptor for self, a KIR whose ligand is a HLA class I group which is absent on allogeneic targets, sense the missing expression of the self-class I KIR ligand and mediate alloreactions ("missing self" recognition).

Combined evidence from in vitro studies, murine models, and clinical trials indicates the ability of NK cells to mediate donor-vs.-recipient alloreactivity rests on "missing self recognition" which, in humans, involves mismatching for each of the 3 KIR ligands (C1, C2, Bw4) in the graft-vs.-host direction. In clinical hematopoietic stem cell transplantation, NK cells mature in a bone marrow microenvironment in which they are predominantly exposed to donor HLA (on hematopoietic cells), which shapes their repertoire to be both self (donor)-tolerant and recipient-alloreactive. In fact, under such mismatch conditions, engrafted stem cells give rise to an NK cell repertoire of donor origin which includes alloreactive clones that kill recipient cryopreserved leukemic cells (see Fig. 1). The beneficial effects of donor-vs.-recipient NK alloreactivity in haploidentical transplants have been confirmed in an updated analysis of 112 high-risk AML patients. The presence of NK alloreactivity was associated with significantly lower relapse rates and better event-free survival (10). NK cell alloreactivity has been shown to provide better protection from leukemia relapse when exerted by maternal donors (14), presumably because of the additive effect of memory T-cell immunity against the child's paternal HLA haplotype that results from maternal exposure to fetal antigens during pregnancy. T-cell-depleted megadose hematopoietic transplantation from NK alloreactive donors has been reported to lower the risk of relapse also in pediatric leukemias (15).

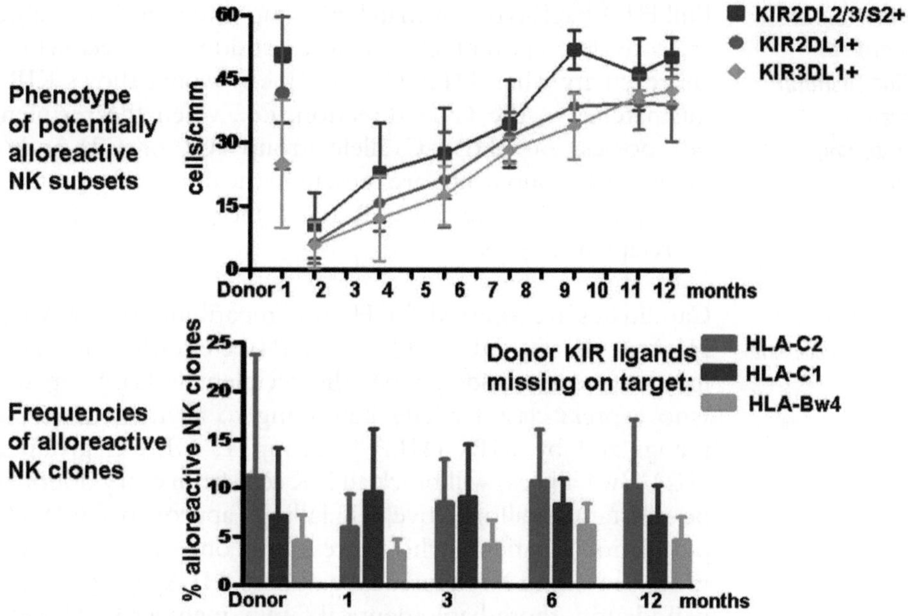


Fig. 1. Posttransplant regeneration of donor-vs.-recipient alloreactive NK cell repertoires. *Top*: absolute numbers of potentially alloreactive NK cells (as evaluated by immune-fluorescence), i.e., of NK cells that express, as their only inhibitory receptor for self, the KIR for which there is no ligand in the recipient (see Subheading 2.3.4). *Bottom*: frequencies of alloreactive NK clones across each one of the three KIR ligand mismatches (C1, C2, Bw4), as documented by limiting dilution cloning and cytotoxicity assays (see Subheading 2.3.5).

## 2. Methods and Key Reagents

### *2.1. Haploidentical Donor HSCT Transplantation Procedures*

Conditioning of the recipient consists of 8 Gy total-body irradiation on day 9 in a single fraction at an instantaneous dose-rate of 0.16 Gy/min; lungs shielded to receive 0.04 Gy; thiotepa (5 mg/kg daily) on days 8 and 7; fludarabine (40 $mg/m^2$ daily) from day 7 to day 3; rabbit anti-thymocyte globulin (ATG) is given at 5 mg/kg daily from days 5 to 2 (4, 8, 10). No immune suppression is given after transplantation as GvHD prophylaxis; no G-CSF is administered posttransplantation.

### *2.2. Graft Processing*

Peripheral-blood hematopoietic progenitor cells from the donor are mobilized and collected as previously described (4, 8, 10). CD34 positive cells are selected using the CliniMacs one-step procedure (Miltenyi Biotech, Bergisch Gladbach, Germany). Flow cytometric analysis quantifies CD34, CD3, and CD20 positive cells before and after selection. G-CSF stem cell mobilization and graft processing. The stem cell "megadose" (i.e., $10 \times 10^6$ cells/kg body weight) is routinely achieved by administering a short course of granulocyte-colony stimulating factor (G-CSF) to the donor, followed by leukapheresis and immunomagnetic-based CD34+ stem cell selection (see Note 1).

### 2.3. Selection of Haploidentical Donors Able to Mount Donor-Versus-Recipient NK Cell Alloreactions

#### 2.3.1. Definition

Full HLA haplotype-mismatched ("haplo-identical") family donors are considered potentially able to exert donor-vs.-recipient NK cell alloreactivity when HLA-C and HLA-B typing shows KIR ligand mismatches in the GvH direction, i.e., when the recipient does not possess one HLA-C allele group (C1 or C2) and/or the HLA-Bw4 group which are present in the donor. Moreover, donors must possess the relevant KIR gene(s) for missing self-recognition on recipient targets.

#### 2.3.2. Identification of Suitable Donor-Recipient Pairs

Candidates are assessed for HLA compatibility by HLA typing at HLA-A, -B, -C, -DR, -DQ, and -DP (see elsewhere in this volume for detailed methods). First, the recipient is HLA typed. Those who express class I alleles belonging to all three class I groups recognized by KIRs (HLA-C group 1, HLA-C group 2, and HLA-Bw4 alleles) will block all NK cells from every donor and will be resistant to alloreactive NK killing (approximately 1/3 of the population). Patients who express only one or two of these allele groups may find NK alloreactive donors. HLA typing on the family will identify those haploidentical family member(s) who expresses the class I group(s) missing in the recipient and who have, therefore, the potential to be a donor whose NK cells exert alloreactivity against the recipient.

#### 2.3.3. KIR Genotyping

Donor KIR genotyping is performed to ensure the donor possesses the relevant inhibitory KIR gene to exert alloreactivity (see Note 2). Moreover, KIR genotyping identifies donors who also possess activating KIR genes (approximately 2/3 of Caucasian population). Studies suggest activating KIRs may play a role in NK cell alloreactivity and haploidentical transplantation (see Note 3). Detailed methods for KIR typing are provided elsewhere in this volume. In our laboratory, KIR typing is performed using a low resolution PCR-SSP assay (KIR Genotyping Kit, Invitrogen, USA) following the manufacturer's instructions. This kit is designed to identify 14 KIR genes (*2DL1, 2DL2, 3DL1, 2DL4, 2DL5, 2DS1, 2DS2, 2DS3, 2DS4, 2DS5, 3DL1, 3DL2, 3DL3, 3DS1*), 2 pseudogenes (2DP1 and 3DP1) and the common variants of *KIR2DL5* (KIR2DL5A, KIR2DL5B), the *KIR2DS4* allele (*001/002 and *003), and *KIR3DP1* allele (*001/002 and *003).

#### 2.3.4. KIR Phenotyping

KIR phenotyping is undertaken to identify potentially alloreactive donor NK cells. Potentially alloreactive donor NK cells are those cells that express, as their only inhibitory receptor for self, the KIR for which there is no ligand in the recipient. Four-color immunofluorescence analysis identifies $KIR^-/NKG2A^+$ vs. $KIR^+/NKG2A^-$, $CD56^+/CD3^-$ NK cells. The following mouse monoclonal antibodies: allophycocyanin (APC)-conjugated anti-CD56 (IgG1; Miltenyi, Bergisch Gladbach, Germany), phycoerythrin (PE)-Cy7-conjugated anti-CD3 (IgG1; BD Bioscience, San Diego,

CA), unconjugated anti-NKG2A (clone Z199, IgG2b) developed with fluorescein isothiocyanate (FITC)-conjugated goat anti-mouse IgG2b antibodies (Southern Biotech, Birmingham, AL), are used in combination with the following PE-conjugated anti-KIR antibodies (Bechman Coulter, Fullerton, CA): either anti-KIR2DL2/3/S2 (clone GL183, IgG1), or anti-KIR2DL1/S1 (clone EB6B, IgG1), or anti-KIR3DL1/S1 (clone Z27, IgG1).

Two-color immunofluorescence analyses are used to visualize NK cells expressing, as their only inhibitory receptor for self, a KIR for which there was no class I ligand in the recipient. KIR2DL2/3/S2 single-positive NK cells are identified with FITC-conjugated anti-KIR2DL2/3/S2 antibody (clone CH-L, IgG2b, BD Bioscience, Franklin Lakes, NJ) in combination with a cocktail of PE-conjugated anti-KIR2DL1 (clone 143211, IgG1, R&D, Minneapolis, MI), anti-KIR3DL1 (clone DX9, IgG1, Miltenyi), and anti-NKG2A (clone Z199, IgG2b, Beckman Coulter, Brea, CA) mouse antibodies. KIR2DL1 single-positive NK cells were identified with PE-conjugated anti-KIR2DL1 (clone 143211, IgG1, R&D, Minneapolis, MI) in combination with a cocktail of FITC-coniugated anti-KIR3DL1 (clone DX9, IgG1, Miltenyi) and anti-KIR2DL2/3S2 (clone CH-L, IgG2b) and anti-NKG2A (clone Z199, IgG2b, Beckman Coulter, Brea, CA) mouse antibodies developed with FITC-conjugated goat anti-mouse IgG2b antibodies (Southern-Biotech). The same assays are used to monitor posttransplant reconstitution of potentially alloreactive NK cells (Fig. 1).

#### 2.3.5. NK Cell Cloning and Cytotoxicity Assay

This analysis aims to confirm donor NK alloreactivity against the recipient by formally identifying donor NK cells which kill allogeneic recipient targets, such as PHA lymphoblasts and/or leukemia cells (see Note 4). Large numbers of donor NK clones are generated by limiting dilution and cytotoxicity assays against recipient target cells are used to detect the frequency of alloreactive NK clones. Peripheral blood mononuclear cells are depleted of T cells by negative anti-CD3 immunomagnetic selection (Miltenyi), are plated under limiting-dilution conditions, activated with phytohemagglutinin (PHA; Biochrom KG, Berlin, Germany), and cultured with interleukin-2 (Chiron BV, Amsterdam, Netherlands) and irradiated feeder cells. Feeder cells are obtained by pooling buffy coats from 5 to 9 healthy donors. Such donors are not HLA typed as PHA + IL2 activation allows efficient NK cell repertoire cloning regardless of feeder cell HLA type. Cloning efficiencies ranges from 1 in 5 to 1 in 10 plated NK cells. Cloned NK cells are screened for alloreactivity by standard 51-Cromium release cytotoxicity at an effector-to-target ratio of 10:1 against recipient PHA lymphoblasts and leukemic cells. Approximately 100 NK clones from each person are screened. Clones exhibiting greater than 30% lysis are scored as alloreactive. The assay is considered positive when the frequency of lytic clones was more than 1 in 50. The same assays are used to monitor posttransplant reconstitution of alloreactive NK cell clones (Fig. 1).

## 3. Notes

1. Median-infused cell doses per kilogram of recipient body weight are as follows: CD34+, $13.8 \times 10^6$/kg (range, 5.1–$29.7 \times 10^6$/kg); CD3+, $1 \times 10^4$/kg (range, 0.04–$3.0 \times 10^4$/kg); and CD20+, $4.1 \times 10^4$/kg (range, 0.4–$22.2 \times 10^4$/kg). The number of infused CD34+ cells per kilogram is generally in the range of 8–$16 \times 10^6$/kg. Median recovery of CD34+ cells is 79%, and purity is 95%. Median T- and B-cell depletion is 4.5 and 3.2 log.
2. Most donors have the potential to exert NK alloreactions as they possess a full complement of inhibitory KIR genes. HLA-C group 1 receptor genes (KIR2DL2 and/or KIR2DL3) are present in 100% of individuals, and the HLA-C group 2 receptor gene (KIR2DL1) in 97%. Therefore, the combination of HLA-C group 2-positive donor/HLA-C group 2-negative recipient which occurs in approximately 1.5% of HLA-C group mismatched transplants, requires donor KIR2DL1 gene typing. The HLA-Bw4 receptor gene (KIR3DL1) is found in approximately 90% of individuals.
3. Studies have suggested the specificity of alloreactive NK cells across C1 mismatching is effected by the activating receptor KIR2DS1 which binds C2 on targets (15–19). Such alloreactive cells are relatively infrequent (approximately 1%) and are only found in C1 homozygous individuals (who lack C2). Patients who have all three KIR ligands (C1, C2, Bw4), who are, therefore, not considered susceptible to donor-vs.-recipient NK cell alloreactivity, might benefit from transplantation from haploidentical C1-homozygous, K2DS1+ donors who possess KIR2DS1 alloreactive cells.

   Additional results in haploidentical transplantation for pediatric acute leukemia have emphasized the role of activating KIR variants in NK cell alloreactivity. While donor KIR2DL1+ NK cells showed good alloreactivity against C2 negative targets, donor KIR2DL2+ and/or 2DL3+ NK cells in most cases showed only poor allorecognition against target cells lacking C1. Allorecognition of these C1 negative (C2 positive) targets depended mainly on the NK cells possessing KIR2DS1 to bind C2. These observations impact on the number of children who might be cured of leukemia. They reduce the pool of NK alloreactive donors because the *KIR2DS1* gene is present in only approximately 1/3 of Caucasians. This genetic restriction does not apply to haploidentical transplantation for AML in adults. In analyzing donor NK cell alloreactivity against C1 missing targets (either PHA blasts or AML cells), frequencies of alloreactive NK cell clones did not differ significantly in KIR2DS1 negative and positive donors, NK alloreactive repertoires in KIR2DS1 positive individuals were largely composed of KIR2DS1-negative clones and, finally, negative clones killed as efficiently as the positive (L. Ruggeri et al., unpublished). Indeed, in an updated analysis of event-free survival of a series of adult AML patients undergoing haploidentical transplantation, each of the 3 KIR ligand mismatches (C1, C2, Bw4) provided a survival advantage over non-NK alloreactive (KIR ligand-matched) transplants regardless of donor activating KIR genetics ((10) and L. Ruggeri et al., unpublished).

4. When tested in large donor cohorts (10), functional analyses detected high-frequency alloreactive NK clones against either HLA-C1 or HLA-C2 group-mismatched allogeneic targets. On the contrary, only 2/3 of HLA-Bw4-positive individuals with the KIR3DL1 gene display alloreactive NK clones against allogeneic HLA-Bw4-negative targets. Failure to detect alloreactive NK clones may be due to their highly variable frequencies, or because certain allelic KIR3DL1 variants do not allow receptor expression at the cell membrane (reviewed in ref. (13)). In donor-recipient pairs that are not KIR ligand-mismatched in the graft-vs.-host direction, no donor alloreactive NK clones are found, indicating that KIR ligand mismatching is a prerequisite for NK cell alloreactivity (10).

## References

1. Reisner Y, Kapoor N, Kirkpatrick D et al (1983) Transplantation for severe combined immunodeficiency with HLA-A, B, D, DR incompatible parental marrow cells fractionated by soybean agglutinin and sheep red blood cells. Blood 61:341–348
2. Bachar-Lustig E, Rachamim N, Li HW et al (1995) Nat Med 1:1268–1273
3. Aversa F, Tabilio A, Terenzi A et al (1994) Successful engraftment of T-cell-depleted haploidentical “three-loci” incompatible transplants in leukemia patients by addition of recombinant human granulocyte colony-stimulating factor-mobilized peripheral blood progenitor cells to bone marrow inoculum. Blood 84:3948–3955
4. Aversa F, Tabilio A, Velardi A et al (1998) Treatment of high-risk acute leukemia with T-cell-depleted stem cells from related donors with one fully mismatched HLA haplotype. N Engl J Med 339:186–193
5. Ciccone E, Pende D, Viale O et al (1992) Evidence of a natural killer (NK) cell repertoire for (allo) antigen recognition: definition of five distinct NK-determined allospecificities in humans. J Exp Med 175:709–718
6. Colonna M, Brooks EG, Falco M et al (1993) Generation of allospecific natural killer cells by stimulation across a polymorphism of HLA-C. Science 260:1121–1124
7. Ruggeri L, Capanni M, Casucci M et al (1999) Role of natural killer cell alloreactivity in HLA-mismatched hematopoietic stem cell transplantation. Blood 94:333–339
8. Ruggeri L, Capanni M, Urbani E et al (2002) Effectiveness of donor natural killer cell alloreactivity in mismatched hematopoietic transplants. Science 295:2097–20100

9. Kärre K (2002) A Perfect Mismatch. Science 295:2029–2031
10. Ruggeri L, Mancusi A, Capanni M et al (2007) Donor natural killer cell allorecognition of missing self in haploidentical hematopoietic transplantation for acute myeloid leukemia: challenging its predictive value. Blood 110: 433–440
11. Velardi A (2008) Role of KIRs and KIR ligands in hematopoietic transplantation. Curr Opin Immunol 20:581–587
12. Christiansen FT, Velardi A (2009) Progress in understanding and exploiting the immune response in solid organ and hemopoietic stem cell transplantation. Curr Opin Immunol 21:522–524
13. Velardi A, Ruggeri L, Mancusi A et al (2009) Natural killer cell allorecognition of missing self in allogeneic hematopoietic transplantation: a tool for immunotherapy of leukemia. Curr Opin Immunol 21:525–530
14. Stern M, Ruggeri L, Mancusi A (2008) Survival after T cell-depleted haploidentical stem cell transplantation is improved using the mother as donor. Blood 112:2990–2995
15. Pende D, Marcenaro S, Falco M et al (2009) Anti-leukemia activity of alloreactive NK cells in KIR ligand-mismatched haploidentical HSCT for pediatric patients: evaluation of the functional role of activating KIR and redefinition of inhibitory KIR specificity. Blood 113:3119–3129
16. Witt CS, Christiansen FT (2006) The relevance of natural killer cell human leucocyte antigen epitopes and killer cell immunoglobulin-like receptors in bone marrow transplantation. Vox Sang 90:10–20
17. Foley BA, De Santis D, Van Beelen E et al (2008) The reactivity of Bw4+ HLA-B and HLA-A alleles with KIR3DL1: implications for patient and donor suitability for haploidentical stem cell transplantations. Blood 112:435–443
18. Foley B, De Santis D, Lathbury L (2008) KIR2DS1-mediated activation overrides NKG2A-mediated inhibition in HLA-C C2-negative individuals. Int Immunol 20:555–563
19. Chewning JH, Gudme CN, Hsu KC (2007) KIR2DS1-positive NK cells mediate alloresponse against the C2 HLA-KIR ligand group in vitro. J Immunol 179:854–868

# Chapter 27

# The Detection of NK Cell Alloreactivity by Flow Cytometric CD107a Assay

Dianne De Santis, Bree Foley, Campbell S. Witt, and Frank T. Christiansen

## Abstract

Natural killer (NK) cell alloreactivity can be exploited in haploidentical (one haplotype mismatched) haematopoietic stem cell transplantation (HSCT) to prevent leukaemia relapse, rejection, and graft-vs-host disease (GVHD) (Blood 94:333–339; Science 295:2097–2100). If NK cell alloreactivity is to be exploited in HSCT, it is important to be able to reliably select donors who have NK alloreactivity towards the patient. The detection of donor NK alloreactivity towards patient target cells has traditionally been evaluated by NK cell cloning and $^{51}$Cr-release cytotoxicity assay. This approach is complex and time consuming with results taking up to 6 weeks. Here, we detail a novel flow cytometric CD107a-based assay capable of detecting NK cell alloreactivity in 14 days.

**Key words:** Natural killer cells, Killer immunoglobulin-like receptors, Alloreactivity, CD107a, Flow cytometry

## 1. Introduction

### 1.1. Background

NK cell cytotoxicity is regulated by a balance of inhibitory and activating signals from receptors expressed on the cell surface. NK cell cytotoxicity is inhibited when inhibitory receptors, such as killer immunoglobulin-like receptors (KIR) interact with self-class I HLA molecules on potential targets (1). The inhibitory KIR recognise allelic epitopes on HLA-B and HLA-C molecules. HLA-C alleles can be divided into two groups based on their amino acid at position 80. C1-group alleles have an asparagine at position 80 and are recognised by the inhibitory receptors KIR2DL2 and KIR2DL3. C2-group alleles have a lysine at position 80 and are recognised by KIR2DL1 (2–5). HLA-B alleles can also be divided into two groups, Bw4 and Bw6, based on the

Frank T. Christiansen and Brian D. Tait (eds.), *Immunogenetics: Methods and Applications in Clinical Practice*, Methods in Molecular Biology, vol. 882, DOI 10.1007/978-1-61779-842-9_27, © Springer Science+Business Media New York 2012

amino acids 77–83. KIR3DL1 recognise HLA-B and some HLA-A alleles with the Bw4 epitope (6–8). The range of different KIR receptors expressed by NK clones in an individual is primarily determined by the KIR genotype but an individual's HLA genotype determines which KIR can be expressed as the only inhibitory receptor on individual NK cell clones (9). Receptor selection occurs during NK cell development to ensure only NK cells with an inhibitory receptor for a self-ligand are permitted to become armed for cytotoxicity (10).

### 1.2. Role of NK Alloreactivity in the Clinical Setting

In a series of studies Ruggeri and colleagues showed that donor-vs-recipient NK cell alloreactivity resulted in less relapse, rejection, GVHD, and increased survival in human haploidentical transplants and murine transplant models (11, 12). Most importantly in haploidentical transplants, NK cells were shown to mediate GVL effects without GVHD (11). Since the initial studies of Ruggeri et al., a number of retrospective studies have been performed in haploidentical and unrelated HSCT. However, many of the studies failed to confirm the findings published by Ruggeri et al. The extensive T-cell depletion used in Perugia compared to the other studies has been considered as a possible explanation for the differences observed. However, other differences in transplant protocols, such as conditioning regimen or stem cell source, or heterogeneous cohorts with differences in the proportions of disease type could also be responsible for the differences observed between the studies. If the findings of Ruggeri et al. can be confirmed in other transplant settings using the same transplant protocol allowing NK cell alloreactivity to be exploited in stem cell transplants, it will be important to be able to reliably select donors who are alloreactive towards the patient.

Donor NK alloreactivity towards a recipient can largely be predicted if the recipient lacks one of the C1, C2, or Bw4 epitopes that is present in the donor. However, this assumes that all HLA-C and HLA-B alleles interact with the appropriate inhibitory KIR receptors as predicted by the presence of the relevant amino acid and that all alleles of the inhibitory KIR receptors interact the same way with the HLA epitopes. Recently, these assumptions have been shown not to be always true. The Bw4-associated HLA-B13 allele has been shown not to interact with KIR3DL1 (13) while KIR2LD2 and KIR2DL3 may interact with both C1- and C2-group HLA-C alleles (14–16). As there has been no comprehensive study to determine which of the HLA alleles interact with KIR receptors, it is not possible to reliably predict alloreactivity from the HLA and KIR genotype. A functional assay is therefore required to confirm NK alloreactivity.

### 1.3. Assays for the Detection of NK Cell Alloreactivity

#### 1.3.1. NK Cloning and Chromium-Release Cytotoxicity

NK cloning and $^{51}$chromium (Cr)-release cytotoxicity assay has been used to detect potential NK alloreactivity. NK clones are used in the cytotoxicity assay as effector cells. Briefly, enriched NK cells are serially diluted (40, 20, 10, 5, 2 cells/100 μL) and cultured with irradiated pooled allogeneic PBMC feeder cells. Following 14–20 days of culture with IL-2 supplemented medium, each NK clone is subcultured and grown further to numbers sufficient for use in cytotoxicity assays to determine NK cell cytotoxicity. As only a few percent of NK clones are expected to demonstrate alloreactivity, 200 clones must be tested in order to be confident of detecting the alloreactive clones. Traditionally, a $^{51}$chromium (Cr)-release cytotoxicity assay is used in which each NK clone is tested for the ability to kill a range of allogeneic targets. These methods are labour intensive and time consuming with results available in around 6 weeks.

#### 1.3.2. The Flow Cytometric CD107a Assay

NK cells have a large number of preformed cytolytic granules in their cytoplasm. Following activation, NK cells release these granules to the site of cell–cell contact (immunological synapse). These granules contain cytolytic proteins, such as perforin and granzyme, that are involved in inducing target cell death (17). Lining the membrane of the granules is the lysosomal-associated membrane protein, LAMP-1 or CD107a (18). CD107a is a glycoprotein representing approximately 50% of the proteins in the lysosomal membrane. During degranulation, CD107a on the luminal membrane is exposed in the immunological synapse and therefore accessible for antibody binding. Betts et al. (19) showed CD107a expression on the cell surface was a marker of cytotoxic CD8+ T cell degranulation. Alter et al. (20) showed that CD107a can also be detected on the surface of NK cells following stimulation with target cells lacking HLA ligands. By modifying the method described by Alter et al. we have developed a rapid flow cytometric assay to detect KIR-dependent alloreactive NK cells. Here, we provide a detailed protocol for the rapid, efficient detection of donor NK alloreactivity by a flow cytometric, CD107a-based assay.

## 2. Materials

1. Target EBV-transformed BLCL (Table 1) (see Note 1).
2. Peripheral blood lymphocyte (PBMC) feeder cells (Subheading 3.1).
3. 1× PBS—17 g NaCl, 2.68 g $Na_2HPO_4 2H_2O$ (disodium hydrogen orthophosphate) and 0.78 g $NaH_2PO_4 2H_2O$ (sodium dihydrogen orthophosphate) were dissolved in 2 L Milli-Q water and the pH adjusted to 7.2.

**Table 1**
**HLA types and KIR epitopes of BLCL used as target cells used in the CD107a assay**

| | KIR epitopes | | | | | |
|---|---|---|---|---|---|---|
| Identifier | C1 | C2 | BW4 | HLA-A | HLA-B | HLA-C |
| "721.221" | – | – | – | – | – | – |
| "All" | + | + | + | 01, 03 | 27, 44 | 01, 04 |
| "C1" | – | + | + | 02 | 57 | 06 |
| "C2" | + | – | + | 33 | 58 | 03 |
| "Bw4" | + | + | – | 03, 11 | 07, 35 | 04, 07 |

4. Heat inactivated foetal calf serum (HIFCS) (see Note 2). Foetal calf serum (Thermo Trace, Melbourne, Australia) was incubated at 56°C with shaking for 30 min, aliquotted and stored at –20°C.
5. Ficoll-Paque Plus (Pharmacia, Uppsala, Sweden).
6. RPMI 1640 medium (Invitrogen, Carlsbad, USA) supplemented with 500 IU/mL penicillin, 500 μg/mL streptomycin, 2 mM L-glutamine, and 10% sterile FCS.
7. DMSO (BDH, Poole, UK).
8. GammaCell 3000 ELAN gamma irradiator (MDS Nordion, Canada).
9. Rosette-Sep Human NK enrichment cocktail (StemCell Technologies, Canada).
10. 2-ME (ICN Biochemicals, OH, USA)—dilute 1:250 in RPMI and store at –20°C. A 1:1,000 dilution of this stock is then added to NK cell culture medium.
11. NK culture medium—RPMI 1640 medium supplemented with penicillin (100 IU/mL), streptomycin (100 μg/mL), L-glutamine (2 mM), 10% HIFCS, 1% non-essential amino acids, 1% pyruvate, and 2-mercaptoethanol.
12. Centrifuge (Multifuge 3, Heraeus).
13. IL-2 (Chiron, Emeryville. USA).
14. 96-well round bottom culture plates (BD, Franklin Lakes, USA).
15. Antibodies (see Table 2).
16. Monensin (6 μg/mL), (BD GolgiStop BD Biosciences).
17. Paraformaldehyde (Sigma P6148)—Dissolve 2 g paraformaldehyde in 100 mL PBS and heat solution to 56°C with

**Table 2**
**Antibodies used in the CD107a experiments**

| Antibody | Fluorochrome | Isotype | Clone | Dilution | Supplier |
|---|---|---|---|---|---|
| CD56 | PeCy7 | IgG1 | B159 | 1/40 | BD Biosciences |
| CD158a | PE | IgG1 | EB6B | 1/10 | Beckman Coulter |
| CD158b | PE | IgG1 | GL183 | 1/10 | Beckman Coulter |
| CD158a | APC | IgG1 | EB6B | 1/25 | Beckman Coulter |
| CD158b | APC | IgG1 | GL183 | 1/25 | Beckman Coulter |
| CD158e | PE | IgG1 | z27.3.7 | 1/10 | Beckman Coulter |
| NKB1(CD158e) | PE | IgG1 | DX9 | 1/10 | BD Biosciences |
| CD107a | FITC | IgG1 | H4A3 | 1/20 | BD Biosciences |

gently shaking. Cool solution and adjust pH to 7.4. Store solution at 4°C wrapped in foil.

18. Trypan blue (ICN Biochemicals, Ohio USA)—Dissolve 0.5 g trypan blue in 100 mL 1× PBS. Sterilise solution using a 0.22-μM filter and store at room temperature.
19. Freezing medium—RPMI 1640, 20% HIFCS, and 10% DMSO.
20. Flow buffer—add 2% HIFCS and 0.1% sodium azide to 1× PBS and store at 4°C.
21. BD FACSCanto Flow Cytometer with BD FACSDiva Software.
22. Adjustable pipettes (2, 10, 20, 100, and 200 μL).

## 3. Methods

### 3.1. Preparation of Peripheral Blood Lymphocytes Feeder Cells

1. PBMC are isolated from ten random buffy coats. From the ten random donors, centrifuge 10 mL of acid citrate dextrose (ACD) blood at 300×*g* for 10 min and harvest 1 mL of buffy coat from each donor (see Note 3).
2. Dilute each buffy coat 1:3 in PBS containing 2% HIFCS (see Note 2), overlay diluted buffy coat onto Ficoll-paque™ PLUS and centrifuge at 1,200×*g* for 20 min with no brake (see Note 4).
3. Harvest the cells from the interface and wash 3 times with PBS/2% HIFCS at 300×*g* for 7 min.
4. Resuspend the cell pellet in 1 mL RPMI/10% HIFCS, count and adjust to $10^6$/mL.

5. Each of the donor's cells at $10^6$/mL should be pooled in equal volumes. The total number of cells from each donor must be the same. Any remaining donor cells can be stored in liquid nitrogen for later use.
6. Irradiate pooled allogeneic PBMC at 30 Gy (see Note 5). After irradiation, wash cells twice with RPMI/10% HIFCS at $300 \times g$ for 7 min to remove any free radicals in cell suspension generated by the irradiation process.
7. Following final wash, resuspend cell pellet in 1-mL NK cell culture medium, count and adjust to $3 \times 10^6$/mL ready for use. Irradiated feeder cells can also be stored in liquid nitrogen for later use (see Note 6).

#### 3.2. Enrichment of NK Cells and Preparation of 12-Day Polyclonal NK Cultures

1. To 4 mL of donor ACD blood add 200 μL of Rosette-Sep Human NK cell enrichment cocktail (50-μL cocktail mix/mL ACD blood) and incubate for 20 min at room temperature with gentle mixing (see Note 7).
2. Following incubation, dilute with equal volume of PBS/2% HIFCS and overlay onto 4 mL of Ficoll-paque™ PLUS. Centrifuge at $1{,}200 \times g$ for 20 min with no brake.
3. Following centrifugation, harvest the cell interface and wash cell pellet 3 times with PBS/2% HIFCS at $300 \times g$ for 7 min (see Note 8).
4. During washing steps, prepare NK medium supplemented with IL-2 to a final concentration of 200 IU/mL.
5. Resuspend the cell pellet in 1 mL NK cell medium supplemented with IL-2 (as prepared in step 4), count and adjust to a final concentration of $3 \times 10^5$/mL with supplemented NK medium.
6. To prepare polyclonal NK cultures, to each well of a 96-well plate, add 100 μL of NK cell suspension from step 5 and 100 μL of the irradiated PBMC feeder cells from Subheading 3.1, step 7. The ratio of NK cells:PBMC feeder cells should be 1:10.
7. On day 3 and every third day, remove 100 μL of supernatant from each well without disturbing the cell pellet and replace with 100 μL of fresh NK culture medium supplemented with 200 IU IL-2/mL. Resuspend the cell pellet, cover the plate, and incubate at 37°C 5% $CO_2$.
8. After 12 days, pool the polyclonal NK cells into a tube, count and adjust to a working cultured polyclonal NK cells can also be frozen and stored in liquid nitrogen for later use (see Note 6).

#### 3.3. Preparation of EBV-Transformed BLCL Target Cells

EBV-transformed BLCL expressing the HLA alleles that encode the presence or absence of the C1, C2, and Bw4 epitopes are used as target cells in the CD107a assay. The 721.221 cell line, a class I negative human BLCL, is also used as a positive control (see Table 1, Note 1).

1. Maintain cell lines in NK cell culture medium and subculture every 2–3 days to $1 \times 10^5$ cells/mL.
2. Subculture and feed target BLCL the day before use. On the day of the assay, count the cells and adjust to $1 \times 10^6$/mL ready for use.

### 3.4. CD107a Cytotoxicity Assay

1. Before use in the CD107a assay, 12-day cultured polyclonal NK cells are activated by further culture for 48 h with NK medium supplemented with 400 IU IL-2/mL (see Note 10). To each well of a 96-well plate, add 100 μL of the cultured polyclonal NK cells from Subheading 3.2, step 8 and 100 μL of IL-2 supplemented NK medium. Incubate for 48 h at 37°C 5% $CO_2$.
2. After the 48-h incubation, pool cells from each well, count and adjust to $1 \times 10^6$/mL in fresh NK cell culture medium.
3. Activated cultured polyclonal NK cells from each donor should be incubated alone (background control), with the HLA class I negative 721.221 target (positive control), a target expressing all epitopes (negative control), target cells expressing C2 and Bw4 and lacking only C1 ($C1^-$), target cells expressing C1 and Bw4 and lacking only C2 ($C2^-$), and target cells expressing both C1 and C2 but not Bw4 ($Bw4^-$) and if available transformed EBV-BLCL from the recipient of HSCT. In duplicate wells, add 100 μL of $1 \times 10^6$/mL EBV-BLCL target cells to wells of a 96-well culture plate followed by 100 μL of $1 \times 10^6$/mL activated cultured polyclonal NK cells (1:1 ratio).
4. To the effector/target mix, add 5 μL of anti-CD107a-FITC (see Table 2) antibody and incubate at 37°C in 5% $CO_2$ for 1 h.
5. After the hour incubation, add 20 μL of monensin (6 μg/mL) at 1/15 dilution to the cells and further incubate for 5 h at 37°C in 5% $CO_2$ (see Note 11).
6. Following the incubation, wash the cells by adding 100 μL of flow buffer to each well followed by centrifugation at $200 \times g$ for 5 min and then incubate with an antibody cocktail of a 1/40 dilution of anti-CD56-PECy7 and 1/20 dilution of the appropriate KIR antibodies (see Tables 2 and 3) to a total volume of 50 μL in the dark for 15 min at 4°C (see Note 12).
7. Wash cells twice in 100 μL flow buffer by centrifugation at $200 \times g$ for 5 min.
8. Finally, resuspend the cells in 180-μL flow buffer containing 1% paraformaldehyde and analyse.

**Table 3**
**KIR antibody combinations and BLCL target cells to be used to detect NK alloreactivity by the flow cytometric CD107a assay**

| NK cell alloreactivity (relevant KIR receptor) | BLCL target cell | KIR antibody combinations | NK cell gating |
|---|---|---|---|
| C1 (2DL2) | C1$^-$ | CD158b-APC, CD158a-PE, CD158e-PE | CD158a$^-$/CD158b$^+$/CD158e$^-$ |
| C2 (2DL1) | C2$^-$ | CD158a-APC, CD158b-PE, CD158e-PE | CD158a$^+$/CD158b$^-$/CD158e$^-$ |
| Bw4 (3DL1) | Bw4$^-$ | CD158e-PE, CD158a-APC, CD158b-APC | CD158a$^-$/CD158b$^-$/CD158e$^+$ |

### 3.5. Data Analysis

The analysis method is critical in the detection of NK alloreactivity. To minimise the effect of irrelevant receptors, it is important to restrict the analysis to only NK cells expressing the inhibitory KIR receptor relevant to the missing epitope against the relevant target cell. An example of the analysis method used for the detection of potential C1 alloreactive NK cells in a C1$^+$, C2$^+$ NK donor tested against a C1$^-$ target is shown in Fig. 1. The analysis method is described below with reference to Fig. 1.

1. Analyse the duplicate tubes on a BD FACSCanto™ flow cytometer using BD FACSDiva software (or similar). The final percentage of cells is an average of the duplicate tubes.
2. Gate events initially on forward (FSC) and side scatter (SSC) to identify lymphocytes. In the example shown in Fig. 1a, 16,217 out of 96,301 events were identified as viable lymphocytes (P1).
3. Then, gate CD56 vs. SSC to acquire at least 10,000 CD56$^+$ cells. Fig. 1b identifies 11,084 events corresponding to CD56 cells (P2).
4. Further gate these CD56$^+$ cells and examine for KIR expression to identify cells expressing the KIR phenotype of interest, e.g. CD158a$^+$/158b$^-$ or CD158b$^+$/158a$^-$. In the example shown in Fig. 1c gate P4 (upper left quadrant) identifies cells expressing CD158b but not CD158a (2,129 events, 19.2%) while gate P5 identifies cells expressing CD158a but not CD158b (1,410 events, 12.7%).
5. To determine the percentage of cells with the KIR phenotype of interest that also express CD107a$^+$, use the gates generated in step 4 (P4 and P5) and analyse in separate bivariate plots the

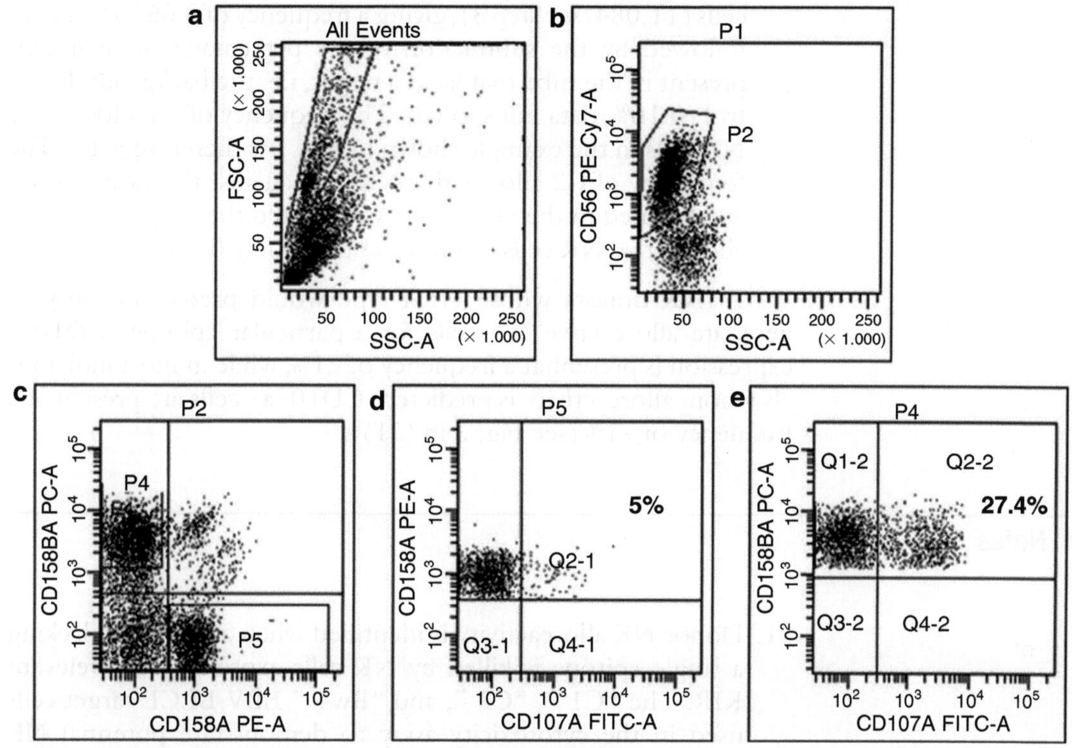


Fig. 1. Flow cytometric histograms showing the detection of potential C1 alloreactive NK cells in a $C1^+$, $C2^+$ NK donor tested against a $C1^-$ target. (**a**) Data gated on forward (FSC) and side scatter (SSC) to identify lymphocytes (16,217 events). (**b**) Data gated on CD56 vs. SSC to acquire at least 10,000 $CD56^+$ cells (11,084 events). (**c**) $CD56^+$ cells expressing the KIR phenotype of interest, e.g. $CD158a^+/158b^-$ or $CD158b^+/158a^-$. Gate P4 (*upper left quadrant*) identifies cells expressing CD158b but not CD158a (2,129 events, 19.2%) while gate P5 identifies cells expressing CD158a but not CD158b (1,410 events, 12.7%). (**d, e**) The number of cells in gates P4 and P5, respectively, that express CD107a. The number of $CD158a^+/CD158b^-/CD107a^+$ cells is 71 (5%) (**d**, Q2-1) while the number of $CD158b^+/CD158a^-/CD107a^+$ cells is 583 (27.4%) (**e**, Q2-2). The frequency of C1 alloreactive NK cells is calculated by dividing the number of $CD158b^+/CD158a^-/CD107a^+$ cells (583) by the total number of $CD56^+$ cells (11,084), giving a frequency of 0.0526 (5.26%), followed by the subtraction of the percentage of such cells present in the tube that lacks a target, i.e. the background control (0.16%, data not shown). The frequency of C1 alloreactive NK cells in the example shown in figure is therefore 5.1%. The frequency of C2 alloreactive NK cells against this target ($C1^-$) is calculated in the same way, as expected the frequency of C2 alloreactive NK cells in this example is low, 0.0056 (0.56%).

cells expressing the receptor of interest (e.g. CD158a) on one axis and CD107a on the other axis. In the example shown in Fig. 1, the number of $CD158a+/CD158b^-/CD107a+$ cells is 71 (5%) (Fig. 1d, Q2-1) while the number of $CD158b+/CD158a^-/CD107a+$ cells is 583 (27.4%) (Fig. 1e, Q2-2).

6. To predict the potential for NK alloreactivity, determine the number of $CD56^+$ cells that express the relevant inhibitory receptor to the missing epitope on target cells and lack other inhibitory KIR and that are $CD107a^+$ as a percentage of all NK cells. For example in Fig. 1, the frequency of C1 alloreactive NK cells is calculated by dividing the number of $CD158b+/CD158a^-/CD107a+$ cells (583) by the total number of $CD56^+$

cells (11,084, see step 3), giving a frequency of 0.0526 (5.26%), followed by the subtraction of the percentage of such cells present in the tube that lacks a target, i.e. the background control (0.16%, data not shown). The frequency of C1 alloreactive NK cells in the example shown in Fig. 1 is therefore 5.1%. The frequency of C2 alloreactive NK cells against this target (C1$^-$) is calculated in the same way. As expected the frequency of C2 alloreactive NK cells in this example is only 0.0056 (0.56%).

In NK donors whose HLA type would predict inability to generate alloreactive NK cells for a particular epitope, CD107a expression is present at a frequency of <1%, while in most individuals whom alloreactivity is predicted, CD107a+ cells are present at a frequency of >1% (see Fig. 3 in (21)).

## 4. Notes

1. Donor NK alloreactivity is identified when a target cell lacking a single epitope is killed by NK cells expressing the relevant KIR. The "C1$^-$", "C2$^-$", and "Bw4$^-$" EBV-BLCL target cells used in the cytotoxicity assay to demonstrate potential NK alloreactivity were selected based on the absence of a single HLA epitope as defined by the HLA type of each cell. The particular cells in Table 1 are suggestions only which we find useful and the use of these particular cells are not essential; however, the absence of a single epitope is crucial. In addition to the target cells used here, transformed EBV-BLCL cells from a recipient of HSCT could also be used in the cytotoxicity assay.
2. HIFCS was prepared by heating foetal calf serum (FCS) for 30 min at 56°C. Heating serum inactivates protease and complement proteins which historically were thought to inhibit or destroy cells under certain culture conditions. The use of FCS (without heat inactivation) in the protocols described here was not evaluated and therefore testing is recommended before FCS is substituted for HIFCS.
3. In our initial experiments, ten random buffy coats were selected to prepare the pooled PBMC feeders; however, in subsequent experiments it was shown that alloreactive polyclonal NK cultures could be successfully grown using feeder cells prepared from at least five buffy coats.
4. The ficoll gradient should be centrifuged with no brake to ensure that the cell interface layer is not disturbed while the centrifuge slows down.

5. To ensure irradiation of PBMC feeder cells is successful, that is, cells are sufficiently irradiated to inhibit cell growth but the production of important growth factors is not, PBMC preparations should be adjusted to no more than $10^6$/mL. The amount of irradiation or the time of irradiation may need to be adjusted in individual laboratories depending on instrumentation used. Initial experiments using 20 Gy was insufficient to prevent PBMC growth and therefore the amount of irradiation was increased to 30 Gy.
6. Cultured polyclonal NK cells can be stored in liquid nitrogen for later use. To prepare cells for freezing, count and adjust the cells to a final concentration of $10 \times 10^6$/mL in freezing medium. Freezing medium should be made fresh and added to the cells drop-wise on ice. To prepare frozen cells for use, remove cells from liquid nitrogen and thaw quickly in a 37°C waterbath and immediately transfer to RPMI/10%HIFCS. Pellet cells by centrifugation at $300 \times g$ for 7 min and resuspended in 1 mL RPMI/10% HIFCS or NK cell medium. Dilute cells either in 1/2 or 1/5 in trypan blue, count and check cell morphology using a Neubauer haemocytometer and adjust to $3 \times 10^6$/mL for use.
7. Rosette-Sep has been optimised for use with whole blood; however, cells can be enriched from buffy coat or isolated PBMC. The concentration of nucleated cells in the sample should not exceed $5 \times 10^7$ cells/mL, and red blood cells should be present at a ratio of at least 30–50 RBCs per nucleated cell.
8. The NK cell interface following centrifugation during the NK cell enrichment process is often not clearly visible. To ensure all NK cells are harvested take up interface layer along with the ficoll from just beneath the NK cell layer.
9. Polyclonal NK cultures should be harvested just before the cultures reach the end of their growth cycle. The culture time may vary between NK cell donors, some NK donors reach the end of their growth cycle around day 11 while others at day 14.
10. It is important that the NK polyclonal cultures are activated by incubating for 48 h with 400 IU IL-2/mL before use in the CD107a assay. We have shown that very few freshly isolated NK cells which have not been cultured for 12 days expressed CD107a in response to BLCL targets.
11. BD GolgiStop™ which contains monensin, blocks the intracellular protein transport processes resulting in the accumulation of CD107a in the cell allowing the glycoprotein to be detected by flow cytometric analysis.
12. We used an antibody cocktail that included the antibodies CD107a, CD56, CD158a, CD158b, and NKB1 which detect

the receptors of interest in our experiments, however, other or additional antibodies can be used. We have noted in our experiments that when using CD158-PE antibody obtained from BD Biosciences at least a 1/5 dilution of antibody is required.

## References


1. Valiante NM, Uhrberg M, Shilling HG, Lienert-Weidenbach K, Arnett KL, D'Andrea A, Phillips JH, Lanier LL, Parham P (1998) Functionally and structurally distinct NK cell receptor repertoires in the peripheral blood of two human donors. Immunity 7:739–751
2. Colonna M, Spies T, Strominger JL, Ciccone E, Moretta A, Moretta L, Pende D, Viale O (1992) Alloantigen recognition by two human natural killer cell clones is associated with HLA-C or a closely linked gene. Proc Natl Acad Sci USA 89:7983–7985
3. Colonna M, Brooks EG, Falco M, Ferrara GB, Strominger JL (1993) Generation of allospecific natural killer cells by stimulation across a polymorphism of HLA-C. Science 260: 1121–1124
4. Moretta A, Vitale M, Bottino C, Orengo AM, Morelli L, Augugliaro R, Barbaresi M, Ciccone E, Moretta L (1993) P58 molecules as putative receptors for major histocompatibility complex (MHC) class I molecules in human natural killer (NK) cells. Anti-p58 antibodies reconstitute lysis of MHC class I-protected cells in NK clones displaying different specificities. J Exp Med 178:597–604
5. Vales-Gomez M, Reyburn HT, Erskine RA, Strominger J (1998) Differential binding to HLA-C of p50-activating and p58-inhibitory natural killer cell receptors. Proc Natl Acad Sci USA 95:14326–14331
6. Cella M, Longo A, Ferrara GB, Strominger JL, Colonna M (1994) NK3-specific natural killer cells are selectively inhibited by Bw4-positive HLA alleles with isoleucine 80. J Exp Med 180:1235–1242
7. Litwin V, Gumperz JE, Parham P, Phillips JH, Lanier LL (1994) NKB1: a natural killer cell receptor involved in the recognition of polymorphic HLA-B molecules. J Exp Med 180:537–543
8. Gumperz JE, Litwin V, Phillips JH, Lanier LL, Parham P (1995) The Bw4 public epitope of HLA-B molecules confers reactivity with natural killer cell clones that express NKB1, a putative HLA receptor. J Exp Med 181:1133–1144
9. Uhrberg M, Valiante NM, Shum BP, Shilling HG, Lienert-Weidenbach K, Corliss B, Tyan D, Lanier LL, Parham P (1997) Human diversity in killer cell inhibitory receptor genes. Immunity 7:753–763
10. Kim S, Poursine-Laurent J, Truscott SM, Lybarger L, Song YJ, Yang L, French AR, Sunwoo JB, Lemieux S, Hansen TH, Yokoyama WM (2005) Licensing of natural killer cells by host major histocompatibility complex class I molecules. Nature 436:709–713
11. Ruggeri L, Capanni M, Casucci M, Volpi I, Tosti A, Perruccio K, Urbani E, Negrin RS, Martelli MF, Velardi A (1999) Role of natural killer cell alloreactivity in HLA-mismatched hematopoietic stem cell transplantation. Blood 94:333–339
12. Ruggeri L, Capanni M, Urbani E, Perruccio K, Shlomchik WD, Tosti A, Posati S, Rogaia D, Frassoni F, Aversa F, Martelli MF, Velardi A (2002) Effectiveness of donor natural killer cell alloreactivity in mismatched hematopoietic transplants. Science 295:2097–2100
13. Foley BA, De Santis D, Van Beelen E, Lathbury LJ, Christiansen FT, Witt CS (2008) The reactivity of Bw4+ HLA-B and HLA-A alleles with KIR3DL1: implications for patient and donor suitability for haploidentical stem cell transplantations. Blood 112:435–443
14. Winter CC, Gumperz JE, Parham P, Long EO, Wagtmann N (1998) Direct binding and functional transfer of NK cell inhibitory receptors reveal novel patterns of HLA-C allotype recognition. J Immunol 161:571–577
15. Moesta AK, Norman PJ, Yawata M, Yawata N, Gleimer M, Parham P (2008) Synergistic polymorphism at 2 positions distal to the ligand-binding site makes KIR2DL2 a stronger receptor for HLA-C than KIR2DL3. J Immunol 180:3969–3979
16. Pende D, Marcenaro S, Falco M et al (2008) Anti-leukemia acitivity of alloreactive NK cells in KIR ligand-mismatched haploidentical HSCT for pediatric patients: evaluation of the functional role of activating KIR and re-definition of inhibitory KIR specificity. Blood 113:3119–3129
17. Djeu JY, Jiang K, Wei S (2002) A view to a kill: signals triggering cytotoxicity. Clin Cancer Res 8:636–640

18. Fukuda M (1991) Lysosomal membrane glycoproteins. Structure, biosynthesis, and intracellular trafficking. J Biol Chem 266:21327–21330
19. Betts MR, Brenchley JM, Price DA, De Rosa SC, Douek DC, Roederer M, Koup RA (2003) Sensitive and viable identification of antigen-specific CD8+ T cells by a flow cytometric assay for degranulation. J Immunol Methods 281: 65–78
20. Alter G, Malenfant JM, Altfeld M (2004) CD107a as a functional marker for the identification of natural killer cell activity. J Immunol Methods 294:15–22
21. De Santis D, Foley BA, John E, Senitzer D, Christiansen FT, Witt CS (2010) Rapid, flow cytometric assay for NK alloreactivity reveals exceptions to rules governing alloreactivity. Biol Blood Marrow Transplant 16(2):179–191

# Chapter 28

# Clinical Production and Therapeutic Applications of Alloreactive Natural Killer Cells

**David H. McKenna, Diane M. Kadidlo, Sarah Cooley, and Jeffrey S. Miller**


## Abstract

Recent advances have improved our understanding of natural killer (NK) cell-mediated alloreactivity after hematopoietic cell transplantation (HCT) or with adoptive transfer. NK cells contribute to a graft-versus-leukemia effect and may play a role in preventing graft-versus-host disease or controlling infectious diseases after allogeneic HCT. New discoveries in NK cell biology, including characterization of NK cell receptors and their interactions with self-HLA molecules and a better understanding of the mechanism of NK cell education have led to the development of novel strategies to exploit NK cell alloreactivity against tumors. While early studies using autologous NK cells lacked efficacy, the use of adoptively transferred NK cells to treat hematopoietic malignancies has been expanding. The production of allogeneic donor NK cells requires efficient removal of T- and B cells from clinical-scale leukapheresis collections. The goal of this chapter is to review NK cell biology, NK cell receptors, the use of NK cells as therapy and then to discuss the clinical decisions resulting in our current good manufacturing practices processing and activation of human NK cells for therapeutic use.


**Key words:** NK cells, Immunotherapy, Cell processing, Current good manufacturing practices

## 1. Introduction

### *1.1. NK Cell Biology*

NK cells are large granular lymphocytes that were first described in the 1970s for their ability to lyse virally infected and tumor target cells without MHC-restriction or prior sensitization (1, 2). Human NK cells are found in the bone marrow, spleen, lymph nodes, and peripheral blood (PB), where they comprise ~10–15% of the lymphocyte pool. NK cells play an important role in immune surveillance and response to infections and link the innate and adaptive immune systems (3, 4). Activated NK cells produce cytokines and chemokines, including granulocyte colony stimulatory factor (G-CSF), TNF, interferon gamma (IFN-γ), and transforming

Frank T. Christiansen and Brian D. Tait (eds.), *Immunogenetics: Methods and Applications in Clinical Practice*, Methods in Molecular Biology, vol. 882, DOI 10.1007/978-1-61779-842-9_28, © Springer Science+Business Media New York 2012

growth factor beta (TGF-β). The approximately 10% of NK cells that are CD56$^{bright}$ proliferate better and produce more cytokines (especially IFN-γ) than the more cytotoxic CD56$^{dim}$ subset, which expresses Fc receptors that mediate antibody-dependent cellular cytotoxicity (ADCC) (5–7). Cytokine-activated cells show more expansion potential, increased cytokine production, and higher cytotoxicity against targets than do resting NK cells (8). NK cells respond to IL-2, IL-15, and IL-21, all of which signal via the IL-2 receptor γ chain (9–11), and to the combination of IL-12 and IL-18 which is an especially strong inducer of IFN-γ production (12). IL-2 is the only US Food and Drug Administration (FDA)-approved common γ chain cytokine available to activate NK cells in vivo or ex vivo.

### 1.2. NK Cell Receptors Control Function, Self-Tolerance, and Alloreactivity

In 1985, Ljunggren and Karre described the phenomenon of "missing self recognition," whereby the loss of MHC class I expression renders autologous targets more sensitive to NK-mediated killing. The mechanism by which these innate killer cells recognize class I loss in tumors or virally infected cells (13) was explained with the discovery of killer-cell immunoglobulin-like receptors (KIR). Human KIR gene content can be simplified into two haplotypes, each of which contain the three framework genes (KIR3DL3, KIR2DL4, and KIR3DL2), and a variable number of activating and inhibitory genes from the centromeric (Cen) or telomeric (Tel) ends. KIR A haplotypes contain five inhibitory receptors (2DL1, 2DL3, 3DL1, 3DL2, 3DL3), and just one activating receptor (2DS4). KIR B haplotypes have variable gene content and contain more activating KIR. Binding of higher affinity inhibitory KIR to their cognate ligands, self-class I HLA, suppresses NK cell effector responses, including cell-mediated lysis and cytokine release (14). KIR2DL1, KIR2DL2/KIR2DL3, and KIR3DL1 bind HLA class I C2, C1 and Bw4 alleles, respectively. In contrast, the natural ligands for activating KIR remain unknown.

Several other families of activating and inhibitory receptors affect NK cell function. The NKG2 family of C-type lectin receptors can be inhibitory (NKG2A) or activating (NKG2C/E), and recognize non-classical HLA-E (15). NKG2D recognizes stress-induced molecules, such as MHC class I polypeptide-related sequence A/B (MICA and MICB) or viral particles (16). Other receptors include the natural cytotoxicity receptors (NCR) NKp30, NKp46 and NKp44, DNAM-1, and Nectin-2 (CD122), 2B4, leukocyte-associated immunoglobulin-like receptor-1 (LAIR-1) (17, 18), and Ig-like (ILT) receptors (19–23). NK cell function is determined by the net sum of signals delivered through inhibitory and activating NK cell receptors.

The mechanism by which NK cells acquire self-tolerance and alloreactivity has been referred to as "NK cell education." Several models have been proposed to explain the integration of inhibitory receptor expression with the acquisition of effector functions.

These models show that human NK cells lacking inhibitory receptors are hyporesponsive (24, 25) and therefore self-tolerant. As strategies to use NK cells therapeutically are considered, it is critically important to understand effector function in vivo. For example, although reconstituting NK cells are abundant after transplant, their KIR expression is decreased and dysregulated KIR expression correlates with clinical outcomes (26, 27). As delayed NK cell education may result in NK cells with abnormal function, adoptive transfer of mature NK cells, educated in the donor, may be a more attractive strategy than using NK cells derived from hematopoietic stem cells which must develop in the patient.

### 1.3. Clinical Applications of NK Cells

NK cells mediate lysis of hematologic malignancies and variety of solid tumors, including breast, ovarian, hepatocellular and colon cancers, neuroblastoma, and melanoma (28–33). The therapeutic efficacy of NK cells is primarily controlled by inhibitory receptor interactions and the relative resistance of some tumors may be due to a higher expression of class I HLA. Coengagement of activating NK cell receptors such as NKG2D also plays an important role in immune surveillance and tumor lysis (34, 35).

The two main strategies to harness the therapeutic power of alloreactive NK cells are: (1) hematopoietic cell transplantation (HCT) (36) and (2) adoptive transfer of NK cells (37). The Perugia group first proposed the KIR-ligand incompatibility model, which predicts that donor-derived NK cells will be alloreactive when recipients lack C2, C1, or Bw4 alleles that are present in the donor. Many groups, including our own (38–40), have tested the clinical efficacy of selecting donors for NK cell therapy or transplantation based on their predicted alloreactivity against the host. The potential benefits include: (1) decreased rates of GVHD (41, 42), (2) decreased rates of graft rejection mediated by NK cell lysis of host T cells, (3) better anti-tumor activity via direct cytotoxicity (43), (4) improved engraftment mediated by NK cell release of hematopoietic cytokines (44, 45), and (5) enhanced immune reconstitution and decreased infections (46–48). The main benefit of KIR ligand mismatch is seen in myeloid malignancies (49), but less so after T-cell replete transplants (50, 51). The inconsistent effects of KIR-ligand mismatch and KIR-ligand absence strategies may be due to differences in NK cell development and education based on the stem cell source, conditioning regimen, extent of T-cell depletion, and the use of post-HCT immunosuppression (52–55). Another approach to exploit the beneficial effects of NK cells after HCT is to consider the full KIR genotype of the donors. Donors with certain KIR B haplotypes (defined on http://www.ebi.ac.uk/ipd/kir/donor_b_content.html) are associated with less relapse and improved survival after unrelated donor HCT for AML (56, 57).

The other therapeutic approach is to use NK cells for adoptive transfer. Several studies have shown that activation of autologous

NK cells lacked efficacy (58). Presumably, inhibition of NK cells by "self" HLA molecules expressed by the tumor resulted in poor tumor lysis. Additionally, NK cells from cancer patients exhibit functional defects, which may prevent them from killing targets or producing cytokines capable of mediating an immune response. To overcome limitations of autologous NK cell therapy, in 2005 we pioneered the use of haploidentical NK cells in patients with advanced cancer (37). The safety and success of adoptive NK cell infusions was established in a trial using haploidentical, related-donor NK cell products with subcutaneous IL-2 to induce in vivo expansion of alloreactive NK cells which persisted in vivo for up to 1 month (37). In patients with refractory leukemia, this persistence and expansion correlated with achieving a clinical remission in those treated with refractory disease having failed standard therapy. NK cell expansion is dependent on a lymphodepleting chemotherapy regimen given to create space and on the enhancement of endogenous cytokines to support the expansion of donor NK cells (59). This preparative therapy also has the potential to decrease immune suppressive factors released by tumor cells, which may interfere with adoptive transfer (60, 61). Addition of a nonmyeloablative dose of 400 cGy of TBI followed by a haploidentical CD34-selected stem cell product from the same donor, resulted in improved rates of successful in vivo NK cell expansion and clinical remission, but with late complications including deaths due to infection (62). A similar approach has been used in a pediatric cohort, where haploidentical NK cell infusions were given with T-cell and B-cell deplete haploidentical grafts to treat neuroblastoma (63). Other groups have used NK cell donor lymphocyte infusions (DLI) after haploidentical HCT to consolidate engraftment in adults with AML (64) or children with leukemia and solid tumors (65, 66). Clinically effective strategies exploiting NK cell alloreactivity to treat cancer require robust NK cell development and education. Ex vivo expansion of NK cell products can increase the cell dose and allow for additional activation of the products. Further improvements may be made by selecting donors based on their NK receptor profile, by using concurrent exogenous cytokine therapy with IL-15, which is in phase I testing at the NCI (67), by manipulation of tumor ligand expression or interactions with other immune cells. For example, eliminating host regulatory T cells, which can suppress NK cell proliferation and killing, may also improve the immune effector functions of the expanding NK cells (68). Ultimately, combination therapy using several strategies at once will likely prove most successful.

### 1.4. Clinical Factors Influencing Development of an NK Cell Product

Studies using autologous NK cells did not require extensive processing because the non-NK cells (T cells, B cells, and monocytes), also autologous to the patient, were not felt to pose a significant risk even after ex vivo IL-2 activation. However, when crossing allogeneic barriers, several issues need to be considered. The goal was to collect an adequate NK cell dose from a single leukapheresis product. The primary concern is the known risk of graft-versus-host disease mediated by donor T cells. Even small T-cell numbers in a blood transfusion can mediate potentially lethal graft-versus-host disease if the recipient is immunocompromised by cancer or other pathology (69). Therefore, initial NK cell enrichment strategies used T-cell depletion alone accomplished by removal of CD3+ cells. Using this approach, T cells which comprised 63% cells in the starting product, decreased to <1% after processing, a 2.7 log T-cell depletion (70). Successful adoptive transfer is defined by persistence and in vivo expansion of donor NK cells. Noting variability in the magnitude of NK cell expansion, we hypothesized that contaminating B cells or monocytes might inhibit NK cells after adoptive transfer. We tested a more rigorous processing approach, positively selecting CD56+ NK cells after CD3 depletion. While this processing yielded a highly pure NK cell product, with minimal contaminating B cells, T cells or monocytes, unfortunately the NK cells failed to persist and expand in vivo when tested in patients with refractory AML. This failure may be explained by (1) the importance of monocyte accessory cells for in vivo NK cell expansion, as has been noted in vitro (71) or (2) the approximate 40–50% decrease in NK cell dose in the final product after both CD3 depletion and CD56 selection. Irrespective of the exact reason, the poor clinical results and lack of NK cell expansion prompted us to revert back to T-cell depletion alone for subsequent trials where we have verified the anti-leukemia activity of haploidentical NK cells (72).

We have infused over 100 haploidentical NK cell products and have noted some unusual complications due to allogeneic donor B cells persisting in the recipient. We observed several cases of post-transplant lymphoproliferative disease (PTLD), a potentially lethal complication (73). This Epstein-Barr virus-driven lymphoproliferation was in B cells of donor origin infused with the NK cell product, and patients receiving NK cells as part of a transplant or who had failed a prior transplant were most susceptible to this complication. We have also seen two patients with immune hemolysis (one clinically significant and one clinically silent) as a result of passenger B lymphocyte syndrome (PBLS) (74). Both of these patients received adoptive NK cell therapy for solid tumors and had not had prior transplants. We demonstrated that contaminating B cells in the NK cell product were responsible for PBLS. Therefore, our current GMP processing utilizes immunomagnetic selection to achieve both CD3 and CD19 depletion to minimize these risks while preventing GVHD (75).

There are several ways to manufacture NK cell products using immunomagnetic selection-based methods. The method described below is now our standard practice for processing NK cells for clinical trials in both nontransplant and transplant settings. This method involves CD3 (T cell) and CD19 (B cell)-depletion of a nonmobilized peripheral blood mononuclear cell apheresis collection followed by an overnight culture and activation with IL-2. This process takes approximately 9 h in total [4 h (preculture processing); 3 h (postculture processing); 2 h (lot release testing)].

## 2. Materials

### 2.1. Equipment

1. Miltenyi Biotec CliniMACS Cell Selection System (Miltenyi Biotec, Bergisch Gladbach, Germany).
2. COBE 2991 Cell Processor (CaridianBCT, Lakewood, Colorado, USA).
3. Incubator, 5% $CO_2$/37°C.

### 2.2. Main Supplies and Reagents

#### 2.2.1. Day 1 (Preculture) Processing

1. CliniMACS PBS/EDTA Buffer (Miltenyi Biotec).
2. CliniMACS CD3 and CD19 Microbeads (Miltenyi Biotec).
3. CliniMACS Tubing Set (LS) (Miltenyi Biotec).
4. COBE 2991 Processing Set (CaridianBCT).
5. Human serum albumin (HSA) 25%.
6. Pall SQ40S Filter (Pall Corp., Port Washington, New York, USA).
7. Transfer Bags, 150–2,000 mL.
8. Interleukin-2.
9. Fluorinated ethylene propylene (FEP) Bags: 290, 500, 730 mL (AFC, Gaithersburg, MD, USA).
10. Human AB serum, heat-inactivated.
11. X-VIVO 15 Medium (Lonza Walkersville, Inc., Walkersville, MD, USA).

#### 2.2.2. Day 2 (Postculture) Processing

1. COBE 2991 Processing Set (CaridianBCT).
2. HSA (5%).
3. HSA (25%).
4. Double Coupler Adapter.
5. Transfer Bag (150, 300 mL).

## 3. Methods

### 3.1. cGMP Production of NK Cells

In general, clinical production and administration of novel cell therapies in the USA requires submission to and approval by the FDA for an investigational new drug (IND) application. Further, the manufacturing of such products typically requires the infrastructure of a "cGMP facility" which includes not only the physical structure (e.g., clean rooms, air handlers, etc.), but the appropriate expertise in manufacturing, quality assurance (QA), and materials management (76).

### 3.2. Procurement of the Leukapheresis

1. Prior to leukapheresis, allogeneic donors must undergo a clinical evaluation for donor eligibility, including a medical history screening and testing for transmissible diseases comparable to current standard practice for whole blood donations (see Note 1). We have focused on related donor haploidentical NK cells but it is not known whether matching in the adoptive transfer setting is of benefit. Donors must be in good general health by established criteria (see Note 2).
2. It is not yet known whether donor choice based on KIR-ligand mismatch or KIR genotyping provides any clinical benefit and these strategies are being tested.
3. A nonmobilized mononuclear cell collection (i.e., leukapheresis) is collected with an apheresis instrument using established, standard collection procedures.
4. Aseptic technique is followed to prevent contamination of the collection and infection at the site of the intravenous catheter(s).
5. The leukapheresis is then transported immediately in a validated shipping container to the laboratory. Shipping containers should be durable, leak-proof, resistant to breakage and able to withstand temperature extremes. Container selection will depend upon distance traveled and mode of transportation.

### 3.3. Cell Processing

The apheresis product is T cell (CD3)-depleted and B cell (CD19)-depleted using the Miltenyi Biotec CliniMACS® Cell Selection System and CD3 and CD19 MicroBeads and reagent (Miltenyi Biotec, Bergisch Gladbach, Germany). Up to $2.50 \times 10^{10}$ total nucleated cells (TNC) may be labeled with the MicroBeads and separated on an LS column (Depletion Program 2.1) which is placed in the magnetic field of the CliniMACS® device. Cells are resuspended at $2 \times 10^6$ cells/mL in X-VIVO 15, without gentamicin and phenol red (Cambrex BioScience, Walkersville, Maryland), supplemented with 1,000 U/mL IL-2 (Chiron Corporation, Emeryville, CA) and 10% human AB serum, heat-inactivated (Valley Biomedical Products and Services, Inc., Winchester, VA) in VueLife™ Teflon® (FEP) bags (American Fluoroseal Corporation, Gaithersburg, MD). Cells are then incubated overnight for 8–16 h (37°C/5% $CO_2$). Cells are washed twice with a 5% HSA, and the final formulation consists of nucleated cells in approximately 80–150 mL of 5% HSA solution ($<100 \times 10^6$ NC/mL). The target dose for infusion is $\leq 8 \times 10^7$ NC/kg.

### 3.4. Day 1 (Preculture) Processing

#### 3.4.1. Pre-CD3 Depletion

1. General cleanroom preparation
   (a) Review and documentation of current cleanroom sanitization and biological safety cabinet calibration records.
2. Leukapheresis receipt and inspection
   (a) Documentation of arrival time and collection center.
   (b) Review label information, including: product name, volume, product identifier, and additives used.
   (c) Confirm product identity by
      - Performing ABO/Rh blood typing from sample taken from the product.
      - Verifying product label information corresponds with physician cell processing order.
   (d) Conduct a gross inspection of product/bag ensuring product bag is intact and product is free of clots/discoloration.
   (e) Review of donor infectious disease testing and donor eligibility determination.
3. Sampling for QC testing
   (a) Nucleated cell (NC) count; differential; flow cytometry (CD3, CD20, CD56, 7-AAD viability).
4. Determination of volume and initial NC count
   (a) Calculate the TNC in the product bag.
   (b) If TNC number exceeds the limit, calculate the volume of cells to remove from the bag (see Note 3). The remaining cells may be cryopreserved for future use or discarded.

#### 3.4.2. CD3/CD19 Depletion

1. Culture medium preparation
   (a) Inspect bottles of X-VIVO 15 and heat-inactivated type AB human serum for part number, expiry date, container integrity, and appearance of reagent
   (b) Add 110 mL of heat-inactivated type AB human serum to each 1,000-mL bottle of X-VIVO 15
   (c) Filter prepared medium with a 0.22-μm filter unit, label accordingly, and place into 37°C incubator to warm
2. Supplement CliniMACS buffer with 0.5% HSA
   (a) Add 20 mL of 25% HSA to each buffer bag and label accordingly
3. Wash cells
   (a) Inspect a COBE 2991 processing set for expiry date and integrity
   (b) Load processing set onto COBE 2991 for wash procedure and attach hemostats to all lines

(c) Attach bag of cells and one bag of CliniMACS buffer/0.5% HSA to the processing set

(d) In manual mode, set the COBE 2991 settings as follows: centrifuge speed—1,200 rpm (198 × *g*); super out rate 450 mL/min; minimum agitate time—30 s; super out volume—600 mL

(e) Open hemostat on cell suspension line and transfer the cells to the COBE processing bag

(f) Fill COBE processing bag with CliniMACS buffer/0.5% HSA. Perform one wash (15 min at 1,200 rpm, 198 × *g*), and expel as much supernatant as possible into waste bag

4. Label CD3+ and CD19+ cells

(a) Remove one vial each of CliniMACS CD3 and CD19 Microbeads from refrigerator; inspect vial and 150-mL transfer bag for expiry date and integrity

(b) Label bag appropriately and insert dispensing pin into one port

(c) Add 52 mL CliniMACS buffer/0.5% HSA and entire vials of CD3 and CD19 Microbeads to transfer bag; inject approximately 90 mL of air from biosafety cabinet into bag, and mix well

(d) Attach transfer bag to blue line of COBE processing set; remove hemostat attached to blue line tubing; add Microbeads/buffer solution to processing bag; clear the blue line of as many Microbeads as possible using air from transfer bag. Place hemostat on the blue line

(e) Lift seal weight and open sliding covers to remove the COBE Processing Bag from the instrument

(f) Resuspend cells in bag by gently massaging

(g) Return bag to centrifuge bowl, close sliding covers, and replace seal weight

(h) Push in rapid succession Start/Spin, Super out, and Agitate/Wash In; incubate product with constant agitation for approximately 30 min

(i) Fill COBE Processing bag with CliniMACS buffer/0.5% HSA; remove air from processing bag and hemostat all lines

(j) Press Start/Spin; wash product once at 1,500 rpm (300 × *g*) for 15 min; at end of wash press Super Out; express as much supernatant as possible into waste bag; press Stop

(k) Heat seal all tubing lines except the line attached to the buffer bag

(l) Remove COBE Processing bag and attached buffer bag from COBE 2991 and place into biosafety cabinet; detach and remove remainder of processing set and discard

(m) Transfer cell suspension from COBE Processing bag into transfer bag; rinse COBE Processing bag with small amount of CliniMACS buffer/0.5% HSA and add diluted cells to transfer bag; dilute cell suspension with CliniMACS buffer/0.5% HSA to final volume of approximately 100 mL

(n) Remove sample for NC count

5. CD3/CD19 depletion

(a) Turn on CliniMACS and choose Depletion Program 2.1

(b) When prompted indicate LS tubing set, NC concentration, percentage of labeled cells (70%), and product volume

(c) The CliniMACS program will calculate volume of buffer needed for the depletion process and volumes expected for collection in the negative fraction bag, the buffer waste bag, and cell fraction bag; adjust bags accordingly (if >400 mL)

(d) Inspect CliniMACS LS tubing set and transfer bag for expiry date and integrity

(e) Label bags accordingly; the transfer bag will be the cell collection bag and should be labeled "CD3/CD19 negative"; label the bag on the tubing set designated "negative fraction" as "CD3 positive"

(f) Load the tubing set onto the CliniMACS instrument and attach the required amount of buffer solution

(g) Perform prime and integrity testing following prompts

(h) Connect the bag containing washed cells to the Pall filter and proceed with the cell separation

(i) Once the separation is completed, heat seal and detach both fractions (i.e., CD3−/CD19− and CD3+/CD19+) and set aside for further processing; discard remainder of tubing set

6. Volume reduction of CD3−/CD19− fraction

(a) Weigh, count, and calculate volume and perform NC count (see Note 4)

(b) Inspect COBE processing set for expiry date and integrity

(c) Load set onto COBE 2991; place hemostats on all lines

(d) In manual mode, set the COBE 2991 settings as follows: centrifuge speed—1,500 rpm ($300 \times g$); super out rate 450 mL/min; minimum agitate time—N/A; super out volume—600 mL

(e) Open the hemostat on the cell suspension line and transfer cells to the COBE processing bag

(f) Volume reduce product at 1,500 rpm (300 × *g*) for 3 min per spin; at the end of super out, expel as much supernatant as possible into the waste bag

(g) Remove the COBE processing bag from the COBE 2991 and place in the biosafety cabinet; discard the remainder of the processing set

(h) Transfer the cell suspension into a transfer bag; add warmed cell culture medium (X-VIVO 15) that has been heated in a 37°C incubator to the drained COBE processing bag and add rinse to the transfer bag

7. Culture preparation and QC testing of CD3−/CD19− and CD3+/CD19+ fractions

(a) Weigh and calculate volume. Remove a small aliquot of cells from product bag and perform NC count

(b) Inspect vial of IL-2 for expiry date, integrity, gross appearance. Do not use reagent if it appears cloudy, contains precipitates or clumps.

(c) Add warmed cell culture medium (X-VIVO 15) to obtain a target cell concentration of 2 × 106 nucleated cells/mL

(d) Add IL-2 to obtain a concentration of 1,000 U/mL of culture medium

(e) Remove samples for QC testing of CD3−/CD19− fraction (e.g., flow cytometry, cytotoxicity, sterility) and CD3+/CD19+ fraction (e.g., NC count, flow cytometry)

#### *3.4.3. Overnight Culture in X-VIVO 15/IL-2*

1. Inspect appropriately sized culture bags (FEP) for expiry date and integrity
2. Transfer cells into culture bags and incubate in 37°C/5% $CO_2$ incubator for 8–16 h

### *3.5. Day 2 (Postculture) Processing*

#### *3.5.1. Wash and Resuspension*

1. General cleanroom preparation

(a) Review and documentation of current room sanitization and biological safety cabinet calibration records

2. Volume reduction/wash (2×)

(a) Remove bags of cells from incubator

(b) Inspect an appropriate number of bottles of 5% HSA for expiry date, integrity, and gross appearance

(c) Inspect COBE processing set for expiry date and integrity

(d) Load set onto COBE 2991; place hemostats on all lines

(e) In manual mode, set the COBE 2991 settings as follows: centrifuge speed—1,500 rpm (300 × g); super out rate 450 mL/min; minimum agitate time—30 s; super out volume—600 mL

(f) Open the hemostat on the cell product line and transfer cells to the COBE processing bag

(g) Volume reduce product at 1,500 rpm (300 × g) for 3 min per spin; at the end of super out, expel as much supernatant as possible into the waste bag

(h) Fill the processing bag with 5% HSA; remove air from processing bag; wash product twice at 1,500 rpm (300 × g) for 3 min per spin; expel as much supernatant as possible into the waste bag

(i) Heat seal and remove the processing bag from the COBE 2991; detach and discard the remainder of the processing set

(j) Transfer the cells into an appropriately sized transfer bag; rinse the processing bag with 5% HSA; and add to the transfer bag

(k) Dilute the final product to approximately 100 mL total volume with 5% HSA

3. Dose adjust (if necessary)

(a) Calculate available dose and determine if a portion of cells needs to be removed

### 3.6. Sampling for QC/Lot Release Testing

1. All lot release testing is performed on the final product prior to release of the product for infusion. Lot release criteria are shown in Table 1.

**Table 1**
**Natural killer cells: lot release criteria**

| Assay | Test method | Specification |
|---|---|---|
| Viability | 7-AAD, flow cytometry (see Note 5) | ≥70.0% |
| NK cell (CD56+/CD3−) enumeration (see Notes 6 and 7) | Flow cytometry (see Note 5) | ≥30.0% (see Note 7) |
| T cell (CD3+) enumeration (see Note 8) | Flow cytometry (see Note 5) | $<3.00 \times 10^5$ T cells/kg |
| B cell (CD20+) enumeration (see Note 9) | Flow cytometry (see Note 5) | <3.0% |
| Endotoxin | LAL method per FDA guidance | <5.0 EU/kg |
| Gram stain | Clinical microbiology lab | No organisms |
| NC dose (see Note 10) | Hematology analyzer | $\leq 8.00 \times 10^7$/kg |

2. Sterility testing is performed on the final product; however, it is not completed prior to release of the NK cell product. In the event that sterility testing becomes positive, lab staff immediately notifies QA and the medical director who contacts the patient physician for appropriate clinical action.

### 3.7. Final Labeling and Release

1. Label appropriately and include the following statement: "Caution: New Drug—Limited by Federal Law to Investigational Use" per 21 CFR 312.6
2. Release NK cell product once lot release testing has been completed, passed, and reviewed by Quality Assurance unit.

## 4. Notes

1. Donors are typically related (sibling, parent, offspring, parent or offspring of an HLA identical sibling) HLA-haploidentical (3–5 of 6 HLA-A, B, and C) match to recipient, between 14 and 75 years of age, and not pregnant.
2. Infectious disease testing typically includes assays for the detection of HIV, HCV, and WNV (by nucleic acid testing), anti-HIV I/II, anti-HTLV I/II, anti-HBc Ab, HBsAg, anti-HCV, anti-CMV, Chagas disease, and *Treponema pallidum* (by serology).
3. The maximum number of NCs to be loaded on the CliniMACS is $2.5 \times 10^{10}$. Loading beyond this limit may require a second column.
4. Remove small aliquot of cells from the bag (1 mL) and perform either a manual or automated nucleated cell count.
5. At our institution, all flow cytometry readouts for lot release are performed by a CLIA certified clinical laboratory. Adherence to these lot release criteria depend on the quality of these readouts. Since these lot criteria are for clinical safety, we recommend that these measures be performed in a certified clinical laboratory (where routine quality control is required) rather than a research laboratory.
6. Failure to meet NK cell content lot release in the final product occurs occasionally and is most often a result of a low NK cell content in the starting apheresis product (products containing <5% NK cells) rather than a failure of the CD3 and CD19 depletion. Products with low NK cell content have been infused safely (with FDA communication by PI) but it is still unknown what NK cell content threshold, if any, will correlate with clinical efficacy.

7. Lot release for NK cell purity has been used as 20% in non-transplant settings of NK cell infusion.
8. The average T-cell content of the final product in a recent non-transplant trial contained a median-infused T-cell dose of $5.6 \times 10^4$ CD3+ T cells/kg. Caution should be used in setting this parameter depending on the clinical setting relative to the risk of transfusion-associated graft-versus-host disease. For example, the threshold for T-cell dose may need to be lower when NK cell products are used as a part of haploidentical transplant. Safe T-cell doses may vary based on the clinical setting where the NK cell product is administered.
9. Absolute safe thresholds for B cell content relative to uncommon complications associated with product B cells have not been firmly established. These thresholds may vary depending on the immune competence of the recipient.
10. An upper dose limit has been set but is rarely reached based on the processing of a single apheresis product (15 L processing volume; roughly 5 h collection). Larger or multiple collection above this threshold have not been tested for safety.

## References


1. Herberman RB, Ortaldo JR (1981) Natural killer cells: their roles in defenses against disease. Science 214(4516):24–30
2. Kiessling R, Petranyi G, Klein G, Wigzel H (1975) Genetic variation of in vitro cytolytic activity and in vivo rejection potential of non-immunized semi-syngeneic mice against a mouse lymphoma line. Int J Cancer 15(6):933–940
3. Moretta L, Ferlazzo G, Bottino C, Vitale M, Pende D, Mingari MC et al (2006) Effector and regulatory events during natural killer-dendritic cell interactions. Immunol Rev 214:219–228
4. Walzer T, Dalod M, Robbins SH, Zitvogel L, Vivier E (2005) Natural-killer cells and dendritic cells: "l'union fait la force". Blood 106(7):2252–2258
5. Cooper MA, Fehniger TA, Caligiuri MA (2001) The biology of human natural killer-cell subsets. Trends Immunol 22(11):633–640
6. Fehniger TA, Caligiuri MA (2001) Interleukin 15: biology and relevance to human disease. Blood 97(1):14–32
7. Caligiuri MA (2008) Human natural killer cells. Blood 112(3):461–469
8. Rayner AA, Grimm EA, Lotze MT, Chu EW, Rosenberg SA (1985) Lymphokine-activated killer (LAK) cells. Analysis of factors relevant to the immunotherapy of human cancer. Cancer 55(6):1327–1333
9. Carson WE, Giri JG, Lindemann MJ, Linett ML, Ahdieh M, Paxton R et al (1994) Interleukin (IL) 15 is a novel cytokine that activates human natural killer cells via components of the IL-2 receptor. J Exp Med 180(4): 1395–1403
10. Trinchieri G (2003) Interleukin-12 and the regulation of innate resistance and adaptive immunity. Nat Rev Immunol 3(2):133–146
11. Young HA, Ortaldo J (2006) Cytokines as critical co-stimulatory molecules in modulating the immune response of natural killer cells. Cell Res 16(1):20–24
12. Singh SM, Yanagawa H, Hanibuchi M, Miki T, Okamura H, Sone S (2000) Augmentation by interleukin-18 of MHC-nonrestricted killer activity of human peripheral blood mononuclear cells in response to interleukin-12. Int J Immunopharmacol 22(1):35–43
13. Ljunggren HG, Karre K (1990) In search of the 'missing self': MHC molecules and NK cell recognition. Immunol Today 11(7):237–244
14. Vales-Gomez M, Reyburn HT, Mandelboim M, Strominger JL (1998) Kinetics of interaction of HLA-C ligands with natural killer cell inhibitory receptors. Immunity 9(3):337–344
15. Houchins JP, Yabe T, McSherry C, Bach FH (1991) DNA sequence analysis of NKG2, a family of related cDNA clones encoding type II

integral membrane proteins on human natural killer cells. J Exp Med 173(4):1017–1020

16. Lopez-Botet M, Angulo A, Guma M (2004) Natural killer cell receptors for major histocompatibility complex class I and related molecules in cytomegalovirus infection. Tissue Antigens 63(3):195–203
17. Moretta L, Bottino C, Pende D, Castriconi R, Mingari MC, Moretta A (2006) Surface NK receptors and their ligands on tumor cells. Semin Immunol 18(3):151–158
18. Meyaard L (2008) The inhibitory collagen receptor LAIR-1 (CD305). J Leukoc Biol 83(4):799–803
19. Riteau B, Menier C, Khalil-Daher I, Martinozzi S, Pla M, Dausset J et al (2001) HLA-G1 co-expression boosts the HLA class I-mediated NK lysis inhibition. Int Immunol 13(2): 193–201
20. Riteau B, Rouas-Freiss N, Menier C, Paul P, Dausset J, Carosella ED (2001) HLA-G2, -G3, and -G4 isoforms expressed as nonmature cell surface glycoproteins inhibit NK and antigen-specific CTL cytolysis. J Immunol 166(8): 5018–5026
21. Shiroishi M, Tsumoto K, Amano K, Shirakihara Y, Colonna M, Braud VM et al (2003) Human inhibitory receptors Ig-like transcript 2 (ILT2) and ILT4 compete with CD8 for MHC class I binding and bind preferentially to HLA-G. Proc Natl Acad Sci USA 100):8856–8861
22. Cerboni C, Achour A, Warnmark A, Mousavi-Jazi M, Sandalova T, Hsu ML et al (2006) Spontaneous mutations in the human CMV HLA class I homologue UL18 affect its binding to the inhibitory receptor LIR-1/ILT2/CD85j. Eur J Immunol 36(3):732–741
23. Kirwan SE, Burshtyn DN (2005) Killer cell Ig-like receptor-dependent signaling by Ig-like transcript 2 (ILT2/CD85j/LILRB1/LIR-1). J Immunol 175(8):5006–5015
24. Anfossi N, Andre P, Guia S, Falk CS, Roetynck S, Stewart CA et al (2006) Human NK cell education by inhibitory receptors for MHC class I. Immunity 25(2):331–342
25. Cooley S, Xiao F, Pitt M, Gleason M, McCullar V, Bergmann TL et al (2007) A subpopulation of human peripheral blood NK cells that lacks inhibitory receptors for self MHC is developmentally immature. Blood 110:578–586
26. Shilling HG, McQueen KL, Cheng NW, Shizuru JA, Negrin RS, Parham P (2003) Reconstitution of NK cell receptor repertoire following HLA-matched hematopoietic cell transplantation. Blood 101(9):3730–3740
27. Cooley S, McCullar V, Wangen R, Bergemann TL, Spellman S, Weisdorf DJ et al (2005) KIR reconstitution is altered by T cells in the graft and correlates with clinical outcomes after unrelated donor transplantation. Blood 106(13):4370–4376
28. Bottino C, Castriconi R, Moretta L, Moretta A (2005) Cellular ligands of activating NK receptors. Trends Immunol 26(4):221–226
29. Soriani A, Zingoni A, Cerboni C, Iannitto ML, Ricciardi MR, Di Gialleonardo V et al (2009) ATM-ATR dependent up-regulation of DNAM-1 and NKG2D ligands on multiple myeloma cells by therapeutic agents results in enhanced NK cell susceptibility and is associated with a senescent phenotype. Blood 113(15):3503–3511
30. Stein MN, Shin J, Gudzowaty O, Bernstein AM, Liu JM (2006) Antibody-dependent cell cytotoxicity to breast cancer targets despite inhibitory KIR signaling. Anticancer Res 26(3A):1759–1763
31. Pende D, Spaggiari GM, Marcenaro S, Martini S, Rivera P, Capobianco A et al (2005) Analysis of the receptor-ligand interactions in the natural killer-mediated lysis of freshly isolated myeloid or lymphoblastic leukemias: evidence for the involvement of the Poliovirus receptor (CD155) and Nectin-2 (CD112). Blood 105(5):2066–2073
32. Re F, Staudacher C, Zamai L, Vecchio V, Bregni M (2006) Killer cell Ig-like receptors ligand-mismatched, alloreactive natural killer cells lyse primary solid tumors. Cancer 107(3):640–648
33. Armeanu S, Bitzer M, Lauer UM, Venturelli S, Pathil A, Krusch M et al (2005) Natural killer cell-mediated lysis of hepatoma cells via specific induction of NKG2D ligands by the histone deacetylase inhibitor sodium valproate. Cancer Res 65(14):6321–6329
34. Guerra N, Tan YX, Joncker NT, Choy A, Gallardo F, Xiong N et al (2008) NKG2D-deficient mice are defective in tumor surveillance in models of spontaneous malignancy. Immunity 28(4):571–580
35. Brenner CD, King S, Przewoznik M, Wolters I, Adam C, Bornkamm GW et al (2010) Requirements for control of B-cell lymphoma by NK cells. Eur J Immunol 40(2):494–504
36. Ruggeri L, Capanni M, Urbani E, Perruccio K, Shlomchik WD, Tosti A et al (2002) Effectiveness of donor natural killer cell alloreactivity in mismatched hematopoietic transplants. Science 295(5562):2097–2100
37. Miller JS, Soignier Y, Panoskaltsis-Mortari A, McNearney SA, Yun GH, Fautsch SK et al (2005) Successful adoptive transfer and in vivo expansion of human haploidentical NK cells in patients with cancer. Blood 105(8): 3051–3057

38. Davies SM, Ruggieri L, DeFor T, Wagner JE, Weisdorf DJ, Miller JS et al (2002) Evaluation of KIR ligand incompatibility in mismatched unrelated donor hematopoietic transplants. Killer immunoglobulin-like receptor. Blood 100(10):3825–3827
39. Farag SS, Bacigalupo A, Eapen M, Hurley C, Dupont B, Caligiuri MA et al (2006) The effect of KIR ligand incompatibility on the outcome of unrelated donor transplantation: a report from the center for international blood and marrow transplant research, the European blood and marrow transplant registry, and the Dutch registry. Biol Blood Marrow Transplant 12(8):876–884
40. Miller JS, Cooley S, Parham P, Farag SS, Verneris MR, McQueen KL et al (2007) Missing KIR ligands are associated with less relapse and increased graft-versus-host disease (GVHD) following unrelated donor allogeneic HCT. Blood 109(11):5058–5061
41. Shlomchik WD, Couzens MS, Tang CB, McNiff J, Robert ME, Liu J et al (1999) Prevention of graft versus host disease by inactivation of host antigen-presenting cells. Science 285(5426):412–415
42. Lundqvist A, McCoy JP, Samsel L, Childs R (2007) Reduction of GVHD and enhanced antitumor effects after adoptive infusion of alloreactive Ly49-mismatched NK cells from MHC-matched donors. Blood 109(8):3603–3606
43. Russell JH, Ley TJ (2002) Lymphocyte-mediated cytotoxicity. Annu Rev Immunol 20:323–370
44. Murphy WJ, Keller JR, Harrison CL, Young HA, Longo DL (1992) Interleukin-2-activated natural killer cells can support hematopoiesis in vitro and promote marrow engraftment in vivo. Blood 80(3):670–677
45. Siefer AK, Longo DL, Harrison CL, Reynolds CW, Murphy WJ (1993) Activated natural killer cells and interleukin-2 promote granulocytic and megakaryocytic reconstitution after syngeneic bone marrow transplantation in mice. Blood 82(8):2577–2584
46. Chen C, Busson M, Rocha V, Appert ML, Lepage V, Dulphy N et al (2006) Activating KIR genes are associated with CMV reactivation and survival after non-T-cell depleted HLA-identical sibling bone marrow transplantation for malignant disorders. Bone Marrow Transplant 38(6):437–444
47. Stern M, Elsasser H, Honger G, Steiger J, Schaub S, Hess C (2008) The number of activating KIR genes inversely correlates with the rate of CMV infection/reactivation in kidney transplant recipients. Am J Transplant 8(6): 1312–1317
48. Farrell HE, Vally H, Lynch DM, Fleming P, Shellam GR, Scalzo AA et al (1997) Inhibition of natural killer cells by a cytomegalovirus MHC class I homologue in vivo. Nature 386(6624): 510–514
49. Giebel S, Locatelli F, Lamparelli T, Velardi A, Davies S, Frumento G et al (2003) Survival advantage with KIR ligand incompatibility in hematopoietic stem cell transplantation from unrelated donors. Blood 102(3):814–819
50. Beelen DW, Ottinger HD, Ferencik S, Elmaagacli AH, Peceny R, Trenschel R et al (2005) Genotypic inhibitory killer immunoglobulin-like receptor ligand incompatibility enhances the long-term antileukemic effect of unmodified allogeneic hematopoietic stem cell transplantation in patients with myeloid leukemias. Blood 105(6):2594–2600
51. Lowe EJ, Turner V, Handgretinger R, Horwitz EM, Benaim E, Hale GA et al (2003) T-cell alloreactivity dominates natural killer cell alloreactivity in minimally T-cell-depleted HLA-non-identical paediatric bone marrow transplantation. Br J Haematol 123(2):323–326
52. Clausen J, Kircher B, Auberger J, Schumacher P, Ulmer H, Hetzenauer G et al (2010) The role of missing killer cell immunoglobulin-like receptor ligands in T cell replete peripheral blood stem cell transplantation from HLA-identical siblings. Biol Blood Marrow Transplant 16(2):273–280
53. Linn YC, Phang CY, Lim TJ, Chong SF, Heng KK, Lee JJ et al (2010) Effect of missing killer-immunoglobulin-like receptor ligand in recipients undergoing HLA full matched, non-T-depleted sibling donor transplantation: a single institution experience of 151 Asian patients. Bone Marrow Transplant 45(6):1031–1037
54. Gagne K, Busson M, Bignon JD, Balere-Appert ML, Loiseau P, Dormoy A et al (2009) Donor KIR3DL1/3DS1 gene and recipient Bw4 KIR ligand as prognostic markers for outcome in unrelated hematopoietic stem cell transplantation. Biol Blood Marrow Transplant 15(11): 1366–1375
55. Triplett BM, Horwitz EM, Iyengar R, Turner V, Holladay MS, Gan K et al (2009) Effects of activating NK cell receptor expression and NK cell reconstitution on the outcomes of unrelated donor hematopoietic cell transplantation for hematologic malignancies. Leukemia 23(7):1278–1287
56. Cooley S, Trachtenberg E, Bergemann TL, Saeteurn K, Klein J, Le CT et al (2009) Donors with group B KIR haplotypes improve relapse-free survival after unrelated hematopoietic cell transplantation for acute myelogenous leukemia. Blood 113(3):726–732

57. Cooley S, Weisdorf DJ, Guethlein LA, Klein JP, Wang T, Le CT et al (2010) Donor selection for natural killer cell receptor genes leads to superior survival after unrelated transplantation for acute myelogenous leukemia. Blood 116(14): 2411–2419
58. Burns LJ, Weisdorf DJ, DeFor TE, Vesole DH, Repka TL, Blazar BR et al (2003) IL-2-based immunotherapy after autologous transplantation for lymphoma and breast cancer induces immune activation and cytokine release: a phase I/II trial. Bone Marrow Transplant 32(2):177–186
59. Dudley ME, Wunderlich JR, Robbins PF, Yang JC, Hwu P, Schwartzentruber DJ et al (2002) Cancer regression and autoimmunity in patients after clonal repopulation with antitumor lymphocytes. Science 298(5594):850–854
60. Bachanova V, Burns LJ, McKenna DH, Curtsinger J, Panoskaltsis-Mortari A, Lindgren BR et al (2010) Allogeneic natural killer cells for refractory lymphoma. Cancer Immunol Immunother 59(11):1739–1744
61. Geller MA, Cooley S, Judson PL, Ghebre R, Carson LF, Argenta PA et al (2010) A phase II study of allogeneic natural killer cell therapy to treat patients with recurrent ovarian and breast cancer. Cytotherapy 13(1):98–107
62. Cooley S, Gada P, McKenna D, McCullar V, Fautsch S, Verneris MR et al (2008) Successful haploidentical hematopoietic cell engraftment using a non-myeloablative preparative regimen including natural killer (NK) cells. In: American Society of Hematology 50th annual meeting, San Francisco, CA: Blood, p 827
63. Pfeiffer MM, Feuchtinger T, Teltschik HM, Schumm M, Muller I, Handgretinger R et al (2010) Reconstitution of NK cell receptors influences NK activity and relapse rate after haploidentical transplantation of T and B cell depleted grafts in children. Haematologica 95(8):1381–1388
64. Passweg JR, Tichelli A, Meyer-Monard S, Heim D, Stern M, Kuhne T et al (2004) Purified donor NK-lymphocyte infusion to consolidate engraftment after haploidentical stem cell transplantation. Leukemia 18(11):1835–1838
65. Koehl U, Esser R, Zimmermann S, Tonn T, Kotchetkov R, Bartling T et al (2005) Ex vivo expansion of highly purified NK cells for immunotherapy after haploidentical stem cell transplantation in children. Klin Padiatr 217(6): 345–350
66. Rubnitz JE, Inaba H, Ribeiro RC, Pounds S, Rooney B, Bell T et al (2010) NKAML: a pilot study to determine the safety and feasibility of haploidentical natural killer cell transplantation in childhood acute myeloid leukemia. J Clin Oncol 28(6):955–959
67. Lugli E, Goldman CK, Perera LP, Smedley J, Pung R, Yovandich JL et al (2010) Transient and persistent effects of IL15 on lymphocyte homeostasis in nonhuman primates. Blood 116(17):3238–3248
68. Barao I, Hanash AM, Hallett W, Welniak LA, Sun K, Redelman D et al (2006) Suppression of natural killer cell-mediated bone marrow cell rejection by CD4+CD25+ regulatory T cells. Proc Natl Acad Sci USA 103(14): 5460–5465
69. Bordin JO, Heddle NM, Blajchman MA (1994) Biologic effects of leukocytes present in transfused cellular blood products. Blood 84(6):1703–1721
70. McKenna DH Jr, Sumstad D, Bostrom N, Kadidlo DM, Fautsch S, McNearney S et al (2007) Good manufacturing practices production of natural killer cells for immunotherapy: a six-year single-institution experience. Transfusion 47(3):520–528
71. Miller JS, Oelkers S, Verfaillie C, McGlave P (1992) Role of monocytes in the expansion of human activated natural killer cells. Blood 80(9):2221–2229
72. Godal R, Bachanova V, Gleason M, McCullar V, Yun GH, Cooley S, Verneris MR, McGlave PB, Miller JS (2010) Natural killer cell killing of AML and ALL blasts by killer cell immunoglobulin-like receptor negative natural killer cells after NKG2A and LIR-1 blockade. Biol Blood Marrow Transplant 16(5): 612–621
73. Curtis RE, Travis LB, Rowlings PA, Socie G, Kingma DW, Banks PM et al (1999) Risk of lymphoproliferative disorders after bone marrow transplantation: a multi-institutional study. Blood 94(7):2208–2216
74. Reed M, Yearsley M, Krugh D, Kennedy MS (2003) Severe hemolysis due to passenger lymphocyte syndrome after hematopoietic stem cell transplantation from an HLA-matched related donor. Arch Pathol Lab Med 127(10): 1366–1368
75. Hummon D, Zantek ND, Sumstad D, Miller JS, McKenna DH (2009) Transfusion-associated graft-versus-host disease: a perspective from a cell therapy laboratory. Transfusion 49(5): 1018–1019
76. McKenna DH, Kadidlo DM, Miller JS, Orchard PJ, Wagner JE, McCullough J (2005) The Minnesota molecular and cellular therapeutics facility: a state-of-the-art biotherapeutics engineering laboratory. Transfus Med Rev 19(3): 217–228

# Chapter 29

# Minor Histocompatibility Antigen Typing by DNA Sequencing for Clinical Practice in Hematopoietic Stem-Cell Transplantation

Eric Spierings and Els Goulmy

## Abstract

In HLA-matched stem-cell transplantation (SCT), minor H antigens are key molecules driving allo-immune responses in both graft-versus-host disease (GvHD) and in graft-versus-leukemia (GvL) reactivity. Dissection of the dual function of minor H antigens became evident through their different modes of tissue and cell expression, i.e., hematopoietic system restricted or broad. Broadly expressed minor H antigens are the targets of immune responses in both arms of graft-versus-host (GvH) responses, i.e., both GvHD and GvL, whereas the immune responses against the hematopoietic system-specific minor H antigens are restricted to the GvL arm of SCT. Evidently, it is this latter group of minor H antigens that can function as curative tools for stem-cell (SC)-based immunotherapy of hematological malignancies and disorders. The HLA-matched patient/donor combinations, incompatible for one of the hematopoietic-specific minor H antigens, are suitable for minor H antigen immunotherapy (Goulmy, Immunol Rev 157:125–140, 1997). Information on the minor H antigen phenotype is therefore needed. Hereto, genomic typing for minor H antigens has been implemented in many HLA laboratories. Here, we firstly summarize the relevance of minor H antigens particularly in hematopoietic SCT. Secondly, we describe a method for typing the various polymorphic minor H antigens molecularly identified to date by DNA sequencing.

**Key words:** Minor histocompatibility antigens, Hematopoietic stem-cell transplantation, Graft-versus-host disease, Graft-versus-leukemia, Genotyping, polymorphism, immunogenetics, immunotherapy

## 1. Introduction

### 1.1. Background

Minor H antigens are peptides derived from polymorphic self-proteins that can differ both between unrelated individuals and between related individuals. Minor H peptides are presented by the various MHC class I and class II molecules. Their immune recognition is a

Frank T. Christiansen and Brian D. Tait (eds.), *Immunogenetics: Methods and Applications in Clinical Practice*, Methods in Molecular Biology, vol. 882, DOI 10.1007/978-1-61779-842-9_29, © Springer Science+Business Media New York 2012

typical example of HLA-restricted recognition by T cells in man (2) The MHC-minor H peptide-complexes can function as barriers in allogeneic HLA-matched stem-cell transplantation (SCT) and in solid organ transplantation (2, 3). In man, the impact of the minor H antigenic systems became apparent in 1976 through a serious clinical problems after HLA identical sibling SCT (2). Although in vitro techniques unequivocally showed cellular immunological reactivity between the SC recipient and the HLA identical SC donor (4, 5), it was not until 1995 that the molecular characteristics of human minor H antigens were clarified (6–8). Their chemical identification was instrumental in novel research aimed at understanding the immunobiology of minor H antigenic systems and for exploring their clinical usefulness in SCT. Interestingly, minor H antigenic immune responses are known to occur in the physiological situation of HLA haplo-mismatched pregnancy as well (9). Namely, multiparous women demonstrate that pregnancy can lead to allo-immune responses against the infant's paternal minor H antigens (9). Similarly, minor H antigen-specific CTLs directed at the noninherited maternal minor H antigens have been demonstrated in cord blood (10). Both minor H antigen sensitization and tolerization occur in mothers and in their adult offspring (11). Evidently, this natural allogeneic situation is a most interesting source for studying minor H antigen immunization patterns in all its aspects providing the basic information for transplantation-related reactions and for the development of minor H antigen-based immunotherapeutic strategies.

### 1.2. Minor H Antigen Immunogenetics

Autosomally encoded minor H antigens show different phenotype frequencies; the latter also differ in the various ethnic populations. Evidently, the number of patients eligible for minor H antigen-based immunotherapy depends on their phenotype frequencies in the relevant ethnic population (12). The high phenotype frequency of HLA-A2 in combination with a relatively high disparity rate for HA-1 in all ethnic populations studied, currently mark HA-1 as the most favorable minor H antigen for clinical application in all ethnic populations. Similar results, however limited to only one or two ethnic groups, were obtained for the minor H antigens ACC-1, ACC-2, and HB-1Y. Based upon frequencies, the ACC-1 minor H antigen is applicable in the Asian/Pacific population, with 6.5% disparity in sibling pairs and 12.1% in MUD pairs. Similarly, ACC-2 and HB-1Y can only be applied in a significant proportion of the pairs in the Caucasian and Mulatto population. Finally, the chance of having at least one mismatch for one of the eight hematopoietic system-restricted minor H antigen systems studied herein was calculated as 21.2 and 33.6% for Caucasian sibling and MUD pairs, respectively. In the black population, these numbers were 7.4 and 11.9%, respectively. In all these estimations, the HLA allele frequencies of the respective populations were taken into account.

**Table 1**
**Y-chromosome-encoded minor H antigens order by HLA-restriction molecule**

| Minor H antigen | HLA restriction | Gene | Peptide | References |
|---|---|---|---|---|
| A1/HY | HLA-A1 | USP9Y | IVDCLTEMY | (59, 60) |
| A2/HY | HLA-A2 | KDM5D | FIDSYICQV | (61) |
| A33/HY | HLA-A33 | TMSB4Y | EVLLRPGLHFR | (62) |
| B27/HY | HLA-B27 | DDX3Y | RDSRGKPGY | (63) |
| B52/HY | HLA-B52 | RPS4Y1 | TIRYPDPVI | (64) |
| B60/HY | HLA-B60 | UTY | RESEEESVSL | (65) |
| B7/HY | HLA-B7 | KDM5D | SPSVDKARAEL | (6) |
| B8/HY | HLA-B8 | UTY | LPHNHTDL | (66) |
| DQ5/HY | HLA-DQ5 | DDX3Y | HIENFSDIDMGE | (67) |
| DR15/HY | HLA-DR15 | DDX3Y | SKGRYIPPHLR | (68) |
| DRB3*0301/HY | HLA-DRB3*0301 | RPS4Y1 | VIKVNDTVQI | (69) |

Since this study on ten minor H antigens was reported, 27 novel autosomally encoded minor H antigens have been identified. It is now estimated that the current set of 37 autosomally encoded minor H antigens leads to at least one identifiable disparity in more than 60% of SCT MUD pairs in the Caucasian population.

### *1.3. Minor H Antigen Tissue Distribution in Relation to Their Clinical Relevance*

The Y-chromosome encoded HY antigens (Table 1), most of which are broadly expressed, are reported to clinically contribute to graft-versus-leukemia (GvL) activity (13). Among others, CTLs specific for the broadly expressed HY antigen can be detected in association with leukemia remission (14).

The involvement of broadly expressed minor H antigens in the GvHD arm of SCT was first shown by in vitro functional assays. Namely, broadly expressed minor H antigens, such as the HY antigens, are, among others, expressed on cell types of organs affected by GvHD, such as fibroblasts, melanocytes, and keratinocytes (15). This indicates that CTLs directed to broadly expressed minor H antigens are particularly relevant for the development of GvHD. To further address this issue, skin sections were incubated with CTLs specific for the broadly expressed minor H antigen, HY, or for the hematopoietic system-restricted minor H antigens HA-1 and HA-2. CTLs specific for the HY minor H antigen induced severe GvH reactions of grades III–IV, while CTLs specific for HA-1 and HA-2 induced no or weak GvH reactions (16). We recently developed specific T-cell staining reagents to directly study infiltrating HY-specific T cells in the skin of sex-mismatched SCT recipients. Indeed, these in situ results fortify the presence of HY-specific T cells in fresh/frozen skin samples taken from male patients suffering from acute GvHD after sex-mismatched SCT (17).

Most autosomally encoded minor H antigens demonstrate expression limited to but expressed on all cells of the hematopoietic system, including leukemic cells and leukemic progenitor cells. In vitro experiments have demonstrated that CTLs specific for HA-1 and HA-2 are capable of lysing leukemic cells (18). Clinically, CTLs specific for the hematopoiesis-restricted minor H antigens HA-1 and HA-2 coincide with remission of hematological malignancies after donor lymphocyte infusion (DLI) (19). Since T cells directed to hematopoiesis-restricted minor H antigens do not target the nonhematopoietic skin components, they may not be involved in local GvHD. However, there exist controversial clinical reports on the role of HA-1 in the development of GVHD as well. The skin explant assay, as described and applied above, does not provide a complete picture of GvHD because antigen presenting cells (APCs) migrate out of the skin samples during its in vitro processing. Therefore, we analyzed the behavior of HA-1-specific CTLs in an ex vivo in situ skin explant model wherein HA-1-expressing dendritic cells (DCs) were added as APCs. Infiltration and activation of HA-1 CTLs occurred only in those cases where both HLA-A2 and HA-1 were expressed, either by the skin or by the DCs, or by the combination of HLA-A2$^{+}$ skin and HA-1$^{+}$ DCs. The infiltrated and activated CTLs did not cause skin tissue destruction. These results point towards the role of recipient's HA-1$^{+}$ DCs in the chimeric patient suffering from GvHD after HA-1-mismatched SCT and provide a first step in understanding the reported association of HA-1 mismatching with clinical GvHD (20).

### 1.4. Minor H Antigens as Treatment Modality

Minor H antigens with expression limited to cells of the hematopoietic system are especially relevant for the GvL activity (21–23). The latter type of minor H antigens can be exploited as curative tools for SC-based immunotherapy of hematological malignancies and disorders (Goulmy, Immunol Rev 157:125–140, 1997). Hereto, HLA-matched minor H antigen-mismatched recipient/donor combinations are selected. Two treatment modalities currently exploit minor H antigen disparity between SC donor and recipient. One modality is the adoptive transfer of in vitro generated SC donor-derived minor H antigen-specific CTLs. The other, a more practical and far less laborious strategy, is post-SCT "vaccination." Both strategies, which are briefly discussed below, are currently ongoing in clinical phase I/II studies.

Adoptive transfer of human minor H antigen-specific CTLs has been shown to be successful in the treatment of human leukemia and solid tumors in an experimental nonobese diabetic/severe combined immunodeficiency mouse model (24, 25). Translation of this approach to the human situation is feasible. Namely, minor H antigen-specific CTLs can be generated in large numbers in vitro by co-culture of donor lymphocytes with donor-derived dendritic cells which are minor H peptide-loaded or retrovirally transduced with the minor H gene (26, 27). Artificial APCs coated with HLA-A2/minor H antigen complexes, CD80 and CD54 might help to selectively enrich minor H antigen-specific CTLs for adoptive immunotherapy (28).

Another form of adaptive cellular immunotherapy is the transfer of minor H antigen-specific T-cell receptor (TCR) genes into peripheral blood mononuclear cells of the SCT donor. In vitro, successful transfer for the minor H antigens HA-2 (29) and HA-1 (30) has been demonstrated. Implementation of the TCR gene-transduced cells into clinical trials is currently not opportune. Two crucial barriers still have to be overcome. Firstly, the relatively low avidity of the transferred TCRs is associated with low lysis capacity. Secondly, autoreactivities caused by pairing of the endogenous $\alpha$-chain with the transduced $\beta$-chain and vice versa cannot be excluded.

Interestingly, minor H antigens could potentially be applied in a partly HLA-mismatched setting of SCT. This supposition is based on in vitro results demonstrating the generation of CTLs specific for the self-antigens HLA-A2/cyclin-D1 (31), and the minor H antigen HA-1 (32) in an HLA-mismatched SCT setting. Although really challenging and with a potential broad applicability, undesired alloreactivity is a major problem of this approach. So far no protocols exist that reliably and reproducibly result in clinically graded non-self HLA/minor H antigen-specific CTLs.

In the treatment modality of minor H antigen peptide vaccination, the relevant recipient-specific minor H peptides are administered to the patient after SCT and/or DLI to boost and thus to further enhance the donor-derived minor H antigen-specific T cells in vivo (21). The observation that HA-1 and HA-2 CTLs emerge after DLI following allogeneic SCT underscores the feasibility of this approach (33, 34). Minor H antigen vaccination will boost minor H antigen-specific CTLs in patients with partial or full donor chimerism, i.e., when host APCs are progressively replaced by minor H antigen-negative donor APCs. The optimal protocol of boosting minor H antigen-specific CTLs by vaccination is still unclear with regard to the extent of the immune response and of the avoidance of tolerance. Although variables, such as the delivery system (naked DNA, recombinant vectors, recombinant protein or, dose, route of administration, frequency of vaccination, and immunological adjuvants (35, 36)), still need to be investigated, the preferable peptide length for vaccination has been determined (37).

Recently, a phase I/II clinical minor H peptide vaccination trial has been initiated for multiple myeloma patients who do not respond on the regular allogeneic SCT treatment. Herein, myeloma is targeted after SCT and DLI by patient vaccination with patient-dendritic cells loaded with graft-versus-myeloma-associated minor H antigens (T. Mutis, H. Lokhorst, L. Hambach, E. Goulmy, 2012 still in progress).

A number of methods have been described for allelic typing of minor H antigens, including allele-specific PCR based on sequence specific primers (PCR-SSP; gene-specific PCR; real-time PCR; PCR with melting curve analyses; reference strand conformation analysis (RSCA); sequencing-based typing (SBT) and multiplex PCT-SSO). PCR-SSP for minor H antigens has already been described in great detail and is not described here (38). However, an updated list of primer sets that can be used in this protocol is presented in Tables 2 and 3. Here we focus on an SBT protocol, as this technique allows typing of the largest number of minor H antigens and is the most universally applicable protocol.

## 2. Materials

### *2.1. Materials*

1. PCR primers as listed in Table 4.
2. Standard thin-wall PCR tubes.
3. Amplitaq DNA polymerase (Applied Biosystems).
4. GeneAmp 10× PCR Buffer II (Applied Biosystems).
5. $MgCl_2$ (25 mM; Applied Biosystems).
6. dNTPs (10 mM; Invitrogen).
7. High-performance liquid chromatography (HPLC) water.
8. Agarose, molecular biology grade.
9. Gel Red (Gentaur).
10. Loading buffer (0.5 g Orange G and 40 g sucrose in 100 mL $H_2O$).
11. Tris-acetate EDTA (TAE) buffer.
12. Exonuclease I (Westburg).
13. SAP (GE Healthcare).
14. Sequence primers as listed in Table 4.
15. Big Dye Terminator (BDT) Cycle sequence kit v1.1 (Applied Biosystems).
16. Sephadex G-50 Superfine DNA Grade (GE Healthcare).
17. Sephadex 96 wells matrix plate, (Millipore).
18. 96-Wells MultiScreen filter plate (Millipore).
19. POP7 (Applied Biosystems).

**Table 2**
**Oligonucleotide primers for the uniform allele-specific PCR-SSP**

| Minor H antigen | Allele | Forward primer | Reverse primer | Amplicon size (bp) |
|---|---|---|---|---|
| HA-1 | H | CTTAAGGAGTGTGTGCTGCA | ACTCCTACACATCCCTCAGAG | 190 |
| | R | CTTAAGGAGTGTGTGTTGCG | ACTCCTACACATCCCTCAGAG | 190 |
| HA-2 | V | ACAGTCTCTGAGTGGCTCAG | GCAGCTCCTGGTAGGGGTTAAC | 271 |
| | M | ACAGTCTCTGAGTGGCTCAG | GCAGCTCCTGGTAGGGGTTAAT | 271 |
| HA-3 | M | GTCCTTCAGAGAGACTTGGGCAT | AGACTCAGCAGGTTTGTTAC | 129 |
| | T | GTCCTTCAGAGAGACTTGGGCAC | AGACTCAGCAGGTTTGTTAC | 318 |
| HA-8 | R | TGCAGTCAGCAGATCACCG | CTTCTGGGCAACAGTTATGGA | 186 |
| | P | TGCAGTCAGCAGATCACCC | CTTCTGGGCAACAGTTATGGA | 186 |
| HB-1 | Y | GCCATTCTTTTCTATAGGTTCTTTGT | AGGGCATATGTTCCACTTGCTT | 213 |
| | H | ATTCTTTTCTATAGGTTCTCTGC | AGGGCATATGTTCCACTTGCTT | 210 |
| ACC-1 | Y | CATTGCCTCAACAGCTTCAAG | GGTTGTGGTATCTGTAGGGCGT | 136 |
| | C | CATTGCCTCAACAGCTTCAAG | GGTTGTGGTATCTGTAGGGCGC | 136 |
| ACC-2 | D | GATGGAAAAGGAGTTTGAAGGCGA | CAGCCTCCGTTTTGCCTTATC | 197 |
| | G | GATGGAAAAGGAGTTTGAAGGCGG | CAGCCTCCGTTTTGCCTTATC | 197 |
| SP110 | R | AATGTGGTTTGAAGACCAAAAGT | CTTGTACTCTCATCTTACCTCC | 185 |
| | G | AATGTGGTTTGAAGACCAAAAGT | CTTGTACTCTCATCTTACCTCT | 185 |
| PANE1 | R | AGGCAAGTCCCACACTCG | AATGGGGTAAATGACGTGCTG | 207 |
| | stop | CAGGCAAGTCCCACACTCA | AATGGGGTAAATGACGTGCTG1 | 207 |

(continued)

**Table 2 (continued)**

| Minor H antigen | Allele | Forward primer | Reverse primer | Amplicon size (bp) |
|---|---|---|---|---|
| LB-ECGF | H | CCTGGCTCCGCGTGCACCG | GAGGGGGCGGCGAATG**T**CGT | 105 |
| | R | CCTGGCTCCGCGTGCACCG | AGGGGGCGGCGAATGGCGC | 105 |
| CTSH | R | TGCCGCTGCTCTGCGCCA | CAGAGTTCCTGGCCTCTCAC | 210 |
| | G | TGCCGCTGCTCTGCGCCG | CAGAGTTCCTGGCCTCTCAC | 210 |
| LRH1 | 5C | GCCCACACACACTCTGAGAA | ACCTGATTGTGACCC**A**CAAC | 193 |
| | 4C | GCCCACACACACTCTGAGAA | AACCTGATTGTGACC**A**CAAC | 193 |
| LB-ADIR | F | GCTGAAGAGCGTCCAAGTACC | GCGCCAGCTTTGGCTCTTTT | 183 |
| | S | GCTGAAGAGCGTCCAAGTACC | CGCCAGCTTTGGCTCTTTC | 183 |

Nucleotides in *bold* indicate introduced mismatches with the genomic sequence for improved performance

**Table 3**
**Oligonucleotide primers for gene-specific PCR**

| Minor H antigen | Forward primer | Reverse primer | Size (bp) |
|---|---|---|---|
| UGT2B17 | | | |
| 5′ region | GGCAGTATCTTGCCAATGT | AGACTCCAAGTGCCAGTT | 341 |
| Exon 1a | TGTTGGGAATATTCTGACTATAA | CCCACTTCTTCAGATCATATGC | 352 |
| Exon 1b | AAATGACAGAAAGAAACAA | GCATCTTCACAGAGCTTATAT | 443 |
| Exon 6 | GAATTCATCATGATCAACCG | ACAGGCAACATTTTGTGATC | 201 |
| HY (SRY) | TGGCGATTAAGTCAAATTCGC | CCCCCTAGTACCCTGACAAT GTATT | 136 |

**Table 4**
**Oligonucleotide primers for sequencing-based typing**

| Minor H antigen | Type of primer | Primer sequence | Amplicon size (bp) |
|---|---|---|---|
| HA-1 | Forward PCR | AAGGACCGTTGTTTGTGAAAGC | |
| | Reverse PCR | **CAGGAAACAGCTATGA**CCCGTT GTCATGCCTTCATCCTAC | 523 |
| | Forward sequence | AAGGACCGTTGTTTGTGAAAGC | |
| | Reverse sequence | **CAGGAAACAGCTATGACC** | |
| HA-2 | Forward PCR | CCCCTTCTTCCTTCTCCACT | |
| | Reverse PCR | **CAGGAAACAGCTATGAC**CAGCC AGGTTCGCTCTCTTA | 526 |
| | Forward sequence | CACAGGAGATGCTCTAATGG | |
| | Reverse sequence | TGTGGGTGCCTGTAAG | |
| HA-3 | Forward PCR | GTGACTGACCCACAGGGAGT | |
| | Reverse PCR | CCCAGGTGGGAAAGTACTCA | 498 |
| | Forward sequence | TACCTCTTGATTGGGAGAAA | |
| | Reverse sequence | CTTGACTTGTTCGATGACAG | |
| HA-8 | Forward PCR | GCTACCTCTTCTGGGCAACA | |
| | Reverse PCR | **CAGGAAACAGCTATGAC**GCCTG GCTCTTTAAATGCAC | 402 |
| | Forward sequence | GCCATTGGAGTTAGAATCTG | |
| | Reverse sequence | TCAGCTAATCAGGTTACTCC | |

(continued)

**Table 4 (continued)**

| Minor H antigen | Type of primer | Primer sequence | Amplicon size (bp) |
|---|---|---|---|
| HB-1 | Forward PCR | CCTGAGCCTTCTGACCTCAC | |
| | Reverse PCR | AAACTCTGGGCTTCGAGTCA | 215 |
| | Forward sequence | CACAGTGGAGAAACCAGAAC | |
| | Reverse sequence | AAGAGCTGTGCCTCAGATAC | |
| ACC-1 and-2 | Forward PCR | CATTGCCTCAACAGCTTCAA | |
| | Reverse PCR | **CAGGAAACAGCTATGAC**AGCCT CCGTTTTGCCTTATC | 478 |
| | Forward sequence | CTCAAGACTTTGCTCTCCAC | |
| | Reverse sequence | CATTATGAACTCCGCAAC | |
| PANE1 | Forward PCR | GCAGGCCACGGAGAT | |
| | Reverse PCR | GTCAAGCCCTGACTGGACAT | 308 |
| | Forward sequence | GGAAGGAGGAACAGC | |
| | Reverse sequence | ACCCTCACAGGTCCTCCA | |
| SP110 | Forward PCR | CCATCACCTAAGGTCACCAA | |
| | Reverse PCR | TGAAGAGTGGGCCTTGATTT | 573 |
| | Forward sequence | CAAGATTGGGAGATCAATGT | |
| | Reverse sequence | TAAAATTCAACCCTCCACAG | |
| CTSH | Forward PCR | GAGAACCCCCGCCTATAATG | |
| | Reverse PCR | GCCGACAGGTGAACTAGAGC | 507 |
| | Forward sequence | TCTGCGTACCTAAGGAGTTC | |
| | Reverse sequence | TCCCAGTTGACGCTC | |
| LRH-1 | Forward PCR | CCTTCATTCTGCCAGGAGAG | |
| | Reverse PCR | **CAGGAAACAGCTATGAC**CCTCA GTGCCTCTCTGGTTC | 378 |
| | Forward sequence | AGAATAGGGGTTCTTCTTCG | |
| | Reverse sequence | GGGTTCTTCTTCGCTT | |

(continued)

**Table 4 (continued)**

| Minor H antigen | Type of primer | Primer sequence | Amplicon size (bp) |
|---|---|---|---|
| LB-ADIR-1 | Forward PCR | CTCCTCGTCCTCGTCACAGT | |
| | Reverse PCR | **CAGGAAACAGCTATGAC**AGG ACCCCAGACAGGGTTT | 447 |
| | Forward sequence | GCTGAAGAGCGTCCAGTA | |
| | Reverse sequence | CCACAGCAACACCAAT | |
| CD19 | Forward PCR | CTCTCTCTGCGGGTCTTTGT | |
| | Reverse PCR | **CAGGAAACAGCTATGAC**TTCA GCTCTAGGCTCAGCAA | 557 |
| | Forward sequence | GTGTCTCTGCATTTGGTTCT | |
| | Reverse sequence | CACAGGACAGCCAGAG | |

Sequences in *bold* represent the M13-reverse primer sequence

20. 10× Genetic Analyzer Buffer with EDTA (Applied Biosystems).
21. DNA size marker, ranging from 100 bp to at least 1,000 bp with a size interval of approximately 100 bp, e.g., the 1 kb+ladder from Invitrogen.

### 2.2. Special Equipment

#### 2.2.1. Pre-PCR Area

1. Standard micropipets ranging from 0.2 μL to 1.0 mL.
2. Filter tips (0.5–10; 10–100; 100–1,000 μL).
3. Thin-walled PCR tubes, strips, or individual tubes (Eppendorf).

#### 2.2.2. Thermal Cycler Area

1. Thermal cycler with a 96-well block. We have successfully used the Dyad Disciple (MJ-Research) and the models 2720 and 9700 from Applied Biosystems.

#### 2.2.3. Post-PCR Area

1. Electrophoresis system. A horizontal electrophoresis system for submerged gel electrophoresis with a tray that accommodates six 26-well combs enables genotyping of 150 DNAs in a single run and allows inclusion of one size marker per row.
2. Combs compatible with multichannel pipets facilitate fast loading of a full gel.
3. DNA size marker 1 kb+ladder (Invitrogen).
4. A multichannel pipettor in the 0.5–10.0 μL range for gel loading.
5. Geldoc 2000 (Biorad) or alternative DNA visualization system.

#### 2.2.4. Sequencing Area

1. Plate centrifuge (Beckman Coulter).
2. Automated DNA sequencer and consumables. We use the ABI 3730, 48 capillary sequencer (Applied Biosystems).

*2.2.5. Allele Identification Software*

1. SBTEngine® Software (Genome Diagnostics) for automated allele assignment.
2. If SBTEngine® is not available, general sequence analysis programs as BioEdit can be used for manual analysis.

## 3. Methods

### 3.1. DNA Preparation

1. Different methods for isolation of genomic DNA are available. For optimal results, high-quality DNA is required. The described protocols assume a DNA concentration of 30 ng/μL. If required, dilute the DNA stock solution in HPLC-grade water. Higher or lower concentrations of DNA may lead to unsuccessful amplification.
2. Control DNA can be obtained from the IHW cell panel. A large number of the cell lines in this panel has been typed for minor H antigens (38). See Note 1 for preventing carryover contamination.

### 3.2. PCR Amplification

1. Dilute PCR primers to a concentration of 100 pmol/μL.
2. For each Minor-H antigen to be tested, prepare a master mix (21.75 μL/reaction) containing 2.5 μL GeneAmp 10× PCR Buffer II, 1.5 μL $MgCl_2$, 1 μL dNTPs, 16.55 μL $H_2O$, 0.1 μL of the appropriate 5′ PCR primer, and 0.1 μL of the appropriate 3′ PCR primer.
3. Mix master mix well.
4. Master mixes can be stored at −20°C for later use.
5. Take the appropriate volume of master mix, depending on the number of amplifications (see Note 2).
6. Add Amplitaq (0.25 μL/reaction) to the master mix (see Note 2).
7. Add 22 μL master mix to a thin-wall PCR tube (see Note 3).
8. Add 3 μL (90 ng) of the test DNA to each aliquot of the master mixes. Only samples with the appropriate HLA restriction molecule for each minor H antigen should be tested (see Note 4).
9. Incubate the samples in a thermal cycler according to the following thermal cycler profile (final volume 25 μL): 1 cycle: 95°C, 10 min; 35 cycle: 95°C, 30 s/54°C, 30 s/72°C, 60 s; 1 cycle: 72°C, 10 min; hold: 15°C. This protocol can be applied for all minor H antigens.

10. Analysis of amplification products: apply 5 μL of each amplification reaction with 3 μL loading buffer to a 1.5% agarose gel. Run gel for 30 min at 200 V. Visualize the amplification products with a Geldoc.
11. The expected sizes of the PCR products have been listed for each minor H antigen in Table 4.
12. The DNA size marker can be diluted for semi-quantitative comparison. In our experience, sequencing of PCR products with a lower intensity than the 1/8 dilution of the 1 kb + DNA marker (Invitrogen), in general appears to be unsuccessful. It is therefore advisable to only proceed with the products showing a stronger intensity than the 1/8 diluted marker. See Note 5 for troubleshooting.

### 3.3. Purification of the Amplification Products

Digestion with Exonuclease I and SAP is performed to remove residual PCR primers and dNTPs.

1. Add 1 μL SAP and 0.5 μL Exonuclease I to each amplification product.
2. Incubate the samples in a thermal cycler: 37°C, 15 min/80°C, 20 min/15°C, hold until ready for use in sequencing reaction.

### 3.4. DNA Sequencing Reaction

1. Dilute sequence primers to a concentration of 100 pmol/μL (see Table 4 for sequences).
2. For each sequencing primer, prepare the appropriate amounts of each of the sequencing reaction mixes containing 1 μL BDT Ready Reaction v1.1 mix, 1.5 μL BDT buffer 5×, 0.1 μL of the appropriate sequence primer, and 6.4 μL $H_2O$ per sequencing reaction.
3. Add 9 μL sequencing mix to a thin-wall PCR tube.
4. Add 1 μL of the purified PCR amplification product—see Subheading 3.3, step 2.
5. Incubate the samples in a thermal cycler: 1 cycle: 96°C, 10 s; 25 cycles: 96°C, 10 s/50°C 10 s/60°C, 120 s; 15°C—hold until ready for purification.

### 3.5. Purification of Sequencing Reaction Products

1. Add Sephadex to the matrix plate (Millipore), fill each matrix well to the rim.
2. Place the Millipore Multiscreen plate upside down on top of the filled matrix plate.
3. Transfer the Sephadex from the matrix plate to the Millipore Multiscreen plate by turning the matrix plate to the top position.

4. Add 300 μL $H_2O$ per well of the Millipore Multiscreen plate.
5. Keep at room temperature for 3 h or overnight at 4°C.
6. Put a dummy 96-well flat bottom plate under the Multiscreen plate.
7. Spin down each pair of the stacked plates for 5 min at 670 × *g*, discard the dummy plate.
8. Overlay the sequencing product on top of the packed Sephadex in the Multiscreen plate, one product per well.
9. Put a sequencing product collection plate under the Multiscreen plate.
10. Spin down the plates for 5 min at 670 × *g*.
11. Add a sequencing cover lid to the collection plates or use a plastic seal.
12. Spin down 5 s at 225 × *g* to remove the air bubbles from the sequencing product.

### 3.6. Settings for Capillary Electrophoresis

1. Install your sequencer with a 50-cm capillary.
2. Use liquid polymer POP-7.
3. If your sequencer is not able to perforate the seal or the sequencing cover lid, remove the seal or the cover.
4. Place the sequencing plate in a cassette and load into the automated sequencer.
5. Start the sequencing procedure using the settings given below:

   Run Module: BDx FastSeq50 POP7

   (a) Prerun time: 180 s
   (b) Prerun voltage: 15.0 kV
   (c) Injection time: 3 s
   (d) Injection voltage: 1.0 kV
   (e) Electrophoresis voltage: 13.4 kV
   (f) Temperature: 60°C

### 3.7. Sequence Analysis

Analyses can be performed manually with general sequencing analysis software like BioEdit, or automated with SBTEngine®, which includes data files for a number of minor H antigens. An example of automated allele assignments is depicted in Fig. 1. Homozygosity can be confirmed with PCR-SSP (see Note 6).

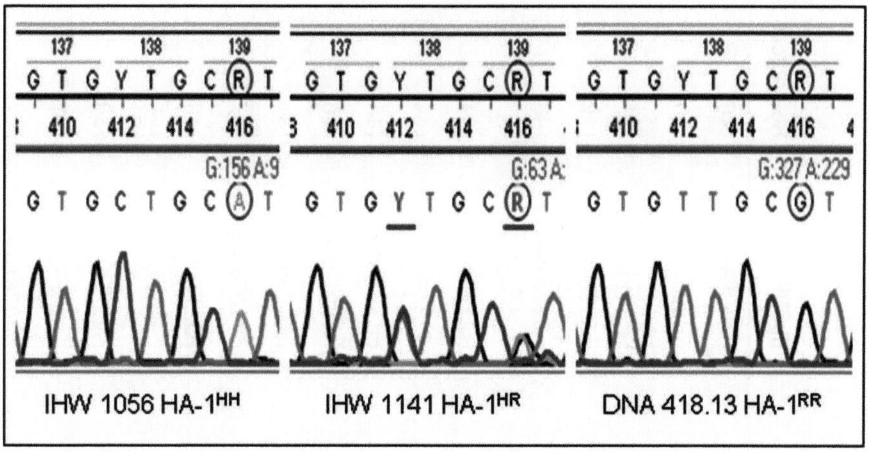


Fig. 1. Sequencing-based typing results for minor H antigen HA-1. The cell-lines used in this validation protocol were previous typed by PCR-SSP. Analyses were performed with SBTEngine© (GenDx BV). *Left panel* shows a reference sample that is homozygous for the HA-1H allele. *Numbers at top* indicate the codon position. The sequence *underneath the codon position* displays the potential nucleic acids and their position, based upon the known HA-1 alleles. The position of the nonsynymous SNP at position 416 has been marked with a *circle*. The *right panel* displays the result for the HA-1R reference sample. In the *middle*, a heterozygous reference sample has been depicted. Both the heterozygous synonymous SNP at position 412 and the nonsynonymous SNP at position 416 have been *underlined*.

## 4. Notes

1. Carryover contamination from previous PCR can be a significant problem due to the abundance of PCR products and to the ideal structure of the contaminant materials for re-amplification. Therefore, controls to detect contamination should always be included. Moreover, a strict physical separation of pre- and post amplification areas is strongly advised. An alternative option to control carryover contamination with PCR products is using uracil DNA glycosylase (UDG) in all PCR samples (39). The procedure requires the following two steps: (1) incorporating dUTP in all PCR products (by substituting dUPT for dTTP), and (2) treating all subsequent fully preassembled starting reactions with UDG, followed by thermal inactivation of UDG. UDG cleaves the uracil base from uracil-containing DNA, but has no effect on thymidine-containing DNA. This cleavage blocks replication by DNA polymerases. UDG does not react with dUTP, and is inactivated during denaturation at 95°C.

**Table 5**
**Autosomally encoded minor H antigens, ordered alphabetically**

| Original name | HLA restriction | Gene | Chrom. | Peptide | dbSNP | References |
|---|---|---|---|---|---|---|
| ACC-1 | HLA-A24 | BCL2A1 | 15 | DYLQYVLQI | rs1138357 | (40) |
| ACC-2 | HLA-B44 | BCL2A1 | 15 | KEFEDDIINW | rs3826007 | (40) |
| ACC-6 | HLA-B44 | HMSD | 18 | MEIFIEVFSHF | rs9945924 | (41) |
| C19orf48 | HLA-B7 | C19orf48 | 19 | TPNQRQNVC | rs5818907 | (42) |
| CD19 | HLA-DQA1*05/B1*02 | CD19 | 16 | RTLDKVLEV | rs2173904 | (43) |
| CTSH/A31 | HLA-A31 | CTSH | 15 | ATLPLLCAR | rs2289702 | (44) |
| CTSH/A33 | HLA-A33 | CTSH | 15 | WATLPLLCAR | rs2289702 | (44) |
| HA-1/A2 | HLA-A2 | HMHA1 | 19 | VLHDDLLEA | rs1801284 | (45) |
| HA-1/B60 | HLA-B60 | HMHA1 | 19 | KECVLHDDLL | rs1801284 | (46) |
| HA-2 | HLA-A2 | MYO1G | 7 | YIGEVLVSV | rs61739531 | (8) |
| HA-3 | HLA-A1 | AKAP13 | 15 | VTEPGTAQY | rs7162168 | (47) |
| HA-8 | HLA-A2 | KIAA0020 | 9 | RTLDKVLEV | rs2173904 | (48) |
| HB-1 | HLA-B44 | HMHB1 | 5 | EEKRGSLHVW | rs161557 | (49) |
| HEATR1 | HLA-B8 | HEATR1 | 1 | ISKERAEAL | rs2275687 | (50) |
| LB-ADIR-1 | HLA-A2 | TOR3A | 1 | SVAPALALFPA | rs2296377 | (51) |
| LB-APOBEC3B-1K | HLA-B7 | APOBEC3B | 22 | KPQYHAEMCF | rs2076109 | (52) |
| LB-ARHGDIB-1R | HLA-B7 | ARHGDIB | 12 | LPRACWREA | rs4703 | (53) |
| LB-BCAT2-1R | HLA-B7 | BCAT2 | 19 | QPRRALLFVIL | rs11548193 | (52) |

| | | | | | | |
|---|---|---|---|---|---|---|
| LB-EBI3-1I | HLA-B7 | EBI3 | 19 | RPRARYYIQV | rs4740 | (52) |
| LB-ECGF-1 | HLA-B7 | TYMP | 22 | RPHAIRRPLAL | n.a. | (52) |
| LB-ERAP1-1R | HLA-B7 | ERAP1 | 5 | HPRQEQIALLA | rs26653 | (52) |
| LB-GEMIN4-1V | HLA-B7 | GEMIN4 | 17 | FPALRFVEV | rs4968104 | (52) |
| LB-LY75-1K | HLA-DRB1*1301 | LY75 | 2 | GITYRNKSLM | rs12692566 | (53) |
| LB-MR1-1R | HLA-DRB3*0202 | MR1 | 1 | YFRLGVSDPIRG | rs2236410 | (53) |
| LB-MTHFD1-1Q | HLA-DRB1*0301 | MTHFD1 | 14 | SSIIADQIALKL | rs2236225 | (53) |
| LB-PDCD11-1F | HLA-B7 | PDCD11 | 10 | GPDSSKTFLCL | rs2986014 | (52) |
| LB-PI4K2B-1 | HLA-DQ6 | PI4K2B | 4 | SRSSSAELDRSR | rs313549 | (54) |
| LB-PRCP-1D | HLA-A2 | PRCP | 11 | FMWDVAEDLKA | rs2298668 | (52) |
| LB-PTK2B-1T | HLA-DRB3*0101 | PTK2B | 8 | VYMNDTSPL | rs751019 | (53) |
| LB-SSR1-1S | HLA-A2 | SSR1 | 6 | SLAVAQDLT | rs10004 | (52) |
| LB-WNK1-1I | HLA-A2 | WNK1 | 12 | RTLSPEIITV | rs12828016 | (52) |
| LRH-1 | HLA-B7 | P2RX5 | 17 | TPNQRQNVC | rs5818907 | (55) |
| PANE1 | HLA-A3 | CENPM | 22 | RVWDLPGVLK | n.a. | (56) |
| SLC1A5 | HLA-B61 | SLC1A5 | 19 | AEATANGGLAL | rs3027956 | (57) |
| SP110 | HLA-A3 | SP110 | 2 | SLPRGTSTPK | rs1365776 | (58) |
| UGT2B17 | HLA-A29/B44 | UGT2B17 | 4 | AELLNIPVLY | n.a. | (59) |
| UGT2B17 | HLA-A2 | UGT2B17 | 4 | CVATMIFMI | n.a. | (57) |

2. Mixes for a maximum of ten samples are optimal in our hands. Master mixes for PCR and sequencing can be stored at −20°C for at least 1 year. Storing of PCR and sequencing reaction mixes after the addition of AmpliTaq or BDT is not advised. Storing mixes after addition of the enzymes results in a rapidly reduction of the PCR yields and sequencing qualities.
3. Preparation of samples for PCR preferentially occurs on ice.
4. Minor H antigens are only relevant when presented in the correct HLA molecule. Check the presence of the HLA-restriction molecule before typing certain minor H antigens. For this purpose, Table 5 can be used.
5. If PCR reactions show a consistently poor result for various samples, adaptations to the protocol should be made. These adaptations could include changes to the PCR temperature profile. For example, PCR yields for HA-1 may improve when increasing the annealing temperature to 56°C. Alternatively, PCR primer concentrations can be doubled.
6. Due to the use of nonpolymorphic amplification primers, SBT has a low risk to miss an allele due to suboptimal amplification conditions. If required, homozygosity may be confirmed using PCR-SSP.

## Acknowledgments

We thank Talitha de Hoop en Walter van Ginkel, University Medical Center Utrecht, for developing and validating the SBT protocols, Jos Pool and Jos Drabbels, Leiden University Medical Center for developing and validating the uniform PCR-SSP protocols, and Erik Rozemuller, Genome Diagnostics BV, Utrecht, for the implementation of automated allele assignment for minor H antigens after SBT in SBTEngine®.

### References

1. Goulmy E (1997) Human minor histocompatibility antigens: new concepts for marrow transplantation and adoptive immunotherapy. Immunol Rev 157:125–140
2. Goulmy E, Termijtelen A, Bradley BA, van Rood JJ (1976) Alloimmunity to human H-Y. Lancet 2:1206
3. Goulmy E, Bradley BA, Lansbergen Q, van Rood JJ (1978) The importance of H-Y incompatibility in human organ transplantation. Transplantation 25:315–319
4. Goulmy E, Gratama JW, Blokland E, Zwaan FE, van Rood JJ (1983) A minor transplantation antigen detected by MHC-restricted cytotoxic T lymphocytes during graft-versus-host disease. Nature 302:159–161
5. van Els CA, D'Amaro J, Pool J, Blokland E, Bakker A, van Elsen PJ et al (1992) Immunogenetics of human minor histocompatibility antigens: their polymorphism and immunodominance. Immunogenetics 35: 161–165

6. Wang W, Meadows LR, den Haan JM, Sherman NE, Chen Y, Blokland E et al (1995) Human H-Y: a male-specific histocompatibility antigen derived from the SMCY protein. Science 269:1588–1590
7. Goulmy E, Pool J, van den Elsen PJ (1995) Interindividual conservation of T-cell receptor beta chain variable regions by minor histocompatibility antigen-specific HLA-A*0201-restricted cytotoxic T-cell clones. Blood 85: 2478–2481
8. den Haan JM, Sherman NE, Blokland E, Huczko E, Koning F, Drijfhout JW et al (1995) Identification of a graft versus host disease-associated human minor histocompatibility antigen. Science 268:1476–1480
9. Verdijk RM, Kloosterman A, Pool J, Van De KM, Naipal AM, Van Halteren AG et al (2004) Pregnancy induces minor histocompatibility antigen-specific cytotoxic T cells: implications for stem cell transplantation and immunotherapy. Blood 103:1961–1964
10. Mommaas B, Stegehuis-Kamp JA, Van Halteren AG, Kester M, Enczmann J, Wernet P et al (2004) Cord blood comprises antigen-experienced T cells specific for maternal minor histocompatibility antigen HA-1. Blood 105: 1823–1827
11. Van Halteren AG, Jankowska-Gan E, Joosten A, Blokland E, Pool J, Brand A et al (2009) Naturally acquired tolerance and sensitization to minor histocompatibility antigens in healthy family members. Blood 114: 2263–2272
12. Spierings E, Hendriks M, Absi L, Canossi A, Chhaya S, Crowley J et al (2007) Phenotype frequencies of autosomal minor histocompatibility antigens display significant differences among populations. PLoS Genet 3:e103
13. Gratwohl A, Hermans J, Niederwieser D, van Biezen A, van Houwelingen HC, Apperley J (2001) Female donors influence transplant-related mortality and relapse incidence in male recipients of sibling blood and marrow transplants. Hematol J 2:363–370
14. Takami A, Sugimori C, Feng X, Yachie A, Kondo Y, Nishimura R et al (2004) Expansion and activation of minor histocompatibility antigen HY-specific T cells associated with graft-versus-leukemia response. Bone Marrow Transplant 34:703–709
15. de Bueger MM, Bakker A, Van Rood JJ, Van der Woude F, Goulmy E (1992) Tissue distribution of human minor histocompatibility antigens ubiquitous versus restricted tissue distribution indicates heterogeneity among human cytotoxic T lymphocyte-defined non-MHC antigens. J Immunol 149:1788–1794
16. Dickinson AM, Wang XN, Sviland L, Vyth-Dreese FA, Jackson GH, Schumacher TN et al (2002) In situ dissection of the graft-versus-host activities of cytotoxic T cells specific for minor histocompatibility antigens. Nat Med 8:410–414
17. Kim YH, Faaij CM, van Halteren AG, Schrama E, de Jong TA, Schøller J, Egeler RM, Pavel S, Vyth-Dreese FA, van Tol MJ, Goulmy E, Spierings E. In situ detection of HY-specific T cells in acute graft-versus-host disease-affected male skin after sex-mismatched stem cell transplantation. Biol Blood Marrow Transplant. 2012 Mar;18(3): 381–7. Epub 2011 Nov 4.
18. van der Harst D, Goulmy E, Falkenburg J, Kooij-Winkelaar Y, van Luxemburg-Heijs S, Goselink H et al (1994) Recognition of minor histocompatibility antigens on lymphocytic and myeloid leukemic cells by cytotoxic T-cell clones. Blood 83:1060–1066
19. Marijt W, Heemskerk M, Kloosterboer F, Goulmy E, Kester M, van der Horn M et al (2003) Hematopoiesis-restricted minor histocompatibilty antigens HA-1- or HA-2-specific T cells can induce complete remissions of relapsed leukemia. Proc Natl Acad Sci USA 100:2742–2747
20. Kim YH, Vyth-Dreese FA, Schrama E, Pavel S, Bajema I, Goulmy E et al (2010) Exogenous addition of minor H antigen HA-1+ dendritic cells to skin tissues ex vivo causes infiltration and activation of HA-1 specific cytotoxic T cells. Biol Blood Marrow Transplant 17(1): 69–77
21. Mutis T, Goulmy E (2002) Hematopoietic system-specific antigens as targets for cellular immunotherapy of hematological malignancies. Semin Hematol 39:23–31
22. Klein CA, Wilke M, Pool J, Vermeulen C, Blokland E, Burghart E et al (2002) The hematopoietic system-specific minor histocompatibility antigen HA-1 shows aberrant expression in epithelial cancer cells. J Exp Med 196:359–368
23. Fujii N, Hiraki A, Ikeda K, Ohmura Y, Nozaki I, Shinagawa K et al (2002) Expression of minor histocompatibility antigen, HA-1, in solid tumor cells. Transplantation 73: 1137–1141
24. Hambach L, Nijmeijer BA, Aghai Z, Schie ML, Wauben MH, Falkenburg JH et al (2006) Human cytotoxic T lymphocytes specific for a single minor histocompatibility antigen HA-1 are effective against human lymphoblastic leukaemia in NOD/scid mice. Leukemia 20:371–374
25. Hambach L, Vermeij M, Buser A, Aghai Z, Van der KT, Goulmy E (2008) Targeting a single mismatched minor histocompatibility antigen

with tumor-restricted expression eradicates human solid tumors. Blood 112:1844–1852

26. Mutis T, Verdijk R, Schrama E, Esendam B, Brand A, Goulmy E (1999) Feasibility of immunotherapy of relapsed leukemia with ex vivo-generated cytotoxic T lymphocytes specific for hematopoietic system- restricted minor histocompatibility antigens. Blood 93:2336–2341
27. Mutis T, Ghoreschi K, Schrama E, Kamp J, Heemskerk M, Falkenburg JH et al (2002) Efficient induction of minor histocompatibility antigen HA-1-specific cytotoxic T-cells using dendritic cells retrovirally transduced with HA-1-coding cDNA. Biol Blood Marrow Transplant 8:412–419
28. Oosten LE, Blokland E, Van Halteren AG, Curtsinger J, Mescher MF, Falkenburg JH et al (2004) Artificial antigen-presenting constructs efficiently stimulate minor histocompatibility antigen-specific cytotoxic T lymphocytes. Blood 104:224–226
29. Heemskerk MH, Hoogeboom M, de Paus RA, Kester MG, van der Hoorn MA, Goulmy E et al (2003) Redirection of antileukemic reactivity of peripheral T lymphocytes using gene transfer of minor histocompatibility antigen HA-2-specific T-cell receptor complexes expressing a conserved alpha joining region. Blood 102:3530–3540
30. Mommaas B, Van Halteren AG, Pool J, Van V, Wieles B, Heemskerk MH et al (2005) Adult and cord blood T cells can acquire HA-1 specificity through HA-1 T-cell receptor gene transfer. Haematologica 90:1415–1421
31. Sadovnikova E, Jopling LA, Soo KS, Stauss HJ (1998) Generation of human tumor-reactive cytotoxic T cells against peptides presented by non-self HLA class I molecules. Eur J Immunol 28:193–200
32. Mutis T, Blokland E, Kester M, Schrama E, Goulmy E (2002) Generation of minor histocompatibility antigen HA-1-specific cytotoxic T cells restricted by nonself HLA molecules: a potential strategy to treat relapsed leukemia after HLA-mismatched stem cell transplantation. Blood 100:547–552
33. Marijt WA, Heemskerk MH, Kloosterboer FM, Goulmy E, Kester MG, van der Hoorn MA et al (2003) Hematopoiesis-restricted minor histocompatibility antigens HA-1- or HA-2-specific T cells can induce complete remissions of relapsed leukemia. Proc Natl Acad Sci USA 100:2742–2747
34. Kircher B, Stevanovic S, Urbanek M, Mitterschiffthaler A, Rammensee HG, Grunewald K et al (2002) Induction of HA-1-specific cytotoxic T-cell clones parallels the therapeutic effect of donor lymphocyte infusion. Br J Haematol 117:935–939
35. Scheibenbogen C, Letsch A, Schmittel A, Asemissen AM, Thiel E, Keilholz U (2003) Rational peptide-based tumour vaccine development and T cell monitoring. Semin Cancer Biol 13:423–429
36. Figdor CG, de Vries I, Lesterhuis WJ, Melief CJ (2004) Dendritic cell immunotherapy: mapping the way. Nat Med 10:475–480
37. Hambach L, Aghai Z, Pool J, Kroger N, Goulmy E (2010) Peptide length extension skews the minor HA-1 antigen presentation toward activated dendritic cells but reduces its presentation efficiency. J Immunol 185: 4582–4589
38. Spierings E, Drabbels J, Hendriks M, Pool J, Spruyt-Gerritse M, Claas F et al (2006) A uniform genomic minor histocompatibility antigen typing methodology and database designed to facilitate clinical applications. PLoS One 1:e42
39. Longo MC, Berninger MS, Hartley JL (1990) Use of uracil DNA glycosylase to control carry-over contamination in polymerase chain reactions. Gene 93:125–128
40. Akatsuka Y, Nishida T, Kondo E, Miyazaki M, Taji H, Iida H et al (2003) Identification of a polymorphic gene, BCL2A1, encoding two novel hematopoietic lineage-specific minor histocompatibility antigens. J Exp Med 197: 1489–1500
41. Kawase T, Akatsuka Y, Torikai H, Morishima S, Oka A, Tsujimura A et al (2007) Alternative splicing due to an intronic SNP in HMSD generates a novel minor histocompatibility antigen. Blood 110:1055–1063
42. Tykodi SS, Fujii N, Vigneron N, Lu SM, Mito JK, Miranda MX et al (2008) C19orf48 encodes a minor histocompatibility antigen recognized by CD8+ cytotoxic T cells from renal cell carcinoma patients. Clin Cancer Res 14: 5260–5269
43. Spaapen RM, Lokhorst HM, Van de OK, Otterud BE, Dolstra H, Leppert MF et al (2008) Toward targeting B cell cancers with CD4+ CTLs: identification of a CD19-encoded minor histocompatibility antigen using a novel genome-wide analysis. J Exp Med 205: 2863–2872
44. Torikai H, Akatsuka Y, Miyazaki M, Tsujimura A, Yatabe Y, Kawase T et al (2006) The human cathepsin H gene encodes two novel minor histocompatibility antigen epitopes restricted by HLA-A*3101 and -A*3303. Br J Haematol 134:406–410
45. den Haan JM, Meadows LM, Wang W, Pool J, Blokland E, Bishop TL et al (1998) The minor histocompatibility antigen HA-1: a diallelic gene with a single amino acid polymorphism. Science 279:1054–1057

46. Mommaas B, Kamp J, Drijfhout JW, Beekman N, Ossendorp F, Van Veelen P et al (2002) Identification of a novel HLA-B60-restricted T cell epitope of the minor histocompatibility antigen HA-1 locus. J Immunol 169: 3131–3136
47. Spierings E, Brickner AG, Caldwell JA, Zegveld S, Tatsis N, Blokland E et al (2003) The minor histocompatibility antigen HA-3 arises from differential proteasome-mediated cleavage of the lymphoid blast crisis (Lbc) oncoprotein. Blood 102:621–629
48. Brickner AG, Warren EH, Caldwell JA, Akatsuka Y, Golovina TN, Zarling AL et al (2001) The immunogenicity of a new human minor histocompatibility antigen results from differential antigen processing. J Exp Med 193:195–206
49. Dolstra H, Fredrix H, Maas F, Coulie PG, Brasseur F, Mensink E et al (1999) A human minor histocompatibility antigen specific for B cell acute lymphoblastic leukemia. J Exp Med 189:301–308
50. Bleakley M, Otterud BE, Richardt JL, Mollerup AD, Hudecek M, Nishida T et al (2010) Leukemia-associated minor histocompatibility antigen discovery using T-cell clones isolated by in vitro stimulation of naive CD8+ T cells. Blood 115:4923–4933
51. van Bergen CA, Kester MG, Jedema I, Heemskerk MH, van Luxemburg-Heijs SA, Kloosterboer FM et al (2007) Multiple myeloma-reactive T cells recognize an activation-induced minor histocompatibility antigen encoded by the ATP-dependent interferon-responsive (ADIR) gene. Blood 109:4089–4096
52. Van Bergen CA, Rutten CE, Van Der Meijden ED, Van Luxemburg-Heijs SA, Lurvink EG, Houwing-Duistermaat JJ et al (2010) High-throughput characterization of 10 new minor histocompatibility antigens by whole genome association scanning. Cancer Res 70: 9073–9083
53. Stumpf AN, van der Meijden ED, van Bergen CA, Willemze R, Falkenburg JH, Griffioen M (2009) Identification of 4 new HLA-DR-restricted minor histocompatibility antigens as hematopoietic targets in antitumor immunity. Blood 114:3684–3692
54. Griffioen M, van der Meijden ED, Slager EH, Honders MW, Rutten CE, van Luxemburg-Heijs SA et al (2008) Identification of phosphatidylinositol 4-kinase type II beta as HLA class II-restricted target in graft versus leukemia reactivity. Proc Natl Acad Sci USA 105: 3837–3842
55. de Rijke B, van Horssens-Zoetbrood A, Beekman JM, Otterrud B, Maas F, Woestenenk R et al (2005) A frame-shift polymorphism in *P2X5* elicits an allogeneic cytotoxic T lymphocyte response associated with remission of chronic myeloid leukemia. J Clin Invest 115: 3506–3516
56. Brickner AG, Evans AM, Mito JK, Xuereb SM, Feng X, Nishida T et al (2006) The PANE1 gene encodes a novel human minor histocompatibility antigen that is selectively expressed in B-lymphoid cells and B-CLL. Blood 107: 3779–3786
57. Kamei M, Nannya Y, Torikai H, Kawase T, Taura K, Inamoto Y et al (2009) HapMap scanning of novel human minor histocompatibility antigens. Blood 113:5041–5048
58. Warren EH, Gavin MA, Xuereb SM, Koo KK, Mito JK, Brown ML et al (2002) A single nucleotide polymorphism in the SP110 nuclear phosphoprotein gene creates a minor histocompatibility antigen whose expression is regulated by interferon-gamma. Blood 100:73A
59. Murata M, Warren EH, Riddell SR (2003) A human minor histocompatibility antigen resulting from differential expression due to a gene deletion. J Exp Med 197:1279–1289
60. Vogt MH, de Paus RA, Voogt PJ, Willemze R, Falkenburg JH (2000) DFFRY codes for a new human male-specific minor transplantation antigen involved in bone marrow graft rejection. Blood 95:1100–1105
61. Pierce RA, Field ED, den Haan JM, Caldwell JA, White FM, Marto JA et al (1999) Cutting edge: the HLA-A*0101-restricted HY minor histocompatibility antigen originates from DFFRY and contains a cysteinylated cysteine residue as identified by a novel mass spectrometric technique. J Immunol 163:6360–6364
62. Meadows L, Wang W, den Haan JM, Blokland E, Reinhardus C, Drijfhout JW et al (1997) The HLA-A*0201-restricted H-Y antigen contains a posttranslationally modified cysteine that significantly affects T cell recognition. Immunity 6:273–281
63. Torikai H, Akatsuka Y, Miyazaki M, Warren EH, Oba T, Tsujimura K et al (2004) A novel HLA-A*3303-restricted minor histocompatibility antigen encoded by an unconventional open reading frame of human TMSB4Y gene. J Immunol 173:7046–7054
64. Rosinski KV, Fujii N, Mito JK, Koo KK, Xuereb SM, Sala-Torra O et al (2008) DDX3Y encodes a class I MHC-restricted H-Y antigen that is expressed in leukemic stem cells. Blood 111: 4817–4826
65. Ivanov R, Aarts T, Hol S, Doornenbal A, Hagenbeek A, Petersen E et al (2005) Identification of a 40S ribosomal protein S4-derived H-Y epitope able to elicit a

lymphoblast-specific cytotoxic T lymphocyte response. Clin Cancer Res 11:1694–1703

66. Vogt MH, Goulmy E, Kloosterboer FM, Blokland E, de Paus RA, Willemze R et al (2000) UTY gene codes for an HLA-B60-restricted human male-specific minor histocompatibility antigen involved in stem cell graft rejection: characterization of the critical polymorphic amino acid residues for T-cell recognition. Blood 96:3126–3132
67. Warren EH, Gavin MA, Simpson E, Chandler P, Page DC, Disteche C et al (2000) The human UTY gene encodes a novel HLA-B8-restricted H-Y antigen. J Immunol 164:2807–2814
68. Vogt MH, van den Muijsenberg J, Goulmy E, Spierings E, Kluck P, Kester M et al (2002) The DBY gene codes for an HLA-DQ5 restricted human male specific minor histocompatibility antigen involved in GvHD. Blood 99: 3027–3032
69. Zorn E, Miklos DB, Floyd BH, Mattes-Ritz A, Guo LX, Soiffer RJ et al (2004) Minor histocompatibility antigen DBY elicits a coordinated B and T cell response after allogeneic stem cell transplantation. J Exp Med 199: 1133–1142
70. Spierings E, Vermeulen C, Vogt MH, Doerner LEE, Falkenburg JHF, Mutis T et al (2003) Identification of HLA class II-restricted H-Y-specific T-helper epitope evoking CD4+ T-helper cells in H-Y-mismatched transplantation. Lancet 362:610–615

# Chapter 30

# Donor Registries and Search Strategies

Carolyn K. Hurley, Machteld Oudshoorn, and Michelle Setterholm

## Abstract

The optimal donor of hematopoietic progenitor cells shares alleles of the major histocompatibility genes with the recipient. This chapter describes the strategies aimed at identifying such a matched donor from registries of volunteers or from umbilical cord blood banks.

**Key words:** Hematopoietic progenitor cell transplantation, Histocompatibility, Human leukocyte antigen, Registries, Cord blood banks, Unrelated donor search

## 1. Introduction

Transplantation of hematopoietic progenitor cells (HPCs) is one therapy for a variety of fatal blood diseases, such as acute myeloid leukemia and aplastic anemia (1). To provide the best chance for an optimal outcome to a transplant, the patient (i.e., the recipient) and the cell donor must express the same histocompatibility molecules on their cell surfaces (i.e., be "matched"). In humans, the major histocompatibility molecules are the human leukocyte antigens (HLA), a highly polymorphic family of six proteins termed HLA-A, HLA-B, HLA-C, HLA-DR, HLA-DQ, and HLA-DP. The genes encoding each HLA protein and their alleles are inherited in traditional Mendelian fashion. Because of the extensive allelic diversity in the human population, a patient requiring an HPC transplant is most likely to find a match among their siblings. However, unrelated donors are the source of HPCs for the approximately 70% of patients who do not have a suitable family donor. To facilitate the search for a matched unrelated donor, many countries have established registries of volunteers who offer to provide HPCs if matched

Frank T. Christiansen and Brian D. Tait (eds.), *Immunogenetics: Methods and Applications in Clinical Practice*, Methods in Molecular Biology, vol. 882, DOI 10.1007/978-1-61779-842-9_30, © Springer Science+Business Media New York 2012

to a searching patient (2, 3). An alternative source of matched HPCs is umbilical cord blood which has been banked for public use (4). This chapter focuses on the procedures for an unrelated donor/umbilical cord blood search and discusses strategies that might be employed to find the optimal HLA matched volunteer donor or umbilical cord blood unit for a specific patient.

## 2. Materials

### *2.1. Web Sites Useful in Search*

1. Bone Marrow Donors Worldwide (BMDW): This Web site (http://www.bmdw.org/) provides a comprehensive listing of almost all registries and cord blood banks in the world and their contact information. It also provides the tools to perform an initial search of a single worldwide database of donors to assess the likelihood of identifying a matched donor (5). This database does not substitute, however, for a search of a specific registry or cord blood bank because it is only a snapshot of each registry/bank at one recent time and does not directly allow access to specific donors/cord blood units for further testing.
2. HLA nomenclature and allele designations: The Web site, http://hla.alleles.org/nomenclature/, is the World Health Organization-designated HLA nomenclature Web site and it includes both current and previous HLA designations (6, 7). The IMmunoGeneTics/HLA Web site (http://www.ebi.ac.uk/imgt/hla/) is a source of information on each HLA allele including whether the sequence has been reported more than once (i.e., has been confirmed) and the race/ethnicity of the individuals in whom the allele was first identified (8). It provides tools to compare HLA sequences and provides a listing of alleles and genotypes that cannot be distinguished from one another (i.e., are ambiguous) based on the nucleotide sequence of their most variable exons. It also provides a tool to link serologic and DNA-based HLA assignments based on an HLA "dictionary" (9).
3. Allele and haplotype frequencies: The frequencies of alleles and haplotypes (see Note 1) within the US National Marrow Donor Program (NMDP) registry can be found at http://bioinformatics.nmdp.org/ (see Note 2) (10). A list of rare alleles identifies alleles that have never been observed or have seldom been observed within the NMDP registry. This site also includes a tool to identify the alleles that are contained within the letter codes used to report HLA types (e.g., DRB1*04:AB where AB indicates 01 or 02 defining the assignment DRB1*04:01 or DRB1*04:02) (7). Two sources of

worldwide allele frequencies are http://www.allelefrequencies.net (11) and http://www.pypop.org/popdata/ (12). Tools to predict the frequencies of specific haplotypes can be found at http://www.hlaexplorer.net and http://bioinformatics.nmdp.org/ under HaploStats.

## 3. Methods

### 3.1. HLA Typing of Patient and Family

1. Obtain a biological sample from the patient and from nuclear family members if transplantation is being considered as a potential treatment option (see Note 3) and perform HLA typing (see Note 4). If available, include parents of the patient, siblings, and biological children. The patient should be typed for HLA-A,-B, -C, -DR, -DQ (see Note 5) at allele or high resolution (see Note 6). The resolution of the typing of the family members should be sufficient to clearly distinguish the HLA types segregating in the family (see Note 7).
2. If sufficient family members are available, confirm the HLA assignments of the patient through observing the same assignments in other family members, identify the HLA types carried by each haplotype segregating in the family (see Note 8), and determine if there is a family member who is HLA matched. The latter should be further evaluated to determine if they might serve as an HPC donor (see Note 9).
3. Perform an unrelated donor and umbilical cord blood search as described below so that these options for treatment of the patient can be considered.

### 3.2. Designing an Unrelated Donor Search Strategy

1. Begin by evaluating whether the patient's HLA assignments are complete. For potential 8/8 matches, the typing must include HLA loci HLA-A, -B, -C, and -DRB1 (see Note 10). In case 10/10 matches are preferred, the typing must include HLA-A, -B, -C, -DRB1, and -DQB1 assignments. Also determine if the level of typing (i.e., the resolution of the typing) of the patient is adequate (see Note 11).
2. Examine the HLA type of the patient to identify any uncommon or unexpected assignments (see Note 12). This step evaluates the accuracy of the HLA assignments.
3. Establish the patient's HLA haplotypes (see Note 13).
4. Determine the frequency of the patient's HLA alleles and haplotypes in various ethnic populations based on Web sites listing the frequencies of alleles and haplotypes. Table 1 provides an example of the evaluation of the patient's HLA assignments in preparation for a search.

**Table 1**
**Example of how a patient typing is evaluated**

| Issue noted | Web site providing information | Action/resolution |
|---|---|---|
| Patient typing: A*02:05, 68:04; B*35:DNXN, 53:01; DRB1*03:01, 13:03; C*04:01; DQB1*02:01, 02:02 | | |
| Is information included on all the loci required for matching? | | If the transplant center would like to search for a 10/10 match, assignments must be included for 5 loci; for a 8/8 match, 4 loci. The typing includes all the required loci for either level of match |
| Evaluate resolution of testing: allele B*35:DNXN has an allele code | http://bioinformatics.nmdp.org DNA type lookup tool | Expand to full allele string. Depending on the assignments, request additional typing to increase the resolution. In this case, the assignment includes only alleles that share the sequence of exons 2 and 3: B*35:01, B*35:40N, B*35:42, B*35:57, B*35:94 |
| Evaluate resolution of testing: C*04:01 allele is at high resolution but this level of resolution required special testing by the HLA laboratory | http://hla.alleles.org/alleles/index.html G groups | Ask the laboratory if it specifically excluded the other alleles that carry the same nucleotide sequence as C*04:01 in the HLA-C exons specifying the peptide binding site. For example, did the laboratory specifically exclude the non-expressed allele C*04:09N? (see Note 46) |
| Evaluate frequency of alleles: allele A*68:04 is uncommon | http://bioinformatics.nmdp.org rare allele list | In family? If yes, acceptable. If no, repeat HLA typing of HLA-A preferably with different reagents/method |
| Investigate B/C and DR/DQ haplotypes: B *35:DNXN with C *04:01, B*53:01 with C*04:01, DRB1*03:01 with DQB1*02:01 or *02:02, DRB1*13:03 with DQB1*02:01 or *02:02 | http://bioinformatics.nmdp.org/ under HaploStats | Concordant with family typing? Common or uncommon? In this case, the B-C associations are common. Both DRB1 alleles are frequently observed with DQB1*02:01 but not with DQB1*02:02 so this is unusual. The laboratory should be asked to confirm the DQB1*02:02 assignment if it is not observed in the family |
| Investigate multilocus haplotypes (A/B/C/DRB1/DQB1) | http://bioinformatics.nmdp.org under HaploStats | Concordant with family typing? Common or uncommon? |

### 3.3. Submitting a Search Request to a National or International Registry

1. An unrelated donor or umbilical cord blood search should be initiated to identify donors and cord blood units whose HLA typing is potentially identical to the patient's (see Notes 14 and 15).
2. Collect the following information about the patient: HLA typing data, preferably including the patient's HLA haplotypes; date of birth; diagnosis date; gender; weight; cytomegalovirus (CMV) status; ethnicity (see Note 16).
3. Determine the parameters of the search, including the type of search to be performed, i.e., adult progenitor cell donor, cord blood unit or both (see Note 17); urgency of the search; the specific HLA loci to be considered during matching; and whether or not mismatches are acceptable. These criteria are found in the transplant center protocol (see Note 18).
4. Perform a search of BMDW which provides you with a comprehensive overview of almost all HPC sources worldwide (see Notes 19 and 20).
5. Complete a search request form and submit the search request form to all registries of interest or electronically enter the patient's information directly using software or Web access where available. A generic form accepted by many registries and cord blood banks (e.g., WMDA Preliminary Search Request Form) can be found under http://www.worldmarrow.org. Alternatively, a search can be started through a registry to registry network, such as the European Marrow Donor Information System (see Note 21).

### 3.4. Reviewing a Search Report to Select Potential Adult Volunteer Donors for Additional HLA Testing

1. Obtain a search report from the registries and banks contacted (see Note 22). Most registries will display adult donor matches based on HLA-A,-B,-DRB1 typing and will list both 6/6 and 5/6 matches. The selection of umbilical cord blood units is described in Subheading 3.6.
2. Ensure that the correct match criteria are known for the patient (whether an 8/8 or 10/10 match is preferred; which and how many mismatches are allowed; and any other donor-specific characteristics that need to be considered, such as gender, age, or CMV status). This will guide the selection of the best potential donors and help to increase the likelihood of a successful transplantation (see Note 23).
3. Expand any donor typing results (see Note 24) that may have letter codes (e.g., A*01:CRY) as necessary to understand the full set of alleles in the assignments. See Note 25 for a tool to assist with this task.
4. Evaluate the donor typing results for completeness according to the transplant center match criteria. For example, if an 8/8 match

is preferred, do the donor typing results include HLA-A, -B, -C, and -DRB1? If incomplete, utilize haplotype frequency data relative to the ethnicity of each donor to help predict the most likely HLA type of the missing loci (see Note 26).

5. Evaluate the donor typing results to determine if the level of resolution at each locus is sufficient in order to make a determination of the likelihood to match the patient's alleles. Utilize allele and haplotype frequency data and the donor's ethnicity to predict the most likely higher resolution types for each locus for the donors of interest on the search report (see Note 27). Table 2 provides an example of the evaluation of a donor's HLA assignments.
6. Prioritize the donors deemed most likely to match the patient's HLA type using all of the information gathered in the analyses above. If multiple, suitably matched donors are available on the search list, apply the additional transplant protocol criteria to the non-HLA information given for each donor to perform a secondary sort. For example, prioritize younger donors over older.
7. Request a biological sample from the selected donors for further typing from the Registry (see Note 28).
8. Perform HLA typing of the samples to obtain more information as to the HLA alleles carried at key loci and to verify the HLA typing assignment (see Note 29).
9. Select the best donor based on the transplant center criteria (see Notes 30 and 31).
10. Contact the registry to request that a specific volunteer be medically evaluated for donation.

### 3.5. Refining the Search Strategy to Identify a Mismatched or Mistyped Donor

1. When the search report or the analyses performed above does not yield donors who potentially match the patient, a strategy to locate the best potential mismatch may need to be implemented. In these instances, a donor with only one mismatch (7/8 or 9/10) may be considered as an alternative depending on the transplant center protocol (see Note 32). The search reports from most registries include 5/6 matched donors (i.e., with one mismatch at one of the three loci, HLA-A, -B, -DRB1). A longer list of potential donors may be needed if the search was initiated through EMDIS since some registries limit the search results to either 50 or 100 donors.
2. Evaluate the patient for the presence of IgG antibodies directed to specific HLA antigens (see Note 33).
3. Evaluate the methodology that may have been utilized to generate the HLA data of the potential donors. Assignments made using older serologic typing techniques have a higher likelihood of appearing falsely disparate than typing techniques that

**Table 2**
**Examples of how potential donor typing is evaluated for patient in Table 1**

| Issue noted | Web site providing information | Action/resolution |
|---|---|---|
| Patient typing: A*02:05, 68:04; B*35:DNXN, 53:01; DRB1*03:01, 13:03; C*04:01 | | |
| Donor 1 typing: A2, 68; B35, 53; DRB1* 03:DHJB, 13:BGTY | | |
| Allele codes need expansion | http://bioinformatics.nmdp.org DNA type lookup tool | DHJB: 03:01/03:06/03:18/03:19/03:22/03:28/03:37 |
| | HaploStats | BGTY: 13:03/13:33/13:66 |
| | | The patient's DR alleles are included in the donor assignments and, based on the frequency of the alleles in the code, are likely to be matched (i.e., DRB1*13:03 is more common than DRB1*13:33 or DRB1*13:66) |
| Determine likelihood for allele match: serologic typing at HLA-A and -B | HaploStats<br>HLA explorer<br>DNA dictionary | Predict higher resolution and likelihood of allele match with patient based on ethnicity. A*02:01 is more frequent than A*02:05; it is unlikely that the donor carries A*68:04. B*35:01 is common and may be present in B35 typed individual although other B*35 alleles (B*35:02, B*35:03) are possible; B*53:01 is likely to be present |
| Evaluate typing for completeness: HLA-C not typed | http://bioinformatics.nmdp.org/index.html, haplotype table | Predict HLA-C alleles that might be present. If B*35:01 and B*53:01 are present, both B alleles are frequently found with C*04:01 |
| Is resolution sufficient to make a determination of match? | | The donor is likely an HLA-A mismatch (i.e., not A*68:04). A donor matched at 7/8 or 9/10 may be acceptable to the transplant center. Depending on other donors available on the search report, determine whether this donor should be typed at higher resolution |

utilize DNA-based methodologies. If the patient carries an antigen that is known to be difficult to distinguish by serologic methods, then donors typed serologically who have a high likelihood of matching the patient may appear as mismatched on the search report (see Note 34). Utilize the HLA dictionary to identify any of these antigens (see Note 35). Perform a new search if needed by substituting the patient's difficult allele or antigen with an alternate choice as indicated by the HLA dictionary "assigned type" field (see Note 36).

4. Evaluate the possibility that allele level differences between a donor and the patient may be permissible mismatches due to the location of the disparity. Some alleles that have different assignments are actually identical, either genotypically or phenotypically, in the region that encodes the peptide binding site and may not impact the transplant outcome (see Notes 37 and 38).
5. Review the patient's HLA assignment to determine if an uncommon haplotype or allele may be present (see Subheading 3.2, step 4). In these cases, it may be possible to substitute a donor with a single mismatched allele at the locus in question and meet the 7/8 or 9/10 transplant center criteria (see Note 39).
6. Prioritize the loci involved and the selection of potentially mismatched donors according to the transplant center criteria and using recommendations given in recent publications (see Note 40). Avoid choosing donors carrying HLA antigens to which the patient is sensitized.

### 3.6. Searching for a Cord Blood Unit

1. Review the cord blood units that have been listed on the patient's search report (see Note 41).
2. Identify units with greater than a minimal required cell dose based on the transplant center protocol (see Note 42).
3. Identify units that may meet the transplant center's HLA matching criteria for a cord blood unit (see Note 43). The units will likely be HLA typed at a low resolution and higher resolution testing may be required for optimal donor selection.
4. Select one or more units that have both an acceptable cell dose and an acceptable HLA match. Request that the Registry/Cord Blood Bank initiate further HLA testing of the selected unit or request a sample for typing at your local HLA laboratory (see Note 44). Also request a Unit Report that gives more information about the unit plus the maternal health history.
5. Consider whether the unit has attached segments for verification typing (see Note 45) in making your decision about whether to request the unit for transplant.
6. Request that the Registry/Cord Blood Bank reserve the unit for your patient until you have completed your evaluation.

## 4. Notes

1. A haplotype is the combinations of HLA alleles that are found on a single copy of chromosome 6. A haplotype may refer to a combination of two or more loci. Some allele combinations such as the combination of DR and DQ alleles found on a haplotype or the combination of HLA-B and HLA-C alleles found on a haplotype can be predicted based on previous population studies. For example, haplotypes with DRB1*01:01 almost always carry DQB1*05:01. Tables of these associations can be found at http://bioinformatics.nmdp.org/ and at http://hlaexplorer.net.
2. The excel files on this Web site can be filtered and sorted.
3. It is important to evaluate the likelihood of finding a suitable HPC donor early during the initial evaluation of the patient when various treatment options are being considered. The outcome of a transplant is more favorable when the patient is transplanted early in the course of their disease (13).
4. See chapters on HLA typing for more information on the methodology. Blood may not be the best sample source for some patients because of the low number of circulating white cells, because of the possibility of mutations in the HLA genes due to the unstable nature of tumors, or because of the presence of transfused cells from another individual. In these cases, a buccal swab or hair follicles might be the preferred sample source.
5. DRB1 and DQB1 genes specify one polypeptide of the DR and DQ heterodimers. These genes are routinely typed during donor selection (14). The DRA and DQA1 genes are not usually typed as they are less polymorphic and provide only limited additional information. The secondary DRB loci, DRB3, DRB4, and DRB5, are often typed. One purpose for typing the HLA loci suggested is to provide further support for the HLA assignments. Specific associations are found between: (1) DRB1 and DQB1 alleles (e.g., DRB1*01:01 is found predominantly associated with DQB1*05:01); (2) HLA-B and -C alleles (e.g., B*07:02 with C*07:02) and (3) DRB1 and the secondary DRB loci (DRB1*15:01 with DRB5 alleles). These associations should be consistent with the HLA assignments.
6. Allelic resolution is defined as a DNA-based typing result that is consistent with a single allele. An allele is defined as a unique nucleotide sequence for a gene as defined by the use of all of the digits in a current allele name. High resolution typing is defined as a typing which includes alternative alleles that specify the same protein sequence for the region of the HLA molecule that forms the peptide binding site. The peptide binding

site is composed of the amino-terminal domains of the HLA proteins (i.e., alpha1 and alpha2 domains for HLA class I molecules and alpha1 and beta1 domains for HLA class II molecules). This is the region that binds self or foreign peptides and that is recognized by T-cell receptors. High resolution also excludes alleles that are not expressed as cell-surface proteins, especially if these null alleles are thought to be common.

7. In general, low resolution HLA typing may be used for typing the patient's family members except in the cases where the parents are not available or where similar alleles are segregating in the family. A low resolution DNA-based typing result is at the level of the digits comprising the first field in the DNA-based nomenclature (e.g., A*11; B*07).
8. Haplotypes are defined by segregation in the family. For example, father is typed as A*01, A*02, B*07, B*08; mother as A*11, A*24, B*18, B*35; sib 1 as A*01, A*24, B*08, B*18; and sib 2 as A*01, A*11, B*08, B*35. Based on segregation, the haplotypes are A*01-B*08, A*02-B*07, A*11-B*35, and A*24-B*18.
9. If there is not a suitable match in the nuclear family, it may be possible to find a match in the extended family (e.g., aunts, uncles, cousins) (15). This is possible if the patient carries a common haplotype which might have been inherited by chance in the extended family. It is also possible if there is a history of consanguinity in the family (e.g., cousin–cousin marriages) or if there are other close family relationships (e.g., two siblings from one family married to two siblings from another family).
10. 8/8 means 2 alleles at 4 loci, usually defined as HLA-A, -B, -C, and -DRB1.
11. Low or intermediate resolution typing will only provide a rough indication of possible donors. Patient typing at this resolution should not be used for an unrelated donor search. Time and money may be wasted if donors with the highest chance of being identical with the patient are not rapidly selected based on the patient's allele/high resolution typing assignment.
12. It can be useful to know whether the patient has an allele that is rare or an unexpected allele combination as this may be a typing error. Rare alleles in patients should always be confirmed either in the family (i.e., by finding another family member carrying the same rare allele) or by using a different typing technique or reagent set. To know whether the patient has a rare allele is also important as it may affect the likelihood of finding a perfectly matched donor. If no potentially identical donor is available, it is best to look for a donor who is identical for all alleles except the one rare allele. It is also important to realize

that there are alleles that may be rare or uncommon in all but one ethnic group. In this case, finding a matched donor can be greatly facilitated by selecting potential donors from the ethnic group in which your patient's allele is less rare or even common.

Furthermore, it may be very difficult to find donors if the patient has a rare HLA association (e.g., HLA-B + HLA-C allele association) and this needs to be identified by using HLA haplotype frequency tables. For example, if the patient has a rare HLA-B + HLA-C association and no potentially identical donors are present, one can substitute the HLA-B allele for another allele that is commonly associated with the patient's HLA-C allele. See Subheading 3.5 for more information on search strategies to find a mismatched donor.

13. Preferentially, family typing is available and the patient's haplotypes can be established through family segregation analyses. If family data are not available, there are haplotype frequency tables that can be used to predict which haplotypes the patient might carry and also to provide information whether or not the patient has common haplotypes. Understanding common haplotype or allele associations can be useful for predicting which alleles are most likely to be present in donors who have only low resolution typing information and no family data to define haplotypes. Two useful Web sites for haplotype analysis are http://bioinformatics.nmdp.org and http://www.hlaexplorer.net.
14. Registries and banks have guidelines for who can submit a search request. Usually, search requests must come from a physician or from a transplant center.
15. Typically, searches are performed in two steps. In the preliminary search, a physician will receive a summary indicating whether or not there are potentially matching donors in a registry or cord blood bank. If the registry appears to include suitable donors, a transplant center will formalize the search. In a formal search, the HLA types of each potentially matching donor/unit will be listed individually and the transplant center can request biologic samples from these donors/units for further HLA and infectious disease testing.
16. It is important to confirm the patient's typing using a second biological sample to ensure that no errors are made in the HLA assignments to be used in the unrelated donor/umbilical cord blood search.
17. It is recommended that the search identify the best unrelated donor and the best umbilical cord blood unit to provide alternatives for the physician. An urgent search might focus only on umbilical cord blood units because they are more rapidly available.

18. The level of matching required for optimal outcome has been discussed in the literature, e.g., (13, 14, 16, 17).
19. Access to the search tool in BMDW requires that a transplant center register with BMDW. The search is submitted online. Matches identified in the BMDW worldwide registry will identify one or more countries where potential donors or cord blood units can be found for the patient. The transplant center can then focus the search on registries and cord blood banks from those countries. Contact information for these registries and banks can be found on the BMDW Web site.
20. The national registry in the country of the transplant center caring for the patient may also assist in contacting multiple registries and banks. For example, a search of the NMDP in the USA will also interrogate the inventory of the BMDW. Any physician may request a search of the NMDP on behalf of a patient through the Office of Patient Advocacy (http://www.bethematch.org). There are also several publicly available Web sites that provide summarized search results (e.g., MatchView at http://www.marrow.org). When using the NMDP, staff will perform all of the contacts and assist with HLA expertise to guide the process of selecting the best potential donor or cord blood unit.
21. Search requests often go from registry to registry using the European Marrow Donor Information System (EMDIS). Transplant centers may have the ability to directly enter the search information into a software application.
22. Searches performed electronically using BMDW or NMDP generate donor lists immediately. Most registries and cord blood banks will provide a search report within 24 h when using the EMDIS system. The matches displayed usually include 6/6 (HLA-A,-B,-DRB1) and 5/6 matched donors but the criteria for the donors displayed on a search should be confirmed with the registry.
23. Non-HLA factors that are often considered in donor selection have been reviewed by Confer et al. (18).
24. The donors/units listed on the report are sorted by the extent of matching with the patient. It is possible, however, that the optimal donor may not appear at the top of the list so it is critical to examine all of the donors on the report.
25. An HLA typing result may include a two or more letter code following the first colon in the allele name (e.g., A*02:AF where AF is a code standing for 01 or 09 indicating that an individual carries A*02:01 or A*02:09). The Web site, http://bioinformatics.nmdp.org, has a tool to define alleles included in any letter codes. Further information on HLA assignments can be found at http://hla.alleles.org and http://www.ebi.ac.uk/imgt/hla/.

26. There are several approaches that can be used to predict the most likely missing data. The HaploStats tool and the HLA Explorer will generate a table of the most frequently seen HLA-C types associated with a known HLA-B and the most frequently seen HLA-DQB1 types associated with a known DRB1 antigen sorted by likelihood and ethnicity. The complete list of HLA-A, -B, -C, -DRB1, and -DQB1 haplotypes found on http://bioinformatics.nmdp.org can be used by searching on the known HLA-A, -B, and DRB1 haplotype and then viewing the possibilities of full haplotype combinations considering the frequencies of each and the racial/ethnic group of the donor (if known).
27. The HaploStats and HLA Explorer tools will each display the possible high resolution types given any low resolution input. The difference in the two tools is that HaploStats requires all known loci to be entered and HLA Explorer will provide data on any single low resolution type. They both sort by frequency within racial/ethnic populations.
28. High or allele resolution typing should be performed to identify those donors who carry the same HLA alleles as the patient. This extended typing should include all loci to be considered for matching. Verification typing using a fresh biological sample from the donor should be performed in order to ensure that this individual was the one with the HLA assignment appearing on the search report. The resolution of verification typing should be sufficient to confirm the original HLA assignments.
29. It is recommended that more than one donor be selected for additional HLA testing. This is because some donors may not carry the same alleles as the patient following higher resolution testing or because some volunteers will be unwilling or unable to donate or cannot be located. The number of donors to select will depend on the likelihood of the patient's alleles and haplotypes being present in the donors. For common alleles and haplotypes, 3–5 donors might be selected for further HLA testing. Uncommon alleles and haplotypes may require 10 or more donors to be selected for extended HLA typing. The registry may have information on the rate of donor availability to help with this decision.
30. The donor's registry or the cord blood bank will request that your extended HLA typing results be provided to them to update the donor/unit file. Follow the policy of the registry for the loci and level of resolution to be tested when reporting the results for each donor.
31. If there are multiple suitable matched donors, HLA assignments at other HLA loci, not routinely considered by the transplant center in determining the match, can be used to select among the donors. For example, if the transplant center requests an 8/8 match and there are several 8/8 matched donors, matching

for HLA-DQB1, HLA-DRB3/DRB4/DRB5, or HLA-DPB1 alleles might be used to prioritize donors.

32. A single mismatched donor is defined as a 7/8 or 9/10 matched donor (14).
33. Prior sensitization to specific HLA antigens may result in rejection of grafts expressing those antigens (19, 20). Antibody assays are described in Chapter 17.
34. For example, if the patient carries A*01:01, A*74:01, it may be possible that those donors typed only as HLA-A1 using serology might actually carry HLA-A74 since HLA-A74 was frequently missed by serology. Lists of frequently missed or misassigned serologic antigens have been reported (21, 22).
35. The HLA dictionary can also be found online at http://www.ebi.ac.uk/imgt/hla/ (9).
36. An example from the HLA dictionary is B*39:20 that has an assigned type of "blank" (67%) or B38 (33%). If the patient carries B*39:20, B*07:02, an alternative phenotype search might be submitted in which the patient's HLA-B assignment is listed as B*38:XX, B*07:02. In some cases, acceptable donors may not appear on the search report because their HLA typing appears to be more mismatched than the registry's minimum criteria. For example, a search report usually lists 6/6 and 5/6 matched donors. A donor who appears as a 4/6 match will not be shown on the report. An example for a patient typed as A*02:01, A*03:01, B*39:20, B*07:02 is a donor typed as A11, A3, B38, B7. Submission of an alternative phenotype search replacing B*39:20 with B38 may yield additional 5/6 donors who did not appear on the initial search.
37. For example, a patient may carry DRB1*14:01 and a potential donor might carry DRB1*14:54. These two alleles specify proteins that are identical in amino acid sequence in the portion of the HLA molecule called the peptide binding site. Note 6 further defines this region of the HLA molecule. Since it is thought that allorecognition focuses on this region of the HLA molecule, the single amino acid difference outside of the peptide binding site that distinguishes these two HLA molecules is thought to be unlikely to trigger allorecognition (23). Thus, differences in HLA molecules that fall outside of the peptide binding site might be considered permissive. A list of alleles that share the sequence of their peptide binding site can be found at http://hla.alleles.org/nomenclature/.
38. Several studies have discussed permissive mismatches (13, 23–26) or have evaluated tools to select these mismatches (27, 28).
39. For example, if the patient carries an uncommon HLA-B locus allele, the search may yield a donor carrying a differing HLA-B locus allele that still matches the patient's HLA-C alleles.

For example, if the patient carries B*35:15-C*07:02, the rare B*35:15 may be substituted by B*07:02, as B*07:02 is strongly associated with C*07:02. Likewise, this strategy can be utilized to identify an HLA-DRB1 mismatched donor who may mismatch the patient's uncommon HLA-DRB1 yet has high potential to match the patient's HLA-DQB1 allele. For example, if the patient carries DRB1*04:07-DQB1*03:01, the rare DRB1*04:07 may be substituted by DRB1*11:01 as DRB1*11:01 is strongly associated with DQB1*03:01.

40. The selection of which locus to mismatch has been discussed in the literature (13, 14, 16). Evidence guiding the selection of a donor with the most permissive mismatch at a locus is limited; most studies have evaluated strategies that ultimately did not predict permissive mismatches (13, 26–28).
41. The units shown on the search report likely meet some minimum HLA match and/or total nucleated cell (TNC) criteria defined by the registry or cord blood bank. The units may be sorted into categories based on the degree of match or size of the unit. It should not be assumed that the optimal unit is found at the top of the list; all units on the report should be evaluated.
42. Cell dose is one of two critical factors in the selection of a unit; HLA match is the second critical factor. The unit selected must contain a minimum of $2.5–3 \times 10^7$ precryopreserved TNC per kilogram of recipient body weight (29). If the possibility of using two cord blood units is being considered, the minimum TNC/kg for a unit as part of a double cord transplantation may be lower, but together the 2 units should have at least $2.5–3 \times 10^7$ TNC/kg.
43. The criteria that are often used for matching is a minimum of a four of six match, two antigen level matches at HLA-A and HLA-B and an allele match at HLA-DRB1. An antigen match is defined as a match at the first two digits of the allele name. For example, a patient typed as A*02:05 and a unit typed as A*02:01 would be considered an antigen match. Matching among B*15 and B*40 alleles is the exception. In these cases, the serologic assignment of the allelic products determines whether the patient and donor are matched at the antigen level. For example, a patient typed as B*15:01 (serologic B62) would not be an antigen match with a donor typed as B*15:03 (serologic B70). Use the HLA dictionary to obtain the serologic types associated with B*15 and B*40 alleles (9).
44. Recent reports suggest that better matching of the patient and the umbilical cord unit may result in better outcome (29). Therefore, it is recommended that the unit be tested at allele to high level resolution at HLA-A, -B, -C, -DRB1 so that the best matched unit can be selected for the patient.

45. It is important to insure that the cord blood unit is the one with the HLA typing found on the search report. This verification typing should be performed on a biological sample found in an aliquot physically attached to the unit.

46. The specifications for the resolution of HLA typing should be established by the transplant center in discussion with the histocompatibility laboratory. The resolution of the patient's typing assignment will determine which donors appear on a search report and may vary among registries. For example, donors listed on a search report for a patient typed as C*04:01 may differ from the donors listed for a patient typed as C*04:01:01G (which includes alternative alleles C*04:01:01:01, C*04:01:01:02, C*04:01:01:03, C*04:01:01:04, C*04:09N, C*04:28, C*04:30, C*04:41, C*04:79, C*04:82, C*04:84) or typed as C*04:FEAS (which includes alternative alleles C*04:01, C*04:09N, C*04:28, C*04:30, C*04:41).

## References

1. Copelan EA (2006) Hematopoietic stem-cell transplantation. N Engl J Med 354: 1813–1826
2. Hurley CK et al (2007) Overview of registries, HLA typing and diversity, and search algorithms. Tissue Antigens 69(Suppl 1):3–5
3. Foeken LM et al (2010) Monitoring the international use of unrelated donors for transplantation: the WMDA annual reports. Bone Marrow Transplant 45:811–818
4. Welte K et al (2010) International exchange of cord blood units: the registry aspects. Bone Marrow Transplant 45:825–831
5. Oudshoorn M et al (1994) Bone Marrow Donors Worldwide: a successful exercise in international cooperation. Bone Marrow Transplant 14:3–8
6. Marsh SG et al (2010) Nomenclature for factors of the HLA system, 2010. Tissue Antigens 75:291–455
7. Bochtler W et al (2007) World Marrow Donor Association guidelines for use of HLA nomenclature and its validation in the data exchange among hematopoietic stem cell donor registries and cord blood banks. Bone Marrow Transplant 39:737–741
8. Robinson J et al (2009) The IMGT/HLA database. Nucleic Acids Res 37:D1013–D1017
9. Holdsworth R et al (2009) The HLA dictionary 2008: a summary of HLA-A, -B, -C, -DRB1/3/4/5, and -DQB1 alleles and their association with serologically defined HLA-A, -B, -C, -DR, and -DQ antigens. Tissue Antigens 73:95–170
10. Maiers M, Gragert L, Klitz W (2007) High-resolution HLA alleles and haplotypes in the United States population. Hum Immunol 68:779–788
11. Middleton D et al (2003) New allele frequency database. Tissue Antigens 61:403–407. http://www.allelefrequencies.net
12. Solberg OD et al (2008) Balancing selection and heterogeneity across the classical human leukocyte antigen loci: a meta-analytic review of 497 population studies. Hum Immunol 69:443–464
13. Lee SJ et al (2007) High-resolution donor-recipient HLA matching contributes to the success of unrelated donor marrow transplantation. Blood 110:4576–4583
14. Bray RA et al (2008) National marrow donor program HLA matching guidelines for unrelated adult donor hematopoietic cell transplants. Biol Blood Marrow Transplant 14:45–53
15. Schipper RF, D'Amaro J, Oudshoorn M (1996) The probability of finding a suitable related donor for bone marrow transplantation in extended families. Blood 87:800–804
16. Petersdorf EW (2008) Optimal HLA matching in hematopoietic cell transplantation. Curr Opin Immunol 20:588–593
17. Shaw BE et al (2010) Diverging effects of HLA-DPB1 matching status on outcome following unrelated donor transplantation depending on disease stage and the degree of matching for other HLA alleles. Leukemia 24:58–65
18. Confer DL et al (2010) Selection of adult unrelated hematopoietic stem cell donors:

beyond HLA. Biol Blood Marrow Transplant 16:S8–S11

19. Spellman S et al (2010) The detection of donor-directed, HLA-specific alloantibodies in recipients of unrelated hematopoietic cell transplantation is predictive of graft failure. Blood 115:2704–2708
20. Ottinger HD et al (2002) Positive serum cross-match as predictor for graft failure in HLA-mismatched allogeneic blood stem cell transplantation. Transplantation 73:1280–1285
21. Lau M, Park MS, Terasaki PI (1997) International cell exchange 1974–1996, a 23-year documentation. (eds. Terasaki PI and Gjertson DW. It was published by the UCLA Tissue Typing Laboratory in Los Angeles California) 85–124
22. Noreen HJ et al (2001) Validation of DNA-based HLA-A and HLA-B testing of volunteers for a bone marrow registry through parallel testing with serology. Tissue Antigens 57:221–229
23. Xiao Y et al (2009) Evaluating the potential impact of mismatches outside the antigen recognition site in unrelated hematopoietic stem cell transplantation: HLA-DRB1*1454 and DRB1*140101. Tissue Antigens 73:595–598
24. Baxter-Lowe LA et al (2009) HLA-A disparities illustrate challenges for ranking the impact of HLA mismatches on bone marrow transplant outcomes in the United States. Biol Blood Marrow Transplant 15:971–981
25. Kawase T et al (2007) High-risk HLA allele mismatch combinations responsible for severe acute graft-versus-host disease and implication for its molecular mechanism. Blood 110:2235–2241
26. Wade JA et al (2007) HLA mismatching within or outside of cross-reactive groups (CREGs) is associated with similar outcomes after unrelated hematopoietic stem cell transplantation. Blood 109:4064–4070
27. Duquesnoy R et al (2008) HLAMatchmaker-defined triplet matching is not associated with better survival rates of patients with class I HLA allele mismatched hematopoietic cell transplants from unrelated donors. Biol Blood Marrow Transplant 14:1064–1071
28. Spellman S, Klein J, Haagenson M, Askar M, Baxter-Lowe LA, He J, et al (2011) Scoring HLA Class I Mismatches by HistoCheck Does Not Predict Clinical Outcome in Unrelated Hematopoietic Stem Cell Transplantation. Biol Blood Marrow Transplant 2011 Sep 29
29. Kamani N et al (2008) State of the art review: HLA matching and outcome of unrelated donor umbilical cord blood transplants. Biol Blood Marrow Transplant 14:1–6

# Chapter 31

# Cytokine Gene Polymorphisms: Methods of Detection and Biological Significance

Gurvinder Kaur and Narinder Mehra



## Abstract

In recent years, several functional polymorphisms, particularly, SNPs have been identified in cytokines and their receptor genes that regulate levels of cytokine expression. These have been implicated as immune prognostic markers in diseases, including differential response to therapy and as biomarkers of graft outcome following organ and stem cell transplantation. Population distribution of cytokine gene polymorphisms (CGPs) reveals significant variations in allele frequencies in different ethnic groups and this might explain, to some extent, the observed differences in SNP associations with various diseases and immune-pathologies. A number of molecular methods are available for defining CGPs. These include PCR-SSP, AFLP, Taqman probe assays as well as sequencing based typing. Of these, the PCR-based sequence-specific primer based test is the most widely accepted technique. This chapter describes steps involved in this procedure along with sources for procuring essential reagents. An important aspect of CGP analyses is the correct interpretation of results particularly determination of their multilocus haplotypes.


**Key words:** Cytokinesm, Single nucleotide polymorphisms, PCR, Population diversity, SSP primers

## 1. Introduction

### *1.1. What Are Cytokines?*

Cytokines (Greek cyto-, cell; and -kinos, movement) are pleiotropic immuomodulatory proteins produced by a wide range of cell types through antigen-specific and nonspecific stimuli. The T-cell subset paradigm and its immunological cytokine networking have attracted much attention over the last decade. With the recent knowledge on cytokine gene polymorphisms (CGPs), differences between individuals have been discovered that influence not only cytokine gene expression, but also susceptibility to diseases, their progression, severity, and clinical outcomes. Ethnic differences

Frank T. Christiansen and Brian D. Tait (eds.), *Immunogenetics: Methods and Applications in Clinical Practice*, Methods in Molecular Biology, vol. 882, DOI 10.1007/978-1-61779-842-9_31, © Springer Science+Business Media New York 2012

observed in patterns of CGPs at the population level are mainly a result of natural selection (1, 2) imposed by invading microbiota, environmental factors, and complex host–pathogen interactions (3). These correlate with population-based variations in the ability to mount an immune response and therefore act as important biomarkers of risk assessment in various diseases as well as for the development of graft- versus host disease (GvHD) or graft rejection following organ and hematopoietic stem cell transplantation (1).

Several studies have examined a possible relationship between CGPs and a variety of diseases, including inflammatory, infectious, autoimmune, malignant, and transplant-related conditions. Online databases of established associations between cytokine gene diversity and disease have been developed (1). The CGP-based studies received a practical boost during the 13th International Histocompatibility Workshop (13IHWC) when specific cytokine genotyping CTS-SSP tray kits were developed for the first time by Joannis Mytilineos and his group for testing by individual participating laboratories. These kits are now made available by the Collaborative Transplant Study (CTS) group led by Gerhard Opelz at the Univ of Heidelberg, Germany and are being used extensively for investigating the role of CGP SNPs in organ and stem cell transplantation (4) (http://www.ctstransplant.org). The main rationale behind this collaborative effort is to encourage investigations on immunogenetic markers for a given disease, ascertain genotype–phenotype correlates and predict clinical responses to therapeutics, vaccines, and transplant outcomes. Data generated over the years has identified several important SNPs in various cytokines that are important markers not only for better understanding of the etiology and pathology of a disease, but also as potential biomarkers of disease susceptibility and severity.

### 1.2. Cytokine Genes Polymorphisms

Genetic polymorphisms are frequently encountered in the 5′ and 3′ regulatory regions or introns of a cytokine and/ or its receptors (Fig. 1) and these have been shown to play an important role in regulating the extent of gene expression through one or more of the following possible mechanisms: (1) by altering the structure of transcription factor binding sites within promoters, (2) manipulating the structure of enhancers or silencers within introns or at distant regions, (3) altering the binding sites within nuclear matrix for architectural transcription factors that modulate promoter activity (1, 5, 6).

Cytokines and their receptor genes are generally conserved in their exonic sequences with a few exceptions like IL4 receptor, TNFβ, TGFβ, GM-CSF, and IL2 receptor-γ gene (6). Most of the observed mutations are synonymous, i.e., do not affect the protein sequences, although they might influence cellular levels of the cytokine expression. Broadly, three different approaches have been employed for the study of CGPs. These include case-control

**Type I (inflammatory)**

| Cytokine | Chromosome | db SNP | position | SNP |
|---|---|---|---|---|
| IL1 α | 2q14 | rs1800587 | -889 | T/C |
| IL1β | 2q14 | rs16944<br>rs1143634 | -511<br>+3962 | T/C<br>T/C |
| γ IFN | 12q14 | rs2430561 | +874 | A/T |
| IL12 | 5p31-33.2 | rs3212227 | -1188 | C/A |
| TNF α | 6p21.3 | rs1800629<br>rs361525 | -308<br>-238 | G/A<br>A/G |

**Type II**

| Cytokine | Chromosome | db SNP | position | SNP |
|---|---|---|---|---|
| TGFβ1 | 19q13.1 | rs1800470<br>rs1800471 | +896 (cdn10)<br>+915 (cdn 25) | C/T Leu/Pro<br>C/G Arg/Pro |
| IL4 | 5q31.1 | rs2243248<br>rs2243250<br>rs2070874 | -1098<br>-590<br>-33 | T/G<br>C/T<br>C/T |
| IL-6 | 7p14-21 | rs1800795<br>rs1800797 | -174<br>+565 | G/C<br>G/A |
| IL10 | 1q31-32 | rs1800896<br>rs1800871<br>rs1800872 | -1082<br>-819<br>-592 | G/A<br>C/T<br>C/A |
| IL 13 | 5q31-33 | rs7719175<br>rs1800925 | -7402<br>-1055 (-1112) | T/G<br>C/T |

**Others**

| Cytokine | Chromosome | db SNP | position | SNP |
|---|---|---|---|---|
| IL1 R | 2q14.2 | rs2234650 | pstI 1970 | C/T |
| IL1RA | 2q14.2 | rs315952 | Mspa1 11100 | T/C |
| IL 2 | 4q26-27 | rs2069762<br>rs2069763 | -330<br>+166 | T/G<br>G/T |
| IL 4Rα | 16p11.2-12.1 | rs1801275 | +1902 | G/A |

Fig. 1. Commonly studied polymorphisms in human type 1, type II, and other cytokines and their receptors. The chromosomal localization, db SNP names, positions of functional polymorphisms in relation to gene start site and the nucleotide substitutions are given.

comparisons, transmission disequilibrium tests, and genome-wide studies. Population-based studies are important for recording the frequency distribution of different cytokine gene variants and for defining differences among various population groups (7–13). Such information is extremely helpful in designing translational studies.

### 1.3. Genotype–Phenotype Correlations

Recent reports have established that some CGPs correlate with the levels of cytokine expression and their phenotypic balance helps to determine and/or predict the type of immune response. Table 1 summarizes the established cytokine genotype–phenotype correlations determined largely on the basis of their in vitro levels of expression (14–24).

### 1.4. Relevance of Cytokine Gene Polymorphisms

Some genetic polymorphisms in cytokine genes affect their transcription levels. Therefore, these polymorphisms may collectively modulate the net magnitude of cytokine-mediated immune responses following transplantation or as a result of infection. This underlies the importance of studying SNPs in relation to CGPs in a variety of situations. Although CGPs play an important role in

**Table 1**
**Established cytokine alleles/genotypes/haplotypes that correlate with their in vitro expression levels[a]**

| Cytokine | Genotype | Expression |
|---|---|---|
| IL1β | +3962 (nt5887)T | Increased |
| TGFβ1 | +896T, +915G | Increased |
| TNFα | −308A | Increased |
| TNFα | −863A | Decreased |
| IFNγ | +874T | Increased |
| IL2 | −330T | Increased |
| IL 6 | −174G | Increased |
| IL6[b] | −597G,−572G,−373A(9)/T(11),−174G | Increased |
| IL6[b] | −597A,−572G,−373A(8)/T(12),−174G | Decreased |
| IL10 | −1082G,−819C,−590C | Increased |
| IL10 | −1082A,−819C,−592C | Decreased |
| IL10 | −1082A,−819T,−592A | Decreased |
| IL13 | −1055T | Increased |
| Fas | −670A | Increased |
| Fas L | −843C | Increased |

[a]Important references (14–24)
[b]In case of IL6, the A(9)/T(11) and A(8)/T(12) represent repeats of A and T nucleotides that constitute a part of the IL6 haplotypes associated with increased and decreased expression, respectively

allograft survival and for evaluating incidence of acute or chronic rejection, the relevance of ethnic differences in their frequencies have not been fully explored yet. Observations based on racial variations in allograft loss, such as a relatively higher rate of renal allograft failure among Blacks could be correlated with ethnic differences in cytokine-mediated immune reactivity through an SNP mapping approach. It has been shown that renal transplant recipients with genotypes predicting high TNFα, IL10, and γIFN are more likely to develop acute chronic rejection (15). Ethnicities of Asian descent as compared to Whites have been documented to possess high frequencies of genotypes that result in low expression of γIFN and IL 10 but high IL6 (12). Similarly, the role of CGPs in infectious or autoimmune diseases has been widely studied and found to correlate with Th1/Th2 dominated immune responses (2, 3, 6, 25).

**1.5. Methods of Detecting Cytokine Gene Polymorphisms**

Several assays are available for defining CGPs or their effects on cytokine expression and these can be prioritized depending on the study design and requirements. Their absolute or relative expression correlates can be estimated using ELISA, CELISA, ELISPOT, real-time RT-PCR, Luminex monitoring, western blotting and immunohistochemistry in conjunction with densitometry, flow cytometry, and microarrays.

Similarly, several techniques are available for studying the biallelic CGPs. These include PCR-SSP (or ARMS PCR), AFLP, Taqman probe assays, microarrays, and sequencing-based typing. Of these, the PCR-SSP is the most widely used and well-established procedure that has been adopted by numerous studies, including the 13IHWC as well as by the CTS, Heidelberg. Cytokine genotyping SSP kits can be procured on request from the CTS, University of Heidelberg or from commercial vendors like One lambda, USA. Primers can also be designed individually using software like the *Primer express* and other online packages and in-house SSP assays can be developed.

Figure 2 describes the basic principle of PCR-SSP procedure. The PCR primers are designed deliberately to include a perfect match with a single allele (i.e., a corresponding mismatch with the other allele). As a result of stringent PCR conditions, allele-specific amplification is initiated with only the perfectly matched primers and continued exponentially during the subsequent PCR cycles.

The amplicons are resolved in agarose gels and interpreted. It is pertinent to include an internal control of reference for amplification in order to rule out amplification failures, if any. An internal control is also needed to check amplification related errors or variations, e.g., quality of template, carryover of salts and other

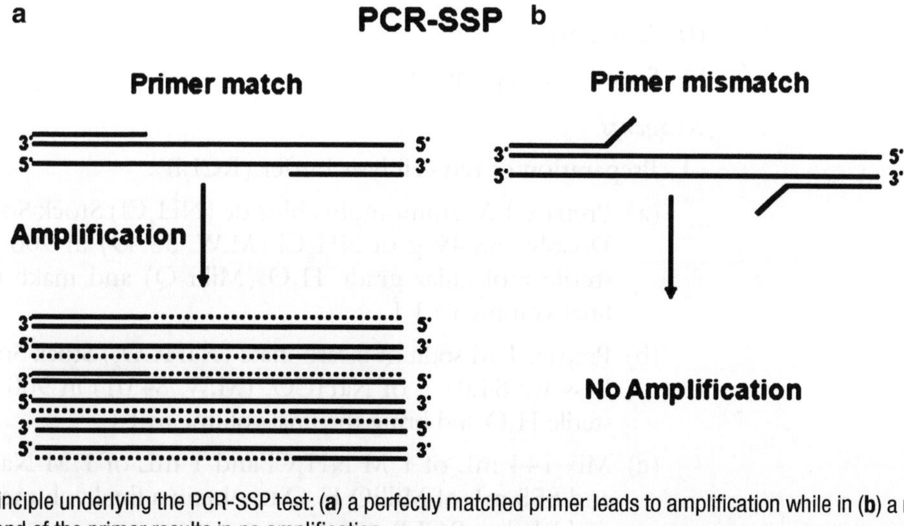


Fig. 2. Principle underlying the PCR-SSP test: (**a**) a perfectly matched primer leads to amplification while in (**b**) a mismatch at the 3′end of the primer results in no amplification.

inhibitors, pippeting errors, etc., and more importantly to avoid interpreting false negative results. The PCR primer mixes are prepared for not only scoring alleles, but also for the identification of genotypes and multilocus haplotypes involving multiple cytokines, e.g., TGFβ, TNFα, IL 2, IL 4, IL 6, and IL 10.

The PCR-SSP technique for cytokine genotyping using kits procured from the CTS (Heidelberg) is described in detail in the following sections. This kit enables detection of SNPs in the promoter regions of IL1α, IL1β, IL1R, IL1RA, IL2, IL4, IL6, IL10, IL12, TNFα, and γIFN genes, as well as in the untranslated regions of TGFβ and IL4Rα genes.

## 2. Materials

### *2.1. Extraction of DNA (Salting-Out Procedure Using Ammonium Acetate)*

Salting out procedure is one of the most commonly employed methods of extraction of DNA and is described in this chapter although a number of commercial kits are also available for DNA extraction from peripheral blood and other tissues.

1. Source of DNA—(see Note 1).
2. Table top Centrifuge.
3. ND-1000 Spectrophotometer (NanoDrop).
4. Incubator/water bath.
5. Vortex mixer.
6. Microfuge.
7. Autopippettes and tips.
8. 1.5-mL polypropylene microfuge tubes.
9. pH meter.
10. Autoclave.
11. Speed-Vac (optional).

*Reagents*

1. Preparation of red cell lysis buffer (RCLB).
   (a) Prepare 1 M ammonium chloride ($NH_4Cl$) Stock Solution: Dissolve 53.49 g of $NH_4Cl$ (M.W. 53.49) in 900 mL of sterile molecular grade $H_2O$ (Milli Q) and make up the final volume to 1 L.
   (b) Prepare 1 M sodium bicarbonate ($NaHCO_3$) Stock Solution: Dissolve 84.01 g of $NaHCO_3$ (M.W. 84.01) in 900 mL of sterile $H_2O$ and bring the final volume to 1 L.
   (c) Mix 144 mL of 1 M $NH_4Cl$ and 1 mL of 1 M $NaHCO_3$ and 855 mL of MilliQ $H_2O$ to obtain a final volume of 1 L and label as RCLB.

2. Nucleus lysis buffer (NLB).
   (a) Prepare 5 M NaCl Stock solution: Dissolve 292.20 g of NaCl (M.W. 58.44) in 700 mL of Milli Q grade water and make the final volume to 1 L.
   (b) Prepare 0.5 M $Na_2EDTA$ Solution (pH 8.0): Dissolve 186.12 g of $Na_2EDTA$ (M.W. 372.24) in 750 mL of MilliQ $H_2O$. Adjust pH to 8 by adding approximately 12 g NaOH pellets and make final volume to 1 L.
   (c) Prepare 2 M Tris–HCl (pH 8.0) Solution: Weigh and dissolve 242.28 g of Tris (M.W. 121.14) in 700 mL of Milli Q grade $H_2O$, adjust the pH to 8 with concentrated HCl, and bring the final volume to 1 L.
   (d) Mix 4 mL of 5 M NaCl + 200 μL of 0.5 M $Na_2EDTA$ (pH 8) + 250 μL of 2 M Tris–HCl (pH 8). Bring the final volume to 50 mL with Milli Q grade $H_2O$ and label as NLB.

   Both RCLB and NLB should be autoclaved and stored at room temperature.
3. Proteinase K solution.
   Dissolve 10 mg proteinase K in 1 mL of sterile water, aliquot into 200 μL fractions in microfuge tubes and store in –20°C.
4. TE solution (1 mM Tris 0.1 mM EDTA pH7.5).
   Dissolve 121.16 mg Tris (MW 121.16) and 37.224 mg EDTA (M.W. 372.24) in 950 mL $dH_2O$, adjust the pH to 7.5 and make the final volume to 1 L with MilliQ $H_2O$ and autoclave.
5. 4 M ammonium acetate.
   Dissolve 154.16 g ammonium acetate (MW 77.08 g) in 500 mL final volume Milli Q water and autoclave.
6. 70% ethanol and isopropyl alcohol.

### 2.2. PCR-SSP Using CTS Kits

1. Thermal cycler (ABI 9700 or equivalent).
2. Sterile molecular grade water.
3. Cytokine CTS-PCR SSP Tray kit (Product no.124) (www.ctstransplant.org). The kit is supplied with 3 mL aliquots of master mix (CYT 5%). It is recommended to prepare further 276 μL aliquots of this mix sufficient for each PCR tray and store frozen at –20°C to avoid repeat thawing.
4. Taq DNA polymerase (5 U/μL) (Fermentas or Inno-Train or Applied Biosystems). Store at –20°C.

### 2.3. Gel Electrophoresis

1. Apparatus for horizontal agarose gel electrophoresis.
2. Power pack for gel electrophoresis apparatus.
3. UV transilluminator (or gel documentation system).
4. Agarose high quality electrophoresis grade and with low electroendosmosis (EEO) (see Note 2).

5. TBE buffer (0.5×):
   (a) Prepare a 10× TBE stock by mixing 108 g Tris base + 55 g boric acid and 40 mL 0.5 M EDTA (pH 8.0) and make up the volume to 1 L with distilled water.
   (b) Autoclave and store at room temperature.
   (c) At the time of use, dilute the stock to 0.5× concentration.
6. Ethidium bromide 10 mg/mL (Caution: Ethidium bromide is a potent carcinogen and must be handled carefully with gloves).

## 3. Methods

### 3.1. Extraction of DNA

#### 3.1.1. Collection of Peripheral Blood

1. Approximately 5 mL of blood is collected by venipuncture in K2-EDTA vacutainer tubes and mixed properly to avoid coagulation. Heparin is not used as an anticoagulant since it has been reported to have a potent inhibitory effect on PCR.

#### 3.1.2. Lysis of RBC

1. Add 40 mL of RCLB to 5 mL of blood sample and mix properly.
2. Incubate the contents at room temperature for 30 min and centrifuge at 1,800 × *g* force for 20 min at room temperature.
3. Drain off the supernatant gently and resuspend the remaining pellet in 40 mL RCLB.
4. Repeat step 2.
5. Drain the supernatant completely and proceed with nucleus lysis steps as described below.

#### 3.1.3. Nucleus Lysis and Protein Digestion

1. Resuspend the pellet obtained in Subheading 3.2, steps 1 and 5 in 3 mL NLB (see Note 3).
2. Add 200 μL of 10% SDS followed by 20 μL (10 mg/mL) of Proteinase-K solution. Mix thoroughly (see Note 4).
3. The mixture is kept at 37–42°C for 6 h to overnight. This is the optimal temperature for maximum digestion. After proper digestion, the solution becomes visibly clear with no debris.

#### 3.1.4. Desalting and Protein Precipitation

A volume of 4 mL of 4 M ammonium acetate is added to the contents obtained in Subheading 3.1.3, step 3 for deproteinization and vortexed extensively. Add 3 mL of chloroform. The high concentration of 4 M ammonium acetate dehydrates proteins and separates them as a precipitate while chloroform helps in removal of lipid contamination.

1. The mixture is vortexed and centrifuged at 1,800 × *g* force for 30 min. Protein settles in between the lower most layer of chloroform and upper aqueous layer.
2. The aqueous layer containing DNA is transferred carefully into another new 50-mL costar centrifuge tube.
3. Add 7 mL of isopropyl alcohol in order to precipitate DNA. Swirl the tube gently until DNA begins to precipitate and appears to float as jelly or whitish mass of thread-like structures.
4. Carefully transfer the visible DNA thread like structure to a 1.5-mL sterile microfuge tube containing 70% ethanol to wash off any salt trapped with DNA.
5. Microfuge the tube for 15 s, drain off the supernatant. Repeat the 70% ethanol wash once more.
6. Add 100 μL TE solution to the DNA pellet and let it dissolve. DNA dissolves better in low concentration salt solution (i.e., TE solution) than in distilled water. Do not use force to dissolve DNA. It should dissolve spontaneously over a few hours.

#### 3.1.5. Quantification of DNA

1. Use 1 μL of DNA to measure optical density (OD) at a wave length of 260λ and 280λ using an ND-1000 spectrophotometer (NanoDrop). Pure DNA preparation gives 260λ/280λ ratio of around 1.8 (between 1.5 and 2.0) (see Note 5). The OD value at 260λ is used to calculate the concentration of DNA. NOTE: 1 OD at 260λ is equivalent to 50 μg DNA.

#### 3.1.6. Storage of DNA

1. DNA is usually stored at 4°C for daily use and at –80°C for several months to years.

### 3.2. PCR-SSP Using CTS Tray Kit

Each 96-well tray supplied by the CTS for cytokine genotyping contains prepipetted lyophilized primer mixes for two DNA , i.e., 48 wells per individual. The PCR mix positions corresponding to every locus specificities in the tray are shown in Fig. 3 and Table 2. A separate master mix (CYT) is also supplied with the kit and contains the reaction buffer but no Taq polymerase. The reader is advised to refer to the procedure manual that is supplied along with the kit and take a note of lot specific differences if any.

1. Program the thermal cycler (ABI 9700) as per following conditions and save the program (see Note 6).

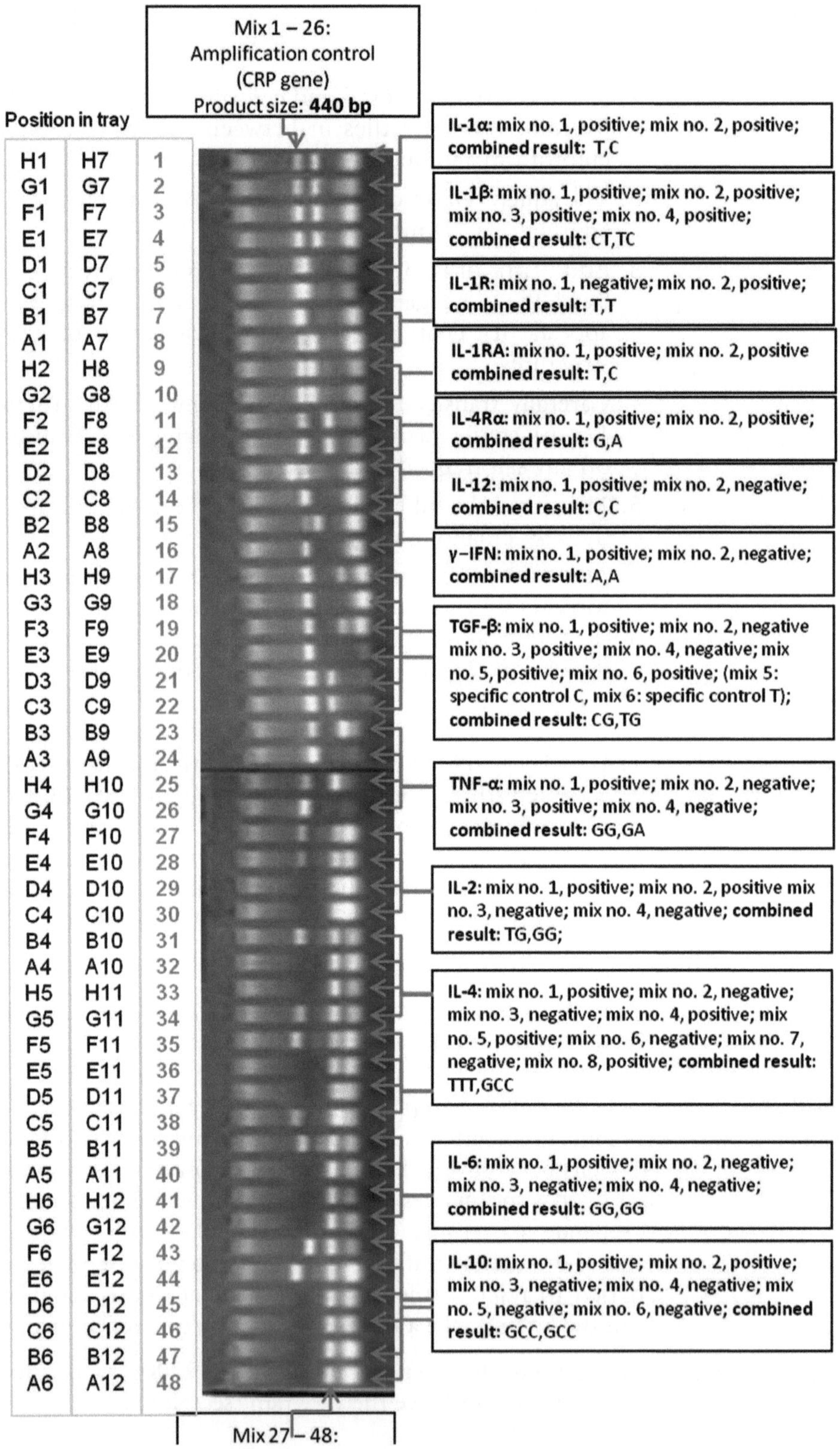


Fig. 3. An example of a 2% agarose gel electrophoregram showing PCR-SSP genotyping for cytokine and receptor genes using the CTS trays obtained from University of Heidelberg, Germany.

**Table 2**
**List of various CGPs, their gene location, allele specificities, and amplicon sizes obtained using CTS PCR-SSP kits**

| Cytokine | Location | SNP-db[a] name | Position on tray | Position on tray | Mix No. | Nucleotide specificity | Corresponding allele/genotype/ haplotype | Size of allele-specific amplicon (bp) | Size of the amplification control |
|---|---|---|---|---|---|---|---|---|---|
| IL 1α | Promoter | rs 1800587 | H1 | H7 | 1 | T at position -889 | T | 220 | 440 |
| | | | G1 | G7 | 2 | C at position -889 | C | 220 | 440 |
| IL 1β | Promoter | rs 16944 | F1 | F7 | 1 | C at position -511 | C | 215 | 440 |
| | | | E1 | E7 | 2 | T at position -511 | T | 215 | 440 |
| | | rs 1143634 | D1 | D7 | 3 | T at position +3962 | T | 340 | 440 |
| | | | C1 | D1 | 4 | C at position +3962 | C | 340 | 440 |
| IL 1R | Promoter | rs 2234650 | B1 | B7 | 1 | C at position pstI 1970 | C | 290 | 440 |
| | | | A1 | A7 | 2 | T at position pstI 1970 | T | 290 | 440 |
| IL 1RA | Promoter | rs 315952 | H2 | H8 | 1 | T at position mspa 11100 | T | 330 | 440 |
| | | | G2 | G8 | 2 | C at position mspa 11100 | C | 330 | 440 |
| IL 4Rα | 1st Exon | rs 1801275 | F2 | F8 | 1 | G at position +1902 | G | 140 | 440 |
| | | | E2 | E8 | 2 | A at position +1902 | A | 140 | 440 |
| IL 12B | Promoter | rs 3212227 | D2 | D8 | 1 | C at position -1188 | C | 800 | 440 |
| | | | C2 | C8 | 2 | A at position -1188 | A | 800 | 440 |
| γIFN | Intron 1 | rs 2430561 | B2 | B8 | 1 | A at position +874 | A | 180 | 440 |
| | | | A2 | A8 | 2 | T at position +874 | T | 180 | 440 |

(continued)

**Table 2 (continued)**

| Cytokine | Location | SNP-db[a] name | Position on tray | Position on tray | Mix No. | Nucleotide specificity | Corresponding allele/genotype/ haplotype | Size of allele-specific amplicon (bp) | Size of the amplification control |
|---|---|---|---|---|---|---|---|---|---|
| TGFβ | 1st Exon | rs 1800470 | H3 | H9 | 1 | C at codon 10 | CG or CC | 195 | 440 |
| | | | G3 | G9 | 2 | T at codon 10 | TG or TC | 195 | 440 |
| | | rs 1800471 | F3 | F9 | 3 | C at codon 10; G at codon 25 | CG | 80 | 440 |
| | | | E3 | E9 | 4 | C at codon 10; C at codon 25 | CC | 80 | 440 |
| | | | D3 | D9 | 5 | T at codon 10; G at codon 25 | TG | 80 | 440 |
| | | | C3 | C9 | 6 | T at codon 10; C at codon 25 | TC | 80 | 440 |
| TNFα | Promoter | rs 1800629 | B3 | B9 | 1 | G at position -308; G at position -238 | GG | 110 | 440 |
| | | rs 361525 | A3 | A9 | 2 | A at position -308; G at position -238 | AG | 110 | 440 |
| | | | H4 | H9 | 3 | G at position -308; A at position -238 | GA | 110 | 440 |
| | | | G4 | G9 | 4 | A at position -308; A at position -238 | AA | 110 | 440 |
| IL 2 | Promoter | rs 2069762 | F4 | F10 | 1 | T at position -330; G at position +166 | TG | 560 | 90 |
| | | rs 2069763 | E4 | E10 | 2 | G at position -330; G at position +166 | GG | 560 | 90 |

| | | | | | | | | | |
|---|---|---|---|---|---|---|---|---|---|
| | | | D4 | D10 | 3 | G at position -330; T at position +166 | GT | 560 | 90 |
| | | | C4 | C10 | 4 | T at position -330; T at position +166 | TT | 560 | 90 |
| IL 4[b] | Promoter | rs 2243248 | B4 | B10 | 1 | T at position -1098; T at position -590 | TT* | 560 | 90 |
| | | rs 2243250 | A4 | A10 | 2 | T at position -1098; C at position -590 | TC* | 560 | 90 |
| | | | H5 | H11 | 3 | G at position -1098; T at position -590 | GT* | 560 | 90 |
| | | | G5 | G11 | 4 | G at position -1098; C at position -590 | GC* | 560 | 90 |
| | | rs 2070874 | F5 | F11 | 5 | T at position -590; T at position -33 | *TT | 610 | 90 |
| | | | E5 | E11 | 6 | T at position -590; C at position -33 | *TC | 610 | 90 |
| | | | D5 | D11 | 7 | C at position -590; T at position -33 | *CT | 610 | 90 |
| | | | C5 | C11 | 8 | C at position -590; C at position -33 | *CC | 610 | 90 |
| IL 6 | Promoter | rs 1800795 | B5 | B11 | 1 | G at position -174; G at position +565 | GG | 430 | 90 |
| | | rs 1800797 | A5 | A11 | 2 | C at position -174; G at position +565 | CG | 430 | 90 |
| | | | H6 | H12 | 3 | G at position -174; A at position +565 | GA | 430 | 90 |
| | | | G6 | G12 | 4 | C at position -174; A at position +565 | CA | 430 | 90 |

(continued)

**Table 2 (continued)**

| Cytokine | Location | SNP-db[a] name | Position on tray | Position on tray | Mix No. | Nucleotide specificity | Corresponding allele/genotype/ haplotype | Size of allele-specific amplicon (bp) | Size of the amplification control |
|---|---|---|---|---|---|---|---|---|---|
| IL 10[b] | Promoter | rs 1800896 | F6 | F12 | 1 | G at position -1082; C at position -819 | GC* (**GCC** or GCA) | 305 | 90 |
| | | rs 1800971 | E6 | E12 | 2 | G at position -1082; C at position -592 | G*C (**GCC** or GAC) | 530 | 90 |
| | | rs 1800872 | D6 | D12 | 3 | A at position -1082; C at position -819 | AC* (**ACC** or ATC) | 305 | 90 |
| | | | C6 | C12 | 4 | A at position -1082; T at position -819 | AT* (ATC or **ATA**) | 305 | 90 |
| | | | B6 | B12 | 5 | A at position -1082; C at position -592 | A*C (**ACC** or ATC) | 530 | 90 |
| | | | A6 | A12 | 6 | A at position -1082; A at position -592 | A*A (ACA or **ATA**) | 530 | 90 |

[a]The reader is advised to refer to Fig. 1 for specific SNP-db names mentioned in this table

[b]In case of IL4 and IL10, it is possible to deduce 3 locus haplotypes where * in the haplotype means any nucleotide at one of the three positions. In case of IL4, these haplotypes refer to -1098,-590, and -33 positions. Similarly, the haplotypes in IL10 encompass the positions -1082,-819, and -592

| | | | |
|---|---|---|---|
| Initial denaturation | 94°C | 2 min | |
| Denaturation | 94°C | 15 s | 10 cycles |
| Annealing + extension | 65°C | 1 min | |
| Denaturation | 94°C | 15 s | 20 cycles |
| Annealing | 61°C | 50 s | |
| Extension | 72°C | 30 s | |
| Hold | 4°C | 15 min | |

2. Prepare the PCR reaction mix for a single DNA sample as shown below:

| Component | Volume (μL) |
|---|---|
| Master mix CYT | 138 |
| Taq Pol (5 U/μL) | 3 |
| Water | 329 |
| DNA (40 ng/μL) | 50 |
| *Final volume* | *520* |

3. Each CTS tray contains primers for genotyping two DNA samples. Use scissors to cut the tray into two halves. The PCR reaction mix can be prepared in volumes depending on the number of samples to be tested (see Notes 7–9).
4. Remove the CTS tray from the 4°C refrigerator. The lower edge of the tray is marked with a black line. The starting position in the tray is H1 and the series is oriented from H1 (bottom) followed by G1, F1, etc., to A1 (top) until the last well A6. The second set of the kit begins from H7 going on to A7 and so on until A12. See Table 2 for all the corresponding positions on the tray.
5. Transfer 10 μL of reaction mix from Subheading 3.2, step 2 into each of the 48 wells (see Note 10).
6. Seal the PCR tray with Strip caps provided with the kit and place in a thermal cycler that preprogrammed as in step 1 above. Ensure the caps completely seal the wells to prevent evaporation.
7. Start thermal cycling, after completion, remove the tray and proceed with gel electrophoresis.
8. A 2% agarose gel can be prepared and kept ready while the PCR is running. To avoid contamination with PCR amplification products, it is necessary to perform the test in two separate working areas: the preamplification and the postamplification areas.

### 3.3. Gel Electrophoresis

1. While the PCR is running (Subheading 3.2, step 7), a 2% agarose gel can be poured and kept ready. For this, boil 25 agarose in 0.5× TBE, cool to ~60°C and add 5 μL ethidium bromide (0.5 μg/mL final concentration). Mix and pour into gel tray prearranged with combs.
2. Allow the gel to set at room temperature for 1 h.
3. After the PCR is over, remove the strip caps carefully from the tray.
4. Remove the combs and ensure that wells are not broken. Place the gel inside and just under the surface of electrophoresis running buffer (0.5× TBE). Load 10 μL amplicons starting from H1 towards A1 as described in Fig. 3.
5. Connect the electrodes in the power-pack and run the electrophoresis at 100 V until just before the tracking dye exits the gel.
6. Visualize the gel under UV illumination (312 nm) and save the image or take a picture for interpretation and documentation.

### 3.4. Interpretation of Results

#### 3.4.1. Positive Internal Control Amplification

Each of the primer mixes contain internal control primer pairs corresponding to either β-globin (90 bp) or CRP gene (440 bp). Note the presence of these internal control bands in all the lanes as per their expected correct band sizes (Table 2 and Fig. 3). The 440 bp band should be visible in lanes corresponding to IL1α, IL1β, IL1R, IL1RA, IL4Rα, IL12, γIFN, TGFβ, and TNFα. Similarly, the 90 bp band should be observed in lanes corresponding to IL 2, IL 4, IL 6, and IL 10.

#### 3.4.2. Allele-Specific Amplification

1. Record the amplification patterns obtained for each of the primer pairs in every well after confirmation of the correct band sizes as shown in Table 2. The wells where allele-specific amplicon is present may show weak or sometimes no internal control band (see Note 11).
2. Some of the cytokine genotyping reagents in the kit allow detection of certain haplotypes depending on characteristic amplification patterns. Refer Table 2 for deducing correct haplotypes.
3. Disregard any products of incorrect size whether strong or weak (see Note 12).
4. A primer dimer diffused band of <80 bp may be observed occasionally but can be distinguished from the allele-specific amplifications which are relatively sharper and usually 80 bp or more in size.
5. False negatives, if any, may be caused by inefficient amplification or poor quality of DNA or variations in thermal cycler and can be ruled out individually.

6. In case of γIFN, mix 1 may yield relatively weaker amplification than mix 2.
7. For TGFβ, a nonspecific smear may be observed but should be discernible from the small sized (80 bp) amplicons.
8. When IL4 amplifications are being interpreted, note that mix 6 may produce faint nonspecific amplification. An allele-specific PCR product is usually strongly positive.
9. The test should be repeated if there is no amplification of control bands as well as allele-specific bands or if reaction pattern is inconclusive.

*3.4.3. An Example of Interpretation of Allele-Specific Amplification for IL 10*

The first observation to look for is an internal control amplification of 90 bp (Fig. 3, lanes 43–48). Now, refer to Table 2 for expected band sizes for allele-specific amplifications relating to IL10 mixes 1–6 corresponding to the same lanes 43–48. As can be seen in Fig. 3, there is a positive band of 305 bp (mix 1) in lane number 43 and a band of size 530 bp (mix 2) in lane 44 while all the remaining lanes 45–48 do not show any allele-specific amplification(s) for IL 10. A combined interpretation of GC* and G*C as suggested against lanes 43 and 44 (Table 2) hence suggests that the individual tested is homozygous for the GCC haplotype.

## 4. Notes

1. EDTA blood is the most widely used material to isolate genomic DNA. A great care needs to be taken to avoid contamination of DNA from another source because PCR technique is a powerful method that would amplify contaminated DNA up to the detection level. White blood cells (WBCs) are used as the major source of DNA and can be easily obtained by removing the red blood cells (RBCs) after lysis from the whole blood.
2. It is advisable to use high quality electrophoresis grade agarose with low EEO (preferably $<0.13$). EEO refers to the flow of liquid under the influence of an electric field due to immobilized charge groups on the matrix. The anionic groups of agarose are affixed to the matrix; however, counter cations tend to migrate towards cathode within the matrix, giving rise to EEO. This movement of water counteracts the otherwise electrophoretic movement of DNA towards anode, hence leads to convection and smearing of bands.
3. The NLB contains Tris, NaCl, and EDTA. Tris and NaCl are used for buffering the reaction (pH-8). Intrinsic DNAse activity is inhibited by EDTA as it chelates the divalent ions ($Mg^{++}$, $Ca^{++}$, $Zn^{++}$) into their respective salts as precipitates. These divalent

ions are cofactors for the DNAse enzyme and by removing them the intrinsic DNAse activity is inhibited and DNA fragmentation avoided. SDS is an ionic detergent which disturbs membranal structure, denatures proteins and can digest the DNAse enzyme.

4. Proteinase-K is a proteolytic enzyme that breaks the peptide bonds and helps to get protein-free DNA.
5. A ratio of 280/260 between 1.5 and 2.0 is acceptable. In case, the DNA isolated does not give this ratio, it is advisable to reextract DNA from a fresh sample.
6. Ensure that thermal cycler is calibrated and verified.
7. Use of excess DNA quantity (>200 ng/μL) may result in nonspecific amplifications, false positives, and smearing in the gel.
8. Use of less DNA (<10 ng/μL) may result in weak amplification bands or false negatives.
9. A poor or no amplification indicates poor quality or degraded DNA. It is advisable to take fresh blood sample and reextract the DNA.
10. When dispensing 10 μL of reaction mix to each well, care should be taken to release the drop onto well side walls near the top and allow it to slide down (you may gently tap the tray). Do not touch the bottom of the well. Make sure that each of the well receives the drop (look for pink color) before proceeding to thermal cycler. Ensure that the caps are sealed completely on top of the wells to avoid evaporation. The time required between addition of samples to wells and initiation of PCR must be minimized and performed as efficiently as possible.
11. In the presence of a positive typing band (specific amplification of a cytokine allele), the product of the internal control primer may be weak or absent due to the difference in concentration and melting temperatures between the specific primer pairs and the internal control primer pair.
12. In a few instances, e.g., if DNA quality is not very good or if there was a delay in starting the thermal cycler etc., non-specific amplifications may occur. Hence, any band (whether strong or weak) that does not correspond to its expected correct size should be ignored.

## Acknowledgements

The authors acknowledge Joannis Mytilineos and his team for developing the Cytokine genotyping reagents and the CTS group at Univ Heidelberg for kindly providing these on regular basis.

The financial support provided by the Indian Council of Medical Research (ICMR) and Department of Biotechnology (DBT), Govt. of India are gratefully acknowledged. The laboratory members, particularly Neeraj Kumar, Chowphi Rapthap, Gaurav Sharma, and Shekhar Neolia are acknowledged for optimizing the above procedures.

## References

1. Hollegaard MV, Bidwell JL (2006) Cytokine gene polymorphism in human disease: on-line databases, supplement 3. Genes Immun 7:269–276
2. Kaur G, Mehra N (2009) Genetic determinants of HIV-1 infection and progression to AIDS: immune response genes. Tissue Antigens 74:373–385
3. Ryan AW, Mapp J, Myna S et al (2006) Levels of interpopulation differentiation among different functional classes of immunologically important genes. Genes and Immunity 7:179–183
4. Mytilineos J, Laux G, Opelz G (2004) Relevance of IL10, TGFb1, TNFa and IL4Ra gene polymorphisms in kidney transplantation: a collaborative transplant study report. Am J Transplant 4:1684–1690
5. Bidwell J, Keen L, Gallagher G et al (1999) Cytokine gene polymorphism in human disease: on-line databases. Genes Immun 1:3–19
6. Bidwell J, Keen L, Gallagher G et al (2001) Cytokine gene polymorphism in human disease: on-line databases, supplement 1. Genes Immun 2:61–70
7. Kaur G, Rapthap CC, Kumar N et al (2007) Frequency distribution of cytokine gene polymorphisms in the healthy North Indian population. Tissue Antigens 69:113–120
8. Pyo CW, Hur SS, Kim YK et al (2003) Polymorphisms of IL1B, IL1RN, IL2, IL4, IL6, IL10 and IFNg genes in the Korean population. Hum Immunol 64:979–989
9. Kurzawski M, Pawlik A, Czerny B et al (2005) Frequencies of the common promoter polymorphisms in cytokine genes in a polish population. Int J Immunogenet 32:285–291
10. Uboldi de Capei MU, Dametto E, Fasano ME et al (2003) Genotyping for cytokine polymorphisms: allele frequencies in the Italian population. Eur J Immunogenet 30:5–10
11. Trajkov D, Arsov T, Petlichkovski A et al (2005) Cytokine gene polymorphisms in population of ethnic Macedonians. Croat Med J 46(4):685–692
12. Costeas PA, Koumas L, Koumouli A et al (2003) Cytokine polymorphism frequencies in the Greek Cypriot population. Eur J Immmunogenet 30:341–343
13. Hoffmann SC, Stanley EM, Cox ED et al (2002) Ethnicity greatly influences cytokine gene polymorphism distribution. Am J Transplant 2(6):560–567
14. Dudler J, Li J, Pagnotta M et al (2006) Gene transfer of programmed death ligand-1.Ig prolongs cardiac allograft survival. Transplantation 82(12):1733–1737
15. Hahn AB, Kasten-Jolly JC, Conctantino DM et al (2001) TNF-alpha, IL-6, IFN-gamma, and IL-10 gene expression polymorphisms and the IL-4 receptor alpha-chain variant Q576R: effects on renal allograft outcome. Transplantation 72(4):660–665
16. Pociot F, Mølvig J, Wogensen L et al (1992) A TaqI polymorphism in the human interleukin-1 beta (IL-1 beta) gene correlates with IL-1 beta secretion in vitro. Eur J Clin Invest 22(6): 396–402
17. Awad MR, El-Gamel A, Hasleton P et al (1998) Genotypic variation in the transforming growth factor-beta1 gene: association with transforming growth factor-beta1 production, fibrotic lung disease, and graft fibrosis after lung transplantation. Transplantation 66(8):1014–1020
18. Pociot F, Wilson AG, Nerup J et al (1993) No independent association between a tumor necrosis factor-alpha promotor region polymorphism and insulin-dependent diabetes mellitus. Eur J Immunol 23(11):3050–3053
19. Fishman D, Faulds G, Jeffery R (1998) The effect of novel polymorphisms in the interleukin-6 (IL-6) gene on IL-6 transcription and plasma IL-6 levels, and an association with systemic-onset juvenile chronic arthritis. J Clin Invest 102(7):1369–1376
20. Terry CF, Loukaci V, Green FR (2000) Cooperative influence of genetic polymorphisms on interleukin 6 transcriptional regulation. J Biol Chem 275(24):18138–18144
21. Turner DM, Williams DM, Sankaran D et al (1997) An investigation of polymorphism in the interleukin-10 gene promoter. Eur J Immunogenet 24(1):1–8

22. Crawley E, Woo P, Isenberg DA et al (1999) Single nucleotide polymorphic haplotypes of the interleukin-10 5′ flanking region are not associated with renal disease or serology in Caucasian patients with systemic lupus erythematosus. Arthritis Rheum 42(9):2017–2018
23. van der Pouw Kraan TC, van Veen A, Boeije LC et al (1999) An IL-13 promoter polymorphism associated with increased risk of allergic asthma. Genes Immun 1(1):61–65
24. Mullighan CG, Marshall SE, Bunce M et al (1999) Variation in immunoregulatory genes determines the clinical phenotype of common variable immunodeficiency. Genes Immun 1:137–148
25. Wang K, Li M, Hakonarson H (2010) Analysing biological pathways in genome-wide association studies. Nat Rev Genet 11:843–854

## Useful Website Links

http://www3.ncbi.nlm.nih.gov/Omim/searchomim.html

http://www.immport.org/immportWeb/queryref/geneListSummary.do

http://snpper.chip.org/

http://genome.cse.ucsc.edu/

http://cmbi.bjmu.edu.cn/cmbidata/cgf/

Chapter 32

# IMGT® Tools for the Nucleotide Analysis of Immunoglobulin (IG) and T Cell Receptor (TR) V-(D)-J Repertoires, Polymorphisms, and IG Mutations: IMGT/V-QUEST and IMGT/HighV-QUEST for NGS

**Eltaf Alamyar, Patrice Duroux, Marie-Paule Lefranc, and Véronique Giudicelli**


## Abstract

IMGT/V-QUEST is the highly customized and integrated online IMGT® tool for the standardized analysis of the immunoglobulin (IG) or antibody and T cell receptor (TR) rearranged nucleotide sequences. The analysis of these antigen receptors represents a crucial challenge for the study of the adaptive immune response in normal and disease-related situations. The expressed IG and TR repertoires represent a potential of $10^{12}$ IG and $10^{12}$ TR per individual. This huge diversity results from mechanisms that occur at the DNA level during the IG and TR molecular synthesis. These mechanisms include the combinatorial rearrangements of the variable (V), diversity (D) and joining (J) genes, the N-diversity (deletion and addition at random of nucleotides during the V-(D)-J rearrangement) and, for IG, somatic hypermutations. IMGT/V-QUEST identifies the V, D, J genes and alleles by alignment with the germline IG and TR gene and allele sequences of the IMGT reference directory. The tool describes the V-REGION mutations and identifies the hot spot positions in the closest germline V gene. IMGT/V-QUEST integrates IMGT/JunctionAnalysis for a detailed analysis of the V-J and V-D-J junctions and IMGT/Automat for a complete annotation of the sequences and also provides IMGT Collier de Perles. IMGT/HighV-QUEST, the high-throughput version of IMGT/V-QUEST, implemented to answer the needs of deep sequencing data analysis from Next Generation Sequencing (NGS), allows the analysis of thousands of IG and TR sequences in a single run. IMGT/V-QUEST and IMGT/HighV-QUEST are available at the IMGT® Home page, http://www.imgt.org.


**Key words:** IMGT, Immunogenetics, Immunoinformatics, Immunoglobulin, Antibody, T cell receptor, Somatic hypermutation, Allelic polymorphism, High-throughput sequencing, IMGT-ONTOLOGY

## 1. Introduction

The efficiency of the adaptive immune response and its capability of recognizing a large number of different antigens depend on the huge diversity of the antigen receptors, antibodies or

Frank T. Christiansen and Brian D. Tait (eds.), *Immunogenetics: Methods and Applications in Clinical Practice*, Methods in Molecular Biology, vol. 882, DOI 10.1007/978-1-61779-842-9_32, © Springer Science+Business Media New York 2012

immunoglobulins (IG) of the B lymphocytes, and T cell receptors (TR) of the T lymphocytes. The genes which code the IG and TR are highly polymorphic and are organized in clusters in several loci (three loci for IG and four for TR in human) located on different chromosomes (four in human) in the genome (1, 2). The molecular synthesis of the IG and TR chains is particularly complex and unique. It includes several mechanisms that occur at the DNA level: combinatorial rearrangements of the variable (V), diversity (D) and joining (J) genes that code the variable domain or V-DOMAIN, exonuclease trimming at the ends of the V, D, and J genes and the random addition of nucleotides by the terminal deoxynucleotidyl transferase (TdT) that create the junction N-diversity, and somatic hypermutations (for IG only) (1, 2). The IG and TR repertoires show an extraordinary diversity with a potential of $10^{12}$ IG and $10^{12}$ TR per individual and the only limiting factor is the number of genetically programmed B and T cells for an organism. Therefore, the analysis of the IG and TR genes and of their expression represents a crucial challenge for the understanding of the immune response in normal and pathological situations.

IMGT/V-QUEST (V-QUEry and STandardization) (3–7) is the IG and TR nucleotide sequence analysis tool of IMGT®, the international ImMunoGeneTics information system® (8) (http://www.imgt.org), created in 1989 at Montpellier, France (CNRS and Université Montpellier 2). IMGT/V-QUEST (Subheading 2) identifies the V, D, and J genes in rearranged IG and TR sequences and, for the IG, the nucleotide (nt) mutations and amino acid (AA) changes resulting from somatic hypermutations. The tool integrates IMGT/JunctionAnalysis (9), for the detailed characterization of the V-D-J or V-J junctions. The standardized analysis is based on the concepts of IMGT-ONTOLOGY, the first ontology in immunogenetics and immunoinformatics, which are generated from the axioms of the Formal IMGT-ONTOLOGY or IMGT-Kaleidoscope (10–13), and more particularly the axioms of CLASSIFICATION (gene and allele nomenclature), DESCRIPTION (standardized labels), and NUMEROTATION (IMGT unique numbering and IMGT Colliers de Perles). That standardization has allowed a considerable upgrade, from IMGT/V-QUEST online analyzing 50 sequences per run, to IMGT/HighV-QUEST (14), the high-throughput version of IMGT/V-QUEST, analyzing up to 150,000 sequences per run, with the same degree of resolution and high quality results. IMGT/HighV-QUEST (Subheading 3) was implemented to answer the needs of data analysis from the Next Generation Sequencing (NGS). The standardized results provided by IMGT/V-QUEST and IMGT/HighV-QUEST are crucial for the analysis of repertoire of IG antibody sites, and TR recognition sites and IG and TR polymorphisms, in normal and pathological situations. IMGT/V-QUEST and IMGT/HighV-QUEST are constantly improved following the results of fundamental and clinical research. New alleles are annotated in IMGT® and integrated in the IMGT/V-QUEST and IMGT/HighV-QUEST reference directories as soon as they are confirmed experimentally and publicly available in the generalist databases and entered in IMGT/GENE-DB (15). Rules for sequence analysis have been improved through scientific collaboration and with the constant feedback of clinicians and scientists. By their wide range of customizable and integrated functionalities and by their high level of standardization, IMGT/V-QUEST and IMGT/HighV-QUEST provide results of much value for the comparative analysis of the IG and TR sequences (including those of the newly sequenced vertebrate genomes), for statistical analysis of the junctions and of the repertoires, for antibody engineering and therapeutic antibodies.

## 2. IMGT/V-QUEST

The link to the IMGT/V-QUEST tool is available from the IMGT® Home page, http://www.imgt.org in the "IMGT tools" section. Clicking on that link gives access to the IMGT/V-QUEST Welcome page (Fig. 1).

### 2.1. IMGT/V-QUEST Welcome Page

1. In the IMGT/V-QUEST Welcome page (Fig. 1), locate the section that corresponds to the receptor type (IG or TR) of your sequences (see Note 1).
2. Locate the species or taxon that corresponds to the IMGT reference directory against which you want your sequences to be analyzed (see Note 2).
3. Click on the species (for instance "Human") or taxon. This will give access to the IMGT/V-QUEST Search page (Fig. 2).

### 2.2. IMGT/V-QUEST Search Page

#### 2.2.1. Entering Nucleotide Sequences for the Analysis

IMGT/V-QUEST can analyze IG and TR rearranged nucleotide sequences from genomic DNA or cDNA, indifferently. Sequences must be submitted in FASTA format (up to 50 sequences per run). The sequences must be copied and pasted in the text area of "Nucleotide sequences," or uploaded as a text file by selecting the option "Or give the path access to a local file containing your sequence(s) in FASTA format" and using the "Browse" button to select the file.

#### 2.2.2. Selection of the Result Display

The user can choose between three types of display for the results: "Detailed view," "Synthesis view," or "Excel file" and the parameters of the analysis can be customized with a large choice of options in "Advanced parameters" (Fig. 2).

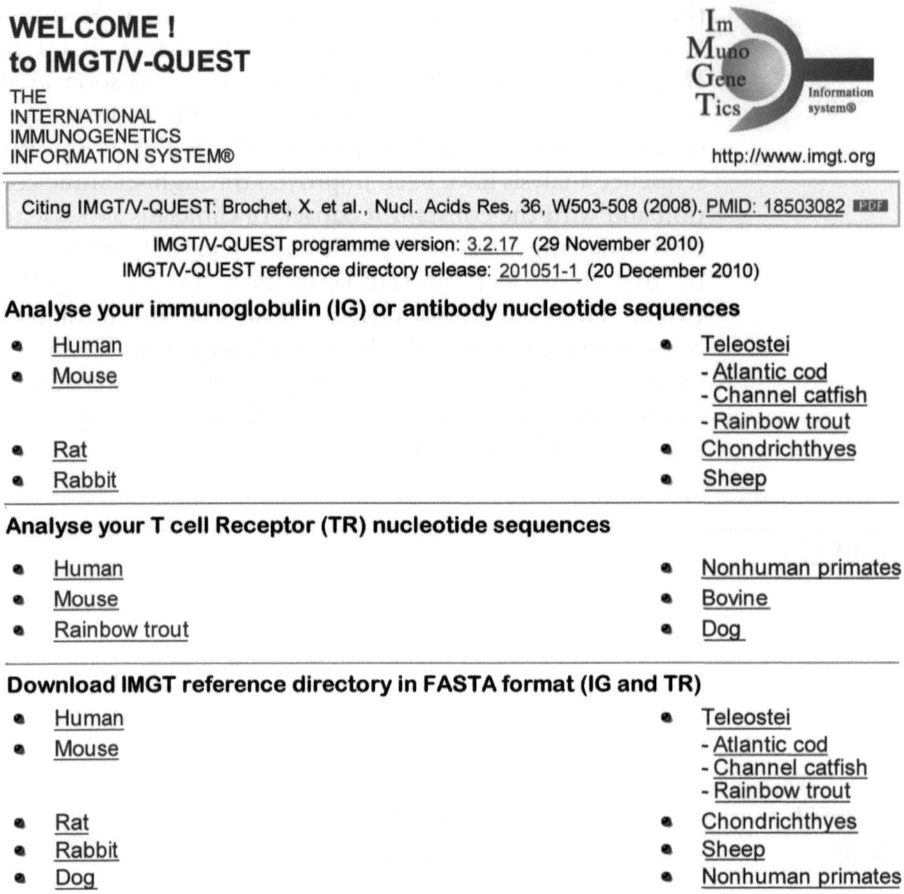


Fig. 1. IMGT/V-QUEST Welcome page. The two upper sections correspond to the immunoglobulin (IG) or antibody and T cell receptor (TR) analyses, respectively. The lowest section is for download of the IMGT reference directory sets.

1. Detailed view.

   "Detailed view" provides the results for each sequence, individually. They may be displayed in HTML (by default) or Text format, with a user-defined number of nucleotides per line in alignments (60 by default). There is a choice of 14 different result displays for the analysis of the V-DOMAIN. The results the most commonly requested are selected by default. You can check or uncheck the result displays as needed:

   (a) Alignment for V-GENE.
   (b) Alignment for D-GENE.
   (c) Alignment for J-GENE.
   (d) "Results of IMGT/JunctionAnalysis" (9) (with or without full list of eligible D-GENEs).
   (e) Sequence of the JUNCTION ("nt" and "AA").

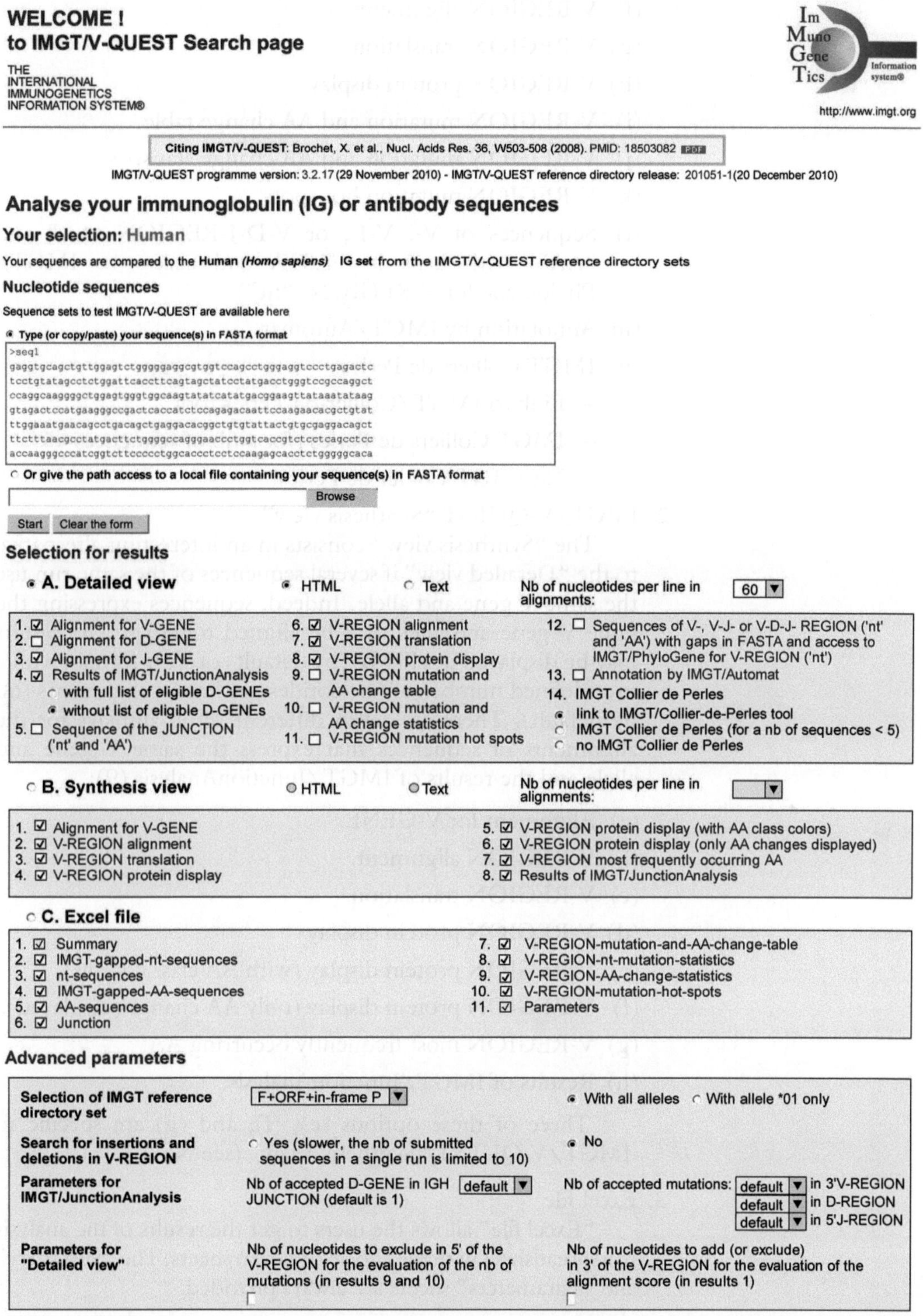
WELCOME !
to IMGT/V-QUEST Search page
THE INTERNATIONAL IMMUNOGENETICS INFORMATION SYSTEM®
Im Muno Gene Tics
Information system®
http://www.imgt.org
Citing IMGT/V-QUEST: Brochet, X. et al., Nucl. Acids Res. 36, W503-508 (2008). PMID: 18503082
IMGT/V-QUEST programme version: 3.2.17 (29 November 2010) - IMGT/V-QUEST reference directory release: 201051-1 (20 December 2010)
Analyse your immunoglobulin (IG) or antibody sequences
Your selection: Human
Your sequences are compared to the Human (Homo sapiens) IG set from the IMGT/V-QUEST reference directory sets
Nucleotide sequences
Sequence sets to test IMGT/V-QUEST are available here
Type (or copy/paste) your sequence(s) in FASTA format
>seq1
gaggtgcagctgttggagtctgggggaggcgtggtccagcctgggaggtccctgagactc
tcctgtatagcctctggattcaccttcagtagctatcctatgacctgggtccgccaggct
ccaggcaaggggctggagtgggtggcaagtatatcatatgacggaagttataaatataag
gtagactccatgaagggccgactcaccatctccagagacaattccaagaacacgctgtat
ttggaaatgaacagcctgacagctgaggacacggctgtgtattactgtgcgaggacagct
ttctttaacgcctatgacttctggggccagggaaccctggtcaccgtctcctcagcctcc
accaagggcccatcggtcttccccctggcaccctcctccaagagcacctctgggggcaca
Or give the path access to a local file containing your sequence(s) in FASTA format
Browse
Start
Clear the form
Selection for results
A. Detailed view
HTML
Text
Nb of nucleotides per line in alignments:
60
1. Alignment for V-GENE
2. Alignment for D-GENE
3. Alignment for J-GENE
4. Results of IMGT/JunctionAnalysis
with full list of eligible D-GENEs
without list of eligible D-GENEs
5. Sequence of the JUNCTION ('nt' and 'AA')
6. V-REGION alignment
7. V-REGION translation
8. V-REGION protein display
9. V-REGION mutation and AA change table
10. V-REGION mutation and AA change statistics
11. V-REGION mutation hot spots
12. Sequences of V-, V-J- or V-D-J- REGION ('nt' and 'AA') with gaps in FASTA and access to IMGT/PhyloGene for V-REGION ('nt')
13. Annotation by IMGT/Automat
14. IMGT Collier de Perles
link to IMGT/Collier-de-Perles tool
IMGT Collier de Perles (for a nb of sequences < 5)
no IMGT Collier de Perles
B. Synthesis view
HTML
Text
Nb of nucleotides per line in alignments:
1. Alignment for V-GENE
2. V-REGION alignment
3. V-REGION translation
4. V-REGION protein display
5. V-REGION protein display (with AA class colors)
6. V-REGION protein display (only AA changes displayed)
7. V-REGION most frequently occurring AA
8. Results of IMGT/JunctionAnalysis
C. Excel file
1. Summary
2. IMGT-gapped-nt-sequences
3. nt-sequences
4. IMGT-gapped-AA-sequences
5. AA-sequences
6. Junction
7. V-REGION-mutation-and-AA-change-table
8. V-REGION-nt-mutation-statistics
9. V-REGION-AA-change-statistics
10. V-REGION-mutation-hot-spots
11. Parameters
Advanced parameters
Selection of IMGT reference directory set
F+ORF+in-frame P
With all alleles
With allele *01 only
Search for insertions and deletions in V-REGION
Yes (slower, the nb of submitted sequences in a single run is limited to 10)
No
Parameters for IMGT/JunctionAnalysis
Nb of accepted D-GENE in IGH JUNCTION (default is 1)
default
Nb of accepted mutations:
default in 3'V-REGION
default in D-REGION
default in 5'J-REGION
Parameters for "Detailed view"
Nb of nucleotides to exclude in 5' of the V-REGION for the evaluation of the nb of mutations (in results 9 and 10)
Nb of nucleotides to add (or exclude) in 3' of the V-REGION for the evaluation of the alignment score (in results 1)

Fig. 2. The IMGT/V-QUEST Search page. The Search page is that for IG: "Analyse your immunoglobulin (IG) or antibody sequences." Your species (or taxon) selection from the IMGT/V-QUEST Welcome page is recalled at the top of the page (here "Human").

(f) V-REGION alignment.

(g) V-REGION translation.

(h) V-REGION protein display.

(i) V-REGION mutation and AA change table.

(j) V-REGION mutation and AA change statistics.

(k) V-REGION mutation hot spots.

(l) Sequences of V-, V-J-, or V-D-J-REGION ("nt" and "AA") with gaps in FASTA and access to IMGT/PhyloGene for V-REGION ("nt").

(m) Annotation by IMGT/Automat.

(n) IMGT Colliers de Perles:

   - Link to IMGT/Collier-de-Perles tool.
   - IMGT Colliers de Perles (for a nb of sequences <5).
   - No IMGT Collier de Perles.

2. IMGT/V-QUEST "Synthesis view"

   The "Synthesis view" consists in an interesting alternative to the "Detailed view" if several sequences of the same run use the same V gene and allele. Indeed, sequences expressing the same V gene and allele will be aligned together. The results may be displayed in HTML (by default) or Text format, with a user-defined number of nucleotides per line in alignments (60 by default). There are seven different result displays for the alignments of sequences that express the same V gene and allele and the results of IMGT/JunctionAnalysis (9):

   (a) Alignment for V-GENE.

   (b) V-REGION alignment.

   (c) V-REGION translation.

   (d) V-REGION protein display.

   (e) V-REGION protein display (with AA class codons).

   (f) V-REGION protein display (only AA changes displayed).

   (g) V-REGION most frequently occurring AA.

   (h) Results of IMGT/JunctionAnalysis.

   Three of these options (e), (f), and (g) are specific to IMGT/V-QUEST "Synthesis View" (see Note 3).

3. Excel file.

   "Excel file" allows the users to get the results of the analysis in a spreadsheet with the choice of eleven sheets. The "Summary" and "Parameters" sheets are always provided.

   (a) Summary.

   (b) IMGT-gapped-nt-sequences.

(c) nt-sequences.
(d) IMGT-gapped-AA-sequences.
(e) AA-sequences.
(f) Junction.
(g) V-REGION-mutation-and-AA-change-table.
(h) V-REGION-nt-mutation-statistics.
(i) V-REGION-AA-change-statistics.
(j) V-REGION-mutation-hot-spots.
(k) Parameters.

*2.2.3. Advanced Parameters*

Default values of "Advanced parameters" have been set for classical analysis. They should be modified for more sophisticated queries or for unusual sequences (e.g., with insertions or deletions). The options include:

1. "Selection of IMGT reference directory set" with a choice of four sets:
   (a) F+ORF.
   (b) F+ORF+in frame P (by default).
   (c) F+ORF including orphons.
   (d) F+ORF+in frame P including orphons.

   Where F is functional, ORF is open reading frame, P is pseudogene. This allows sequences to be compared with only relevant gene sequences (e.g., orphon sequences are relevant for genomic but not for expressed repertoire studies). The selected set can also be chosen either "With all alleles" or "With allele *01 only" (see Note 4).
2. "Search for insertions and deletions in V-REGION" ("Yes" or "No"): somatic hypermutations by nucleotide insertions and deletions in the V-REGION are rare events that are known to occur in normal and malignant cells (16). By default, IMGT/V-QUEST does not search for insertions and deletions. If "Yes" is selected, the analysis is slower and the number of submitted sequences in a single run is limited to ten (see Note 5).
3. Parameters for IMGT/JunctionAnalysis:
   (a) "Nb of accepted D-GENE": this selection is provided for the IGH junctions (for the IG) and for the TRB and TRD junctions (for the TR).
   (b) "Nb of accepted mutations" in 3′V-REGION, D-REGION, and 5′J-REGION (by default, no mutation is accepted for the TR junctions. For IGH, 2, 4, and 2 mutations are accepted in the 3′V-REGION, D-REGION, and 5′J-REGION, respectively. For the IGK and IGL loci,

the maximum number of accepted mutations is 7 in the 3′V-REGION and 7 in the 5′J-REGION).

4. Parameters for "Detailed view":

   (a) "Nb of nucleotides to exclude in 5′ of the V-REGION for the evaluation of the nb of mutations": in case of primer specific nucleotides.

   (b) "Nb of nucleotides to add (or exclude) in 3′ of the V-REGION for the evaluation of the alignment score": in case of low (or high) exonuclease activity.

### 2.3. IMGT/V-QUEST Output for Detailed View

The top of "Detailed view" results are displayed in "A. Detailed results for the IMGT/V-QUEST analyzed sequences." The top of this page indicates the number of analyzed sequences with links to individual results. Use the link associated with a sequence name to go directly to its individual result that comprises the sequence and "Result summary" followed by the different displayed results as selected in the Search page.

#### 2.3.1. Sequence and Result Summary

The sequence and "Result summary" are shown at the top of each individual result (Fig. 3). The IMGT reference directory set against which the sequence was analyzed (e.g., human IG set) is indicated

**Sequence number 1: seq1**

Sequence compared with the human IG set from the IMGT reference directory

```
>seq1
gaggtgcagctgttggagtctggggaggcgtggtccagcctgggaggtccctgagactc
tcctgtatagcctctggattcaccttcagtagctatcctatgacctgggtccgccaggct
ccaggcaaggggctggagtgggtggcaagtatatcatatgacggaagttataaatataag
gtagactccatgaagggccgactcaccatctccagagacaattccaagaacacgctgtat
ttggaaatgaacagcctgacagctgaggacacggctgtgtattactgtgcgaggacagct
ttctttaacgcctatgacttctggggccagggaaccctggtcaccgtctcctcagcctcc
accaagggcccatcggtcttccccctggcaccctcctccaagagcacctctgggggcaca
gcggccctgggctgcctggtcaaggactacttccccgaaccggtgacggtgtcgtggaac
tcaggcgccctgaccagcggcgtgcacaccttcccggctgtcctacagtcctcaggactc
tactccctcagcagcgtggtgaccgtgccctccagcagcttgggcacccagacctacatc
tgcaacgtgaatcacaagcccagcaacaccaaggtggacaagaaagttgagcccaaatct
tgtgacaaaactcacaca
```

| **Result summary:** | **Productive IGH rearranged sequence** (no stop codon and in-frame junction) | | |
|---|---|---|---|
| V-GENE and allele | IGHV3-30*04 | score = 1255 | identity = 93,06% (268/288 nt) |
| J-GENE and allele | IGHJ4*02 | score = 204 | identity = 91,67% (44/48 nt) |
| D-GENE and allele by IMGT/JunctionAnalysis | IGHD5-5*01 | D-REGION is in reading frame 1 | |
| FR-IMGT lengths, CDR-IMGT lengths and AA JUNCTION | [25.17.38.11] | [8.8.11] | CARTAFFNAYDFW |

Fig. 3. IMGT/V-QUEST "Detailed view" result page: Sequence and "Summary." The upper part of an individual result shows the sequence and "Result summary." The seq1 is the human IGH rearranged sequence with the accession number AB012909 in the IMGT/LIGM-DB database (34).

(Fig. 3). A sequence submitted in antisense orientation will be shown as complementary reverse sequence, which is in V gene sense orientation. The "Result summary" provides a crucial feature that is the evaluation of the user sequence functionality performed automatically by IMGT/V-QUEST: productive (if no stop codon and in-frame junction) or unproductive (if stop codons and/or out-of-frame junction) (see Note 6). It also summarizes the main characteristics of the analyzed sequence which include (1) the names of the closest "V-GENE and allele" (e.g., IGHV3-30*04) and "J-GENE and allele" (e.g., IGHJ4*02) (see Note 7) with the alignment score (see Note 8), the percentage of identity and the ratio of the number of identical nucleotides (nt)/number of aligned nt, (2) the name of the closest "D-GENE and allele" (IGHD5-5*01) determined by IMGT/JunctionAnalysis (9) with the D-REGION reading frame, (3) the FR-IMGT lengths (e.g., [25.17.38.11]), the CDR-IMGT lengths (e.g., [8.8.11]), and the amino acid (AA) JUNCTION sequence which characterizes a V domain. The information shown in Fig. 3 (online in orange) "Productive IGH rearranged sequence" and "93.06%" is used by clinicians analyzing the level of mutations in chronic lymphocytic leukemia (CLL) IGHV rearranged sequences as a prognostic criterion (17) (see Note 9). IMGT/V-QUEST provides warnings (not shown) that appear as notes in red to alert the user, if potential insertions or deletions are suspected in the V-REGION (see Note 10), or if other possibilities for the J-GENE and allele names are identified (see Note 11).

#### 2.3.2. Sequence and Result Summary with the Option "Search for Insertions and Deletions"

If insertions and/or deletions are suspected, as mentioned above (Subheading 2.3.1), the user can go back to the IMGT/V-QUEST Search page and select the option "Search for insertions and deletions" in "Advanced parameters." If indeed insertions and/or deletions are detected, they will be described in the "Result summary" row (Fig. 4) with their localization in FR-IMGT or CDR-IMGT, the number of inserted or deleted nucleotides and, for insertions, the inserted nucleotides, the presence or absence of frameshift, the V-REGION codon from which the insertion or deletion starts and the nt position in the user sequence. The insertions are highlighted in capital letters in the user sequence (Fig. 4) and the tool runs a classical IMGT/V-QUEST search after having removed the insertion(s) from the user sequence. In case of deletions, the tool adds gaps to replace the identified deletions before running a classical IMGT/V-QUEST search. Users should be aware that an insertion or a deletion at the beginning of FR1-IMGT or at the end of the FR3-IMGT may not be detected.

#### 2.3.3. Alignments for V, D, and J Genes and Alleles

The alignments for V, D, J genes and alleles, if selected in the Search page, display the alignments with the five closest V, D, and J gene alleles, respectively, with their alignment score and their

**Sequence number 2: seq2**

Sequence compared with the human IG set from the IMGT reference directory

```
>seq2
gaggtgaaggtggtgcagtctggagcagaggtgaaaaagcccggggagtctctgcacatc
tcctgtcagatttctGCAGACGGTggagacgactttaccactctctggatcggctgggtg
cgccagatgcccgggaaagggctggagtggatggggatcatctggcctggtgactctgat
accacatacagtccgtccttccaaggccacgtctccatttcagccgacaagtccaccagt
accgcctaccttcagtggagcagcctgaaggcctcggactccgccatgtattactgtgcg
accaacagtggttattaccccggggatggctttgattactggggccagggaaccctgatc
attgtctcctca
```

Result summary:

Nucleotide insertions have been detected and automatically removed for this analysis: they are displayed as capital letters in the user submitted sequence above.

| localization in V-REGION | nb of inserted nt | inserted nt | causing frameshift | from V-REGION codon | from nt position in user submitted sequence |
|---|---|---|---|---|---|
| CDR1-IMGT | 9 | GCAGACGGT | no | 27 | 76 |

IMGT/V-QUEST results after removal of the insertion(s):
Potentially productive IGH rearranged sequence: no stop codon and in-frame junction
(Check also your sequence with BLAST against IMGT/GENE-DB reference sequences to eventually identify out-of-frame pseudogenes)

| | | | |
|---|---|---|---|
| V-GENE and allele | IGHV5-51*01 | score = 1201 | identity = 90,97%(262/288 nt)[90,62% (261/288 nt)] |
| J-GENE and allele | IGHJ4*02 | score = 172 | identity = 85,11% (40/47 nt) |
| D-GENE and allele by IMGT/JunctionAnalysis | IGHD3-22*01 | D-REGION is in reading frame 2 | |
| FR-IMGT lengths, CDR-IMGT lengths and AA JUNCTION | [25.17.38.11] | [8.8.14] | CATNSGYYPGDGFDYW |

Fig. 4. IMGT/V-QUEST "Detailed view" result page: Sequence and "Result summary" with the option "Search for insertions and deletions." An insertion of 9 nt was detected by IMGT/V-QUEST. The analysis is then performed after having removed the insertion.

identity percentage (Fig. 5). The alignment for D-GENE and allele should be considered with caution since it may show discrepancies with the results obtained by IMGT/JunctionAnalysis (9) (see Note 12).

*2.3.4. "Results of IMGT/JunctionAnalysis" and "Sequence of the JUNCTION ('nt' and 'AA')"*

The results of IMGT/JunctionAnalysis comprise (Fig. 6):

1. "Analysis of the JUNCTION" (top section of Fig. 6): it provides the name of the D gene and allele (for IGH, TRB, and TRD sequences) and shows the details of the junction at the nucleotide level (nucleotides trimmed at the V, D, and J gene ends and N nucleotides added by the TdT) with an accurate delimitation of the 3′V-REGION (from the 2nd-CYS 104 to the 3′ end of the V-REGION), D-REGION, and 5′J-REGION (from the 5′ end of the J-REGION to J-TRP 118 or J-PHE 118) (see Note 13). Dots represent the nucleotides that have been trimmed by the exonuclease. The number of

## 1. Alignment for V-GENE and allele identification

**Closest V-REGIONs** (evaluated from the V-REGION first nucleotide to the 2nd-CYS codon)

```
                                  Score     Identity
L06615 IGHV3-30*04                1255      93,06% (268/288 nt)
M83134 IGHV3-30*01                1246      92,71% (267/288 nt)
M77300 IGHV3-30*09                1246      92,71% (267/288 nt)
M77324 IGHV3-30*14                1246      92,71% (267/288 nt)
X92283 IGHV3-30-3*01              1246      92,71% (267/288 nt)
```

Alignment with FR-IMGT and CDR-IMGT delimitations

```
                        <-------------------------------- FR1-IMGT ---------------------------->____________ CDR1-IMGT ___________<-----
seq1                    gaggtgcagctgttggagtctggggga...ggcgtggtccagcctgggaggtccctgagactctcctgtatagcctctggattcaccttc............agtagctatcctatgacc
L06615 IGHV3-30*04      c-----------g--------------...---------------------------------------gc-------------------............---------g-----ca-
M83134 IGHV3-30*01      c-----------g--------------...---------------------------------------gc-------------------............---------g-----ca-
M77300 IGHV3-30*09      c-----------g--------------...---------------------------------------gc-------------------............---------g-----ca-
M77324 IGHV3-30*14      c-----------g--------------...---------------------------------------gc-------------------............---------g-----ca-
X92283 IGHV3-30-3*01    c-----------g--------------...---------------------------------------gc-------------------............---------g-----ca-

                        -------------- FR2-IMGT ------------------>__________ CDR2-IMGT ________<-----------------------------------------
seq1                    tgggtccgccaggctccaggcaaggggctggagtgggtggcaagtatatcatatgac......ggaagttataaatataaggtagactccatgaag...ggccgactcaccatctccaga
L06615 IGHV3-30*04      ------------------------------------------gt------------t......------a-------ct-c-c-------g-----...------t--------------
M83134 IGHV3-30*01      -----------------------------a------------gt------------t......------a-------ct-c-c-------g-----...------t--------------
M77300 IGHV3-30*09      ------------------------------------------gt------------t......------a-------ct-c-c-------g-----...------t--g-----------
M77324 IGHV3-30*14      ------------------------------------------gt------------t......------a-------ct-c-c-------g-----...------t--------------
X92283 IGHV3-30-3*01    ------------------------------------------gt------------t......-----ca-------ct-c-c-------g-----...------t--------------

                        -------- FR3-IMGT ---------------------------------------------------->___________ CDR3-IMGT __________
seq1                    gacaattccaagaacacgctgtatttggaaatgaacagcctgacagctgaggacacggctgtgtattactgtgcgaggacagctttctttaacgcctatgacttctggggccagggaacc
L06615 IGHV3-30*04      ------------------------c--c---------------g---------------------------------aga
M83134 IGHV3-30*01      ------------------------c--c---------------g---------------------------------aga
M77300 IGHV3-30*09      ------------------------c--c---------------g---------------------------------aga
M77324 IGHV3-30*14      ------------------------c-tc---------------g---------------------------------aga
X92283 IGHV3-30-3*01    ------------------------c--c---------------g---------------------------------a
```

## 3. Alignment for J-GENE and allele identification

**Closest J-REGIONs**

```
                                  Score     Identity
X86355 IGHJ4*02                   204       91,67% (44/48 nt)
J00256 IGHJ4*01                   195       89,58% (43/48 nt)
M25625 IGHJ4*03                   177       85,42% (41/48 nt)
J00256 IGHJ5*01                   174       82,35% (42/51 nt)
X86355 IGHJ5*02                   174       82,35% (42/51 nt)
```

**Alignment**

```
seq1                    gacagctttctttaacgcctatgacttctggggccagggaaccctggtcaccgtctcctcagcctccaccaagggcccatcggtcttcccccctggcaccctcctccaagagcacctctgg
X86355 IGHJ4*02         ..............--ta--t-----a-----------------------------------
J00256 IGHJ4*01         ..............--ta--t-----a---------a-------------------------
M25625 IGHJ4*03         ..............g-ta--t-----a---------a--g----------------------
J00256 IGHJ5*01         ...........ac---tgg-tc----c---------a-------------------------
X86355 IGHJ5*02         ...........ac---tgg-tc---cc-----------------------------------
```

Fig. 5. IMGT/V-QUEST "Detailed view" result page: "Alignment for V-GENE and allele identification" and "Alignment for J-GENE and allele identification." *Dashes* indicate identical nucleotides. *Dots* indicate gaps. FR-IMGT and CDR-IMGT are delimited according to the IMGT unique numbering (19–21). The seq1 is the human IGH rearranged sequence with the accession number AB012909 in the IMGT/LIGM-DB database (34).

## 4. Results of IMGT/JunctionAnalysis

**Maximum number of accepted mutations in:** 3'V-REGION = 2, D-REGION = 4, 5'J-REGION = 2
**Maximum number of accepted D-GENE =** 1

**Analysis of the JUNCTION**

D-REGION is in reading frame 1.
Click on mutated (underlined) nucleotide to see the original one:

| Input | V name | 3'V-REGION | N1 | D-REGION | N2 | 5'J-REGION | J name | D name | Vmut | Dmut | Jmut | Ngc |
|---|---|---|---|---|---|---|---|---|---|---|---|---|
| seq1 | IGHV3-30*04 | tgtgcgag...g | ......acagct<u>t</u>t<u>c</u>tta. | acgc | ....ct<u>a</u>tgact<u>t</u>ctgg | IGHJ4*02 | IGHD5-5*01 | 0 | 3 | 2 | 4/5 | |

**Eligible D genes:**

| D name | D length | tgtgcgaggacagctttctttaacgcctatgacttctgg | Score# | Mutation# | Location |
|---|---|---|---|---|---|
| IGHD1-1*01 | 17 | ---a-- | 5 | 1 | d[4-9],s[10-15] |
| IGHD2-2*01 | 31 | ----- | 5 | 0 | d[19-23],s[11-15] |
| IGHD2-2*02 | 31 | ----- | 5 | 0 | d[19-23],s[11-15] |
| IGHD2-2*03 | 31 | ----- | 5 | 0 | d[19-23],s[11-15] |
| IGHD3-3*01 | 31 | --t-- | 4 | 1 | d[10-14],s[16-20] |
| IGHD3-3*02 | 31 | ---a--t-- | 7 | 2 | d[6-14],s[12-20] |
| IGHD4-4*01 | 16 | ---- | 4 | 0 | d[10-13],s[21-24] |
| IGHD5-5*01 | 20 | ------a-gg--- | 10 | 3 | d[7-19],s[10-22] |
| IGHD6-6*01 | 18 | ----- | 5 | 0 | d[9-13],s[11-15] |
| IGHD1-7*01 | 17 | ---- | 4 | 0 | d[5-8],s[21-24] |
| IGHD2-8*01 | 31 | --a-- | 4 | 1 | d[25-29],s[18-22] |
| IGHD2-8*02 | 31 | --a-- | 4 | 1 | d[25-29],s[18-22] |
| IGHD3-9*01 | 31 | ---g-- | 5 | 1 | d[13-18],s[19-24] |
| IGHD3-10*01 | 31 | ---- | 4 | 0 | d[28-31],s[21-24] |
| IGHD3-10*02 | 30 | --a-g-- | 5 | 2 | d[7-13],s[14-20] |
| IGHD4-11*01 | 16 | ---- | 4 | 0 | d[10-13],s[21-24] |
| IGHD5-12*01 | 23 | ---acga--- | 6 | 4 | d[13-22],s[13-22] |
| IGHD6-13*01 | 21 | ----- | 5 | 0 | d[12-16],s[11-15] |
| IGHD1-14*01 | 17 | ---- | 4 | 0 | d[5-8],s[21-24] |
| IGHD2-15*01 | 31 | ---- | 4 | 0 | d[20-23],s[12-15] |
| IGHD3-16*01 | 37 | --t-a-gc--- | 7 | 4 | d[23-33],s[12-22] |
| IGHD3-16*02 | 37 | --t-a--g--- | 8 | 3 | d[23-33],s[12-22] |
| IGHD5-18*01 | 20 | ------a-gg--- | 10 | 3 | d[7-19],s[10-22] |
| IGHD1-20*01 | 17 | ---- | 4 | 0 | d[5-8],s[21-24] |
| IGHD2-21*01 | 28 | --g-- | 4 | 1 | d[19-23],s[15-19] |
| IGHD2-21*02 | 28 | ---t--- | 6 | 1 | d[17-23],s[9-15] |
| IGHD3-22*01 | 31 | --a-- | 4 | 1 | d[22-26],s[16-20] |
| IGHD4-23*01 | 19 | ---- | 4 | 0 | d[13-16],s[21-24] |
| IGHD5-24*01 | 20 | ---acaa--- | 6 | 4 | d[10-19],s[13-22] |
| IGHD6-25*01 | 18 | ---- | 4 | 0 | d[9-12],s[11-14] |
| IGHD1-26*01 | 20 | ---- | 4 | 0 | d[12-15],s[12-15] |
| IGHD7-27*01 | 11 | ---- | 4 | 0 | d[2-5],s[21-24] |

**Translation of the JUNCTION**

D-REGION is in reading frame 1.
Click on mutated (underlined) amino acid to see the original one:

| | 104 | 105 | 106 | 107 | 108 | 109 | 110 | 113 | 114 | 115 | 116 | 117 | 118 | Frame | CDR3-IMGT length | Molecular mass | pI |
|---|---|---|---|---|---|---|---|---|---|---|---|---|---|---|---|---|---|
| | C | A | R | T | A | <u>F</u> | <u>F</u> | N | A | <u>Y</u> | D | <u>F</u> | W | | | | |
| seq1 | tgt | gcg | agg | aca | gct | <u>t</u>t<u>c</u> | <u>t</u>tt | aac | gcc | t<u>a</u>t | gac | t<u>t</u>c | tgg | + | 11 | 1,611.8 | 6.44 |

## 5. Sequence of the JUNCTION ('nt' and 'AA')

```
104 105 106 107 108 109 110 113 114 115 116 117 118
 C   A   R   T   A   F   F   N   A   Y   D   F   W
tgt gcg agg aca gct ttc ttt aac gcc tat gac ttc tgg
```

**Input for IMGT/JunctionAnalysis**

```
>seq1,IGHV3-30*04,IGHJ4*02
tgtgcgaggacagctttctttaacgcctatgacttctgg
```

Fig. 6. IMGT/V-QUEST "Detailed view" result page: "Results of IMGT/JunctionAnalysis" (with "Analysis of the JUNCTION," "Eligible D genes" and "Translation of the JUNCTION") and "Sequence of the JUNCTION ('nt' and 'AA')." The seq1 is the human IGH rearranged sequence with the accession number AB012909 in the IMGT/LIGM-DB database (34).

mutations in the 3′V-REGION, D-REGION, and 5′J-REGION is indicated, for example Vmut 0, Dmut 3, Jmut 2 (Fig. 6) and the corresponding mutated nucleotides are underlined. Nucleotides of the N-REGION are displayed in N1 and N2. The ratio of the number of g+c nucleotides to the total number of N nucleotides is indicated under "Ngc," for example in Fig. 6 "Ngc" is 4/5 as there are 4 "c" or "g" in N1+N2 and the total of nt is 5 (g (N1), acgc (N2)). By default, the number of allowed mutations in the IG 3′V-REGION, (D-REGION for IGH) and 5′J-REGION is limited (parameters ′2,(4),2′ for IGH, parameters ′7,7′ for IGK and IGL). Moreover, in case of unmutated IGHV genes (no mutation from FR1-IMGT to FR3-IMGT), the tool does not allow any mutation in the 3′V-REGION and 5′J-REGION and automatically limits the number of allowed mutations in the D-REGION to 2 (parameters "0,(2),0") in order to reflect the low probability of somatic hypermutations. By default, mutations are not allowed for the TR (see Note 14).

2. "Eligible D genes" (middle section of Fig. 6): this option allows to compare the IMGT/JunctionAnalysis D gene identification with all D genes which match the junction with their corresponding score. The D gene allele with the best score, selected by IMGT/JunctionAnalysis, is shown in the rectangle in Fig. 6. The location d[7–19]s[10–22] means that the D-REGION nucleotides (d) from positions 7–19 of the germline IGHD5-5*01 match the sequence (s) of the junction from positions 10–22.
3. "Translation of the JUNCTION" (lower section of Fig. 6): it displays the junction with amino acids colored according to the 11 IMGT physicochemical classes (18) (see Note 15), the frame ("+" and "−" indicate in-frame and out-of-frame, respectively), the CDR3-IMGT length, the molecular mass, and the isoelectric point (pI). In case of frameshifts, gaps (represented by one or two dots) are inserted to maintain the J-REGION frame. The corresponding codon which cannot be translated is represented by "#."
4. "Sequence of the JUNCTION ('nt' and 'AA')": this provides the JUNCTION in nucleotides (nt) and amino acids (AA) according to the IMGT unique numbering, and in the FASTA format with the correctly formatted header required as input by IMGT/JunctionAnalysis online (9).

#### 2.3.5. "V-REGION Alignment," "V-REGION Translation," and "V-REGION Protein Display"

The results provide three displays of the V-REGION (Fig. 7):

1. The "V-REGION alignment according to the IMGT unique numbering" displays the nt sequences with the FR-IMGT and CDR-IMGT delimitations according to the IMGT unique numbering (19–21).

**6. V-REGION alignment according to the IMGT unique numbering**

```
                         <------------------------------------------- FR1 - IMGT
                         1               5                  10                15
seq1                     gag gtg cag ctg ttg gag tct ggg gga ... ggc gtg gtc cag cct
L06615 IGHV3-30*04       c-- --- --- --- g-- --- --- --- --- ... --- --- --- --- ---
M83134 IGHV3-30*01       c-- --- --- --- g-- --- --- --- --- ... --- --- --- --- ---
M77300 IGHV3-30*09       c-- --- --- --- g-- --- --- --- --- ... --- --- --- --- ---
M77324 IGHV3-30*14       c-- --- --- --- g-- --- --- --- --- ... --- --- --- --- ---
X92283 IGHV3-30-3*01     c-- --- --- --- g-- --- --- --- --- ... --- --- --- --- ---

                         ----------------------------------------->  ______________
                                         20                  25                30
seq1                     ggg agg tcc ctg aga ctc tcc tgt ata gcc tct gga ttc acc ttc
L06615 IGHV3-30*04       --- --- --- --- --- --- --- --- gc- --- --- --- --- --- ---
M83134 IGHV3-30*01       --- --- --- --- --- --- --- --- gc- --- --- --- --- --- ---
M77300 IGHV3-30*09       --- --- --- --- --- --- --- --- gc- --- --- --- --- --- ---
M77324 IGHV3-30*14       --- --- --- --- --- --- --- --- gc- --- --- --- --- --- ---
X92283 IGHV3-30-3*01     --- --- --- --- --- --- --- --- gc- --- --- --- --- --- ---

                         __  CDR1 - IMGT  ______________  <-------------------------
                                         35                  40                45
seq1                     ... ... ... ... agt agc tat cct atg acc tgg gtc cgc cag gct
L06615 IGHV3-30*04       ... ... ... ... --- --- --- g-- --- ca- --- --- --- --- ---
M83134 IGHV3-30*01       ... ... ... ... --- --- --- g-- --- ca- --- --- --- --- ---
M77300 IGHV3-30*09       ... ... ... ... --- --- --- g-- --- ca- --- --- --- --- ---
M77324 IGHV3-30*14       ... ... ... ... --- --- --- g-- --- ca- --- --- --- --- ---
X92283 IGHV3-30-3*01     ... ... ... ... --- --- --- g-- --- ca- --- --- --- --- ---
```

**7. V-REGION translation**

```
                         <------------------------------------------- FR1 - IMGT
                         1               5                  10                15
                          E   V   Q   L   L   E   S   G   G       G   V   V   Q   P
seq1                     gag gtg cag ctg ttg gag tct ggg gga ... ggc gtg gtc cag cct
                          Q               V
L06615 IGHV3-30*04       c-- --- --- --- g-- --- --- --- --- ... --- --- --- --- ---

                         ----------------------------------------->  ______________
                                         20                  25                30
                          G   R   S   L   R   L   S   C   I   A   S   G   F   T   F
seq1                     ggg agg tcc ctg aga ctc tcc tgt ata gcc tct gga ttc acc ttc
                                                          A
L06615 IGHV3-30*04       --- --- --- --- --- --- --- --- gc- --- --- --- --- --- ---

                         __  CDR1 - IMGT  ______________  <-------------------------
                                         35                  40                45
                                          S   S   Y   P   M   T   W   V   R   Q   A
seq1                     ... ... ... ... agt agc tat cct atg acc tgg gtc cgc cag gct
                                                      A       H
L06615 IGHV3-30*04       ... ... ... ... --- --- --- g-- --- ca- --- --- --- --- ---
```

**8. V-REGION protein display**

```
                                   FR1-IMGT          CDR1-IMGT       FR2-IMGT       CD
                                    (1-26)            (27-38)         (39-55)        (
                         __________________________ ___________ _________________ __
                         1       10        20        30          40        50
                         .........|.........|...... ...|........ .|.........|..... ..
seq1                     EVQLLESGG.GVVQPGRSLRLSCIAS GFTF....SSYP MTWVRQAPGKGLEWVAS IS
L06615 IGHV3-30*04       QVQLVESGG.GVVQPGRSLRLSCAAS GFTF....SSYA MHWVRQAPGKGLEWVAV IS
                         E   L                 I            P   T                S

                         R2-IMGT                FR3-IMGT
                         56-65)                 (66-104)
                         ________ ______________________________________
                                  60        70        80        90        100
                         ..|..... ....|.........|.........|.........|....
seq1                     YD..GSYK YKVDSMK.GRLTISRDNSKNTLYLEMNSLTAEDTAVYYC A
L06615 IGHV3-30*04       YD..GSNK YYADSVK.GRFTISRDNSKNTLYLQMNSLRAEDTAVYYC AR
                               Y  KV  M   L               E     T
```

Fig. 7. IMGT/V-QUEST “Detailed view” result page: Three displays of the V-REGION. The seq1 is the human IGH rearranged sequence with the accession number AB012909 in the IMGT/LIGM-DB database (34). Only a part of each of the three displays is shown.

2. The "V-REGION translation" displays the nt sequence and deduced AA translation of the input sequence, aligned with the closest germline V-REGION, and with the FR-IMGT and CDR-IMGT delimitations.
3. The "V-REGION protein display" displays the deduced AA translation of the input sequence, aligned with the V-REGION translation of the closest germline V-GENE and with the FR-IMGT and CDR-IMGT delimitations, and with the third line of the alignment and shown in bold, the AA of the input sequence which are different from the closest germline V-REGION.

#### 2.3.6. Analysis of the Mutations: "V-REGION Mutation and AA Change Table," "V-REGION Mutation and AA Change Statistics," and "V-REGION Mutation Hot Spots"

The analysis of the mutations in the V-REGION is performed by comparison of the analyzed sequence with the closest germline V gene and allele.

1. The "V-REGION mutation and AA change table" (Fig. 8) lists the nt mutations and the corresponding AA changes if the mutations are not silent. They are described for each FR-IMGT and CDR-IMGT, with their nt and codon position according to the IMGT unique numbering (19–21) and for the AA changes according to the IMGT AA classes (18). For example, c1 > g, Q1 > E (++−) means that the nt mutation (c > g) at nt 1 leads to an AA change (Q > E) at codon 1 with the same hydropathy (+) and volume (+), but with different physicochemical properties (−) classes. It is the first time that such qualification of amino acid replacement is provided. This has led to identify four types of AA changes: very similar (+++), similar (++−, +−+), dissimilar (−−+, −+−, +−−), and very dissimilar (−−−).
2. The "V-REGION mutation and AA change statistics" (Fig. 8) comprises two tables, the first one for "Nucleotide (nt) mutations" described as silent/nonsilent, transitions/transversions, and the second one for "Amino acid (AA) changes." For both tables, results are given for the V-REGION and for FR-IMGT and CDR-IMGT. Statistics are calculated up to the 3′ end of the V-REGION identified in the input sequence (this includes the 3′ last two identical nucleotides with the closest germline V-REGION). The numbers in parentheses, in the V-REGION and CDR3-IMGT columns, correspond to the statistics calculated up to the 3′ end of the closest germline V-REGION and therefore may include nt and AA differences due to the junction diversity.

In order to avoid to count sequence differences due to the 5′ primer in "V-REGION mutation and AA change table" and in "V-REGION mutation and AA change statistics," before launching the analysis it is possible to exclude in 5′ of the V-REGION, a given number of nucleotides, defined by the user, in "Advanced

**9. V-REGION mutation and AA change table**

| FR1-IMGT | CDR1-IMGT | FR2-IMGT | CDR2-IMGT | FR3-IMGT | CDR3-IMGT |
|---|---|---|---|---|---|
| c1>g, Q1>E (+ + -) | g112>c, A38>P (- - -) | c118>a, H40>T (+ - -) | t177>c | c198>t | a318>g |
| g13>t, V5>L (+ - +) | | a119>c, H40>T (+ - -) | a190>t, N64>Y (- - -) | t199>a, Y67>K (- - -) | g319>a |
| g70>a, A24>I (+ - +) | | g163>a, V55>S (- - -) | | c201>g, Y67>K (- - -) | a320>c |
| c71>t, A24>I (+ - +) | | t164>g, V55>S (- - -) | | c203>t, A68>V (+ - +) | |
| | | | | g211>a, V71>M (+ - -) | |
| | | | | t226>c, F76>L (+ - -) | |
| | | | | c265>t | |
| | | | | c268>g, Q90>E (+ + -) | |
| | | | | g284>c, R95>T (- - -) | |

**10. V-REGION mutation and AA change statistics**

**Nucleotide (nt) mutations**

| IMGT labels | | V-REGION | FR1-IMGT | CDR1-IMGT | FR2-IMGT | CDR2-IMGT | FR3-IMGT | CDR3-IMGT |
|---|---|---|---|---|---|---|---|---|
| Nb of positions including IMGT gaps (nt) | | **317** (320) | 78 | 36 | 51 | 30 | 117 | 5 (8) |
| Nb of nucleotides | | **293** (296) | 75 | 24 | 51 | 24 | 114 | 5 (8) |
| Nb of identical nucleotides | | **273** | 71 | 23 | 47 | 22 | 105 | 5 |
| Nb of mutations | | **20** (23) | 4 | 1 | 4 | 2 | 9 | 0 (3) |
| Mutations | Silent | **3** (6) | 0 | 0 | 0 | 1 | 2 | 0 (3) |
| | Nonsilent | **17** | 4 | 1 | 4 | 1 | 7 | 0 |
| Transitions | a>g | **0** (1) | 0 | 0 | 0 | 0 | 0 | 0 (1) |
| | g>a | **3** (4) | 1 | 0 | 1 | 0 | 1 | 0 (1) |
| | c>t | **4** | 1 | 0 | 0 | 0 | 3 | 0 |
| | t>c | **2** | 0 | 0 | 0 | 1 | 1 | 0 |
| Transversions | a>c | **1** (2) | 0 | 0 | 1 | 0 | 0 | 0 (1) |
| | c>a | **1** | 0 | 0 | 1 | 0 | 0 | 0 |
| | a>t | **1** | 0 | 0 | 0 | 1 | 0 | 0 |
| | t>a | **1** | 0 | 0 | 0 | 0 | 1 | 0 |
| | g>c | **2** | 0 | 1 | 0 | 0 | 1 | 0 |
| | c>g | **3** | 1 | 0 | 0 | 0 | 2 | 0 |
| | g>t | **1** | 1 | 0 | 0 | 0 | 0 | 0 |
| | t>g | **1** | 0 | 0 | 1 | 0 | 0 | 0 |

**Amino acid (AA) changes**

| IMGT labels | | | V-REGION | FR1-IMGT | CDR1-IMGT | FR2-IMGT | CDR2-IMGT | FR3-IMGT | CDR3-IMGT |
|---|---|---|---|---|---|---|---|---|---|
| Nb of positions including IMGT gaps (AA) | | | **105** (106) | 26 | 12 | 17 | 10 | 39 | 1 (2) |
| Nb of AA | | | **97** (98) | 25 | 8 | 17 | 8 | 38 | 1 (2) |
| Nb of identical AA | | | **84** (85) | 22 | 7 | 15 | 7 | 32 | 1 (2) |
| Nb of AA changes | | | **13** | 3 | 1 | 2 | 1 | 6 | 0 |
| AA changes | Very similar | (+ + +) | **0** | 0 | 0 | 0 | 0 | 0 | 0 |
| | Similar | (+ + -) | **2** | 1 | 0 | 0 | 0 | 1 | 0 |
| | | (+ - +) | **3** | 2 | 0 | 0 | 0 | 1 | 0 |
| | | (+ - -) | **3** | 0 | 0 | 1 | 0 | 2 | 0 |
| | | (- + -) | **0** | 0 | 0 | 0 | 0 | 0 | 0 |
| | Dissimilar | (- - +) | **0** | 0 | 0 | 0 | 0 | 0 | 0 |
| | Very dissimilar | (- - -) | **5** | 0 | 1 | 1 | 1 | 2 | 0 |

Fig. 8. IMGT/V-QUEST "Detailed view" result page: "V-REGION mutation and AA change table" and "V-REGION mutation and AA change statistics." Results are for the human IGH rearranged sequence AB012909 of the IMGT/LIGM-DB database (34) by comparison with the germline IGHV3-30*04.

parameters" (Parameters for "Detailed view" in the IMGT/V-QUEST Search page).

The positions of the mutations have been correlated with the presence of specific patterns in the germline V gene and allele

**11. V-REGION mutation hot spots (motifs and localizations in germline V-REGION)**

**(a/t)a**
**wa**

| Motif | Localization |
|---|---|
| ta | 105-106 (CDR1) |
| ta | 109-110 (CDR1) |
| ta | 114-115 (CDR1) |
| aa | 142-143 (FR2) |
| ta | 165-166 (FR2-CDR2) |
| ta | 167-168 (CDR2) |
| ta | 172-173 (CDR2) |
| aa | 186-187 (CDR2) |
| ta | 189-190 (CDR2) |
| ta | 192-193 (CDR2) |
| aa | 194-195 (CDR2) |
| ta | 196-197 (FR3) |
| ta | 199-200 (FR3) |
| aa | 214-215 (FR3) |
| aa | 244-245 (FR3) |
| aa | 250-251 (FR3) |
| aa | 253-254 (FR3) |
| ta | 262-263 (FR3) |
| aa | 269-270 (FR3) |
| aa | 274-275 (FR3) |
| ta | 304-305 (FR3) |
| ta | 307-308 (FR3) |

**t(a/t)**
**tw**

| Motif | Localization |
|---|---|
| tt | 82-83 (CDR1) |
| tt | 88-89 (CDR1) |
| ta | 105-106 (CDR1) |
| ta | 109-110 (CDR1) |
| ta | 114-115 (CDR1) |
| tt | 164-165 (FR2) |
| ta | 167-168 (CDR2) |
| ta | 172-173 (CDR2) |
| ta | 189-190 (CDR2) |
| ta | 192-193 (CDR2) |
| ta | 196-197 (FR3) |
| ta | 199-200 (FR3) |
| tt | 226-227 (FR3) |
| tt | 246-247 (FR3) |
| ta | 262-263 (FR3) |
| ta | 304-305 (FR3) |
| tt | 306-307 (FR3) |

**(a/g)g(c/t)(a/t)**
**rgyw**

| Motif | Localization |
|---|---|
| agct | 8-11 (FR1) |
| agta | 103-106 (CDR1) |
| ggct | 132-135 (FR2) |
| ggca | 139-142 (FR2) |
| ggct | 146-149 (FR2) |
| ggca | 159-162 (FR2) |
| agta | 187-190 (CDR2) |
| agct | 285-288 (FR3) |
| ggct | 297-300 (FR3) |

**(a/t)(a/g)c(c/t)**
**wrcy**

| Motif | Localization |
|---|---|
| agct | 8-11 (FR1) |
| agcc | 41-44 (FR1) |
| agcc | 72-75 (FR1) |
| agct | 106-109 (CDR1) |
| tgct | 111-114 (CDR1) |
| tact | 196-199 (FR3) |
| agcc | 277-280 (FR3) |
| agct | 285-288 (FR3) |
| tact | 307-310 (FR3) |

Fig. 9. IMGT/V-QUEST "Detailed view" result page: "V-REGION mutation hot spots (motifs and localization of hot spots in germline V-REGION)." Mutation hot spots are those of the human IGHV3-30*04 allele.

(see Somatic hypermutations, in IMGT Education: http://www.imgt.org/IMGTeducation/Tutorials/IGandBcells/_UK/SomaticHypermutations/). The "V-REGION mutation hot spots" table (Fig. 9) shows the localization of the hot spot patterns (a/t)a (or wa) and (a/g)g(c/t)(a/t) (or rgyw) and their complementary reverse motifs t(a/t) (or tw) and (a/t)(a/g)c(c/t) (or wrcy) in the closest germline V gene and allele.

*2.3.7. Sequences of V-, V-J- or V-D-J-REGION ("nt" and "AA") with Gaps in FASTA and Access to IMGT/PhyloGene for V-REGION ("nt")*

This result provides nt and AA sequences with gaps according to the IMGT unique numbering (19–21) and includes (Fig. 10) the "V-REGION nucleotide sequence in FASTA format" with access to the IMGT/PhyloGene tool (22), "V-REGION amino acid in FASTA format," "V-REGION amino acid on one line," V-J or V-D-J-REGION nt and AA sequences in FASTA format, and V-J or V-D-J-REGION AA sequence on one line. In that option, the J reading frame of sequences with an out-of-frame junction is not restored (the sequence does not include "#") and a note alerts the user.

*2.3.8. Annotation by IMGT/Automat*

The results of the analysis of the input sequence by IMGT/Automat (23, 24) provide a full automatic annotation for the V-J-REGION or V-D-J-REGION using IMGT® standardized labels (Fig. 11).

## 12. 'AB012909' V-REGION and V-D-J-REGION

**V-REGION nucleotide sequence in FASTA format**

```
>AB012909
gaggtgcagctgttggagtctgggga...ggcgtggtccagcctgggaggtccctgaga
ctctcctgtatagcctctggattcaccttc............agtagctatcctatgacc
tgggtccgccaggctccaggcaaggggctggagtgggtggcaagtatatcatatgac...
...ggaagttataaatataaggtagactccatgaag...ggccgactcaccatctccaga
gacaattccaagaacacgctgtatttggaaatgaacagcctgacagctgaggacacggct
gtgtattactgtgcgag
```

Analyse this sequence with IMGT/PhyloGene

**V-REGION amino acid sequence in FASTA format**

```
>AB012909
EVQLLESGG.GVVQPGRSLRLSCIASGFTF....SSYPMTWVRQAPGKGLEWVASISYD.
.GSYKYKVDSMK.GRLTISRDNSKNTLYLEMNSLTAEDTAVYYCA
```

**V-REGION amino acid sequence on one line**

```
>AB012909
EVQLLESGG.GVVQPGRSLRLSCIASGFTF....SSYPMTWVRQAPGKGLEWVASISYD..GSYKYKVDSMK.GR
```

**V-D-J-REGION nucleotide sequence in FASTA format**

```
>AB012909
gaggtgcagctgttggagtctgggga...ggcgtggtccagcctgggaggtccctgaga
ctctcctgtatagcctctggattcaccttc............agtagctatcctatgacc
tgggtccgccaggctccaggcaaggggctggagtgggtggcaagtatatcatatgac...
...ggaagttataaatataaggtagactccatgaag...ggccgactcaccatctccaga
gacaattccaagaacacgctgtatttggaaatgaacagcctgacagctgaggacacggct
gtgtattactgtgcgaggacagctttctttaacgcctatgacttctggggccagggaacc
ctggtcaccgtctcctcag
```

**V-D-J-REGION amino acid sequence in FASTA format**

```
>AB012909
EVQLLESGG.GVVQPGRSLRLSCIASGFTF....SSYPMTWVRQAPGKGLEWVASISYD.
.GSYKYKVDSMK.GRLTISRDNSKNTLYLEMNSLTAEDTAVYYCARTAFFNAYDFWGQGT
LVTVSS
```

**V-D-J-REGION amino acid sequence on one line**

```
EVQLLESGG.GVVQPGRSLRLSCIASGFTF....SSYPMTWVRQAPGKGLEWVASISYD..GSYKYKVDSMK.GR
```

Fig. 10. IMGT/V-QUEST "Detailed view" result page: V-REGION and V-(D)-J-REGION sequences with IMGT gaps. Sequences ("nt" and "AA") are for the human IGH rearranged sequence AB012909 of the IMGT/LIGM-DB database (34). The 3′ end of the "on one line" sequences are not shown owing to the figure format.

*2.3.9. IMGT Colliers de Perles*

The "IMGT Collier de Perles" (25–27) can be displayed either as a "link to IMGT/Collier-de-Perles tool" or as a direct "IMGT Collier de Perles (for a number of sequences <5)" representation integrated in IMGT/V-QUEST results (Fig. 12), depending on the user selection in the IMGT/V-QUEST Search page (see Note 16).

### 2.4. IMGT/V-QUEST Output for "Synthesis View"

The "Synthesis view" results are displayed in "B. Synthesis for the IMGT/V-QUEST analyzed sequences." At the top of the page, the number of analyzed sequences is indicated.

*2.4.1. Summary Table*

The "Summary table" (Fig. 13) displays one row for each input sequence with the corresponding results, including: (1) the name of the sequence (Sequence ID), (2) the name of the closest

## 13. Annotation by IMGT/Automat

```
        Label       Location/Qualifiers
V-D-J-REGION        1..355
                    /CDR_length="[8.8.11]"
                    /FR_length="[25.17.38.11]"
                    /nucleotide sequence
                    gaggtgcagctgttggagtctgggggaggcgtggtccagcctgggaggtccctgagactc
                    tcctgtatagcctctggattcaccttcagtagctatcctatgacctgggtccgccaggct
                    ccaggcaaggggctggagtgggtggcaagtatatcatatgacggaagttataaatataag
                    gtagactccatgaagggccgactcaccatctccagagacaattccaagaacacgctgtat
                    ttggaaatgaacagcctgacagctgaggacacggctgtgtattactgtgcgaggacagct
                    ttctttaacgcctatgacttctggggccagggaaccctggtcaccgtctcctcag
                    /translation
                    EVQLLESGGGVVQPGRSLRLSCIASGFTFSSYPMTWVRQAPGKGLEWVASISYDGSYKYK
                    VDSMKGRLTISRDNSKNTLYLEMNSLTAEDTAVYYCARTAFFNAYDFWGQGTLVTVSS
V-REGION            1..293
                    /allele="IGHV3-30*04"
                    /gene="IGHV3-30"
                    /nucleotide sequence
                    gaggtgcagctgttggagtctgggggaggcgtggtccagcctgggaggtccctgagactc
                    tcctgtatagcctctggattcaccttcagtagctatcctatgacctgggtccgccaggct
                    ccaggcaaggggctggagtgggtggcaagtatatcatatgacggaagttataaatataag
                    gtagactccatgaagggccgactcaccatctccagagacaattccaagaacacgctgtat
                    ttggaaatgaacagcctgacagctgaggacacggctgtgtattactgtgcgag
                    /translation
                    EVQLLESGGGVVQPGRSLRLSCIASGFTFSSYPMTWVRQAPGKGLEWVASISYDGSYKYK
                    VDSMKGRLTISRDNSKNTLYLEMNSLTAEDTAVYYCA
FR1-IMGT            1..75
                    /AA_IMGT="AA 1 to 26, AA 10 is missing"
                    /nucleotide sequence
                    gaggtgcagctgttggagtctgggggaggcgtggtccagcctgggaggtccctgagactc
                    tcctgtatagcctct
                    /translation
                    EVQLLESGGGVVQPGRSLRLSCIAS
1st-CYS             64..66
                    /nucleotide sequence
                    tgt
                    /translation
                    C
CDR1-IMGT           76..99
```

Fig. 11. IMGT/V-QUEST "Detailed view" result page: "Annotation by IMGT/Automat." Results are for the human IGH rearranged sequence AB012909 of the IMGT/LIGM-DB database (34). Only a part of the annotation is shown.

V-GENE and allele (see Note 7), (3) the functionality of the sequence (when found, the presence of stop codons is indicated), (4) the V-REGION score (see Note 8), (5) the V-REGION percentage of identity with, between parentheses, the ratio of number of identical nucleotides (nt)/number of aligned nt (see Note 17), (6) the name of the closest J-GENE and allele (see Note 18), (7) and, provided according to the IMGT/JunctionAnalysis results, the D-GENE and allele name, the D reading frame, the CDR-IMGT lengths, the AA JUNCTION, and the JUNCTION frame. In the absence of results of IMGT/JunctionAnalysis, only the AA JUNCTION defined by IMGT/V-QUEST is displayed.

*2.4.2. Results of IMGT/JunctionAnalysis*

Below the "Summary table," use the links associated to the locus name(s) (e.g., IGH) to display "Results of IMGT/JunctionAnalysis" for sequences identified by the tool as belonging to the same locus

**14. IMGT Collier de Perles for seq1**

IMGT/V-QUEST identified region: V-D-J-REGION

CDR-IMGT lengths: [8.8.11]
FR-IMGT lengths: [25.17.38.11]

CDR-IMGT and FR-IMGT lengths are based on the IMGT unique numbering for V-DOMAIN

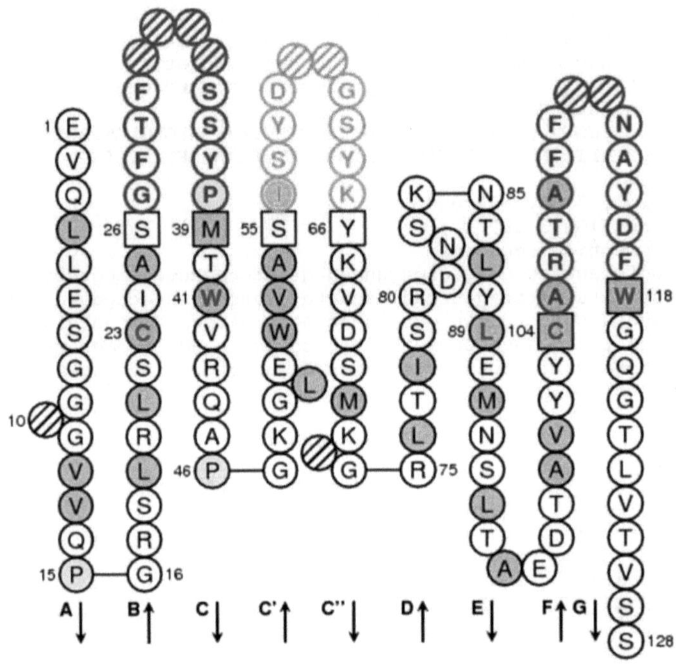


Fig. 12. IMGT/V-QUEST "Detailed view" result page: IMGT Collier de Perles. The IMGT Collier de Perles was obtained with the option "IMGT Collier de Perles (for a nb of sequences <5)" of the human IGH rearranged sequence AB012909 of the IMGT/LIGM-DB database (34). Anchor positions are shown as *squares*. In FR-IMGT, the hydrophobic amino acids (hydropathy index with positive value) and tryptophan (W) found at a given position in more than 50% of sequences are displayed (online with a blue background color).

(Fig. 14). Results are displayed for the IGH, IGK, or IGL locus for IG sequences, and for the TRA, TRB, TRG, or TRD locus for TR sequences. They are similar to those obtained for individual sequences detailed in Subheading 2.3.4.

*2.4.3. Alignment with the Closest Alleles*

The synthesis results provide six different displays (if all were selected): "Alignment for V-GENE," "V-REGION alignment according to the IMGT unique numbering" and "V-REGION translation" (Fig. 15), and "V-REGION protein display" in three different formats (Fig. 16).

*2.4.4. V-REGION Most Frequently Occurring AA Per Position and Per FR-IMGT and CDR-IMGT*

This section shows, for each FR-IMGT and CDR-IMGT, and for each position according to the IMGT unique numbering (19–21), the most frequently occurring amino acid (AA) (Fig. 17).

**B. Synthesis for the IMGT/V-QUEST analysed sequences**

**Number of analysed sequences:** 7

Sequences compared with the human IG set from the IMGT reference directory

**Summary table:**

| Sequence ID | V-GENE and allele | Functionality | V-REGION score | V-REGION identity % (nt) | J-GENE and allele | D-GENE and allele | D-REGION reading frame | CDR-IMGT lengths | AA JUNCTION | JUNCTION frame |
|---|---|---|---|---|---|---|---|---|---|---|
| seq1 | IGHV1-69*01 | Productive | 1273 | 93,75% (270/288 nt) | IGHJ4*01 or IGHJ4*02 or IGHJ4*03 | IGHD3-22*01 | 2 | [8.8.12] | CARQYGSSGYYAYW | in-frame |
| seq2 | IGHV3-30*03, or IGHV3-30*18 | Productive | 1417 | 99,31% (286/288 nt) | IGHJ6*02 | IGHD3-16*02 | 2 | [8.8.23] | CAKDLDDYVWGSYRHSRYYYGMDFW | in-frame |
| seq3 | IGHV3-30*04 | Productive | 1255 | 93,06% (268/288 nt) | IGHJ4*02 | IGHD5-5*01 | 1 | [8.8.11] | CARTAFFNAYDFW | in-frame |
| seq4 | IGHV3-30*04 | Productive | 1435 | 100,00% (288/288 nt) | IGHJ4*02 | IGHD6-19*01 | 2 | [8.8.15] | CARDRSIAVAQYYFDYW | in-frame |
| seq5 | IGHV3-30*04 | Productive | 1408 | 98,96% (285/288 nt) | IGHJ4*02 | IGHD6-13*01 | 2 | [8.8.17] | CARDSSYPPGIAAAGVXYW | in-frame |
| seq6 | IGHV3-30*04 | Productive | 1426 | 99,65% (287/288 nt) | IGHJ1*01 | IGHD3-10*01 | 2 | [8.8.16] | CARGRTKGSGRPGYFQHW | in-frame |
| seq7 | IGHV3-9*01 | Unproductive (stop codons) | 1417 | 99,31% (286/288 nt) | IGHJ4*02 | IGHD3-10*01 | 2 | [8.8.17] | CAKDIGGKYGSGGSGLD*W | in-frame |

- **Results of IMGT/JunctionAnalysis for:** IGH **junctions**
- **Alignment with the closest alleles:**

**The analysed sequences are aligned with the closest allele (with number of aligned sequences in parentheses):**

IGHV1-69*01(1) IGHV3-30*03(1) IGHV3-30*04(4) IGHV3-9*01(1)

Fig. 13. IMGT/V-QUEST "Synthesis view" result page: Top of the page: The seq1, seq2, seq3, seq4, seq5, seq6, and seq7 correspond to the DQ100777, AB021524, AB012909, AB021511, AB021516, AB021514, and AB021539 accession numbers, respectively, from the IMGT/LIGM-DB database (34).

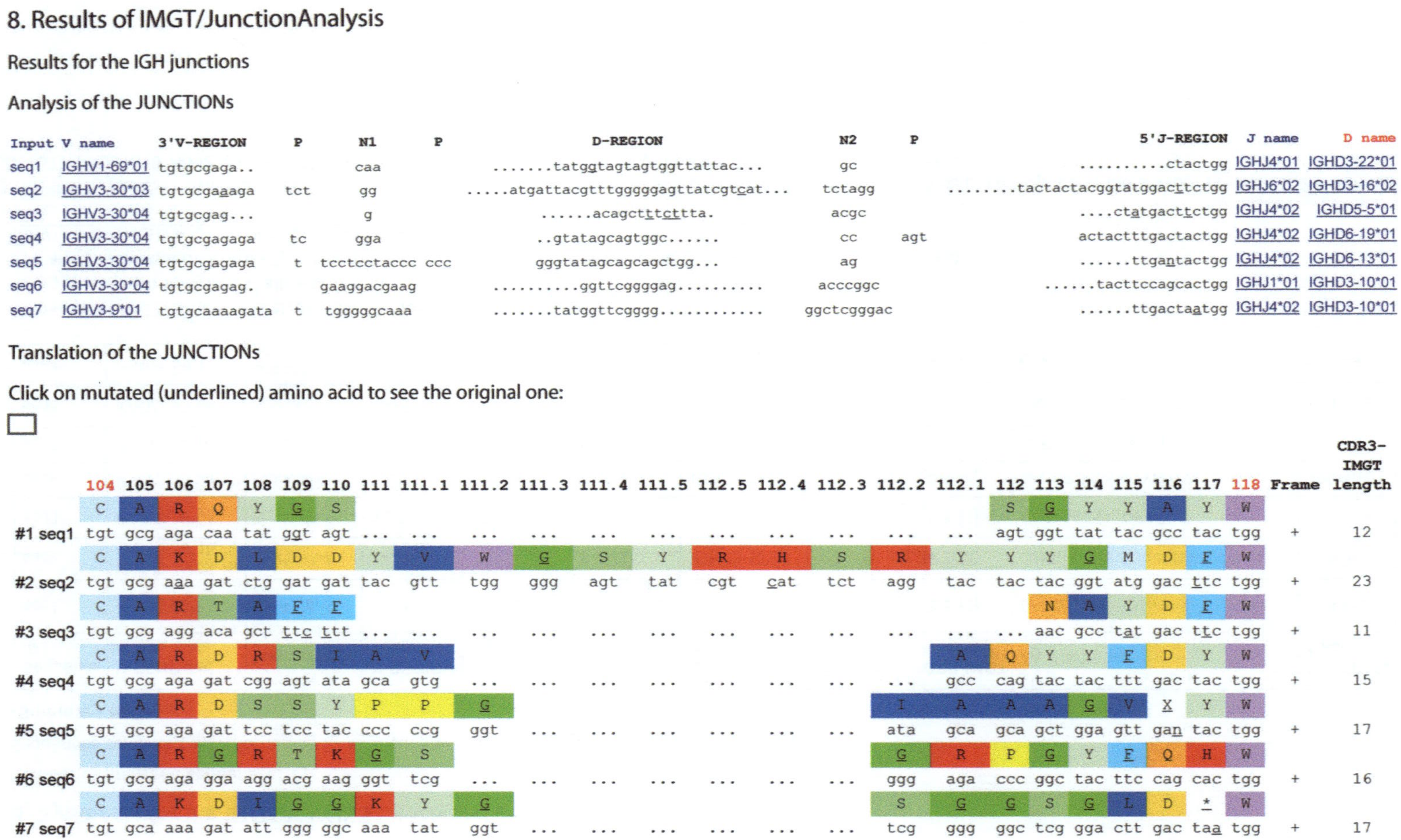

## 8. Results of IMGT/JunctionAnalysis

Results for the IGH junctions

Analysis of the JUNCTIONs

| Input | V name | 3'V-REGION | P | N1 | P | D-REGION | N2 | P | 5'J-REGION | J name | D name |
|---|---|---|---|---|---|---|---|---|---|---|---|
| seq1 | IGHV1-69*01 | tgtgcgaga.. | | caa | | .......tatggtagtagtggttattac... | gc | | ..........ctactgg | IGHJ4*01 | IGHD3-22*01 |
| seq2 | IGHV3-30*03 | tgtgcgaaaga | tct | gg | | .....atgattacgtttggggggagttatcgtcat... | tctagg | | ........tactactacggtatggacttctgg | IGHJ6*02 | IGHD3-16*02 |
| seq3 | IGHV3-30*04 | tgtgcgag... | | g | | ......acagctttcttta. | acgc | | ....ctatgacttctgg | IGHJ4*02 | IGHD5-5*01 |
| seq4 | IGHV3-30*04 | tgtgcgagaga | tc | gga | | ..gtatagcagtggc...... | cc | agt | actactttgactactgg | IGHJ4*02 | IGHD6-19*01 |
| seq5 | IGHV3-30*04 | tgtgcgagaga | t | tcctcctaccc | ccc | gggtatagcagcagctgg... | ag | | ......ttgantactgg | IGHJ4*02 | IGHD6-13*01 |
| seq6 | IGHV3-30*04 | tgtgcgagag. | | gaaggacgaag | | ..........ggttcggggag.......... | acccggc | | ......tacttccagcactgg | IGHJ1*01 | IGHD3-10*01 |
| seq7 | IGHV3-9*01 | tgtgcaaaagata | t | tgggggcaaa | | .......tatggttcgggg............ | ggctcgggac | | ......ttgactaatgg | IGHJ4*02 | IGHD3-10*01 |

Translation of the JUNCTIONs

Click on mutated (underlined) amino acid to see the original one:

| | 104 | 105 | 106 | 107 | 108 | 109 | 110 | 111 | 111.1 | 111.2 | 111.3 | 111.4 | 111.5 | 112.5 | 112.4 | 112.3 | 112.2 | 112.1 | 112 | 113 | 114 | 115 | 116 | 117 | 118 | Frame | CDR3-IMGT length |
|---|---|---|---|---|---|---|---|---|---|---|---|---|---|---|---|---|---|---|---|---|---|---|---|---|---|---|---|
| | C | A | R | Q | Y | G | S | | | | | | | | | | | | S | G | Y | Y | A | Y | W | | |
| #1 seq1 | tgt | gcg | aga | caa | tat | ggt | agt | ... | ... | ... | ... | ... | ... | ... | ... | ... | ... | ... | agt | ggt | tat | tac | gcc | tac | tgg | + | 12 |
| | C | A | K | D | L | D | D | Y | V | W | G | S | Y | R | H | S | R | Y | Y | Y | G | M | D | F | W | | |
| #2 seq2 | tgt | gcg | aaa | gat | ctg | gat | gat | tac | gtt | tgg | ggg | agt | tat | cgt | cat | tct | agg | tac | tac | tac | ggt | atg | gac | ttc | tgg | + | 23 |
| | C | A | R | T | A | F | F | | | | | | | | | | | | | N | A | Y | D | F | W | | |
| #3 seq3 | tgt | gcg | agg | aca | gct | ttc | ttt | ... | ... | ... | ... | ... | ... | ... | ... | ... | ... | ... | ... | aac | gcc | tat | gac | ttc | tgg | + | 11 |
| | C | A | R | D | R | S | I | A | V | | | | | | | | | A | Q | Y | Y | F | D | Y | W | | |
| #4 seq4 | tgt | gcg | aga | gat | cgg | agt | ata | gca | gtg | ... | ... | ... | ... | ... | ... | ... | ... | gcc | cag | tac | tac | ttt | gac | tac | tgg | + | 15 |
| | C | A | R | D | S | S | Y | P | P | G | | | | | | | I | A | A | A | G | V | X | Y | W | | |
| #5 seq5 | tgt | gcg | aga | gat | tcc | tcc | tac | ccc | ccg | ggt | ... | ... | ... | ... | ... | ... | ata | gca | gca | gct | gga | gtt | gan | tac | tgg | + | 17 |
| | C | A | R | G | R | T | K | G | S | | | | | | | | G | R | P | G | Y | F | Q | H | W | | |
| #6 seq6 | tgt | gcg | aga | gga | agg | acg | aag | ggt | tcg | ... | ... | ... | ... | ... | ... | ... | ggg | aga | ccc | ggc | tac | ttc | cag | cac | tgg | + | 16 |
| | C | A | K | D | I | G | G | K | Y | G | | | | | | | S | G | G | S | G | L | D | * | W | | |
| #7 seq7 | tgt | gca | aaa | gat | att | ggg | ggc | aaa | tat | ggt | ... | ... | ... | ... | ... | ... | tcg | ggg | ggc | tcg | gga | ctt | gac | taa | tgg | + | 17 |

Fig. 14. IMGT/V-QUEST "Synthesis view" result page: Results of IMGT/JunctionAnalysis. The results show the "Analysis of the JUNCTIONs" and the "Translation of the JUNCTIONs" for the IGH sequences of the submitted analysis. Owing to the figure format, Vmut, Dmut, Jmut, Ngc, molecular mass, and pI are not shown.

## 1. Alignment for V-GENE

```
                         <---------------------------------- FR1-IMGT --------------
L06615 IGHV3-30*04       caggtgcagctggtggagtctgggggga...ggcgtggtccagcctgggaggtccctgaga
seq3                     g-----------t--------------...------------------------------
seq4                     ---------------------------...------------------------------
seq5                     ---------------------------...----------------------------a-
seq6                     ---------------------------...------------------------------

                         ----------------->_____________ CDR1-IMGT ___________<-----
L06615 IGHV3-30*04       ctctcctgtgcagcctctggattcaccttc............agtagctatgctatgcac
seq3                     ---------at-------------------............---------c-----ac-
seq4                     ------------------------------............------------------
seq5                     ------------------------------............------------------
seq6                     ------------------------------............------------------
```

## 2. V-REGION alignment according to the IMGT unique numbering

```
                         <--------------------------------------------  FR1 - IMGT
                         1           5                   10                  15
L06615 IGHV3-30*04       cag gtg cag ctg gtg gag tct ggg gga ... ggc gtg gtc cag cct
seq3                     g-- --- --- --- t-- --- --- --- --- ... --- --- --- --- ---
seq4                     --- --- --- --- --- --- --- --- --- ... --- --- --- --- ---
seq5                     --- --- --- --- --- --- --- --- --- ... --- --- --- --- ---
seq6                     --- --- --- --- --- --- --- --- --- ... --- --- --- --- ---

                         ------------------------------------------> _______________
                                         20                  25                  30
L06615 IGHV3-30*04       ggg agg tcc ctg aga ctc tcc tgt gca gcc tct gga ttc acc ttc
seq3                     --- --- --- --- --- --- --- --- at- --- --- --- --- --- ---
seq4                     --- --- --- --- --- --- --- --- --- --- --- --- --- --- ---
seq5                     --- --- --- --- -a- --- --- --- --- --- --- --- --- --- ---
seq6                     --- --- --- --- --- --- --- --- --- --- --- --- --- --- ---
```

## 3. V-REGION translation

```
                         <--------------------------------------------  FR1 - IMGT
                         1           5                   10                  15
                          Q   V   Q   L   V   E   S   G   G       G   V   V   Q   P
L06615 IGHV3-30*04       cag gtg cag ctg gtg gag tct ggg gga ... ggc gtg gtc cag cct
                          E               L
seq3                     g-- --- --- --- t-- --- --- --- --- ... --- --- --- --- ---

seq4                     --- --- --- --- --- --- --- --- --- ... --- --- --- --- ---

seq5                     --- --- --- --- --- --- --- --- --- ... --- --- --- --- ---

seq6                     --- --- --- --- --- --- --- --- --- ... --- --- --- --- ---


                         ------------------------------------------> _______________
                                         20                  25                  30
                          G   R   S   L   R   L   S   C   A   A   S   G   F   T   F
L06615 IGHV3-30*04       ggg agg tcc ctg aga ctc tcc tgt gca gcc tct gga ttc acc ttc
                                                          I
seq3                     --- --- --- --- --- --- --- --- at- --- --- --- --- --- ---

seq4                     --- --- --- --- --- --- --- --- --- --- --- --- --- --- ---
                                          K
seq5                     --- --- --- --- -a- --- --- --- --- --- --- --- --- --- ---

seq6                     --- --- --- --- --- --- --- --- --- --- --- --- --- --- ---
```

Fig. 15. IMGT/V-QUEST "Synthesis view" result page: "Alignment for V-GENE," "V-REGION alignment according to the IMGT unique numbering," and "V-REGION translation." Displayed sequences are those of the input set, which have been identified as using the same closest germline V gene and allele (here IGHV3-30*04). *Dashes* indicate identical nucleotides. *Dots* indicate gaps. FR-IMGT and CDR-IMGT are delimited according to the IMGT unique numbering (19–21). The sequence of the V-REGION of the closest germline V is shown on the first line and the input sequences are aligned, with nt mutations indicated by comparison. *Underlined* nucleotides in the closest germline V correspond to mutation hot spot motif localizations. Only a part of each of the three displays is shown.

## 4. V-REGION protein display

```
                         FR1-IMGT              CDR1-IMGT      FR2-IMGT       CDR2-IMGT              FR3-IMGT
                          (1-26)                (27-38)        (39-55)        (56-65)               (66-104)
                     ___________________________ ___________ ____________________ __________ _________________________________________
                     1        10        20       30          40        50          60         70        80        90        100
                     .........|.........|......  ...|........ .|.........|.....   ....|.....  ....|.........|.........|.........|....
L06615 IGHV3-30*04   QVQLVESGG.GVVQPGRSLRLSCAAS  GFTF....SSYA MHWVRQAPGKGLEWVAV   ISYD..GSNK  YYADSVK.GRFTISRDNSKNTLYLQMNSLRAEDTAVYYC AR
seq3                 EVQLLESGG.GVVQPGRSLRLSCIAS  GFTF....SSYP MTWVRQAPGKGLEWVAS   ISYD..GSYK  YKVDSMK.GRLTISRDNSKNTLYLEMNSLTAEDTAVYYC AR
seq4                 QVQLVESGG.GVVQPGRSLRLSCAAS  GFTF....SSYA MHWVRQAPGKGLEWVAV   ISYD..GSNK  YYADSVK.GRFTISRDNSKNTLYLQMNSLRAEDTAVYYC AR
seq5                 QVQLVESGG.GVVQPGRSLKLSCAAS  GFTF....SSYA MHWVRQAPGKGLEWVAV   ISYD..GSNK  YYANSVK.GRFTISRDNSKNTLYLQMNSLRAEDTAVYYC AR
seq6                 QVQLVESGG.GVVQPGRSLRLSCAAS  GFTF....SSYA MHWVRQAPGKGLEWVAV   ISYD..GSNK  YYADSVK.GRFTISRDNSKNTLYLQMNSLRAEDTAVYYC AR
```

## 5. V-REGION protein display with colored AA according to the AA IMGT classes

```
                         FR1-IMGT              CDR1-IMGT      FR2-IMGT       CDR2-IMGT              FR3-IMGT
                          (1-26)                (27-38)        (39-55)        (56-65)               (66-104)
                     ___________________________ ___________ ____________________ __________ _________________________________________
                     1        10        20       30          40        50          60         70        80        90        100
                     .........|.........|......  ...|........ .|.........|.....   ....|.....  ....|.........|.........|.........|....
L06615 IGHV3-30*04   QVQLVESGG.GVVQPGRSLRLSCAAS  GFTF....SSYA MHWVRQAPGKGLEWVAV   ISYD..GSNK  YYADSVK.GRFTISRDNSKNTLYLQMNSLRAEDTAVYYC AR
seq3                 EVQLLESGG.GVVQPGRSLRLSCIAS  GFTF....SSYP MTWVRQAPGKGLEWVAS   ISYD..GSYK  YKVDSMK.GRLTISRDNSKNTLYLEMNSLTAEDTAVYYC AR
seq4                 QVQLVESGG.GVVQPGRSLRLSCAAS  GFTF....SSYA MHWVRQAPGKGLEWVAV   ISYD..GSNK  YYADSVK.GRFTISRDNSKNTLYLQMNSLRAEDTAVYYC AR
seq5                 QVQLVESGG.GVVQPGRSLKLSCAAS  GFTF....SSYA MHWVRQAPGKGLEWVAV   ISYD..GSNK  YYANSVK.GRFTISRDNSKNTLYLQMNSLRAEDTAVYYC AR
seq6                 QVQLVESGG.GVVQPGRSLRLSCAAS  GFTF....SSYA MHWVRQAPGKGLEWVAV   ISYD..GSNK  YYADSVK.GRFTISRDNSKNTLYLQMNSLRAEDTAVYYC AR
```

## 6. V-REGION protein display (only AA changes displayed)

```
                         FR1-IMGT              CDR1-IMGT      FR2-IMGT       CDR2-IMGT              FR3-IMGT
                          (1-26)                (27-38)        (39-55)        (56-65)               (66-104)
                     ___________________________ ___________ ____________________ __________ _________________________________________
                     1        10        20       30          40        50          60         70        80        90        100
                     .........|.........|......  ...|........ .|.........|.....   ....|.....  ....|.........|.........|.........|....
L06615 IGHV3-30*04   QVQLVESGG.GVVQPGRSLRLSCAAS  GFTF....SSYA MHWVRQAPGKGLEWVAV   ISYD..GSNK  YYADSVK.GRFTISRDNSKNTLYLQMNSLRAEDTAVYYC AR
seq3                 E---L----.-------------I--  ----....---P -T--------------S   ----..--Y-  -KV--M-.--L------------E----T--------- --
seq4                 ---------.----------------  ----....---- -----------------   ----..----  -------.------------------------------ --
seq5                 ---------.---------K------  ----....---- -----------------   ----..----  ---N---.------------------------------ --
seq6                 ---------.----------------  ----....---- -----------------   ----..----  -------.------------------------------ --
```

Fig. 16. IMGT/V-QUEST "Synthesis view" result page. V-REGION protein displays: Three different displays are shown. "V-REGION protein display," "V-REGION protein display with colored AA according to the AA IMGT classes," (online colored AA) and "V-REGION protein display (only AA changed displayed)." The first line shows the AA sequence of the closest V-REGION allele against which are aligned the translations of the input sequences identified by IMGT/V-QUEST as using the same V gene and allele (here IGHV3-30*04).

## 7. V-REGION most frequently occurring AA per position and per FR-IMGT and CDR-IMGT

**FR1-IMGT**

| Position | 1 | 2 | 3 | 4 | 5 | 6 | 7 | 8 | 9 | 10 | 11 | 12 | 13 | 14 | 15 | 16 | 17 | 18 | 19 | 20 | 21 | 22 | 23 | 24 | 25 | 26 |
|---|---|---|---|---|---|---|---|---|---|---|---|---|---|---|---|---|---|---|---|---|---|---|---|---|---|---|
| AA | Q | V | Q | L | V | E | S | G | G | | G | V | V | Q | P | G | R | S | L | R | L | S | C | A | A | S |
| Occurrence nb | 3/4 | 4/4 | 4/4 | 4/4 | 3/4 | 4/4 | 4/4 | 4/4 | 4/4 | . | 4/4 | 4/4 | 4/4 | 4/4 | 4/4 | 4/4 | 4/4 | 4/4 | 4/4 | 3/4 | 4/4 | 4/4 | 4/4 | 3/4 | 4/4 | 4/4 |
| Frequency | 75% | 100% | 100% | 100% | 75% | 100% | 100% | 100% | 100% | | 100% | 100% | 100% | 100% | 100% | 100% | 100% | 100% | 100% | 75% | 100% | 100% | 100% | 75% | 100% | 100% |

**CDR1-IMGT**

| Position | 27 | 28 | 29 | 30 | 31 | 32 | 33 | 34 | 35 | 36 | 37 | 38 |
|---|---|---|---|---|---|---|---|---|---|---|---|---|
| AA | G | F | T | F | | | | | S | S | Y | A |
| Occurrence nb | 4/4 | 4/4 | 4/4 | 4/4 | . | . | . | . | 4/4 | 4/4 | 4/4 | 3/4 |
| Frequency | 100% | 100% | 100% | 100% | | | | | 100% | 100% | 100% | 75% |

**FR2-IMGT**

| Position | 39 | 40 | 41 | 42 | 43 | 44 | 45 | 46 | 47 | 48 | 49 | 50 | 51 | 52 | 53 | 54 | 55 |
|---|---|---|---|---|---|---|---|---|---|---|---|---|---|---|---|---|---|
| AA | M | H | W | V | R | Q | A | P | G | K | G | L | E | W | V | A | V |
| Occurrence nb | 4/4 | 3/4 | 4/4 | 4/4 | 4/4 | 4/4 | 4/4 | 4/4 | 4/4 | 4/4 | 4/4 | 4/4 | 4/4 | 4/4 | 4/4 | 4/4 | 3/4 |
| Frequency | 100% | 75% | 100% | 100% | 100% | 100% | 100% | 100% | 100% | 100% | 100% | 100% | 100% | 100% | 100% | 100% | 75% |

**CDR2-IMGT**

| Position | 56 | 57 | 58 | 59 | 60 | 61 | 62 | 63 | 64 | 65 |
|---|---|---|---|---|---|---|---|---|---|---|
| AA | I | S | Y | D | | | G | S | N | K |
| Occurrence nb | 4/4 | 4/4 | 4/4 | 4/4 | . | . | 4/4 | 4/4 | 3/4 | 4/4 |
| Frequency | 100% | 100% | 100% | 100% | | | 100% | 100% | 75% | 100% |

**FR3-IMGT**

| Position | 66 | 67 | 68 | 69 | 70 | 71 | 72 | 73 | 74 | 75 | 76 | 77 | 78 | 79 | 80 | 81 | 82 | 83 | 84 | 85 | 86 | 87 | 88 | 89 | 90 | 91 | 92 |
|---|---|---|---|---|---|---|---|---|---|---|---|---|---|---|---|---|---|---|---|---|---|---|---|---|---|---|---|
| AA | Y | Y | A | D | S | V | K | | G | R | F | T | I | S | R | D | N | S | K | N | T | L | Y | L | Q | M | N |
| Occurrence nb | 4/4 | 3/4 | 3/4 | 3/4 | 4/4 | 3/4 | 4/4 | . | 4/4 | 4/4 | 3/4 | 4/4 | 4/4 | 4/4 | 4/4 | 4/4 | 4/4 | 4/4 | 4/4 | 4/4 | 4/4 | 4/4 | 4/4 | 4/4 | 3/4 | 4/4 | 4/4 |
| Frequency | 100% | 75% | 75% | 75% | 100% | 75% | 100% | | 100% | 100% | 75% | 100% | 100% | 100% | 100% | 100% | 100% | 100% | 100% | 100% | 100% | 100% | 100% | 100% | 75% | 100% | 100% |

**CDR3-IMGT**

| Position | 105 |
|---|---|
| AA | A |
| Occurrence nb | 4/4 |
| Frequency | 100% |

Fig. 17. IMGT/V-QUEST "Synthesis view" result page: "V-REGION most frequently occurring AA per position and per FR-IMGT and CDR-IMGT." Results are for a set of four sequences expressing IGHV3-30*04 (accession numbers AB012909, AB021511, AB021516, AB021514 from IMGT/LIGM-DB database (34)). For each set of user sequences that express the same closest germline V gene and allele, the most frequently occurring amino acid is shown per amino acid (or codon) position and per FR-IMGT and CDR-IMGT. The display highlights the conserved as well as the polymorphic positions.

#### 2.5. IMGT/V-QUEST Output for Excel File

"Excel file" allows the users to open and save a spreadsheet including the results of the IMGT/V-QUEST analysis. The file contains 11 sheets (if all were selected in the IMGT/V-QUEST Search page, see Subheading 2.2.2). The "Summary" and "Parameters" are always selected.

The content of the eleven sheets is detailed in the IMGT/HighV-QUEST "Download" (Subheading 3.4).

## 3. IMGT/HighV-QUEST

IMGT/HighV-QUEST, the high-throughput version of IMGT/V-QUEST, can analyze large numbers of IG and TR-rearranged sequences (up to 150,000) in a single run.

#### 3.1. IMGT/HighV-QUEST Welcome Page

As for the other IMGT® databases and tools, IMGT/HighV-QUEST is freely available for academics. However, the IMGT/HighV-QUEST Welcome page requires user identification and provides, for new users, a link to register. User identification has been set to avoid nonrelevant use and overload of the server and to contact the user if needed.

#### 3.2. IMGT/HighV-QUEST Search Page

1. After user identification, a unique IMGT/HighV-QUEST Search page is displayed (Fig. 18). It is very similar to the classical IMGT/V-QUEST Search page with however, at the top, four additional fields:
   (a) The analysis title (which must be provided by the user).
   (b) The selection of the species.
   (c) The selection of the receptor type or locus. IMGT/HighV-QUEST allows the user to restrict the analysis to a particular locus, for example, "IGH" or "TRA." Values for receptor type or locus are displayed only if the corresponding IMGT reference directory is available.
   (d) The choice of e-mail notifications. Because of their large number of sequences, the analyses are first queued on the IMGT® server and they are performed depending on the available resources. Therefore, the results are not displayed immediately and users may choose to be notified by e-mail: when analysis is queued, when analysis is submitted, when analysis is completed (selected by default), and/or before the results are removed (always selected). These choices are not exclusive.
2. The sequences must be uploaded using the simple text formatted file (the copy and paste option is not available). Then, the customization for the "Detailed View" (except for IMGT

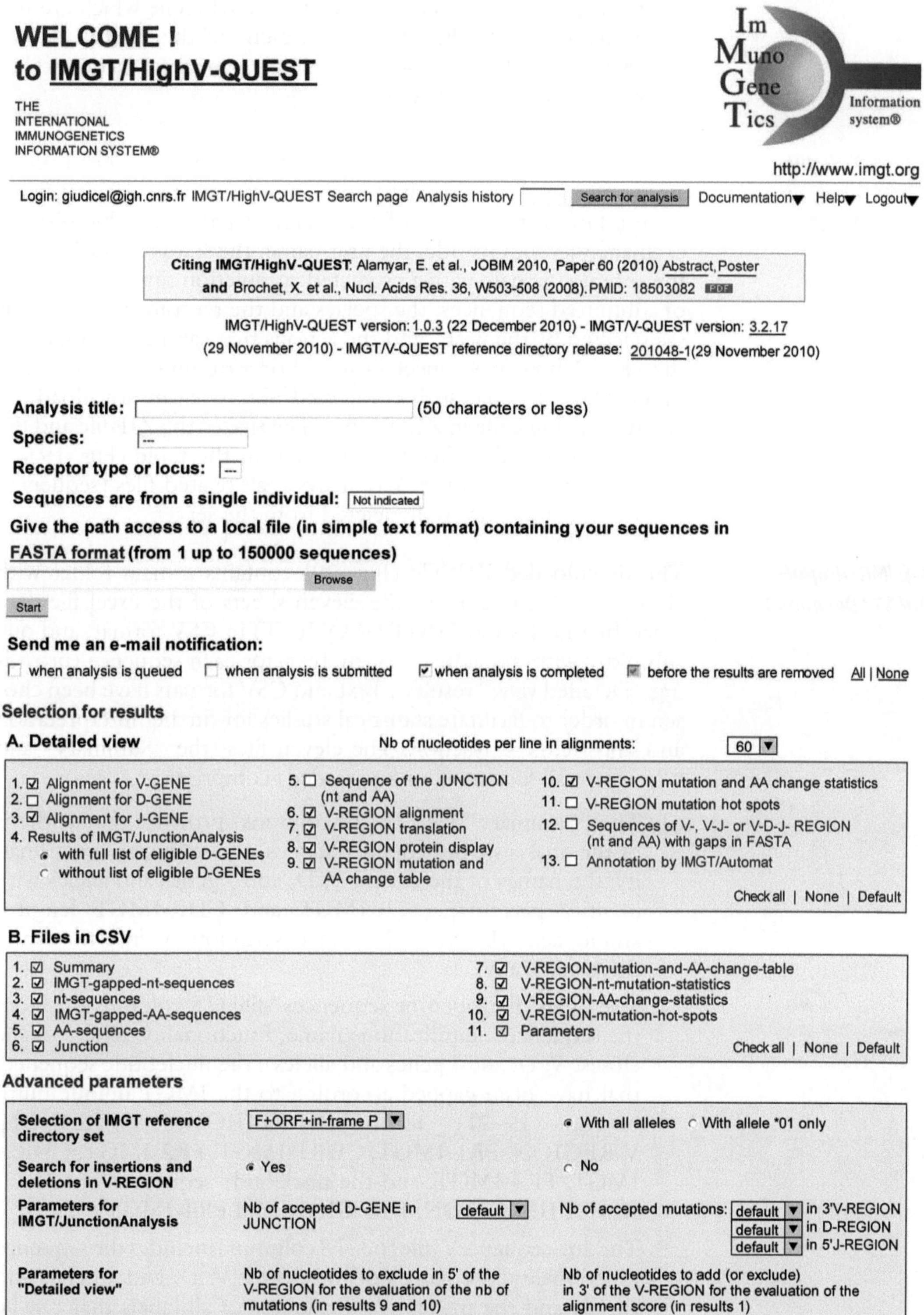


Fig. 18. IMGT/HighV-QUEST Search page.

Collier de Perles results and IMGT/Phylogene which are not available), "Files in CSV" (equivalent of the "Excel file" of IMGT/V-QUEST) and "Advanced parameters" is identical to those of IMGT/V-QUEST.

### 3.3. IMGT/HighV-QUEST "Analysis History Page"

From their account, the user can check the status of his/her analyses at any time by displaying the "Analysis history" (Fig. 19) (available from a link from the top of the Search page). The table displays each analysis with its title, the user name, the status of the analysis, the submission date with a predicted completion time, the number of submitted sequences, the species and the receptor type or locus (as selected by the user), and the actions that can be performed by the user. A user may cancel a queued or a running analysis at any time. When the analysis is completed, the user can download the results as a single file in ZIP format. The size of the ZIP file and the number of included files are indicated in the table (Fig. 19). If the user removes a completed analysis, all related files (sequences and results) are definitively deleted from the server.

### 3.4. IMGT/HighV-QUEST "Download"

The downloaded ZIP file (Fig. 20) contains a main folder with eleven files (equivalent to the eleven sheets of the excel file provided by the classical IMGT/V-QUEST) in CSV format, and one subfolder with individual files, in Text, for each sequence (providing "Detailed view" results). Text and CSV formats have been chosen in order to facilitate statistical studies for further interpretation and knowledge extraction. The eleven files (the "Summary" and "Parameters" files are always provided) comprise:

1. The "Summary" file (25–29 columns) provides the synthesis of the analysis (the sequence names, the sequence functionality, the names of the closest V, D, and J genes and alleles with identity percentage, FR-IMGT and CDR-IMGT lengths, amino acid JUNCTION, the description of insertions and deletions if any ...).
2. The "IMGT-gapped-nt-sequences" file (18 columns) includes the sequence identification (name, functionality, names of the closest V, D, and J genes and alleles), the nucleotide sequences that have been gapped according to the IMGT unique numbering (19–21) for V-D-J-REGION, V-J-REGION, V-REGION, FR1-IMGT, CDR1-IMGT, FR2-IMGT, CDR2-IMGT, FR3-IMGT, and the nucleotide sequences of CDR3-IMGT, JUNCTION, J-REGION, and FR4-IMGT.
3. The "nt-sequences" file (63–78 columns) includes the sequence functionality, the names of the closest V, D, and J genes and alleles, and the nucleotide sequences of all labels that can be automatically annotated by IMGT/Automat (23, 24) in the analyzed sequences.

| Title | User | Status | Submission Date | N° of sequences | Species | Receptor type | Actions |
|---|---|---|---|---|---|---|---|
| test-human-TR | Giudi VÉRONIQUE | queued | 2011-01-19 15:44:26 CET **predicted completion time: 2011-01-19 at 17:37:34 CET** | 3000 | Homo_sapiens | TR | **Not completed** Cancel |
| test-mouse-TRA | Giudi VÉRONIQUE | running | 2011-01-19 15:43:22 CET **predicted completion time: 2011-01-19 at 17:37:34 CET** | 3575 | Mus_musculus | TRA | **Not completed** Cancel |
| test_human_IGK | Giudi VÉRONIQUE | completed | 2011-01-19 15:42:07 CET | 272 | Homo_sapiens | IGK | Download (462.52 KB , 284 Files) Remove |

**Note:** this table is not dynamic, please click here to Refresh the table

Fig. 19. IMGT/HighV-QUEST “Analysis history” page.

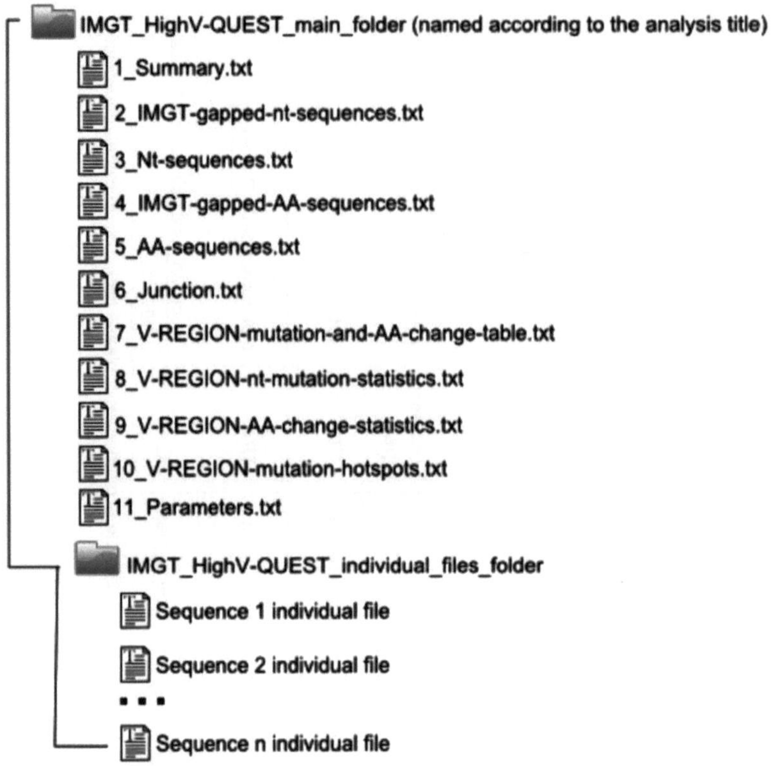


Fig. 20. IMGT/HighV-QUEST content of a results ZIP file.

4. The "IMGT-gapped-AA-sequences" file (18 columns) includes the sequence identification, the amino acid sequences that have been gapped according to the IMGT unique numbering for V-D-J-REGION, V-J-REGION, V-REGION, FR1-IMGT, CDR1-IMGT, FR2-IMGT, CDR2-IMGT, FR3-IMGT, and the amino acid sequences of CDR3-IMGT, JUNCTION, J-REGION and FR4-IMGT.
5. The "AA-sequences" file (18 columns) includes the same columns as the "IMGT-gapped-AA-sequences" file, but sequences are without IMGT gaps.
6. The "Junction" file includes the sequence identification and the results of IMGT/JunctionAnalysis (9) (33 columns for IGL, IGK, TRA and TRG sequences, 46 (if one D), 66 (if two D) or 77 (if 3 D) columns for IGH, TRB and TRD sequences).
7. The "V-REGION-mutation-and-AA-change table" file (11 columns) includes the sequence name, the functionality, the name of the closest V gene and allele, and list of mutations (nucleotide mutation, AA change, AA class identity or change for V-REGION, FR1-IMGT, CDR1-IMGT, FR2-IMGT, CDR2-IMGT, FR3-IMGT and CDR3-IMGT).

8. The "V-REGION-nt-mutation-statistics" file (130 columns) includes the sequence name, the sequence functionality, the name of the closest V gene and allele, then the number of positions including IMGT gaps, the number of nucleotides, the number of identical nucleotides, the total number of mutations, the number of silent mutations, the number of nonsilent mutations, the number of transitions (a>g, g>a, c>t, t>c), and the number of transversions (a>c, c>a, a>t, t>a, g>c, c>g, g>t, t>g) for V-REGION, FR1-IMGT, CDR1-IMGT, FR2-IMGT, CDR2-IMGT, FR3-IMGT, and CDR3-IMGT.
9. The "V-REGION-AA-change-statistics" file (189 columns) includes the sequence name, the sequence functionality, the name of the closest V gene and allele, then the number of AA positions including IMGT gaps, the number of AA, the number of identical AA, the total number of AA changes, the number of AA changes according to AAclassChangeType (+++, ++–, +–+, +––, –+–, ––+, –––), and the number of AA class changes according to AAclassSimilarityDegree (number of Very similar, number of Similar, number of Dissimilar, number of Very dissimilar) for V-REGION, FR1-IMGT, CDR1-IMGT, FR2-IMGT, CDR2-IMGT, FR3-IMGT, and CDR3-IMGT.
10. The "V-REGION-mutation-hot-spots" file (eight columns) includes the sequence functionality, the name of the closest V gene and allele, and the hot spots motifs (a/t)a, t(a/t), (a/g)g(c/t)(a/t), (a/t)(a/g)c(c/t) identified in the closest germline V-REGION and with CDR-IMGT and FR-IMGT localizations.
11. The "Parameters" file includes the date of the analysis, the IMGT/V-QUEST programme version, the IMGT/V-QUEST reference directory release, and the parameters used for the analysis: the species, the receptor type or locus, the IMGT reference directory set, "with allele *01" (if selected), "Search for insertions and deletions," the number of nucleotides to add (or exclude) in 3′ of the V-REGION for the evaluation of the alignment score, and the number of nucleotides to exclude in 5′ of the V-REGION for the evaluation of the number of mutations, if these 2 numbers are not 0 (default value).

## 4. Notes

1. The tool will automatically identify the locus (IGH, IGK, or IGL for IG sequences, or TRA, TRB, TRG, or TRD for TR sequences).
2. The IMGT/V-QUEST reference directory sets include IMGT reference sequences from all functional genes and alleles, all

open reading frame (ORF) and all in-frame pseudogenes (P) alleles. By definition, these sets contain one sequence for each allele. IMGT reference directories have been set up for species which have been extensively studied, such as human and mouse. This also holds for the other species or taxons with incomplete IMGT reference directory sets. In those cases, results should be interpreted considering the status of the IMGT reference directory (information on the updates on the IMGT® Web site). Links to the IMGT/V-QUEST reference directory sets are available from the IMGT/V-QUEST Welcome page.

3. The options (e) and (f) provide different displays of the results shown in option (d), whereas the option (g) allows to evaluate the occurrence of amino acids changes at each position.

4. By default, the user sequences are compared with all genes and alleles. However, the option "With allele *01 only" is useful if the user sequences need to be compared in "Detailed view" with different genes. In "Synthesis view," this option allows to align all user sequences that express the same gene independently of the allelic polymorphism.

5. This option is usually selected in a second step after a first analysis by IMGT/V-QUEST that provided warnings for potential insertions or deletions (Subheading 2.3.1).

6. The "Functionality" is an important concept for IG and TR nucleotide sequence identification, as it allows to distinguish on the one hand the functionality of germline and conventional genes: functional, ORF (open reading frame), or pseudogene, and on the other hand the functionality of IG and TR rearranged sequences: productive or unproductive. An IG or a TR rearranged sequence is productive if no stop codon has been detected in the V-D-J-REGION or in the V-J-REGION, and if the junction is in-frame. An IG or a TR rearranged sequence is unproductive if stop codons are detected in the V-D-J-REGION or in the V-J-REGION and/or if the junction is out-of-frame.

7. The IMGT® IG and TR gene names (1, 2, 28, 29) were approved by the Human Genome Organization (HUGO) Nomenclature Committee (HGNC) in 1999 (30) and are the official references for the World Health Organization-International Union of Immunological Societies (WHO-IUIS) Nomenclature Subcommittee for IG and TR (31, 32). The complete list of the human IG and TR gene names has been entered in IMGT/GENE-DB (15), the IMGT® gene database, and in Entrez Gene at the National Center for Biotechnology Information (NCBI) (33). IMGT® IG and TR gene and allele names are based on the concepts of classification

of IMGT-ONTOLOGY (CLASSIFICATION axiom) (10–13). IMGT® reference sequences have been defined for each allele of each gene based on one or, whenever possible, several of the following criteria: germline sequence, first sequence published, longest sequence, mapped sequence (34, 35). IMGT® IG gene and allele names are used for the antibody description in the WHO International Nonproprietary Name (INN) programme (36).

8. The score of the alignment for 2 sequences is calculated by counting +5 for each position where nucleotides are identical (match) and −4 for each position with different nucleotides (mismatch).
9. In addition to the analysis of the somatic mutations, results of IMGT/V-QUEST, frequently used by clinicians, also include the sequences of the V-(D)-J junctions which are used in the synthesis of specific probes for the follow-up of residual diseases in leukemias and lymphomas.
10. Potential insertions or deletions are suspected by IMGT/V-QUEST when the V-REGION score is very low (less than 200), and/or the percentage of identity is less than 85%, and/or when the input sequence has different CDR1-IMGT and/or CDR2-IMGT lengths, compared to those of the closest germline V.
11. The note (in red online) indicates the additional J-GENE and allele names and the criterion used for their identification (usually highest number of consecutive identical nucleotides).
12. The way to identify the closest germline D is different between IMGT/V-QUEST and IMGT/JunctionAnalysis since the evaluation of the alignment score is different. In case of discrepancy, the results of IMGT/JunctionAnalysis are the most accurate. However, the alignment provided by IMGT/V-QUEST that is less stringent and displays several D genes and alleles may be helpful to solve ambiguous cases when IMGT/JunctionAnalysis does not provide results for the D gene and allele.
13. Amino acids of the V-DOMAIN are numbered according to the IMGT unique numbering (19–21). Position 104 (second-CYS) and position 118 (J-PHE or J-TRP) that belong to the FR3-IMGT and FR4-IMGT, respectively, are the anchors of the CDR3-IMGT. They correspond to the 5′ and 3′ ends of the JUNCTION.
14. The default can be modified in "Advanced parameters," but only for TR with mutations in the V-REGION (between positions 1 and 104).
15. The 20 amino acids have been classified in eleven IMGT "Physicochemical" classes which are based on "Hydrophathy,"

"Volume," and "Chemical" characteristics (http://www.imgt.org/, section "Amino acids" in IMGT Education > Aide-mémoire).

16. The IMGT Colliers de Perles (25–27) allows the user to bridge the gap between sequences and structures (37, 38) and is widely used in the protocol for antibody humanization or for the evaluation of therapeutic monoclonal antibodies (39, 40): the provided information is useful to localize the amino acids of the loops CDR1-IMGT, CDR2-IMGT, CDR3-IMGT that are involved in the contacts with the antigen. It allows study of the physicochemical properties of the amino acids at a given position in a pool of sequences. IMGT/Collier-de-Perles tool can be customized to display the amino acids colored according to their hydropathy, volume, or IMGT physicochemical classes (18). By default, the IMGT Colliers de Perles are displayed on one layer. They can also be displayed on two layers in order to get a graphical representation closer to the 3D structure. In the case of sequences with an out-of-frame junction, the J reading frame is not restored (the sequence does not include "#").
17. A note (in red online) may appear with the V-GENE and allele name when potential insertions or deletions are suspected (criteria detailed in Note 10). In those cases, the alignment for this sequence has to be checked in "A. Detailed view," using the advanced parameters "Search for insertions and deletions in V-REGION" (Subheading 2.2.3).
18. A note (in red online) may appear to inform on other possibilities for the J-GENE and allele name as described in Note 11.

## Acknowledgements

We are grateful to Gérard Lefranc for helpful discussion and to the IMGT® team for its expertise and constant motivation. IMGT® received funding from Centre National de la Recherche Scientifique CNRS, Ministère de l'Enseignement Supérieur et de la Recherche MESR (University Montpellier 2), Région Languedoc-Roussillon (GPTR, GEPETOS), Agence Nationale de la Recherche ANR (ANR-06-BYOS-0005-01), and European Community (ImmunoGrid, FP6-2004-IST-4). This work was granted access to the HPC resources of CINES under the allocations 2010-036029 and 2011-036029 made by GENCI (Grand Equipement National de Calcul Intensif).

## References


1. Lefranc M-P, Lefranc G (2001) The immunoglobulin FactsBook. Academic Press, London, UK, pp 1–458
2. Lefranc M-P, Lefranc G (2001) The T cell receptor FactsBook. Academic Press, London, UK, pp 1–398
3. Giudicelli V, Chaume D, Lefranc M-P (2004) IMGT/V-QUEST, an integrated software program for immunoglobulin and T cell receptor V-J and V-D-J rearrangement analysis. Nucleic Acids Res 32:W435–W440
4. Lefranc M-P (2004) IMGT, the international ImMunoGeneTics information system. Methods Mol Biol 248:27–49
5. Giudicelli V, Lefranc M-P (2005) Interactive IMGT on-line tools for the analysis of immunoglobulin and T cell receptor repertoires. In: Veskler BA (ed) New research on immunology. Nova Science Publishers, Inc., New York, pp 77–105
6. Brochet X, Lefranc M-P, Giudicelli V (2008) IMGT/V-QUEST: the highly customized and integrated system for IG and TR standardized V-J and V-D-J sequence analysis. Nucleic Acids Res 36:W503–W508
7. Giudicelli V, Lefranc M-P (2008) IMGT® standardized analysis of immunoglobulin rearranged sequences. In: Ghia P, Rosenquist R, Davi F (eds) Immunoglobulin gene analysis in chronic lymphocytic leukemia (chapter 2). Wolters Kluwer Health, Italy, pp 33–52
8. Lefranc M-P, Giudicelli V, Ginestoux C, Jabado-Michaloud J, Folch G, Bellahcene F, Wu Y, Gemrot E, Brochet X, Lane J, Regnier L, Ehrenmann F, Lefranc G, Duroux P (2009) IMGT®, the international ImMunoGeneTics information system®. Nucleic Acids Res 37:D1006–D1012
9. Yousfi Monod M, Giudicelli V, Chaume D, Lefranc M-P (2004) IMGT/JunctionAnalysis: the first tool for the analysis of the immunoglobulin and T cell receptor complex V-J and V-D-J JUNCTIONs. Bioinformatics 20:i379–i385
10. Giudicelli V, Lefranc M-P (1999) Ontology for immunogenetics: the IMGT-ONTOLOGY. Bioinformatics 15:1047–1054
11. Lefranc M-P, Giudicelli V, Ginestoux C, Bosc N, Folch G, Guiraudou D, Jabado-Michaloud J, Magris S, Scaviner D, Thouvenin V, Combres K, Girod D, Jeanjean S, Protat C, Yousfi-Monod M, Duprat E, Kaas Q, Pommié C, Chaume D, Lefranc G (2004) IMGT-ONTOLOGY for immunogenetics and immunoinformatics. In Silico Biol 4:17–29
12. Lefranc M-P, Giudicelli V, Regnier L, Duroux P (2008) IMGT, a system and an ontology that bridge biological and computational spheres in bioinformatics. Brief Bioinform 9:263–275
13. Duroux P, Kaas Q, Brochet X, Lane J, Ginestoux C, Lefranc M-P, Giudicelli V (2008) IMGT-Kaleidoscope, the formal IMGT-ONTOLOGY paradigm. Biochimie 90:570–583
14. Alamyar E, Giudicelli V, Duroux P, Lefranc M-P (2010) IMGT/HighV-QUEST: a high-throughput system and web portal for the analysis of rearranged nucleotide sequences of antigen receptors-high-throughput version of IMGT/V-QUEST. Journées Ouvertes en Biologie, Informatique et Mathématiques, September 7-9, 2010, Montpellier, France (JOBIM 2010), Poster #60, http://www.jobim2010.fr/?q=fr/node/55. Accessed 31 Jan 2011
15. Giudicelli V, Chaume D, Lefranc M-P (2005) IMGT/GENE-DB: a comprehensive database for human and mouse immunoglobulin and T cell receptor genes. Nucleic Acids Res 33:D256–D261
16. Belessi C, Davi F, Stamatopoulos K, Degano M, Andreou TM, Moreno C, Merle-Béral H, Crespo M, Laoutaris NP, Montserrat E, Caligaris-Cappio F, Anagnostopoulos AZ, Ghia P (2006) IGHV gene insertions and deletions in chronic lymphocytic leukemia: "CLL-biased" deletions in a subset of cases with stereotyped receptors. Eur J Immunol 36:1963–1974
17. Ghia P, Stamatopoulos K, Belessi C, Moreno C, Stilgenbauer S, Stevenson F, Davi F, Rosenquist R (2007) ERIC recommendations on IGHV gene mutational status analysis in chronic lymphocytic leukemia. Leukemia 21:1–3
18. Pommié C, Levadoux S, Sabatier R, Lefranc G, Lefranc M-P (2004) IMGT standardized criteria for statistical analysis of immunoglobulin V-REGION amino acid properties. J Mol Recognit 17:17–32
19. Lefranc M-P (1997) Unique database numbering system for immunogenetic analysis. Immunol Today 18:509
20. Lefranc M-P (1999) The IMGT unique numbering for Immunoglobulins, T cell receptors and Ig-like domains. Immunologist 7: 132–136
21. Lefranc M-P, Pommié C, Ruiz M, Giudicelli V, Foulquier E, Truong L, Thouvenin-Contet V, Lefranc G (2003) IMGT unique numbering for immunoglobulin and T cell receptor variable domains and Ig superfamily V-like domains. Dev Comp Immunol 27:55–77

22. Elemento O, Lefranc M-P (2003) IMGT/PhyloGene: an on-line tool for comparative analysis of immunoglobulin and T cell receptor genes. Dev Comp Immunol 27:763–779
23. Giudicelli V, Chaume D, Jabado-Michaloud J, Lefranc M-P (2005) Immunogenetics sequence annotation: the Strategy of IMGT based on IMGT-ONTOLOGY. Stud Health Technol Inform 116:3–8
24. Giudicelli V, Protat C, Lefranc M-P (2003) The IMGT strategy for the automatic annotation of IG and TR cDNA sequences: IMGT/Automat. In: INRIA (DISC/Spid), Paris, DKB-31. Proceedings of the European Conference on Computational Biology (ECCB 2003), pp 103–104
25. Ruiz M, Lefranc M-P (2002) IMGT gene identification and Colliers de Perles of human immunoglobulins with known 3D structures. Immunogenetics 53:857–883
26. Kaas Q, Lefranc M-P (2007) IMGT Colliers de Perles: standardized sequence-structure representations of the IgSF and MhcSF superfamily domains. Curr Bioinform 2:21–30
27. Kaas Q, Ehrenmann F, Lefranc M-P (2007) IG, TR and IgSF, MHC and MhcSF: what do we learn from the IMGT Colliers de Perles? Brief Funct Genomic Proteomic 6:253–264
28. Lefranc M-P (2001) Nomenclature of the human immunoglobulin genes. In: Coligan JE, Bierer BE, Margulies DH, Shevach EM, Strober W (eds) Current protocols in immunology. Wiley, Hoboken, NJ, USA, pp A.1P.1–A.1P.37
29. Lefranc M-P (2001) Nomenclature of the human T cell receptor genes. In: Coligan JE, Bierer BE, Margulies DH, Shevach EM, Strober W (eds) Current protocols in immunology. Wiley, Hoboken, NJ, USA, pp A.1O.1–A.1O.23
30. Wain HM, Bruford EA, Lovering RC, Lush MJ, Wright MW, Povey S (2002) Guidelines for human gene nomenclature. Genomics 79:464–470
31. Lefranc M-P (2007) WHO-IUIS nomenclature subcommittee for immunoglobulins and T cell receptors report. Immunogenetics 59:899–902
32. Lefranc M-P (2008) WHO-IUIS nomenclature subcommittee for immunoglobulins and T cell receptors report August 2007, 13th International Congress of Immunology, Rio de Janeiro, Brazil. Dev Comp Immunol 32:461–463
33. Maglott D, Ostell J, Pruitt KD, Tatusova T (2011) Entrez gene: gene-centered information at NCBI. Nucleic Acids Res 39:D52–D57
34. Giudicelli V, Duroux P, Ginestoux C, Folch G, Jabado-Michaloud J, Chaume D, Lefranc M-P (2006) IMGT/LIGM-DB, the IMGT comprehensive database of immunoglobulin and T cell receptor nucleotide sequences. Nucleic Acids Res 34:D781–D784
35. Lefranc M-P (1998) IMGT (ImMunoGeneTics) locus on focus. A new section of experimental and clinical immunogenetics. Exp Clin Immunogenet 15:1–7
36. Lefranc M-P (2011) Antibody nomenclature: from IMGT-ONTOLOGY to INN definition. MAbs 3:1
37. Kaas Q, Ruiz M, Lefranc M-P (2004) IMGT/3Dstructure-DB and IMGT/Structural Query, a database and a tool for immunoglobulin. T cell receptor and MHC structural data. Nucleic Acids Res 32:D208–D210
38. Ehrenmann F, Kaas Q, Lefranc M-P (2010) IMGT/3Dstructure-DB and IMGT/DomainGapAlign: a database and a tool for immunoglobulins or antibodies, T cell receptors, MHC, IgSF and MhcSF. Nucleic Acids Res 38:D301–D307
39. Lefranc M-P (2009) Antibody databases and tools: the IMGT® experience. In: Zhiqiang An (ed) Therapeutic monoclonal antibodies: from bench to clinic (chapter 4). Wiley, Hoboken, NJ, USA, pp 91–114
40. Ehrenmann F, Duroux P, Giudicelli V, Lefranc M-P (2010) Standardized sequence and structure analysis of antibody using IMGT®. In: Kontermann R, Dübel S (eds) Antibody engineering (chapter 2), vol 2, Springer. Berlin, Heidelberg, pp 11–31

# Chapter 33

# IMGT/DomainGapAlign: The IMGT® Tool for the Analysis of IG, TR, MH, IgSF, and MhSF Domain Amino Acid Polymorphism

**François Ehrenmann and Marie-Paule Lefranc**

## Abstract

IMGT/DomainGapAlign is the online tool of IMGT®, the international ImMunoGeneTics information system®, for the analysis of amino acid sequences and two-dimensional (2D) structures of domains. IMGT/DomainGapAlign allows the analysis of the closest variable (V) and constant (C) domains of immunoglobulins (IG) or antibodies, T cell receptors (TR), and immunoglobulin superfamily (IgSF) proteins, and of the groove (G) domains of major histocompatibility (MH; in humans, HLA for human leukocyte antigen) and MH superfamily proteins. IMGT/DomainGapAlign aligns the user own sequences against the IMGT domain reference directory, displays amino acid changes, creates IMGT gaps, and delimits the domain strands and loops (and helix for G domain) according to the IMGT unique numbering. IMGT/DomainGapAlign is coupled to the IMGT/Collier-de-Perles tool that draws standardized IMGT Colliers de Perles. The analysis is based on the IMGT-ONTOLOGY concepts of identification, classification, description, and numerotation generated from the axioms of the Formal IMGT-ONTOLOGY or IMGT-Kaleidoscope. IMGT/DomainGapAlign provides an invaluable help for antibody engineering and antibody humanization as it precisely defines the standardized framework regions (FR-IMGT) and complementarity determining regions (CDR-IMGT) to be grafted. IMGT/DomainGapAlign is freely available at http://www.imgt.org.

**Key words:** IMGT, Immunoglobulin, Antibody, T cell receptor, IMGT-ONTOLOGY, Immunoglobulin superfamily, Major histocompatibility, HLA, MH superfamily, Antibody humanization

## 1. Introduction

### *1.1. Overview*

IMGT®, the international ImMunoGeneTics information system® (1), http://www.imgt.org, is specialized in the sequences, structures, and genetic data of the immunoglobulins (IG) or antibodies, T cell receptors (TR), major histocompatibility (MH; in humans, HLA for human leukocyte antigen), proteins of the immunoglobulin superfamily (IgSF) and MH superfamily (MhSF), and related

Frank T. Christiansen and Brian D. Tait (eds.), *Immunogenetics: Methods and Applications in Clinical Practice*, Methods in Molecular Biology, vol. 882, DOI 10.1007/978-1-61779-842-9_33, 

proteins of the immune system (RPI) (1). IMGT® comprises databases, online tools, and more than 15,000 pages of Web resources (1). IMGT/DomainGapAlign (2) is the IMGT® online tool for the analysis of amino acid sequences and two-dimensional (2D) structures of domains. IMGT/DomainGapAlign standardization is based on the IMGT-ONTOLOGY concepts of identification, classification, description, and numerotation generated from the axioms of the Formal IMGT-ONTOLOGY or IMGT-Kaleidoscope (3–6). IMGT/DomainGapAlign provides the standardized IMGT gene and allele names (CLASSIFICATION axiom), the standardized IMGT labels (DESCRIPTION axiom), and the IMGT unique numbering (NUMEROTATION axiom).

Three types of domains can be analyzed by IMGT/DomainGapAlign: the variable (V) (7–9) and constant (C) (10) domains of the IG and TR and other IgSF proteins, and the groove (G) (11) domain of MH and other MhSF proteins. IMGT/DomainGapAlign identifies domains in terms of sequence identity and aligns the user amino acid (AA) sequences with the closest V, C, or G domain from the IMGT domain reference directory. For the IG and TR V domains (V-DOMAIN) which result from V-(D)-J rearrangements (12, 13), the tool displays alignments with the translation of the germline V and joining (J) genes from IMGT/GENE-DB (14). IMGT/DomainGapAlign creates gaps in the user amino acid sequences, delimits domains, strands, turns and loops, helix for G, framework regions (FR-IMGT) and complementarity determining regions (CDR-IMGT) for V-DOMAIN, according to the IMGT unique numbering (7–11). IMGT/DomainGapAlign also displays the amino acid changes, highlights them in IMGT Colliers de Perles (15–17) generated using the IMGT/Collier-de-Perles tool, and provides tables with their detailed description, according to the eleven IMGT amino acid physicochemical classes (18). The IMGT/DomainGapAlign tool allows analysis of several sequences simultaneously (up to 50) and users can choose how many alignments to display for each sequence. IMGT/DomainGapAlign is freely available at http://www.imgt.org.

### 1.2. Basic Information for IMGT/DomainGapAlign

Basic information related to domain types, IMGT domain reference directory, IMGT unique numbering, and IMGT Collier de Perles, necessary for an effective use of IMGT/DomainGapAlign, is briefly reviewed.

#### 1.2.1. Domain Types

1. V domain.

   A V domain (8, 9) comprises about 100 amino acids and is made of nine antiparallel beta strands (A, B, C, C′, C″, D, E, F, and G) linked by beta turns (AB, CC′, C″D, DE, and EF) or loops (BC, C′C″ and FG) and forming a sandwich of two sheets

**Table 1**
**V domain strands and loops, IMGT positions and lengths, based on the IMGT unique numbering for V domain (V-DOMAIN and V-LIKE-DOMAIN) (7–9)**

| V domain strands and loops[a] | IMGT positions | Lengths[b] | Characteristic Residue@Position[c] | V-DOMAIN FR-IMGT and CDR-IMGT |
|---|---|---|---|---|
| A-STRAND | 1–15 | 15 (14 if gap at 10) | | FR1-IMGT |
| B-STRAND | 16–26 | 11 | 1st-CYS 23 | |
| BC-LOOP | 27–38 | 12 (or less) | | CDR1-IMGT |
| C-STRAND | 39–46 | 8 | CONSERVED-TRP 41 | FR2-IMGT |
| C′-STRAND | 47–55 | 9 | | |
| C′C″-LOOP | 56–65 | 10 (or less) | | CDR2-IMGT |
| C″-STRAND | 66–74 | 9 (or 8 if gap at 73) | | FR3-IMGT |
| D-STRAND | 75–84 | 10 (or 8 if gaps at 81, 82) | | |
| E-STRAND | 85–96 | 12 | Hydrophobic 89 | |
| F-STRAND | 97–104 | 8 | 2nd-CYS 104 | |
| FG-LOOP | 105–117 | 13 (or less, or more) | | CDR3-IMGT |
| G-STRAND | 118–128 | 11 (or 10) | V-DOMAIN J-PHE 118 or J-TRP 118[d] | FR4-IMGT |

[a]IMGT® labels (concepts of description) are written in capital letters
[b]In number of amino acids (or codons)
[c]Residue@Position is an IMGT® concept of numerotation that numbers the position of a given residue (or that of a conserved property amino acid class), based on the IMGT unique numbering
[d]In the IG and TR V-DOMAIN, the G-STRAND (or FR4-IMGT) is the C-terminal part of the J-REGION, with J-PHE or J-TRP 118 and the canonical motif F/W-G-X-G at positions 118–121. The JUNCTION refers to the CDR3-IMGT plus the two anchors 2nd-CYS 104 and J-PHE or J-TRP 118

(see Table 1). The sheets are closely packed against each other through hydrophobic interactions giving a hydrophobic core and joined together by a disulfide bridge between 1st-CYS at position 23 in the B-STRAND in the first sheet and the 2nd-CYS 104 in the F-STRAND in the second sheet. The V domain type (8, 9) includes the V-DOMAIN of the IG and TR, which corresponds to the V-J-REGION or V-D-J-REGION encoded by V-(D)-J rearrangements (12, 13), and the V-LIKE-DOMAIN of the IgSF other than IG and TR (19–21).

2. C domain.

   A C domain (10) comprises about 100 amino acids and is made of seven antiparallel beta strands (A, B, C, D, E, F, and G) linked by beta turns, a transversal strand (CD) and loops (BC and FG), on two sheets (see Table 2). A C domain has a topology and a three-dimensional structure similar to that of a V

**Table 2**
**C domain strands, turns, and loops, IMGT positions and lengths, based on the IMGT unique numbering for C domain (C-DOMAIN and C-LIKE-DOMAIN) (10)**

| C domain strands, turns, and loops[a] | IMGT positions | Lengths[b] | Characteristic Residue@ Position[c] |
|---|---|---|---|
| A-STRAND | 1–15 | 15 (14 if gap at 10) | |
| AB-TURN | 15.1–15.3 | 0–3 | |
| B-STRAND | 16–26 | 11 | 1st-CYS 23 |
| BC-LOOP | 27–31, 34–38 | 10 (or less) | |
| C-STRAND | 39–45 | 7 | CONSERVED-TRP 41 |
| CD-STRAND | 45.1–45.9 | 0–9 | |
| D-STRAND | 77–84 | 8 (or 7 if gap at 82) | |
| DE-TURN | 84.1–84.7, 85.1–85.7 | 0–14 | |
| E-STRAND | 85–96 | 12 | Hydrophobic 89 |
| EF-TURN | 96.1–96.2 | 0–2 | |
| F-STRAND | 97–104 | 8 | 2nd-CYS 104 |
| FG-LOOP | 105–117 | 13 (or less, or more) | |
| G-STRAND | 118–128 | 11 (or less) | |

[a]IMGT® labels (concepts of description) are written in capital letters
[b]In number of amino acids (or codons)
[c]Residue@Position is an IMGT® concept of numerotation that numbers the position of a given residue (or that of a conserved property amino acid class), based on the IMGT unique numbering

domain, but without the C′ and C″ strands and the C′C″ loop. The C domain type (10) includes the C-DOMAIN of the IG and TR (12, 13) and the C-LIKE-DOMAIN of the IgSF other than IG and TR (19–23).

3. G domain.

   A G domain (11) comprises about 90 amino acids and is made of four antiparallel beta strands linked by turns and a helix that sits on the beta strands, its axis forming an angle of about 40° with the strands (see Table 3). Two G domains are needed to form the MhSF groove made of a "floor" and two "walls." Each G domain contributes groove structure by its four strands and turns to half of the groove floor and by its helix to one wall of the groove (11). The G domain type includes the G-DOMAIN of the MH (11) and the G-LIKE-DOMAIN of the MhSF other than MH (22, 24).

*1.2.2. IMGT Domain Reference Directory*

The IMGT domain reference directory is the IMGT reference directory for V, C, and G domains (2). It is manually curated and

**Table 3**
**G domain strands, turns, and helix, IMGT positions and lengths, based on the IMGT unique numbering for G domain (G-DOMAIN and G-LIKE-DOMAIN) (11)**

| G domain strands, turns, and helix[a] | IMGT positions | Lengths[b] | Characteristic Residue@Position[c] and additional positions[d] |
|---|---|---|---|
| A-STRAND | 1–14 | 14 | 7A, CYS-11 |
| AB-TURN | 15–17 | 3 (or 2 or 0) | |
| B-STRAND | 18–28 | 11 (or 10[e]) | |
| BC-TURN | 29–30 | 2 | |
| C-STRAND | 31–38 | 8 | |
| CD-TURN | 39–41 | 3 (or 1[f]) | |
| D-STRAND | 42–49 | 8 | 49.1–49.5 |
| HELIX | 50–92 | 43 (or less or more) | 54A, 61A, 61B, 72A, CYS-74, 92A |

[a]IMGT® labels (concepts of description) are written in capital letters
[b]In number of amino acids (or codons)
[c]Residue@Position is an IMGT® concept of numerotation that numbers the position of a given residue (or that of a conserved property amino acid class), based on the IMGT unique numbering
[d]For details on the characteristic Residue@Position and additional positions, see ref. (11)
[e]Or 9 in some G-BETA (11)
[f]Or 0 in some G-ALPHA2-LIKE (11)

contains the amino acid sequences of the domains delimited according to the IMGT rules (based on the exon delimitations) (10). Sequences are from the IMGT Repertoire (1) or from IMGT/GENE-DB (14) (see Note 1). Owing to the particularities of the V-DOMAIN synthesis (12, 13), there is no V-DOMAIN in the IMGT reference directory. Instead, the directory comprises the translation of the IG and TR germline V and J genes (V-REGION and J-REGION, respectively). The IMGT domain reference directory provides the IMGT "gene" and "allele" names ("CLASSIFICATION" axiom) (see Note 2). Data are comprehensive for human and mouse IG and TR and human MH, whereas for other species and IgSF and MhSF they are added progressively.

*1.2.3. IMGT Unique Numbering*

1. IMGT unique numbering for V domain.

   The V domain strands and loops and their delimitations and lengths are based on the IMGT unique numbering for V domain (V-DOMAIN and V-LIKE-DOMAIN) (7–9) (Table 1). In the IG and TR V-DOMAIN, the G-STRAND is the C-terminal part of the J-REGION, with J-PHE or J-TRP 118 and the canonical motif F/W-G-X-G at positions 118–121 (8, 9). The loop length (number of amino acids (or codons), that is number of occupied positions) is a crucial and original concept of IMGT-ONTOLOGY. The lengths of the loops BC (or CDR1-IMGT for V-DOMAIN), C′C″ (or CDR2-IMGT for V-DOMAIN), and FG (or CDR3-IMGT for V-DOMAIN) characterize the V domain. The lengths of the three loops BC, C′C″, and FG are shown in number of amino acids (or codons), into brackets and separated by dots. For example, [9.6.9] means that the BC, C′C″, and FG loops (or CDR1-IMGT, CDR2-IMGT, and CDR3-IMGT for a V-DOMAIN) have a length of 9, 6, and 9 amino acids (or codons), respectively.

2. IMGT unique numbering for C domain.

   The C domain strands, turns, and loops, and their delimitations and lengths are based on the IMGT unique numbering for C domain (C-DOMAIN and C-LIKE-DOMAIN) (10) (Table 2).

3. IMGT unique numbering for G domain.

   The G domain strands, turns, and helix and their delimitations and lengths are based on the IMGT unique numbering for G domain (G-DOMAIN and G-LIKE-DOMAIN) (11) (Table 3).

#### 1.2.4. IMGT Colliers de Perles

IMGT Colliers de Perles are standardized IMGT 2D graphical representations of protein domains (15–17) that can be obtained using the IMGT/Collier-de-Perles tool available from the IMGT® Home Page at http://www.imgt.org (for sequences already gapped according to the IMGT unique numbering) or using the IMGT/Collier-de-Perles tool integrated in IMGT/V-QUEST (25) (starting from V-(D)-J nucleotide sequences) or integrated in IMGT/DomainGapAlign (2) (starting from V, C, or G domain amino acid sequences).

## 2. IMGT/DomainGapAlign

### 2.1. IMGT/DomainGapAlign Welcome Page

1. The IMGT/DomainGapAlign Welcome page is accessed by clicking the link IMGT/DomainGapAlign ("IMGT tools" section) in the IMGT® Home page at http://www.imgt.org.
2. In the IMGT/DomainGapAlign Welcome page (Fig. 1), locate the text area and paste your amino acid sequences in FASTA format. Alternatively, you can upload a file. A precise delimitation of the domain sequences is not required; however, if the sequence contains several domains, the sequence should be split between the different domains. Several domain amino acid sequences can be analyzed simultaneously (up to 50), but each sequence must have a distinct name and belong to the

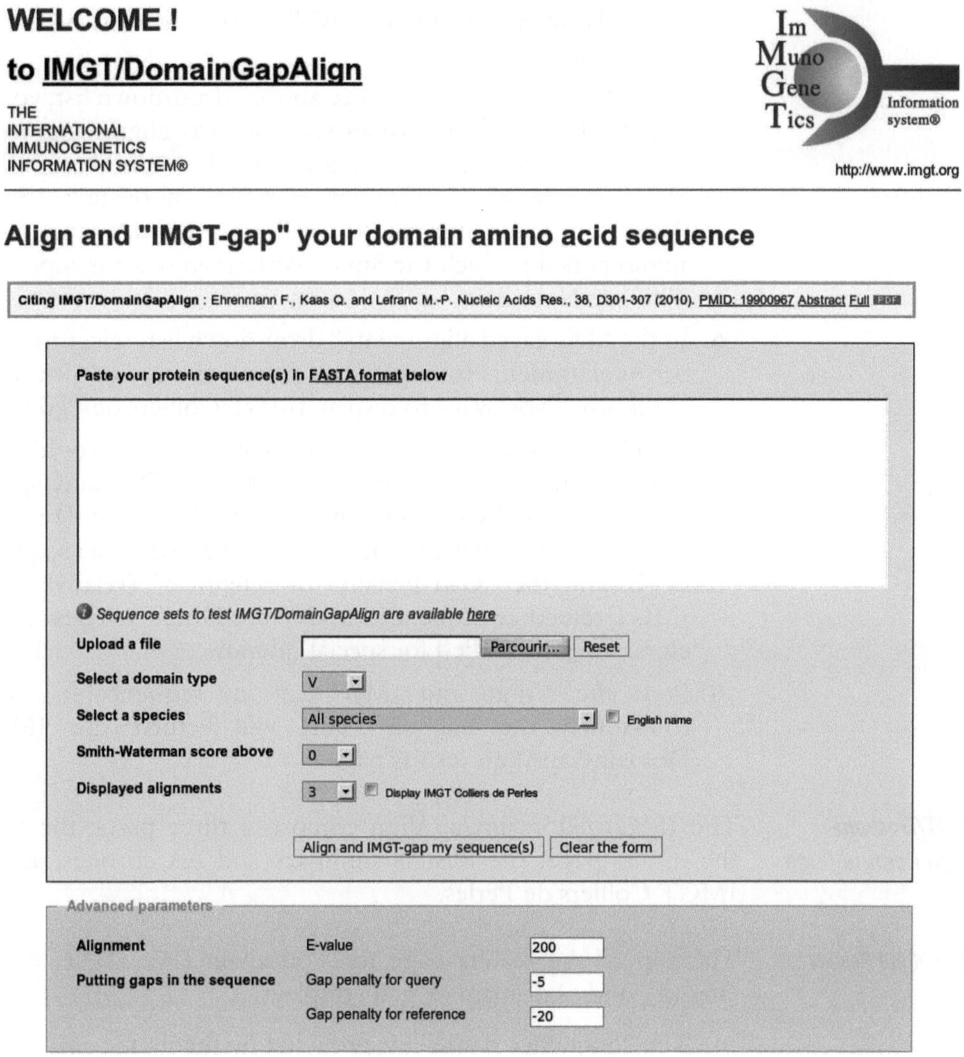


Fig. 1. IMGT/DomainGapAlign Welcome page.

same domain type. If not, the query needs to be launched for each domain type, successively. If the limits and the numbers of domains of an amino acid sequence are unknown, you can progressively analyze the protein, shortening the sequence once a domain has been identified by the tool (it should be reminded that the first domain identified by the tool is not necessarily the first one in the protein). Sequences to test IMGT/DomainGapAlign are available by clicking on the link "here."

3. In the "Select a Domain type" drop-down list, select a domain type V, C, or G (detailed in Subheading 1.2.1).
4. In the "Select a Species" drop-down list, select a Species. If the selection is "All species," the IMGT/DomainGapAlign tool will compare your sequence with all sequences available for the

selected domain type in the IMGT reference directory (detailed in Subheading 1.2.2).

5. In the "Smith-Waterman score above" drop-down list, you can modify the Smith-Waterman score for the alignments to display. Selecting a higher score corresponds to a higher selection of the results to display. For example, choosing a "Smith-Waterman score above 200" will only provide and display alignments for which the Smith-Waterman score is superior to 200 (see Note 3).
6. In the "Displayed alignments" drop-down list, select the number of alignments to display (by default three) and tick off the checkbox if you want to display IMGT Colliers de Perles.
7. Check the "Advanced parameters" section if you would like to modify parameters. For alignment, IMGT/DomainGapAlign use parameters by default: The E-value (see Note 4) is set to 200, the "Gap penalty for query" (relative to the user sequence) is −5, and the "Gap penalty for reference" (relative to the IMGT reference sequence) is −20 (see Note 5). These parameters can be modified for special queries.
8. Press the "Align and IMGT-gap my sequence(s)" button to launch the analysis. This will return the IMGT/DomainGapAlign results page.

### 2.2. IMGT/DomainGapAlign Results Page

The IMGT/DomainGapAlign comprises three parts: the top of the results page, the Results summary and AA changes, and the IMGT Colliers de Perles.

#### 2.2.1. Top of the Results Page

The top of the results page for V domain (Fig. 2), C domain (Fig. 3), and G domain (Fig. 4) displays:

1. The "Sequence name" (as provided by the user).
2. The "Closest reference gene and allele(s) from the IMGT domain directory" section. The domain type (V, C or G) and the species as selected by the user are indicated in the section title (online in orange). The following results are displayed: "Gene and allele name" (see Note 2), "Species," "Domain number," "Smith-Waterman Score" (online in orange), label of the domain (online in color) as identified in the closest reference gene and allele domain with its "percentage of identity" and "Overlap" score. If several closest gene and alleles are displayed, the user can select "Align your sequence with" to display the corresponding alignment. For V-DOMAIN (Fig. 2a), the closest reference gene and alleles section shows the results for the V-REGION and J-REGION of the V and J genes and alleles, respectively.
3. The Alignment(s) with the domain of the closest gene and allele from the IMGT domain directory. The domain type (V, C or G) and the species as selected by the user as indicated in

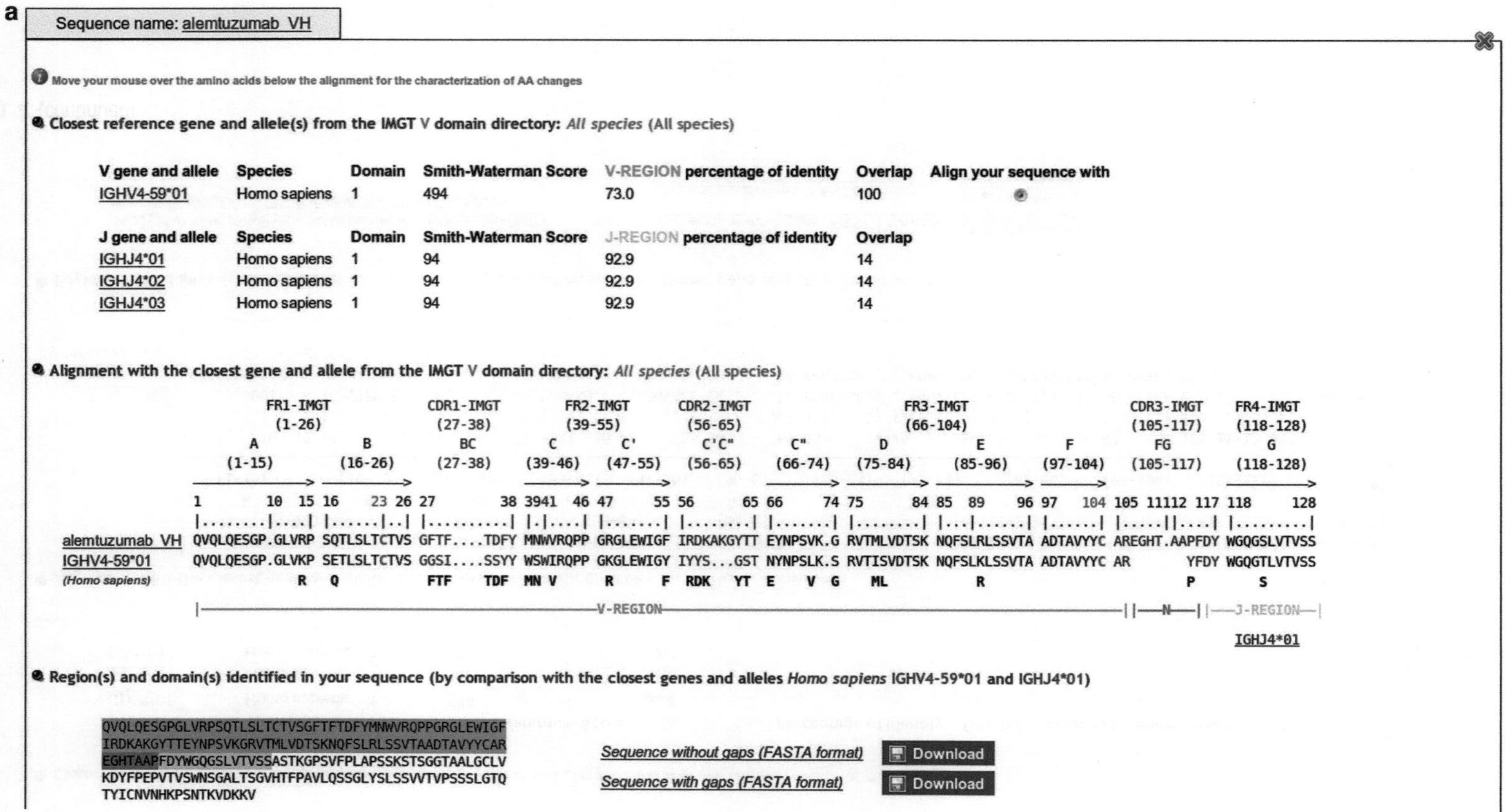


Fig. 2. IMGT/DomainGapAlign top of the results page for a V domain. (**a**) V-DOMAIN. The user amino acid (AA) sequence is aligned with the closest germline V-REGION and J-REGION, with IMGT gaps and delimitations of the FR-IMGT and CDR-IMGT according to the IMGT unique numbering (8, 9). In this example, the user sequence is the V-DOMAIN of the heavy chain (VH) of the monoclonal antibody (mAb) alemtuzumab (2). The V-REGION and J-REGION of the alemtuzumab (2) VH is identified as having 73 and 92.9% identity with the *Homo sapiens* IGHV4-59*01 and IGHJ4*01, respectively. The alemtuzumab domain, an antibody humanized before the IMGT standardized delimitations of the FR-IMGT and CDR-IMGT, shows 14 AA changes in the FR-IMGT, which most probably explains the immunogenicity of that antibody. (**b**) V-LIKE-DOMAIN. The CD58 domain is a V-LIKE-DOMAIN. The domain AA sequence of the 3D structure 1ci5 from IMGT/3Dstructure-DB (2) shows four AA changes compared to the CD58*01 allele.

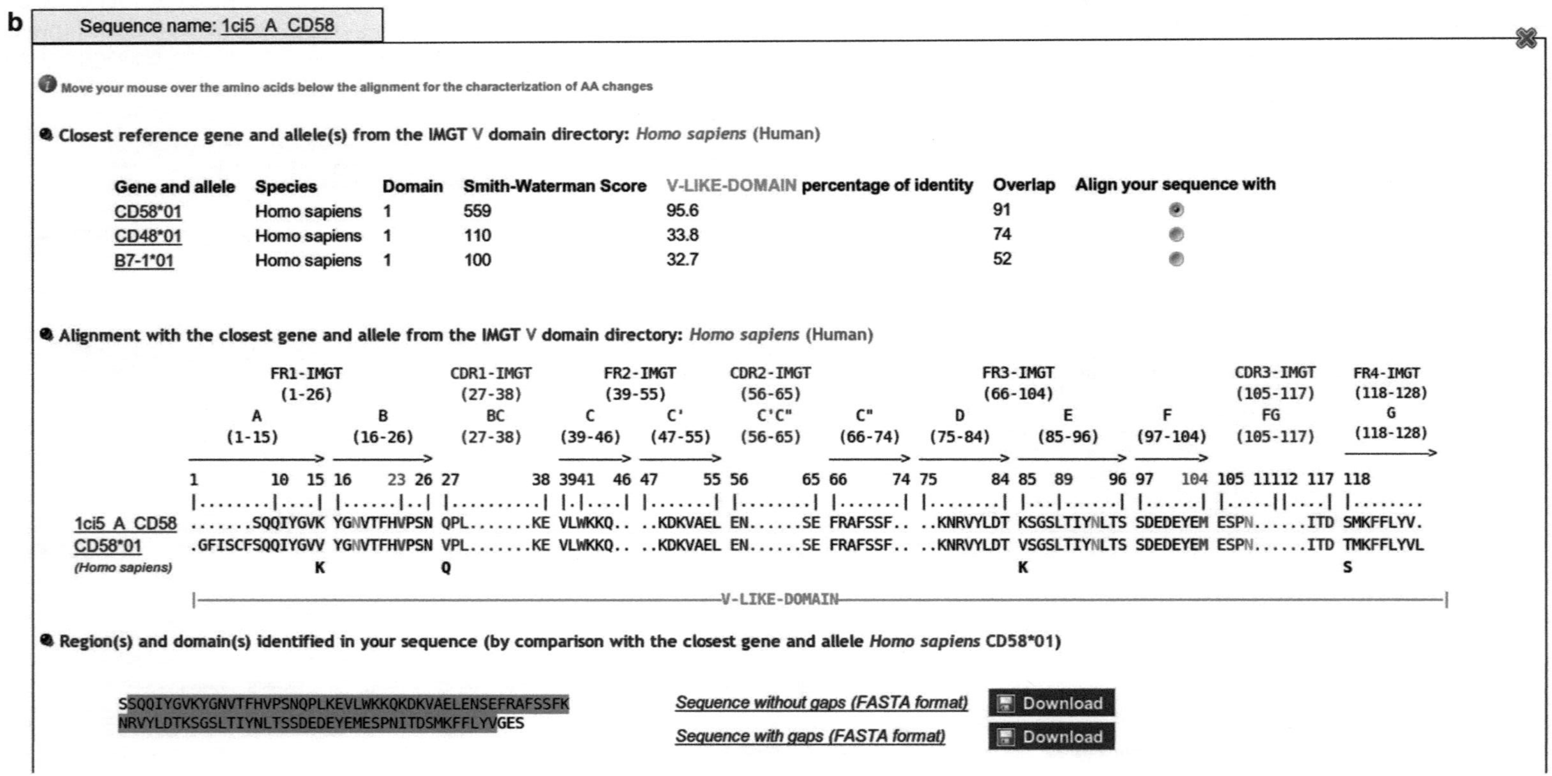


Fig. 2. (continued)

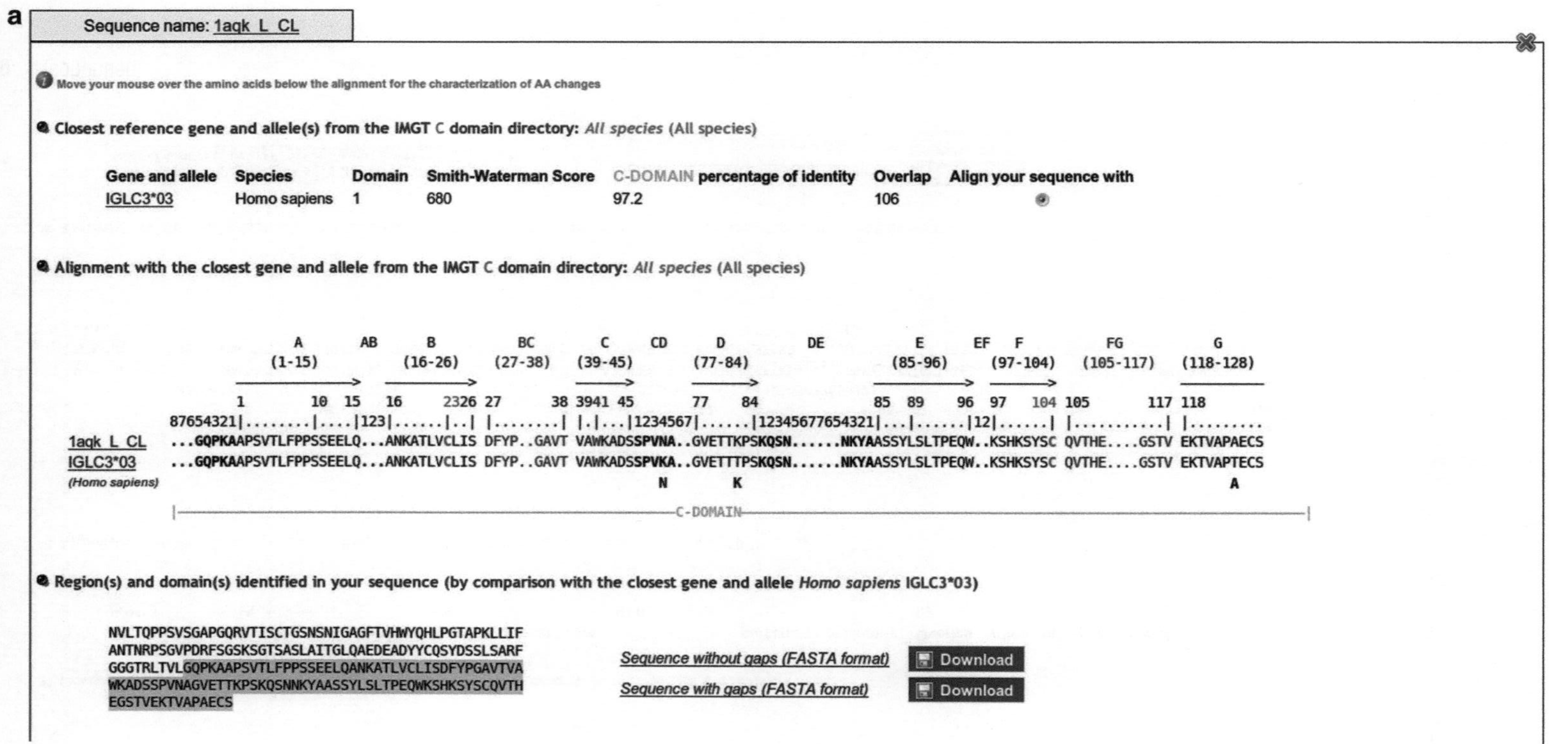


Fig. 3. IMGT/DomainGapAlign top of the results page for a C domain. (**a**) C-DOMAIN. The C domain of an IG lambda chain (or C-LAMBDA) is a C-DOMAIN. The domain AA sequence of the 3D structure 1aqk from IMGT/3Dstructure-DB (2) shows 3 AA changes with the closest allele IGLC3*03. (**b**) C-LIKE-DOMAIN. The beta2 microglobulin domain is a C-LIKE-DOMAIN. The AA sequence of the 3D structure 2d4d from IMGT/3Dstructure-DB (2) shows 3 AA changes compared to the B2M*01 allele.

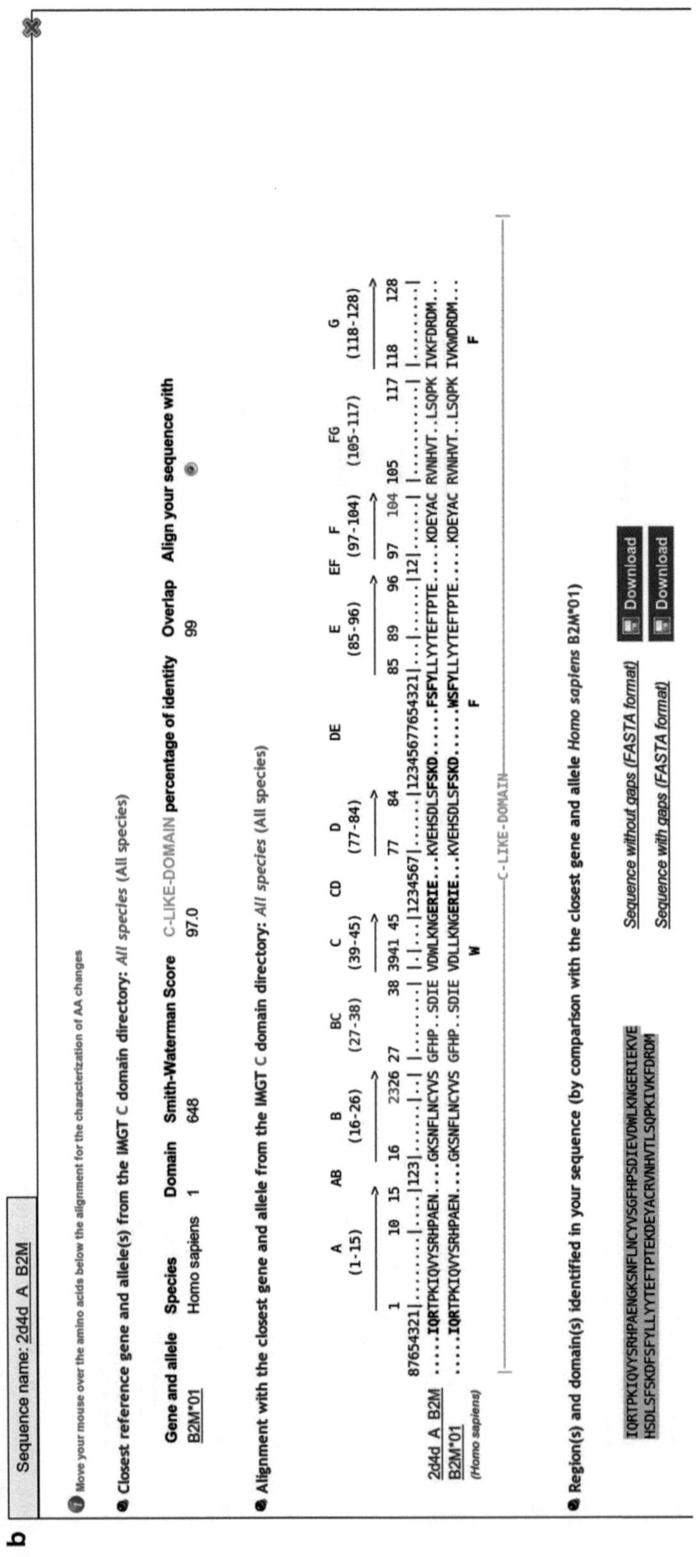


Fig. 3. (continued)

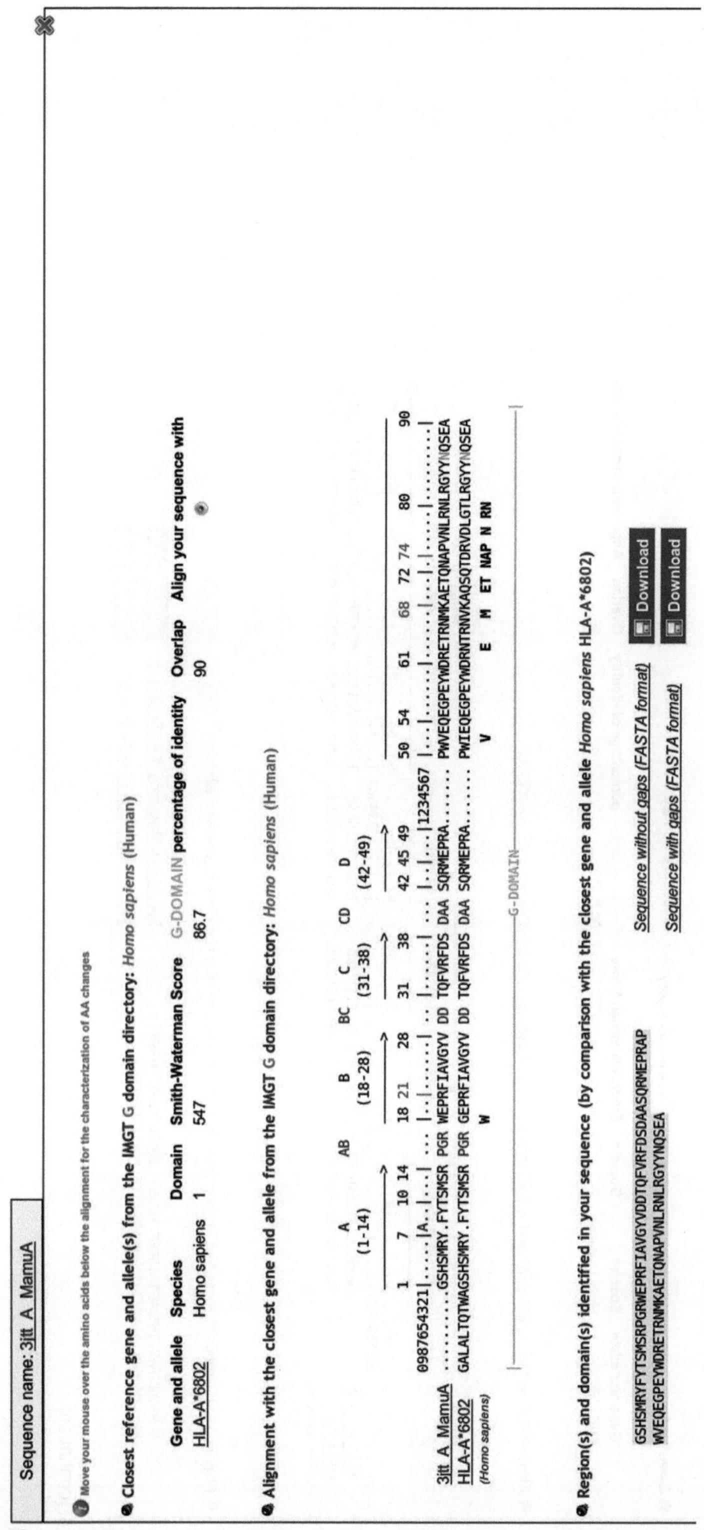


Fig. 4. IMGT/DomainGapAlign top of the results page for a G domain. (**a**) G-DOMAIN. The first G domain of a MH1 chain is a G-DOMAIN (more precisely G-ALPHA1) (11). In this example, the user sequence MamuA is the G-ALPHA1 of a MH1 protein of the rhesus monkey *Macaca mulatta* (2) aligned with the G-ALPHA1 of the closest human HLA-A allele. The query was with a selection of "Homo sapiens" as a species. (**b**) G-LIKE-DOMAIN. MICA is a member of the MhSF (11). The alignment identifies the closest domain as being [D2] (G-ALPHA2-LIKE) of MICA*65 (24).

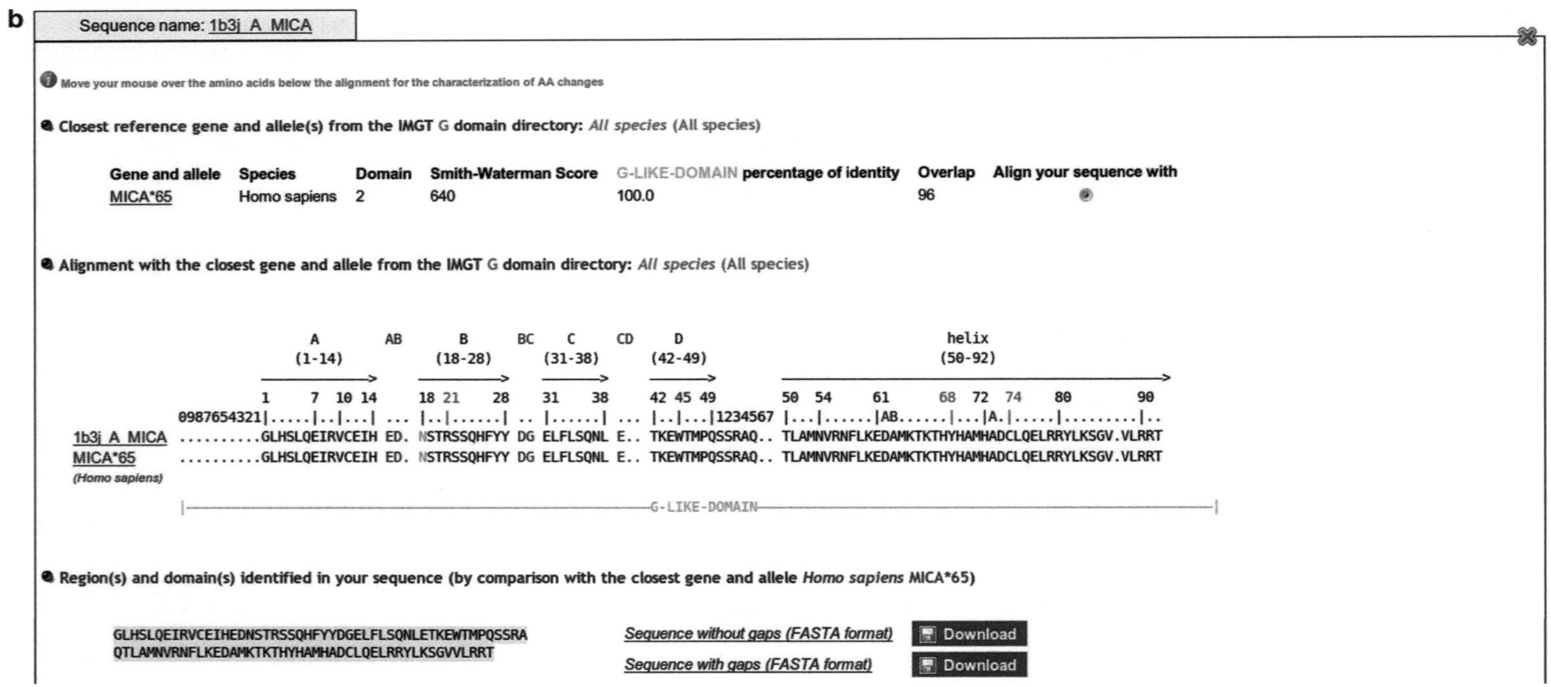


Fig. 4. (continued)

the section title (online in orange). The alignments are shown, based on the IMGT unique numberings for V domain (7–9) (Fig. 2), C domain (10) (Fig. 3), and G domain (11) (Fig. 4). Below the alignment, the label of the domain (online in color), as identified by the tool for the closest reference gene and allele, is indicated with a horizontal line. For the V-DOMAIN (Fig. 2a), the V-REGION, N (for (N-D)-REGION), and J-REGION are delimited by IMGT/DomainGapAlign.

4. The Region(s) and domain(s) identified in your sequence (by comparison with the closest genes and alleles). The species and gene and allele name identified by IMGT/DomainGapAlign are recalled (online in dark red). The domains (or regions for the V-DOMAIN) identified by the tool are colored according to the IMGT color menu.
5. The links to the sequence, with or without gaps, in FASTA format (HTML page or downloadable).

#### 2.2.2. Results Summary and AA Changes

The Results summary (by comparison with the closest gene and allele) and AA changes for V domain (Fig. 5), C domain (Fig. 6), and G domain (Fig. 7) are shown as tables:

1. The Results summary table has three columns that are common to the V, C, and G domains; and four additional columns for the V domain. The three common columns are:
   - Sequence name.
   - Domain (V-REGION for V-DOMAIN, V-LIKE-DOMAIN, C-DOMAIN, C-LIKE-DOMAIN, G-DOMAIN, G-LIKE-DOMAIN) identity percentage.
   - Total number of AA changes in the domain.

   The four additional columns for the V domain (Fig. 5) are: "CDR-IMGT lengths," "Number of different AA in CDR1-IMGT and CDR2-IMGT," "FR-IMGT lengths," and "Number of different AA in FR-IMGT" (V-DOMAIN) (Fig. 5a). "Loop lengths," "Number of different AA in loops," "Strand lengths," and "Number of different AA in strands" (V-LIKE-DOMAIN) (Fig. 5b).

2. The tables for AA changes are located below the Results summary and provide AA changes in:
   - Strands and Loops (for V domain) (Fig. 5).
   - Strands, Turns, and Loops (for C domain) (Fig. 6).
   - Strands, Turns, and Helix (for G domain) (Fig. 7).

   In these tables, IMGT amino acid (AA) changes are described according to the IMGT AA hydropathy, volume, and physicochemical classes (18) (see Note 6).

**a**

**Results summary (by comparison with the closest genes and alleles *Homo sapiens* IGHV4-59*01 and IGHJ4*01)**

| Sequence name | V-REGION identity percentage | CDR-IMGT lengths | Number of different AA in CDR1- and CDR2-IMGT | FR-IMGT lengths | Number of different AA in FR-IMGT | Total number of AA changes in V-DOMAIN |
|---|---|---|---|---|---|---|
| alemtuzumab_VH | 73.0% | [8.10.12] | 11 | [25.17.38.11] = 91 AA | 14 | 25 |

**AA changes in strands and loops**

| Strands | Number of different AA | AA changes |
|---|---|---|
| A strand (1-15) | 1 | K14>R (+ + +) very similar |
| B strand (16-26) | 1 | E17>Q (+ + -) similar |
| C strand (39-46) | 3 | W39>M (+ - -) dissimilar<br>S40>N (- - -) very dissimilar<br>I42>V (+ - +) similar |
| C' strand (47-55) | 2 | K48>R (+ + +) very similar<br>Y55>F (- + -) dissimilar |
| C" strand (66-74) | 3 | N66>E (+ - -) dissimilar<br>L71>V (+ - +) similar<br>S74>G (+ + -) similar |
| D strand (75-84) | 2 | I78>M (+ + -) similar<br>S79>L (- - -) very dissimilar |
| E strand (85-96) | 1 | K90>R (+ + +) very similar |
| F strand (97-104) | 0 | - |
| G strand (118-128) | 1 | T122>S (+ - +) similar |

| Loops | Number of different AA | AA changes |
|---|---|---|
| BC loop (27-38) | 6 | G28>F (- - -) very dissimilar<br>S29>T (+ - +) similar<br>I30>F (+ - -) dissimilar<br>S35>T (+ - +) similar<br>S36>D (- - -) very dissimilar<br>Y37>F (- + -) dissimilar |
| C'C" loop (56-65) | 5 | Y57>R (- - -) very dissimilar<br>Y58>D (- - -) very dissimilar<br>S59>K (- - -) very dissimilar<br>G63>Y (+ - -) dissimilar<br>S64>T (+ - +) similar |
| FG loop (105-117,111.1-111.6,112.1-112.6) | 1 | Y114>P (+ - -) dissimilar |

**AA changes in FR-IMGT and CDR-IMGT**

| FR-IMGT | Number of different AA | AA changes |
|---|---|---|
| FR1-IMGT (1-26) | 2 | K14>R (+ + +) very similar<br>E17>Q (+ + -) similar |
| FR2-IMGT (39-55) | 5 | W39>M (+ - -) dissimilar<br>S40>N (- - -) very dissimilar<br>I42>V (+ - +) similar<br>K48>R (+ + +) very similar<br>Y55>F (- + -) dissimilar |
| FR3-IMGT (66-104) | 6 | N66>E (+ - -) dissimilar<br>L71>V (+ - +) similar<br>S74>G (+ + -) similar<br>I78>M (+ + -) similar<br>S79>L (- - -) very dissimilar<br>K90>R (+ + +) very similar |
| FR4-IMGT (118-129) | 1 | T122>S (+ - +) similar |

| CDR-IMGT | Number of different AA | AA changes |
|---|---|---|
| CDR1-IMGT (27-38) | 6 | G28>F (- - -) very dissimilar<br>S29>T (+ - +) similar<br>I30>F (+ - -) dissimilar<br>S35>T (+ - +) similar<br>S36>D (- - -) very dissimilar<br>Y37>F (- + -) dissimilar |
| CDR2-IMGT (56-65) | 5 | Y57>R (- - -) very dissimilar<br>Y58>D (- - -) very dissimilar<br>S59>K (- - -) very dissimilar<br>G63>Y (+ - -) dissimilar<br>S64>T (+ - +) similar |

**b** ❷ **Results summary (by comparison with the closest gene and allele *Homo sapiens* CD58*01)**

| Sequence name | V-LIKE-DOMAIN identity percentage | Loop lengths | Number of different AA in loops | Strand lengths | Number of different AA in strands | Total number of AA changes in V-LIKE-DOMAIN |
|---|---|---|---|---|---|---|
| 1ci5_A_CD58 | 95.6% | [5.4.7] | 1 | [19.13.35.8] = 75 AA | 3 | 4 |

▸ **AA changes in strands and loops**

| Strands | Number of different AA | AA changes |
|---|---|---|
| A strand (1-15) | 1 | V15>K (- - -) very dissimilar |
| B strand (16-26) | 0 | - |
| C strand (39-46) | 0 | - |
| C' strand (47-55) | 0 | - |
| C" strand (66-74) | 0 | - |
| D strand (75-84) | 0 | - |
| E strand (85-96) | 1 | V85>K (- - -) very dissimilar |
| F strand (97-104) | 0 | - |
| G strand (118-128) | 1 | T118>S (+ - +) similar |

| Loops | Number of different AA | AA changes |
|---|---|---|
| BC loop (27-38) | 1 | V27>Q (- + -) dissimilar |
| C'C" loop (56-65) | 0 | - |
| FG loop (105-117,111.1-111.6,112.1-112.6) | 0 | - |

Fig. 5. IMGT/DomainGapAlign Results summary for a V domain. (**a**) V-DOMAIN. The results summary provides sequence name, V-REGION identity percentage, CDR-IMGT lengths, number of different AA in CDR1- and CDR2-IMGT, FR-IMGT lengths, number of different AA in FR-IMGT, and total number of AA changes. AA changes are shown for strands and loops, and for FR-IMGT and CDR-IMGT (8, 9). (**b**) V-LIKE-DOMAIN. The results summary provides sequence name, V-LIKE-DOMAIN, identity percentage, loop lengths, number of different AA in loops, strand lengths, number of different AA in strands, and the total number of AA changes in V-LIKE-DOMAIN. Loop lengths are those of [BC.C′C″.FG] that correspond to the CDR-IMGT of the V-DOMAIN. Strand lengths are those of [(A + B).(C + C′).(C″ + D + E + F).G] that correspond to the FR-IMGT of the V-DOMAIN (8, 9). AA changes are shown for strands and loops (9).

**Results summary (by comparison with the closest gene and allele *Homo sapiens* IGLC3*03)**

| Sequence name | C-DOMAIN identity percentage | Total number of AA changes in C-DOMAIN |
|---|---|---|
| 1aqk_L_CL | 97.2% | 3 |

| Strands | Number of different AA | AA changes |
|---|---|---|
| A strand (1.9-1.1,1-15) | 0 | - |
| B strand (16-26) | 0 | - |
| C strand (39-45) | 0 | - |
| CD strand (45.1-45.7) | 1 | K45.4>N (+ - -) dissimilar |
| D strand (77-84) | 1 | T82>K (- - -) very dissimilar |
| E strand (85-96) | 0 | - |
| F strand (97-104) | 0 | - |
| G strand (118-128) | 1 | T124>A (- - -) very dissimilar |

| Turns | Number of different AA | AA changes |
|---|---|---|
| AB turn (15.1-15.3) | 0 | - |
| DE turn (84.1-84.7, 85.7-85.1) | 0 | - |
| EF turn (96.1-96.2) | 0 | - |

| Loops | Number of different AA | AA changes |
|---|---|---|
| BC loop (27-36) | 0 | - |
| FG loop (105-117,111.1-111.6,112.1-112.6) | 0 | - |

Fig. 6. IMGT/DomainGapAlign Results summary for a C domain. Results summary are similar for a C-DOMAIN or a C-LIKE-DOMAIN. A C-DOMAIN (1aqk_L_CL, same sequence as in Fig. 3a) is shown as an example. The Results summary provides sequence name, C-DOMAIN (or C-LIKE-DOMAIN), identity percentage, and total number of AA changes. AA changes are shown for strands (A, B, C, CD, D, E, F, and G), turns (AB, DE, EF), and loops (BC and FG) (10).

**Results summary (by comparison with the closest gene and allele *Homo sapiens* HLA-A*6802)**

| Sequence name | G-DOMAIN identity percentage | Total number of AA changes in G-DOMAIN |
|---|---|---|
| 3jtt_A_MamuA | 86.7% | 12 |

| Turns | Number of different AA | AA changes |
|---|---|---|
| AB turn (15-17) | 0 | - |
| BC turn (29-30) | 0 | - |
| CD turn (39-41) | 0 | - |

| Strands | Number of different AA | AA changes |
|---|---|---|
| A strand (1.9-1.1,1-14) | 0 | - |
| B strand (18-28) | 1 | G19>W (- - -) very dissimilar |
| C strand (31-38) | 0 | - |
| D strand (42-49,49.1-49.5) | 0 | - |

| Helix | Number of different AA | AA changes |
|---|---|---|
| Helix (50-92) | 11 | I53>V (+ - +) similar<br>N62>E (+ - -) dissimilar<br>V66>M (+ - -) dissimilar<br>Q69>E (+ + -) similar<br>S70>T (+ - +) similar<br>T72>N (- + -) dissimilar<br>D72.>A (- - -) very dissimilar<br>R73>P (- - -) very dissimilar<br>D75>N (+ + -) similar<br>G77>R (- - -) very dissimilar<br>T78>N (- + -) dissimilar |

Fig. 7. IMGT/DomainGapAlign Results summary for a G domain. Results summary are similar for a G-DOMAIN or a G-LIKE-DOMAIN. A G-DOMAIN (G-ALPHA, same sequence as in Fig. 4a) is shown as an example. The results summary provides sequence name, G-DOMAIN (or G-LIKE-DOMAIN), identity percentage, and total number of AA changes. AA changes are shown for strands (A, B, C and D), turns (AB, BC and CD), and helix (11).

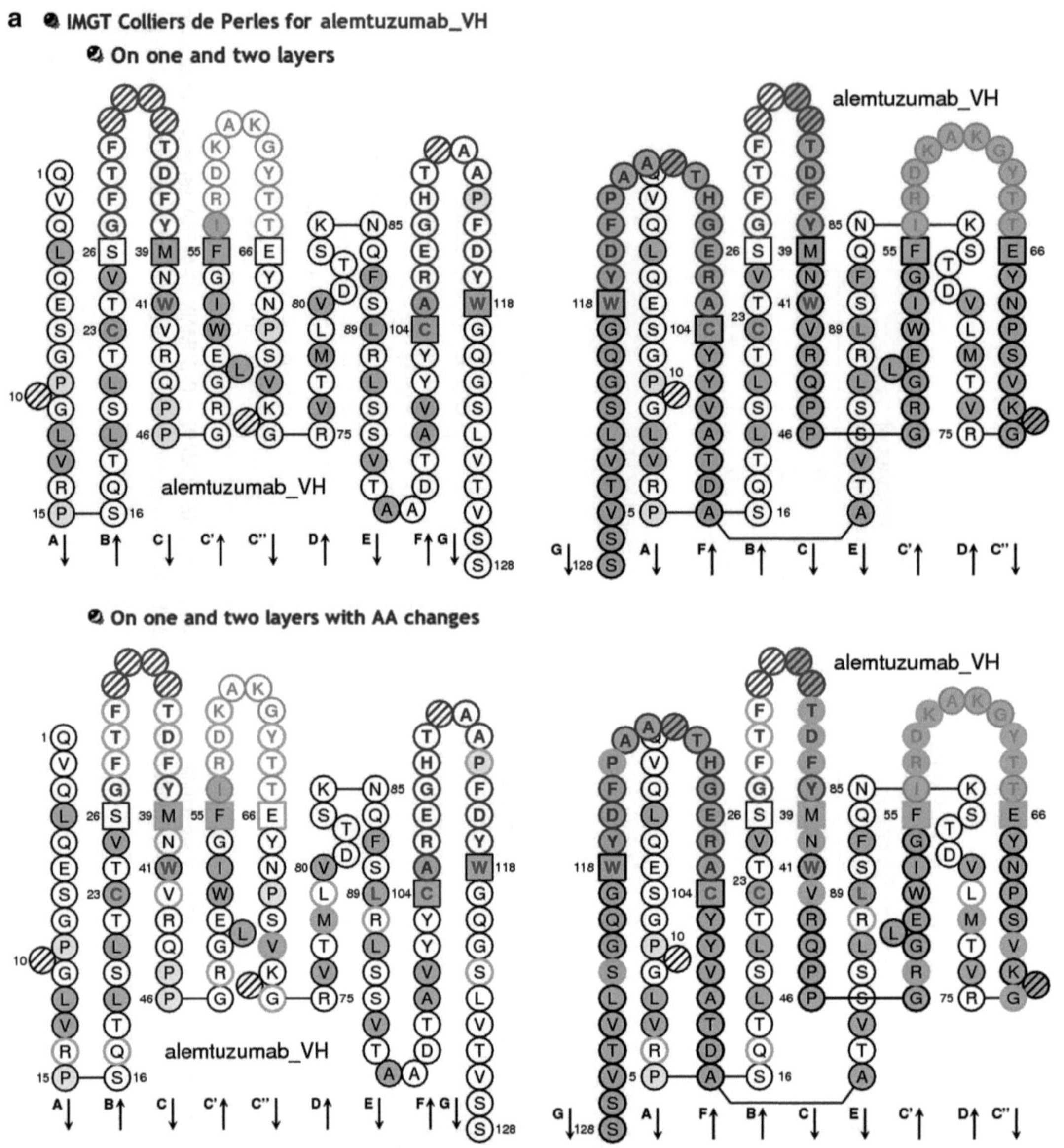


Fig. 8. IMGT Collier de Perles for V domain. IMGT Collier de Perles on one and two layers are on the *left* hand side and *right* hand side of the figure, respectively. IMGT Colliers de Perles on one and two layers with AA changes (online pink border) are shown in the lower section of the figure. (**a**) V-DOMAIN. In an IG or TR V-DOMAIN, the G-STRAND (or FR4-IMGT) is the C-terminal part of the J-REGION. The FR4-IMGT is at least composed of 9 or 10 amino acids beyond the phenylalanine F (J-PHE 118) or tryptophan W (J-TRP 118) of the motif F/W-G-X-G that characterizes the J-REGION. The example is the VH of alemtuzumab (as in Figs. 2a and 5a). The CDR-IMGT lengths are [8.10.12]. (**b**) V-LIKE-DOMAIN. The example is the V-LIKE-DOMAIN of *Homo sapiens* CD58 (same sequence as in Figs. 2b and 5b). The loop lengths are [5.4.7].

*2.2.3. IMGT Colliers de Perles*

If selected in the IMGT/DomainGapAlign Welcome page (step 6 in Subheading 2.1), IMGT Colliers de Perles on one and two layers, and with or without amino acid (AA) changes are displayed. IMGT Colliers de Perles for the V domain, C domain, and G domain are shown in Figs. 8–10, respectively. In IMGT Colliers de

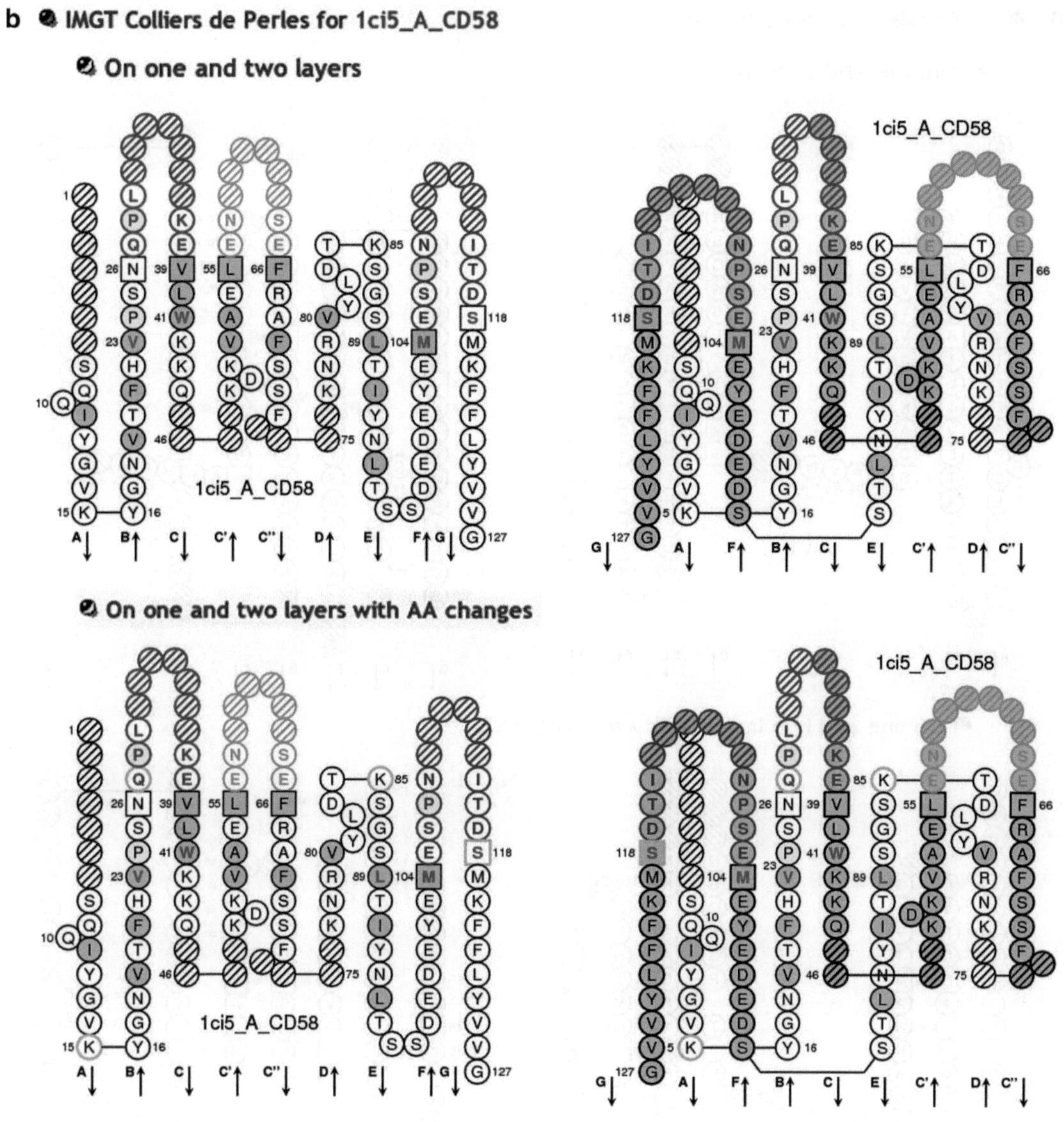


Fig. 8. (continued)

Perles for V and C domains (15–17), highlighted positions (online in blue) mean that the AA of the user sequence at these positions is hydrophobic (hydropathy index with positive value) or is a tryptophan (W), like in 50% or more of analyzed V domains. Anchor positions are in square (see Note 7). Hatched positions correspond to gaps according to the IMGT unique numbering (7–10). Proline are shown in yellow. Positions with bold (online red) letters indicate the four conserved positions that are common to a V domain and to a C domain: 1st-CYS 23, CONSERVED-TRP 41, hydrophobic 89, 2nd-CYS 104, and a fifth conserved position that is specific to the V-DOMAIN: J-TRP or J-PHE 118 (Table 1).

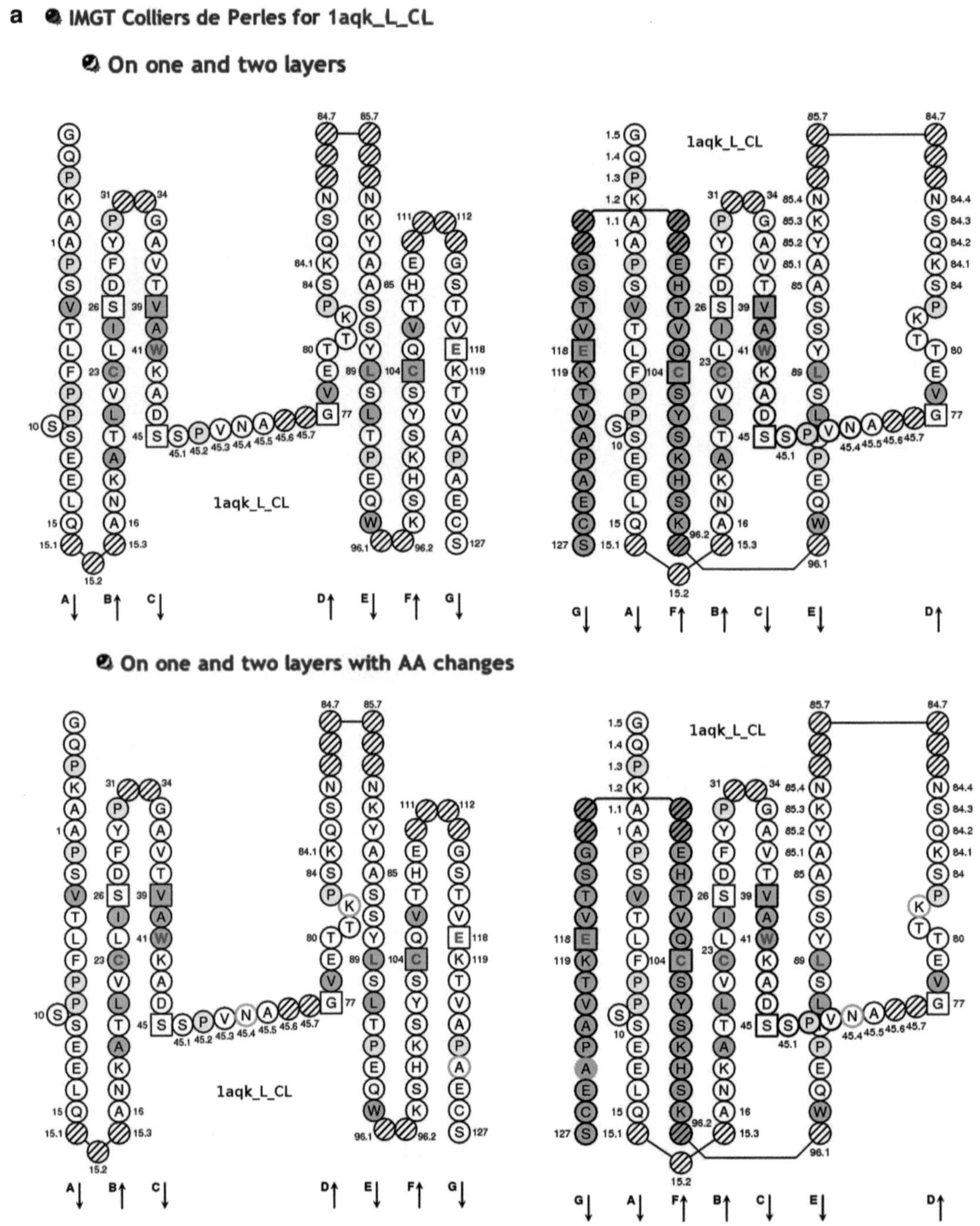


Fig. 9. IMGT Collier de Perles for C domain. IMGT Collier de Perles on one and two layers are on the *left* hand side and *right* hand side of the figure, respectively. IMGT Colliers de Perles on one and two layers with AA changes (online pink border) are shown in the lower section of the figure. (**a**) C-DOMAIN. The example is the *Homo sapiens* C-LAMBDA of 1aqk (1aqk_L_CL) as in Figs. 3a and 6. (**b**) C-LIKE-DOMAIN. The example is the B2M C-LIKE-DOMAIN of 2d4d (same sequence as in Fig. 3b).

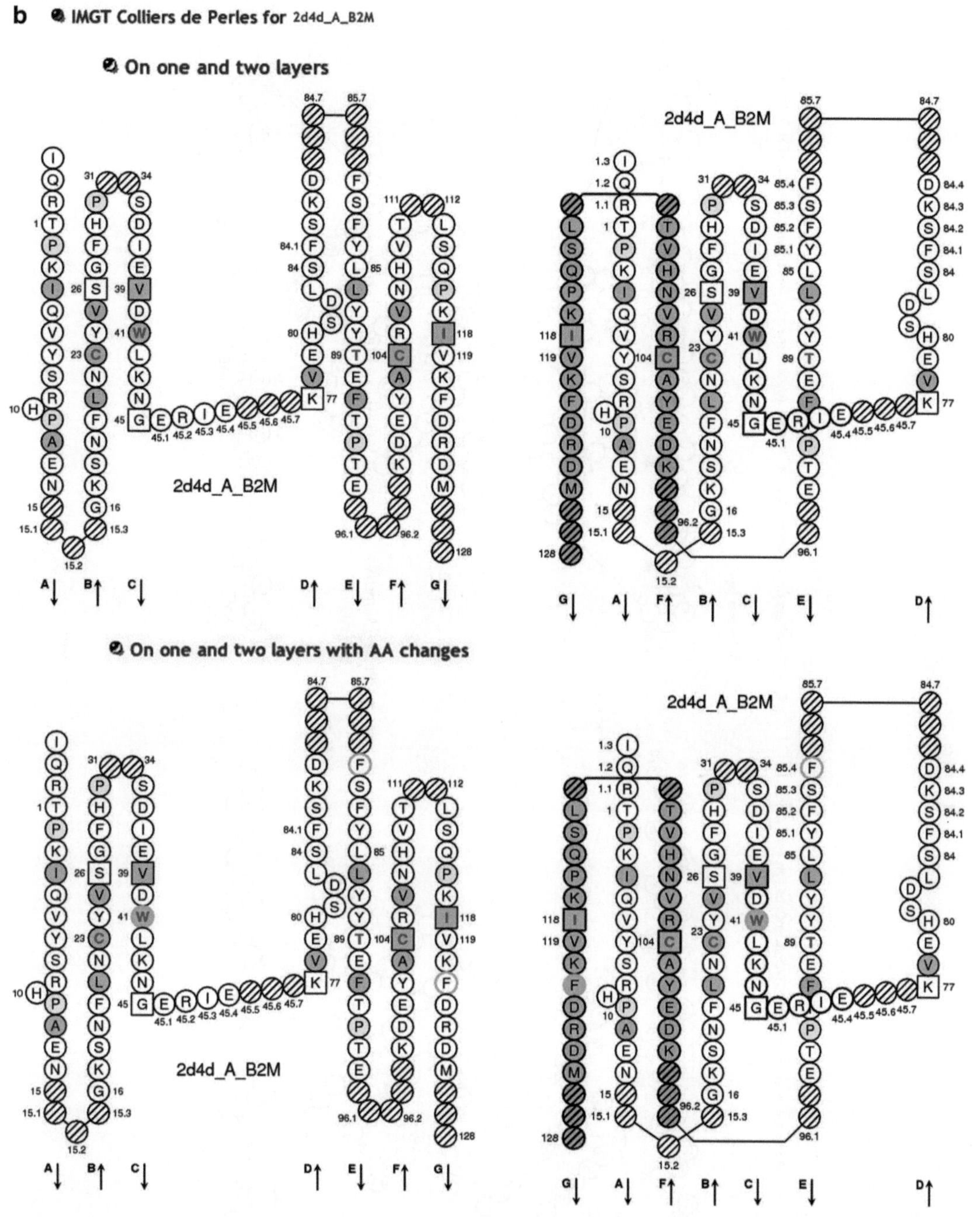


Fig. 9. (continued)

The MH groove (16, 17) which binds peptide consists of two G domains, belonging to the same chain (MH1-ALPHA) for MH class I (MH1) or to two different chains (MH2-ALPHA and MH2-BETA) for MH class II (MH2) (11). For the MhSF other than MH (or RPI-MH1Like) (see Note 8), the two G domains

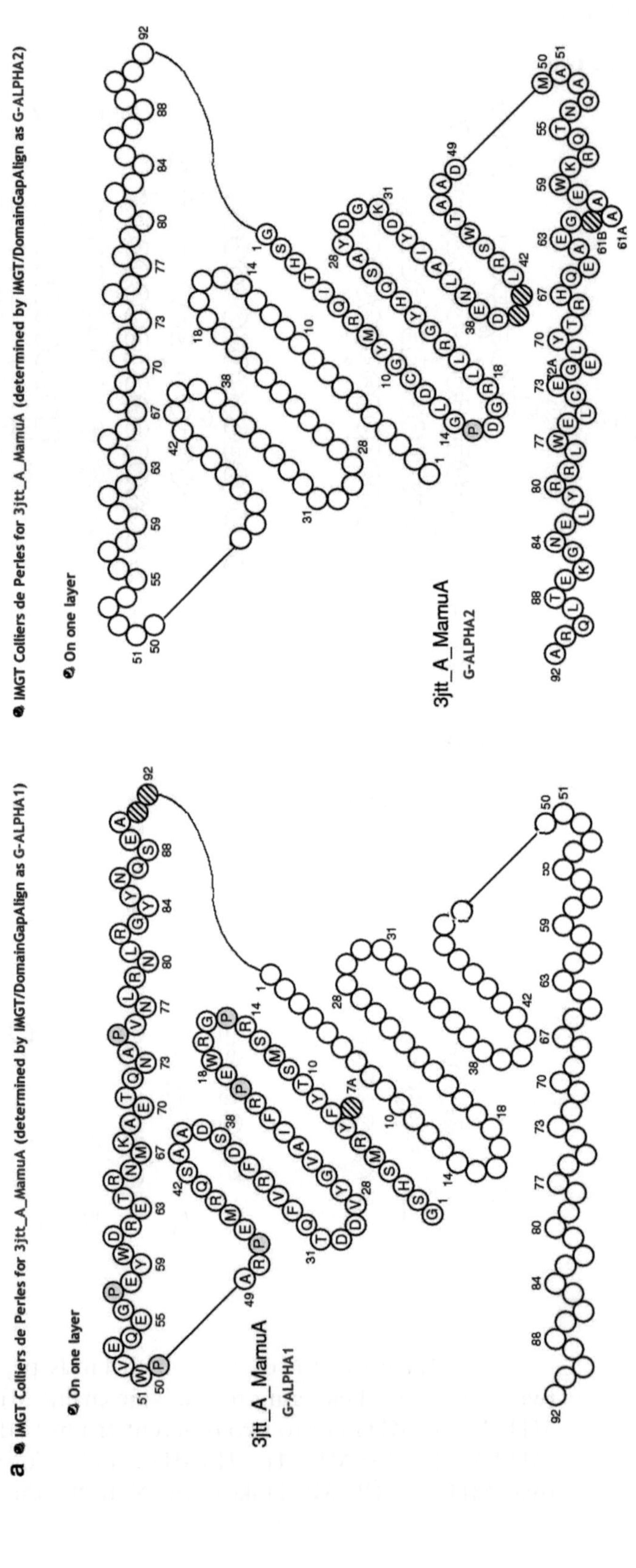
a
IMGT Colliers de Perles for 3jtt_A_MamuA (determined by IMGT/DomainGapAlign as G-ALPHA1)
On one layer
3jtt_A_MamuA
G-ALPHA1
IMGT Colliers de Perles for 3jtt_A_MamuA (determined by IMGT/DomainGapAlign as G-ALPHA2)
On one layer
3jtt_A_MamuA
G-ALPHA2

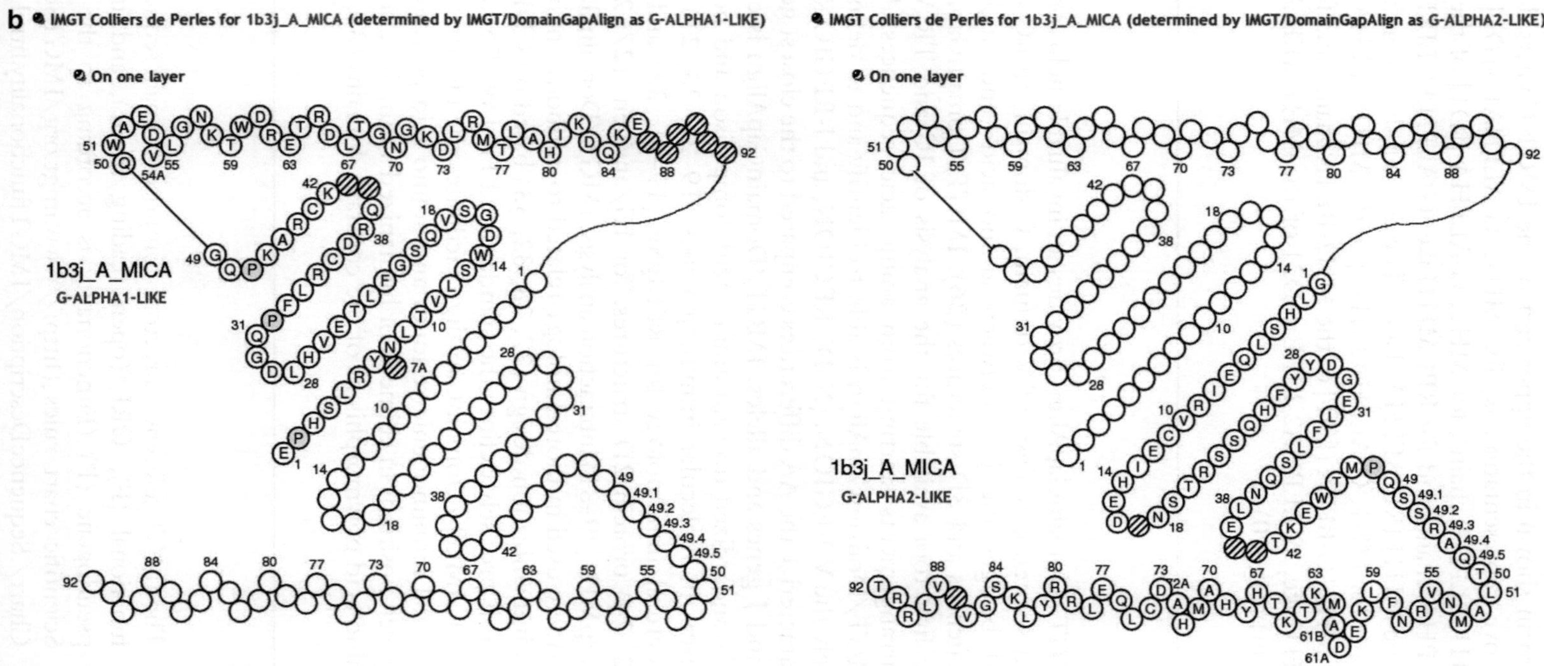


Fig. 10. IMGT Collier de Perles for G domain. IMGT/DomainGapAlign works per domain. IMGT Collier de Perles of the MH groove are shown separately (2). (**a**) G-DOMAIN. The example is a MH1 groove. The domain G-ALPHA1 ([D1] of the MH1-ALPHA chain) is automatically located by the tool in the upper part of the IMGT Collier de Perles groove representation (the example is G-ALPHA1 of MamuA, 3jtt_A_MamuA, *left* hand side of the figure), whereas the domain G-ALPHA2 ([D2] of the MH1-ALPHA chain) is automatically located in the lower part of the groove (the example is G-ALPHA2 of MamuA, 3jtt_A_MamuA, *right* hand side of the figure). (**b**) G-LIKE-DOMAIN. The domain G-ALPHA1-LIKE ([D1] of the MH1LIKE-ALPHA chain) is automatically located in the upper part (G-ALPHA1-LIKE, 1b3j_A_MICA, *left* hand side of the figure) where the domain G-ALPHA2-LIKE ([D2] of the MH1LIKE-ALPHA chain) is automatically located in the lower part (G-ALPHA2-LIKE, 1b3j_A_MICA, *right* hand side of the figure) (same sequence as in Fig. 4b). Note that in IMGT/3Dstructure-DB (2), the two G domains are displayed together.

also belong to the same chain (MH1LIKE-ALPHA) (11, 24). The domain shown in the upper part of the IMGT Colliers de Perles groove representation is, for MH1, G-ALPHA1 ([D1] of the MH1-ALPHA chain), for MH2, G-ALPHA ([D1] of the MH2-ALPHA chain) and for RPI-MH1Like, G-ALPHA1-LIKE ([D1] of the MH1LIKE-ALPHA chain). The domain shown in the lower part is for MH1, G-ALPHA2 ([D2] of the MH1-ALPHA chain), for MH2, G-BETA ([D1] of the MH2-BETA chain), and for RPI-MH1Like, G-ALPHA2-LIKE ([D2] of the MH1LIKE-ALPHA chain) (Fig. 10).

## 3. Conclusion

IMGT/DomainGapAlign provides an invaluable help for amino acid sequence analysis of V domain, C domain, and G domain and bridges the gap between amino acid (and nucleotide) sequences and 3D structures (26). IMGT/DomainGapAlign is the first tool available for the analysis of IG and TR V-(D)-J rearrangements starting from amino acid sequences. Indeed, IMGT/DomainGapAlign is able to identify and to delimit precisely the V-REGION, (N-D)-REGION, and J-REGION and to characterize the AA differences compared to the closest germline V and J genes and alleles. IMGT/DomainGapAlign is essential for standardized domain amino acid comparison and polymorphisms in molecular immunogenetics (19–21, 23, 24) and in structural immunology for RPI.IgSF (19–21, 23) and MhSF (22, 24) protein 2D structures, for IG/antigen (27, 28) and TR/pMH (29–31) interaction analysis. IMGT/DomainGapAlign is widely used in biotechnology related to antibody engineering and humanization design (27, 28, 32, 33) based on CDR grafting as it precisely defines the standardized FR-IMGT and CDR-IMGT. IMGT/DomainGapAlign facilitates the identification of potential immunogenic residues and amino acid polymorphism at given positions in chimeric or humanized antibodies, including amino acid polymorphisms of the constant domains (34, 35).

## 4. Notes

1. The IMGT reference directory comprises domain sequences of functional (F), ORF (open reading frame), and in-frame pseudogene (P) (Functionality is according to the IMGT Scientific chart rules (http://www.imgt.org/IMGTScientificChart/ SequenceDescription/IMGTfunctionality.html), based on the concepts of identification, generated from the IDENTIFICATION axiom) (3–6).

2. In IMGT, an allele is a polymorphic variant of a gene, which is characterized by the mutations of its sequence at the nucleotide level, identified in its core coding sequence and compared to the gene reference sequence designated as allele *01. Identical sequences at the amino acid level may therefore correspond to different alleles in the IMGT domain reference directory.
3. The Smith-Waterman algorithm is a well-known algorithm for performing local sequence alignment (36). The algorithm determines identical regions between two nucleotide or protein sequences. Instead of looking at the complete sequence, the Smith-Waterman algorithm compares segments of all possible lengths and optimizes the similarity measure. The higher the score, the better the alignment in a series of results. Selecting a higher score in IMGT/DomainGapAlign corresponds to a display of higher sequence similarities.
4. The Expect value (E-value) is a parameter that describes the number of hits one can "expect" to see by chance, for a given score of the match, when searching a database of a particular size. Each hit is associated to a score and an E-value. For example, an E-value of 1 assigned to a match "means" that in a database of a particular size one can expect 1 hit with a similar score simply by chance. The lower the E-value, or the closer it is to zero, the more "significant" the match is. A way of measuring the significance of a score of an alignment is to consider its E-value. Decreasing the E-value parameter for the alignment corresponds to a higher selection of the results to display.
5. The alignment is performed by a modified Smith-Waterman algorithm that considers the IMGT gap as a full amino acid and which discriminates the creation of gaps in the IMGT reference sequence. The asymmetry management of insertions between the user query and the reference sequences allows the user to modify one or the other gap penalty.
6. The amino acid (AA) changes are described according to the IMGT AA hydropathy, volume, and physicochemical classes (18). For example, Q1 > E (++−) means that in the AA change (Q > E), the two amino acids belong to the same hydropathy (+) and volume (+) classes but to different physicochemical properties (−) classes. Four types of AA changes are identified in IMGT: very similar (+++), similar (++−, +−+), dissimilar (−−+, −+−, +−−) and very dissimilar (−−−).
7. Anchors are positions that belong to strands and represent anchors for the loops of the V and C domains (and by extension to the transverse CD strand of the C domain that does not have the C′-C″ loop). Positions 26 and 39 are anchors of the BC-LOOP (CDR1-IMGT in V-DOMAIN). Positions 55

and 66 are anchors of the C′-C″ loop (CDR2-IMGT in V-DOMAIN), whereas positions 45 and 77 are anchors of the CD-STRAND of the C domain. Positions 104 and 118 are anchors of the FG-LOOP (CDR3-IMGT in V-DOMAIN). Anchor positions are shown as squares in IMGT Colliers de Perles.

8. MhSF proteins other than MH only include RPI-MH1Like proteins (there is no "RPI-MH2Like" identified so far) (11, 22, 24). The RPI-MH1Like proteins in humans comprise: AZGP1, CD1A to CD1E, FCGRT, HFE, MICA and MICB, MR1, PROCR (previously EPCR), RAET1E, RAETG, and RAET1L (22, 24).

## References


1. Lefranc M-P, Giudicelli V, Ginestoux C, Jabado-Michaloud J, Folch G, Bellahcene F, Wu Y, Gemrot E, Brochet X, Lane J, Regnier L, Ehrenmann F, Lefranc G, Duroux P (2009) IMGT®, the international ImMunoGeneTics information system®. Nucleic Acids Res 37:D1006–D1012
2. Ehrenmann F, Kaas Q, Lefranc M-P (2010) IMGT/3Dstructure-DB and IMGT/DomainGapAlign: a database and a tool for immunoglobulins or antibodies, T cell receptors, MHC, IgSF and MhcSF. Nucleic Acids Res 38:D301–D307
3. Giudicelli V, Lefranc M-P (1999) Ontology for immunogenetics: IMGT-ONTOLOGY. Bioinformatics 15:1047–1054
4. Lefranc M-P, Giudicelli V, Ginestoux C, Bosc N, Folch G, Guiraudou D, Jabado-Michaloud J, Magris S, Scaviner D, Thouvenin V, Combres K, Girod D, Jeanjean S, Protat C, Yousfi Monod M, Duprat E, Kaas Q, Pommié C, Chaume D, Lefranc G (2004) IMGT-ONTOLOGY for Immunogenetics and Immunoinformatics. In Silico Biol 4:17–29. http://www.imgt.org
5. Lefranc M-P (2004) IMGT-ONTOLOGY and IMGT databases, tools and web resources for immunogenetics and immunoinformatics. Mol Immunol 40:647–660
6. Duroux P, Kaas Q, Brochet X, Lane J, Ginestoux C, Lefranc M-P, Giudicelli V (2008) IMGT-Kaleidoscope, the formal IMGT-ONTOLOGY paradigm. Biochimie 90: 570–583
7. Lefranc M-P (1997) Unique database numbering system for immunogenetic analysis. Immunol Today 18:509
8. Lefranc M-P (1999) The IMGT unique numbering for immunoglobulins, T cell receptors and Ig-like domains. Immunologist 7:132–136
9. Lefranc M-P, Pommié C, Ruiz M, Giudicelli V, Foulquier E, Truong L, Thouvenin-Contet V, Lefranc G (2003) IMGT unique numbering for immunoglobulin and T cell receptor variable domains and Ig superfamily V-like domains. Dev Comp Immunol 27:55–77
10. Lefranc M-P, Pommié C, Kaas Q, Duprat E, Bosc N, Guiraudou D, Jean C, Ruiz M, Da Piedade I, Rouard M, Foulquier E, Thouvenin V, Lefranc G (2005) IMGT unique numbering for immunoglobulin and T cell receptor constant domains and Ig superfamily C-like domains. Dev Comp Immunol 29:185–203
11. Lefranc M-P, Duprat E, Kaas Q, Tranne M, Thiriot A, Lefranc G (2005) IMGT unique numbering for MHC groove G-DOMAIN and MHC superfamily (MhcSF) G-LIKE-DOMAIN. Dev Comp Immunol 29:917–938
12. Lefranc M-P, Lefranc G (2001) The immunoglobulin FactsBook. Academic Press, London, UK, pp 1–458
13. Lefranc M-P, Lefranc G (2001) The T cell receptor FactsBook. Academic Press, London, UK, pp 1–398
14. Giudicelli V, Chaume D, Lefranc M-P (2005) IMGT/GENE-DB: a comprehensive database for human and mouse immunoglobulin and T cell receptor genes. Nucleic Acids Res 33:D256–D261
15. Ruiz M, Lefranc M-P (2002) IMGT gene identification and Colliers de Perles of human immunoglobulins with known 3D structures. Immunogenetics 53:857–883
16. Kaas Q, Lefranc M-P (2007) IMGT Colliers de Perles: standardized sequence-structure representations of the IgSF and MhcSF superfamily domains. Curr Bioinform 2:21–30

17. Kaas Q, Ehrenmann F, Lefranc M-P (2007) IG, TR and IgSf, MHC and MhcSF: what do we learn from the IMGT Colliers de Perles? Brief Funct Genomic Proteomic 6:253–264
18. Pommié C, Levadoux S, Sabatier R, Lefranc M-P (2004) IMGT standardized criteria for statistical analysis of immunoglobulin V-REGION amino acid properties. J Mol Recognit 17:17–32
19. Duprat E, Kaas Q, Garelle V, Lefranc G, Lefranc M-P (2004) IMGT standardization for alleles and mutations of the V-LIKE-DOMAINs and C-LIKE-DOMAINs of the immunoglobulin superfamily. In: Pandalai SG (ed) Recent research developments in human genetics Research Signpost, Trivandram, Kerala, vol 2. pp 111–136
20. Garapati VP, Lefranc M-P (2007) IMGT Colliers de Perles and IgSF domain standardization for T cell costimulatory activatory (CD28, ICOS) and inhibitory (CTLA4, PDCD1 and BTLA) receptors. Dev Comp Immunol 31:1050–1072
21. Bernard D, Hansen JD, du Pasquier L, Lefranc M-P, Benmansour A, Boudinot P (2005) Costimulatory receptors in jawed vertebrates: conserved CD28, odd CTLA4 and multiple BTLAs. Dev Comp Immunol 31:255–271
22. Duprat E, Lefranc M-P, Gascuel O (2006) A simple method to predict protein binding from aligned sequences-application to MHC superfamily and beta2-microglobulin. Bioinformatics 22:453–459
23. Bertrand G, Duprat E, Lefranc M-P, Marti J, Coste J (2004) Characterization of human FCGR3B*02 (HNA-1b, NA2) cDNAs and IMGT standardized description of FCGR3B alleles. Tissue Antigens Cover 64:119–131
24. Frigoul A, Lefranc M-P (2005) MICA: standardized IMGT allele nomenclature, polymorphisms and diseases. In: Pandalai SG (ed) Recent research developments in human genetics, vol 3. Research Signpost, Trivandrum, Kerala, pp 95–145
25. Brochet X, Lefranc M-P, Giudicelli V (2008) IMGT/V-QUEST: the highly customized and integrated system for IG and TR standardized V-J and V-D-J sequence analysis. Nucleic Acids Res 36:W503–W508
26. Lefranc M-P, Giudicelli V, Regnier L, Duroux P (2008) IMGT®, a system and an ontology that bridge biological and computational spheres in bioinformatics. Brief Bioinform 9:263–275
27. Lefranc M-P (2009) Antibody databases and tools: The IMGT® experience. In: Zhiqiang An (ed) Therapeutic monoclonal antibodies: from bench to clinic (chapter 4). John Wiley & Sons, Inc., Hoboken, NJ, USA, pp 91–114
28. Ehrenmann F, Duroux P, Giudicelli V, Lefranc M-P (2010) Standardized sequence and structure analysis of antibody using IMGT®. In: Kontermann R, and Dübel S (eds) Antibody engineering (chapter 2), vol 2, Springer-Verlab, Berlin, Heidelberg, pp 11–31
29. Kaas Q, Ruiz M, Lefranc M-P (2004) IMGT/3Dstructure-DB and IMGT/StructuralQuery, a database and a tool for immunoglobulin, T cell receptor and MHC structural data. Nucleic Acids Res 32:D208–D210
30. Kaas Q, Lefranc M-P (2005) T cell receptor/peptide/MHC molecular characterization and standardized pMHC contact sites in IMGT/3Dstructure-DB. In Silico Biol 5: 505–528
31. Kaas Q, Duprat E, Tourneur G, Lefranc M-P (2008) IMGT standardization for molecular characterization of the T cell receptor/peptide/MHC complexes. In: Schoenbach C, Ranganathan S, Brusic V (eds) Immunoinformatics. Immunomics Reviews, Series of Springer Science and Business Media LLC (chapter 2). Springer, New York, USA, pp 19–49
32. Lefranc M-P (2009) Antibody databases: IMGT®, a French platform of world-wide interest. Bases de données anticorps: IMGT®, une plate-forme française d'intérêt mondial "Anticorps monoclonaux en thérapeutique". Med Sci 25:1020–1023
33. Lefranc M-P (2011) Antibody nomenclature: from IMGT-ONTOLOGY to INN definition. MAbs 3:1–2
34. Jefferis R, Lefranc M-P (2009) Human immunoglobulin allotypes: possible implications for immunogenicity. MAbs 1(4):332–338
35. Lefranc M-P, Lefranc G (2012) Human Gm, Km and Am allotypes and their molecular characterization: a remarkable demonstration of polymorphism. In: Tait B, Christiansen F (eds) Methods in Molecular Biology – Immunogenetics, Chapter 34
36. Smith TF, Waterman MS (1981) Identification of common molecular subsequences. J Mol Biol 147(1):195–197

# Chapter 34

# Human Gm, Km, and Am Allotypes and Their Molecular Characterization: A Remarkable Demonstration of Polymorphism

**Marie-Paule Lefranc and Gérard Lefranc**

## Abstract

Human immunoglobulin allotypes are antigenic determinants (or "markers") determined serologically, classically by hemagglutination inhibition, on the human immunoglobulin (IG) heavy and light chains. The allotypes have been identified on the gamma1, gamma2, gamma3, and alpha2 heavy chains (they are designated as G1m, G2m, G3m, and A2m allotypes, respectively), and on the kappa light chain (Km allotypes). Gm-Am allotypes are inherited in fixed combinations, or Gm-Am haplotypes, owing to the linkage of the human IGHC genes (IGHG3, IGHG1, IGHA1, IGHG2, IGHG4, IGHE, and IGHA2 from 5′ to 3′ in the IGH locus on chromosome 14). Gm and Am allotypes have been one of the most powerful tools in population genetics and very instrumental in molecular characterization of the human IGHC genes (gene conversion, copy number variation, gene order). They represent a major system for understanding immunogenicity of the polymorphic IG chains, in relation with amino acid and conformational changes. The correlation between G3m allotypes and amino acid changes has been possible with the sequencing of many alleles of the IGHG3 gene, from individuals from different populations and with known allotypes. In this chapter, we integrate genetics and sequence data and provide an updated overview of the Gm-Am haplotypes and Km allotypes. We propose, for the first time, a complete elucidation of the G3m allotypes, illustrated by the "IMGT G3m allele butterfly" concept that allows a graphical representation of the G3m alleles (variants of a gene expressing a given set of allotypes). Knowledge of allotypes is important in antibody engineering and humanization of monoclonal antibodies to improve immunotherapy.

**Key words:** IMGT, Immunogenetics, Allotype, Haplotype, Gm, Km, Am, Gm-Am, Immunoinformatics, Immunoglobulin, Antibody, Allelic polymorphism, IMGT-ONTOLOGY

## 1. Introduction

Allotypes are allelic antigenic determinants identified in humans on the immunoglobulin (IG) gamma1, gamma2, gamma3, and alpha2 heavy chains (they are designated as G1m, G2m, G3m, and A2m allotypes, respectively), and on the kappa light chain (Km allotypes) (1).

Frank T. Christiansen and Brian D. Tait (eds.), *Immunogenetics: Methods and Applications in Clinical Practice*, Methods in Molecular Biology, vol. 882, DOI 10.1007/978-1-61779-842-9_34, © Springer Science+Business Media New York 2012

Recently, allotypes regained a lot of attention, owing to the development of therapeutical monoclonal antibodies (2) and their potential immunogenicity (3, 4). IMGT®, the international ImMunoGeneTics information system® (http://www.imgt.org) (5, 6), was built on the concepts of IMGT-ONTOLOGY (7–9), providing a standardized characterization of the allotypes. The concepts of classification (nomenclature of genes and alleles (10–13)) and the concepts of numerotation (IMGT unique numbering for constant (C) domains (14)) are used in the IMGT gene database, IMGT/GENE-DB (15), the three-dimensional (3D) database, IMGT/3Dstructure-DB (16, 17), the IMGT online tools, IMGT/Collier-de-Perles (18, 19), IMGT/DomainGapAlign (17), and the IMGT Repertoire Web resources ("Protein displays," "Alignments of alleles," "Allotypes," etc.) (5, 6).

The first allotype was identified by Grubb in 1956 (20, 21), and for a period of 20 years, Gm, Am, and Km allotypes were discovered and characterized (20–46). Currently, 26 allotypes are known. Gm and Am allotypes are inherited in fixed combinations, or Gm-Am haplotypes (47–53), owing to the linkage of the corresponding encoding human IG heavy constant (IGHC) genes (IGHG3, IGHG1, IGHG2, IGHA2, respectively, from 5′ to 3′ in the IGH locus on chromosome 14) (1, 11). This system is unique in its ability to characterize human populations by specific sets of haplotypes, and for years, the Gm haplotypes have been the most powerful tools for the characterization of different populations (47–87). The Gm system is very instrumental for population genetics research, as it is highly polymorphic and unbalanced with respect to linkage. Interestingly also, it is one of the cheapest and one of the most informative systems. Vast screenings of human populations worldwide have uncovered considerable variability both in the contents of Gm haplotypes and in their frequencies, which enabled the investigators to examine valuable data with regard to gene admixture, genogeography, ethnoanthropology, evolutionary, and population genetics. It is one of the most powerful tools to characterize the polymorphism between individuals. Prior to the development of DNA fingerprinting techniques, Gm haplotypes were used for follow-up of bone marrow transplants (88), forensic medicine, and paternity testing.

Gm analysis has thrown light on the molecular characterization and evolution of the human IGHC genes (1, 47–53, 89–113), including evidence for "silent" IGHG3 on three exceptional haplotypes, in seven homozygous individuals in two related Lebanese and Syrian families (48), gene conversion (100, 102, 103, 106), gene duplications and deletions, and gene copy number variations (CNV) (97–99, 102, 105, 107, 108, 110, 111). It is worthwhile to note that it is the absence of the G1m allotypes in a healthy consanguineous Tunisian woman that led to the first description of a large deletion of 150 kilobases encompassing several IGHC genes on both chromosomes 14 and of the simultaneous and complete absence of the IgG1, IgG2, IgG4 and IgA2 subclasses in a healthy individual (97–99). This multigene deletion contributed to the identification of the order of the human IGHC genes (114, 115) and was the first demonstration of a CNV of the IGHC genes in humans (97–99). Correlations between Gm and restriction fragment length polymorphism (RFLP) have been carried out for haplotypes from diverse populations (1, 116–122). In this chapter, we first present an overview on the basic information on allotypes and isoallotypes, then we describe Gm, Am, and Km allotypes with their localization in the C domains and correlation with amino acid changes, and Gm, Am, and Km alleles with their correspondence to the IGHG, IGHA, and IGKC gene alleles. The first complete molecular characterization of the G3m alleles, illustrated by the "IMGT G3m allele butterfly" representation, is provided. This information confirms the importance of conformational configuration in the expression of allotypes and will be useful for understanding immunogenicity of therapeutical antibodies that may be used with various isotypes and allotypes in different populations.

## 2. Basic Information on Allotypes and Isoallotypes

### 2.1. Human IG Allotype Discovery

Allotypy within IgG was first described by Grubb who showed that certain human sera would agglutinate erythrocytes sensitized with human "incomplete" anti-Rh antibody (20, 21) (see Note 1). Polymorphism of the C region of human IG heavy gamma and alpha and light kappa chains was subsequently recognized by serological typing using the classical reaction of inhibition of hemagglutination (20–46). Thus, the discovery of this polymorphism demonstrated that exposure of an individual to IgG or IgA of a nonself allotype can induce an anti-allotype response.

### 2.2. Gm, Am, and Km Allotype and Allele Definition

Allotypes of IG are unique antigenic determinants recognized by specific antibodies. They are IG markers that, in terms of immunogenicity, represent B cell epitopes. Allotypes correspond to serologically detected amino acid changes that characterize the polymorphism of a chain within a given isotype. By definition, allotypes are shared among individuals within populations. Allotypes have been identified on the C region of the human IG heavy gamma1, gamma2, gamma3, and alpha2 chains of the IgG1, IgG2, IgG3, and IgA2 subclasses, respectively, and on the C region of the human IG light kappa chains (see Note 2). They are designated as Gm (Gamma marker), Am (Alpha marker), and Km (Kappa marker), with a number for the subclass: G1m, G2m, and G3m for allotypes of the gamma1, gamma2, and gamma3 chains, and A2m for allotypes of the alpha2 chains (1).

A combination of allotypes, encoded by one or several alleles of a given gene (IGHG1, IGHG2, IGHG3, IGHA2, or IGKC) (see Note 3), is defined as a G1m, G2m, G3m, A2m, or Km allele, respectively.

### 2.3. Gm-Am Haplotype Definition

Gm allotypes are inherited in fixed combinations called "Gm haplotypes" (see Subheading 7) or "Gm-Am haplotypes" (if A2m allotypes are tested), owing to the linkage of the IGHC genes within a cluster in the IGH locus (47–53). Haplotypes have a low frequency of crossovers; however, crossover events and gene conversions (100, 102, 103, 106) have occurred during evolution resulting in characteristic haplotypes present in diverse populations, hence the usefulness of the allotype system in population studies. Equal or unequal crossovers, the later generating gene duplication (or expansion) or, in contrast, gene deletion (or contraction) in the IGH locus has been demonstrated (97–99, 102, 105, 107, 108, 110, 111) and they are now commonly named CNV.

### 2.4. Allotype Determination

#### 2.4.1. Hemagglutination Inhibition Methodology

Allotypes are determined by serological typing using a classical reaction of inhibition of hemagglutination. The methodology uses human O Rh+ erythrocytes (red blood cells) sensitized (coated) with "incomplete" anti-Rh IgG antibodies of known allotypes (e.g., G1m1), and human reagents (polyclonal IgG specific for a given allotype, e.g., anti-G1m1). The polyclonal IgG reagents are obtained from multiparous women, multiple transfused individuals, and normal blood donors. If the tested serum is G1m1-negative, the anti-G1m1 reagent binds the G1m1-positive antibodies coating the erythrocytes and the hemagglutination occurs. In contrast, if the tested serum is G1m1-positive, the anti-G1m1 reagent binds the G1m1-positive antibodies contained in the serum, and the hemagglutination is inhibited. The reactions are performed with different dilutions of the reagents and of the tested sera (47, 48, 52, 53). The determination of some allotypes (G2m23, A2m1, and A2m2) is more delicate owing to the rarity of the reagents and, in particular, the absence of available anti-Rh antibodies for the coating. In those cases, myeloma proteins are coupled using chromic chloride (123). It is highly recommended to provide the list and source of the anti-Rh, myeloma proteins, polyclonal IgG, and eventually their dilutions, the list of tested allotypes, and the number of individuals tested for each allotype, for allowing standardized result comparison.

#### 2.4.2. Phenotype and Genotype Deduction

Positive results (corresponding to a hemagglutination inhibition) and negative results (corresponding to a hemagglutination) obtained for the tested allotypes allow assignment of the "Gm phenotype" (or "Gm-Am phenotype," if the A2m allotypes are tested) of an individual (see Subheading 7.3). In populations where the main Gm (or Gm-Am) haplotypes are already known, it is usually possible to deduce, from the phenotype the Gm (or Gm-Am) genotype that is the two haplotypes that contribute to it (47–53). However, it is not always possible to deduce the genotype. In those cases, familial studies with allotype typing of several members are needed.

*2.4.3. Other Methodologies*

To compensate for the rarity of some reagents, attempts were made to obtain monoclonal antibodies; however, the main difficulty resides in the characterization of their specificity (124, 125). Molecular biology was first used for the determination of A2m2 by RFLP (101) (see Subheading 8.3). This method is particularly interesting given the rarity of the reagents and was the first protocol to determine allotypes in the absence of serum (e.g., from cell lines). Polymerase chain reaction (PCR) amplification methods, using allele-specific oligonucleotides (ASO) or specific restriction sites, were subsequently developed for the determination of the Km allotypes (126) and of some Gm allotypes (4, 127–130), but their application remains limited.

## 2.5. Allotype Characterization

*2.5.1. Allotype Nomenclature*

At present, 26 human allotypes are known, 20 Gm (18 "classical" ones and two "surnumerary" ones), three A2m, and three Km allotypes (Table 1). The 18 "classical" Gm allotypes comprise four G1m, G1m (1, 2, 3, 17), one G2m, G2m (23), and thirteen G3m, G3m (5, 6, 10, 11, 13, 14, 15, 16, 21, 24, 26, 27, 28). The two "surnumerary" allotypes, G1m27 and G1m28, correspond to allotypes demonstrated to be on gamma1 chains in Negroid populations, instead of being on gamma3, as expected (96). The A2m and Km comprise A2m (1, 2, 3) and Km (1, 2, 3), respectively.

*2.5.2. Allotype Localization*

The localization of the allotypes has been determined by inhibition studies with Fab and Fc fragments (obtained by papain digestion), and with pF'c fragments (obtained by pepsin digestion) of Gm-positive or Gm-negative myeloma proteins (131–136). Amino acid sequence analysis of peptides obtained from Fd (part of the heavy chain from a Fab) and from pF'c have revealed amino acid changes, allowing establishment of correlations between serologically defined allotypes and amino acid sequences. Except for G1m3 and G1m17 located on the CH1 of gamma1, all other Gm allotypes are localized on the Fc (on CH2 or on CH3) (Table 1). Thus, for example, the G3m21 allotype was detectable on the Fc fragment of gamma3 chains but not on isolated CH3 domains, and therefore was localized on the CH2 (134). G3m10, G3m11, and G3m13 were localized on the CH3 domain of the gamma3 chain (134). G3m28 was localized on the CH3 domain of a G3m28 myeloma protein (38). However, the first detailed correlation between G3m allotypes and amino acid changes has only been possible following the complete nucleotide sequencing of many IGHG3 alleles from individuals homozygous for well-characterized G3m alleles (104, 106, 113). G3m allotypes and their localization, and correspondence with G3m alleles, illustrated by the "IMGT G3m allele butterfly" representation, are further defined in this chapter (see Subheading 5.2).

**Table 1**
**Nomenclature of the Gm and Km allotypes**

| Localization[a] | | Nomenclature | | |
| --- | --- | --- | --- | --- |
| IG heavy chain | Domain | WHO nomenclature[b] | Previous designation | |
| H-GAMMA1 | CH3 | G1m1 | G1m(a) | Grubb (20), Grubb and Laurell (21) |
| | CH3 | G1m2 | (x) | Harboe and Lundevall (22) |
| | CH1 | G1m3 | (f) | Steinberg and Wilson (23), Gold et al. (24, 25) |
| | CH1 | G1m17 | (z) | Litwin and Kunkel (26) |
| | CH3 | G1m27[c] | | van Loghem et al. (96) |
| | CH3 | G1m28[c] | | van Loghem et al. (96) |
| H-GAMMA2 | CH2 | G2m23 | G2m(n) | Kunkel et al. (27) |
| H-GAMMA3 | CH3 | G3m5 | G3m(b1) | Harboe (28) |
| | CH3 | G3m6 | (c3) | Steinberg et al. (29) |
| | CH3 | G3m10 | (b5) | Ropartz et al. (30) |
| | CH3 | G3m11 | (b0) | Ropartz et al. (30) |
| | CH3 | G3m13 | (b3) | Steinberg and Goldblum (31) |
| | CH3 | G3m14 | (b4) | Steinberg and Goldblum (31) |
| | CH3 | G3m15 | (s) | Martensson et al. (32) |
| | CH2 | G3m16 | (t) | Martensson et al. (32) |
| | CH2 | G3m21 | (g1) | Natvig (33) |
| | CH3 | G3m24 | (c5) | van Loghem and Martensson (34) |
| | CH3 | G3m26 | (u) | van Loghem and Grobbelaar (35) |
| | CH3 | G3m27[d] | (v)[d] | Schanfield and Fudenberg (36) |
| | CH3 | G3m28[d] | (g5)[d] | Blanc et al. (37) |
| H-ALPHA2 | CH1 | A2m1 | A2m1 | Vyas and Fudenberg (39), Kunkel et al. (40) |
| | CH1 | A2m2 | A2m2 | van Loghem et al. (41) |
| | CH3 | A2m3[e] | | |

(continued)

**Table 1 (continued)**

| Localization[a] | | Nomenclature | | |
|---|---|---|---|---|
| IG light chain | Domain | WHO nomenclature[b] | Previous designation | |
| L-KAPPA | C-KAPPA | Km1 | Km1 | Ropartz et al. (43) |
| | C-KAPPA | Km2 | Km2 | Ropartz et al. (42) |
| | C-KAPPA | Km3 | Km3 | Steinberg et al. (44) |

[a]IMGT® labels for chains and domains are written in capital letters (concepts of description of IMGT-ONTOLOGY) (7, 8)
[b]The World Health Organization (WHO) nomenclature (45, 46) has been adopted by the WHO/International Union of Immunological Societies (IUIS)/IMGT nomenclature (12, 13) (see Note 4)
[c]Observed in Negroid populations (96) and in rare unusual haplotypes with "surnumerary" Gm27 and Gm28 in other populations (52, 53, 94, 95, 102). G1m27 and G1m28 are detected with the same reagents as G3m27 and G3m28 (see Subheading 5.1.7)
[d]In Caucasoid and Mongoloid populations, Gm27 and Gm28 are on gamma3 (G3m27 and G3m28); however, in rare unusual haplotypes, "surnumerary" Gm27 and Gm28 may be explained by the presence of G1m27 and G1m28 (52, 53, 94, 95, 102). In Negroid populations, Gm27 can be on the gamma3 chains (G3m27), but also on the gamma1 chains (G1m27), Gm28 is always "surnumerary" and on the gamma1 chains (G1m28) (96)
[e]Identified with TOU II-5 sera (IGHA2*02 allele) (98, 100, 101) (unpublished data, van Loghem, GL and MPL) (see Subheading 8.5)

**Table 2**
**Nomenclature and distribution of the isoallotypes**

| Nomenclature | | Distribution on IG heavy chains | | | | | |
|---|---|---|---|---|---|---|---|
| WHO nomenclature | Previous designation | gamma1 | gamma2 | gamma3 | gamma4 | alpha1 | alpha2 |
| nG1m1 | nG1m(a) | Allo | Iso | Iso | Iso[a] | – | – |
| nG1m17 | nG1m(z) | Allo | – | Iso | Iso | – | – |
| nG3m5 | nG3m(b1) | Iso[b] | Iso | Allo | – | – | – |
| nG3m11 | nG3m(b0) | Iso | Iso | Allo | – | – | – |
| nG3m21 | nG3m(g) | – | Iso | Allo | – | – | – |
| nG4m(a) | nG4m(a) | Iso | – | Iso | Allo | – | – |
| nG4m(b) | nG4m(b) | – | Iso | – | Allo | – | – |
| nA2m3[c] | nA2m(2) | – | – | – | – | Iso | Allo |

[a]Isoallotype only detected by some antisera
[b]In Negroid populations, the G1m28 allotype can be expressed instead of nG3m5 (see Subheading 5.1.7)
[c]nA2m3 has been renamed as this isoallotype is located on the CH3 domain and is antithetical to the A2m3 allele (it is not antithetical to A2m2 located on the CH1) (see Subheading 8.5)

### 2.6. Isoallotypes

By definition, allotypes are found on chains within one IG isotype (encoded by one given IG gene). However, the same amino acids may be found in chains of other isotypes (encoded by other IG genes), but without being polymorphic in these isotypes. If these amino acids are detected *in vitro* by antibody reagents, they are referred as "isoallotypes" (designated with the letter "n" preceding the allotype name, e.g., nG1m1). Seven isoallotypes have been identified for the gamma chains (137–141) and one for the alpha chains identified on the CH3 domain (142) (Table 2) (see Note 5).

### 2.7. Protein Displays and IMGT Colliers de Perles

Protein displays are standardized IMGT representations of the amino acid sequences of the coding regions of the genes (11). Protein displays of C domains show the sequences per domain, using the IMGT unique numbering for C domain (14). They allow a standardized localization of the amino acids involved in the allotypes in relation to the strands and loops of the domains. Figure 1 provides the Protein displays of the C domains (CH1, CH2, and CH3) of the IGHG and IGHA genes (5, 6, 17). Only the first allele is shown. Other alleles are available in IMGT/DomainDisplay (5, 6) and in IMGT/GENE-DB (15) (IMGT®, http://www.imgt.org). IMGT/DomainGapAlign (17) allows gaps to be inserted in C domains of the IGHG, IGHA, and IGKC genes according to the IMGT unique numbering (14). Correspondences with other numberings are available in the IMGT Scientific chart (http://www.imgt.org). Standardized representations or IMGT Colliers de Perles of the C domains can be obtained using the IMGT/Collier-de-Perles tool (18, 19).

## 3. G1m

### 3.1. G1m Allotypes and nG1m Allotypes

#### 3.1.1. G1m1 and nG1m1

G1m1 (previously G1m(a)) was the first discovered allotype (20). In 1956, Grubb noticed that 60% of normal human sera could inhibit the agglutination of human O Rh+ erythrocytes sensitized by means of certain "incomplete" anti-Rh sera, the factor responsible for the inhibition was called Gm(a) (now G1m1 allotype). Grubb and Laurel demonstrated that Gm(a) was transmitted as a dominant autosomal Mendelian trait (21).

By inhibition studies with IgG1 fragments, it was established that G1m1 is located on the CH3 domain and was associated with aspartate 356 and leucine 358 (Eu numbering) (131). According to the IMGT unique numbering for C domain (14), the G1m1 allotype corresponds to IGHG1 CH3 Asp D12 and Leu L14 (Table 3) (Figs. 2 and 3).

In the G1m1-negative gamma1 chains and in the gamma chains of the other IgG subclasses, glutamate (E) and methionine (M) are found, respectively, at positions 12 and 14 of the CH3

**a**

| Species | Gene | Allele | AccNum | Domain label | Domain | Sequence |
|---|---|---|---|---|---|---|
| | | | | | | A (1-15) AB B (16-26) BC (27-38) C (39-45) CD D (77-84) DE E (85-96) EF F (97-104) FG (105-117) G (118-128) |
| | | | | | | 1 10 15 16 2326 27 38 3941 45 77 84 85 89 96 97 104 105 117 118 128 |
| | | | | | | 87654321\|........\|....\|123\|......\|..\| \|.........\| \|.\|...\|1234567\|......\|12345677654321\|...\|......\|12\|......\| \|...........\| \|.........\| |
| *Homsap* | IGHG1 | IGHG1*01 | J00228 | CH1 | [D2] | ....ASTKGPSVFPLAPSSKSTS...GGTAALGCLVK DYFP..EPVT VSWNSGALTS....GVHTFPAVLQSS......GLYSLSSVVTVPSSSL...GTQTYIC NVNHKP..SNTKV DKKV....... |
| *Homsap* | IGHG2 | IGHG2*01 | J00230 | CH1 | [D2] | ....ASTKGPSVFPLAPCSRSTS...ESTAALGCLVK DYFP..EPVT VSWNSGALTS....GVHTFPAVLQSS......GLYSLSSVVTVPSSNF...GTQTYTC NVDHKP..SNTKV DKTV....... |
| *Homsap* | IGHG3 | IGHG3*01 | X03604 | CH1 | [D2] | ....ASTKGPSVFPLAPCSRSTS...GGTAALGCLVK DYFP..EPVT VSWNSGALTS....GVHTFPAVLQSS......GLYSLSSVVTVPSSSL...GTQTYTC NVNHKP..SNTKV DKRV....... |
| *Homsap* | IGHG4 | IGHG4*01 | K01316 | CH1 | [D2] | ....ASTKGPSVFPLAPCSRSTS...ESTAALGCLVK DYFP..EPVT VSWNSGALTS....GVHTFPAVLQSS......GLYSLSSVVTVPSSSL...GTKTYTC NVDHKP..SNTKV DKRV....... |
| *Homsap* | IGHG1 | IGHG1*01 | J00228 | CH2 | [D3] | ..APELLGGPSVFLFPPKPKDTLMI.SRTPEVTCVVV DVSHEDPEVK FNWYVDGVEVH...NAKTKPREEQYN......STYRVVSVLTVLHQDW..LNGKEYKC KVSNKA..LPAPI EKTISKAK... |
| *Homsap* | IGHG2 | IGHG2*01 | J00230 | CH2 | [D3] | ..AP.PVAGPSVFLFPPKPKDTLMI.SRTPEVTCVVV DVSHEDPEVQ FNWYVDGVEVH...NAKTKPREEQFN......STFRVVSVLTVVHQDW..LNGKEYKC KVSNKG..LPAPI EKTISKTK... |
| *Homsap* | IGHG3 | IGHG3*01 | X03604 | CH2 | [D3] | ..APELLGGPSVFLFPPKPKDTLMI.SRTPEVTCVVV DVSHEDPEVQ FKWYVDGVEVH...NAKTKPREEQYN......STFRVVSVLTVLHQDW..LNGKEYKC KVSNKA..LPAPI EKTISKTK... |
| *Homsap* | IGHG4 | IGHG4*01 | K01316 | CH2 | [D3] | ..APEFLGGPSVFLFPPKPKDTLMI.SRTPEVTCVVV DVSQEDPEVQ FNWYVDGVEVH...NAKTKPREEQFN......STYRVVSVLTVLHQDW..LNGKEYKC KVSNKG..LPSSI EKTISKAK... |
| *Homsap* | IGHG1 | IGHG1*01 | J00228 | CH3 | [D4] | ....GQPREPQVYTLPPSRDELT...KNQVSLTCLVK GFYP..SDIA VEWESNGQPEN...NYKTTPPVLDSD......GSFFLYSKLTVDKSRW..QQGNVFSC SVMHEA.LHNHYT QKSLSLSP... |
| *Homsap* | IGHG2 | IGHG2*01 | J00230 | CH3 | [D4] | ....GQPREPQVYTLPPSREEMT...KNQVSLTCLVK GFYP..SDIA VEWESNGQPEN...NYKTTPPMLDSD......GSFFLYSKLTVDKSRW..QQGNVFSC SVMHEA.LHNHYT QKSLSLSP... |
| *Homsap* | IGHG3 | IGHG3*01 | X03604 | CH3 | [D4] | ....GQPREPQVYTLPPSREEMT...KNQVSLTCLVK GFYP..SDIA VEWESSGQPEN...NYNTTPPMLDSD......GSFFLYSKLTVDKSRW..QQGNIFSC SVMHEA.LHNRFT QKSLSLSP... |
| *Homsap* | IGHG4 | IGHG4*01 | K01316 | CH3 | [D4] | ....GQPREPQVYTLPPSQEEMT...KNQVSLTCLVK GFYP..SDIA VEWESNGQPEN...NYKTTPPVLDSD......GSFFLYSRLTVDKSRW..QEGNVFSC SVMHEA.LHNHYT QKSLSLSL... |

**b**

| Species | Gene | Allele | AccNum | Domain label | Domain | Sequence |
|---|---|---|---|---|---|---|
| | | | | | | A (1-15) AB B (16-26) BC (27-38) C (39-45) CD D (77-84) DE E (85-96) EF F (97-104) FG (105-117) G (118-128) |
| | | | | | | 1 10 15 16 2326 27 38 3941 45 77 84 85 89 96 97 104 105 117 118 |
| | | | | | | 87654321\|........\|....\|123\|......\|..\| \|.........\| \|.\|...\|1234567\|......\|12345677654321\|...\|......\|12\|......\| \|...........\| \|....... |
| *Homsap* | IGHA1 | IGHA1*01 | J00220 | CH1 | [D2] | ....ASPTSPKVFPLSLCSTQP....DGNVVIACLVQ GFFPQ.EPLS VTWSESGQGV....TARNFPPSQDASG.....DLYTTSSQLTLPATQC..LAGKSVTC HVKHY...TNPSQ DVTVPCP. |
| *Homsap* | IGHA2 | IGHA2*01 | J00221 | CH1 | [D2] | ....ASPTSPKVFPLSLDSTPQ....DGNVVVACLVQ GFFPQ.EPLS VTWSESGQNV....TARNFPPSQDASG.....DLYTTSSQLTLPATQC..PDGKSVTC HVKHY...TNPSQ DVTVPCP. |
| *Homsap* | IGHA1 | IGHA1*01 | J00220 | CH2 | [D3] | ......CCHPRLSLHRPALEDLLL..GSEANLTCTLT GLRDA.SGVT FTWTPSSGKS.....AVQGPPERDLCG......CYSVSSVLPGCAEPW..NHGKTFTC TAAYPE..SKTPL TATLSKS. |
| *Homsap* | IGHA2 | IGHA2*01 | J00221 | CH2 | [D3] | ......CCHPRLSLHRPALEDLLL..GSEANLTCTLT GLRDA.SGAT FTWTPSSGKS.....AVQGPPERDLCG......CYSVSSVLPGCAQPW..NHGETFTC TAAHPE..LKTPL TANITKS. |
| *Homsap* | IGHA1 | IGHA1*01 | J00220 | CH3 | [D4] | ....GNTFRPEVHLLPPPSEELAL..NELVTLTCLAR GFSP..KDVL VRWLQGSQELPRE.KYLTWASRQEPSQG...TTTFAVTSILRVAAEDW..KKGDTFSC MVGHEA.LPLAFT QKTIDRLA |
| *Homsap* | IGHA2 | IGHA2*01 | J00221 | CH3 | [D4] | ....GNTFRPEVHLLPPPSEELAL..NELVTLTCLAR GFSP..KDVL VRWLQGSQELPRE.KYLTWASRQEPSQG...TTTFAVTSILRVAAEDW..KKGDTFSC MVGHEA.LPLAFT QKTIDRLA |

Fig. 1. Protein display of the human IGHG and IGHA constant (C) domains. (**a**) Human IGHG CH domains. (**b**) Human IGHA CH domains. Only allele *01 is shown (see Note 3). Other alleles are available in IMGT/DomainGapAlign (5, 6) and in IMGT/GENE-DB (15) (IMGT®, http://www.imgt.org). The alignments are based on the IMGT unique numbering for C domain (14). Hinge and CHS regions are not shown. Domains are numbered with [D1] being the variable domain (not shown).

## Table 3
## G1m allotypes and isoallotypes

| G1m allotypes and isoallotypes | Amino acid positions[a] | | | | |
|---|---|---|---|---|---|
| | Domain | CH1 | CH3[b] | | |
| | IMGT<br>Eu | **120**<br>*214* | **12**<br>*356* | **14**<br>*358* | **110**<br>*431* |
| G1m1 | | | Asp D12 | Leu L14 | |
| nG1m1 | | | Glu E12 | Met M14 | |
| G1m2 | | | | | Gly G110 |
| G1m3 | | Arg R120 + Ileu I103 | | | |
| G1m17 | | Lys K120 | | | |
| nG1m17 | | Arg R120 | | | |

[a]Positions in bold are according to the IMGT unique numbering for C domain (14), and in italics, Eu numbering (IMGT Scientific chart, http://www.imgt.org) (5, 6)

[b]G1m27 and G1m28 found in Negroid populations (96) are not shown. G1m27 most probably corresponds to IGHG1 CH3 Ileu I101, and G1m28 to IGHG1 CH3 Arg R115, Tyr Y116

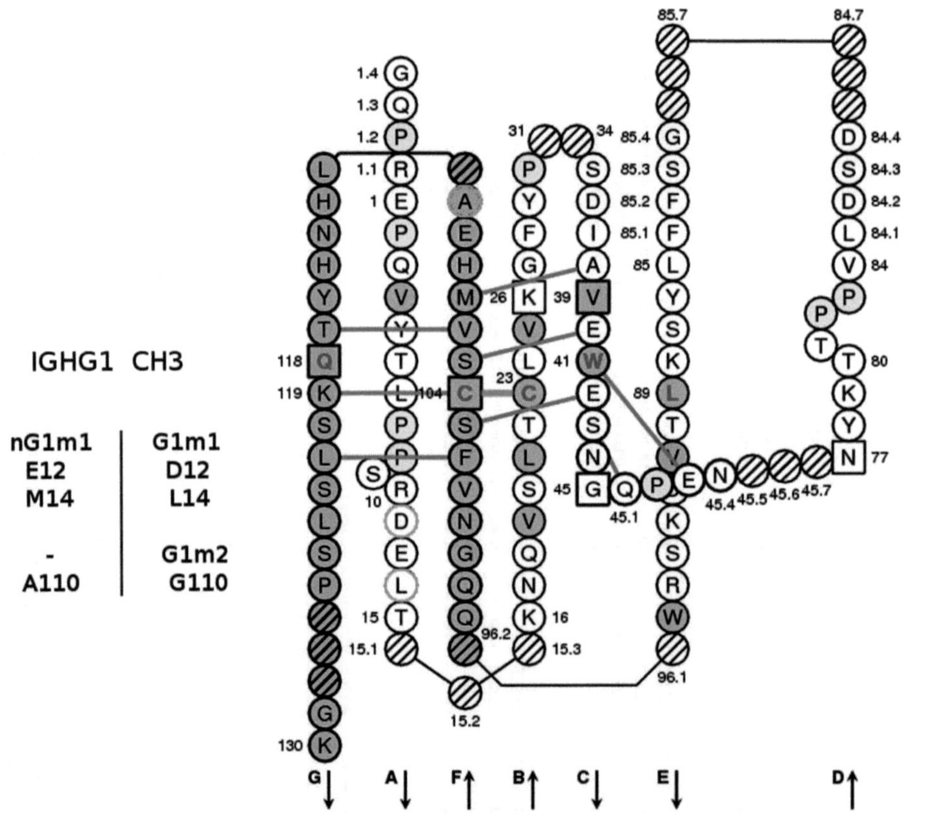


Fig. 2. IMGT Collier de Perles of the IGHG1 CH3 domain. The CH3 domain is from the b12 antibody (IMGT/3Dstructure-DB, code PDB:1hzh, http://www.imgt.org) (16, 17). The IMGT Collier de Perles is shown on two layers, with hydrogen bonds shown as *green lines* online. Hatched positions correspond to gaps according to the IMGT unique numbering (14). The aspartate D12 and leucine L14 (strand A) correspond to G1m1, whereas E12 and methionine M14 (not shown) correspond to nG1m1. In G1m2-negative chain, as that of b12, there is an alanine at position 110. A glycine at position 110 would correspond to G1m2. The amino acids glycine (G)-lysine (K) at positions 129 and 130 represent the CHS in secreted IG.

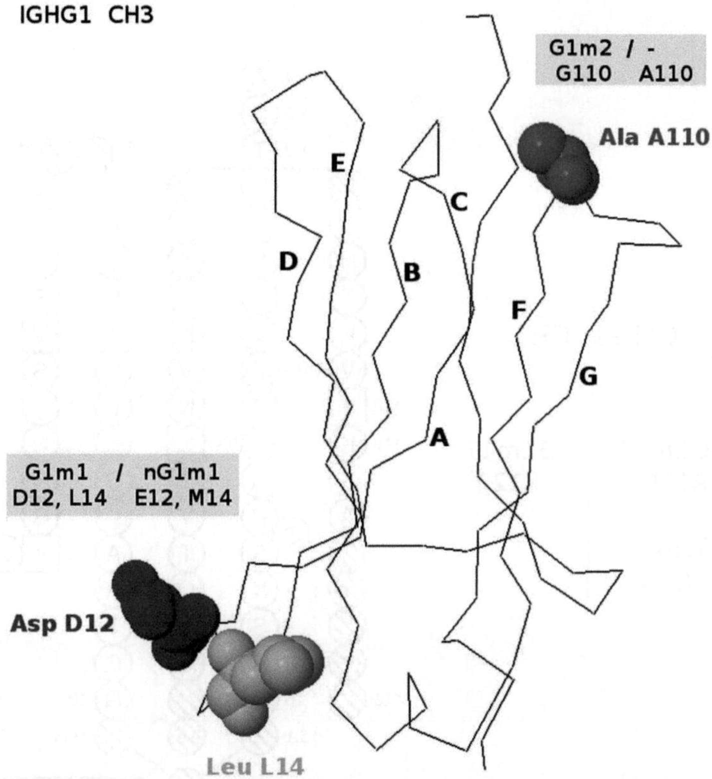


Fig. 3. Three-dimensional structure of the IGHG1 CH3 domain. The CH3 domain is from the b12 antibody (IMGT/3Dstructure-DB, code PDB:1hzh, http://www.imgt.org) (16, 17). Positions 12 and 14 of the G1m1/nG1m1 allotype, and position 110 of the G1m2/- allotype in the IGHG1 CH3 domain are shown. The aspartate D12 and leucine L14 correspond to G1m1, whereas alanine A110 corresponds to nG1m2. Glutamate E12 and methionine M14 correspond to nG1m1, whereas a glycine G110 corresponds to G1m2.

domain (131). These amino acid changes can be determined, by specific antisera, on the G1m1-negative gamma1, gamma2, and gamma3 chains (Table 2). This epitope corresponds to the isoallotype nG1m1. The gamma4 chains also express CH3 E12 and M14, but the corresponding epitope is only detected by certain antisera (143). This restricted accessibility of the nG1m1 epitope of the gamma4 chains has been correlated with the presence, at position 11 of CH3, of a glutamine (Q) instead of an arginine (R) as found in the other subclasses (11, 15) (Fig. 1a). In Old World Monkeys (OWM) (144), the IGHG1 CH3 sequence contains E12 and L14 and it has therefore be postulated that two independent single amino acid changes may have led to the G1m1 allotype (CH3 E12 > D) and to the nG1m1 isoallotype (CH3 L14 > M).

*3.1.2. G1m2*

The G1m2 allotype was discovered in 1959 by Harboe and Lundevall (22). The G1m2 allotype was detected on the CH3 domain (134). It corresponds to a glycine at position 110 (IGHG1 CH3 Gly G110), whereas the absence of the allotype correlates to alanine at that position (145) (see Note 6) (Table 3) (Figs. 2 and 3).

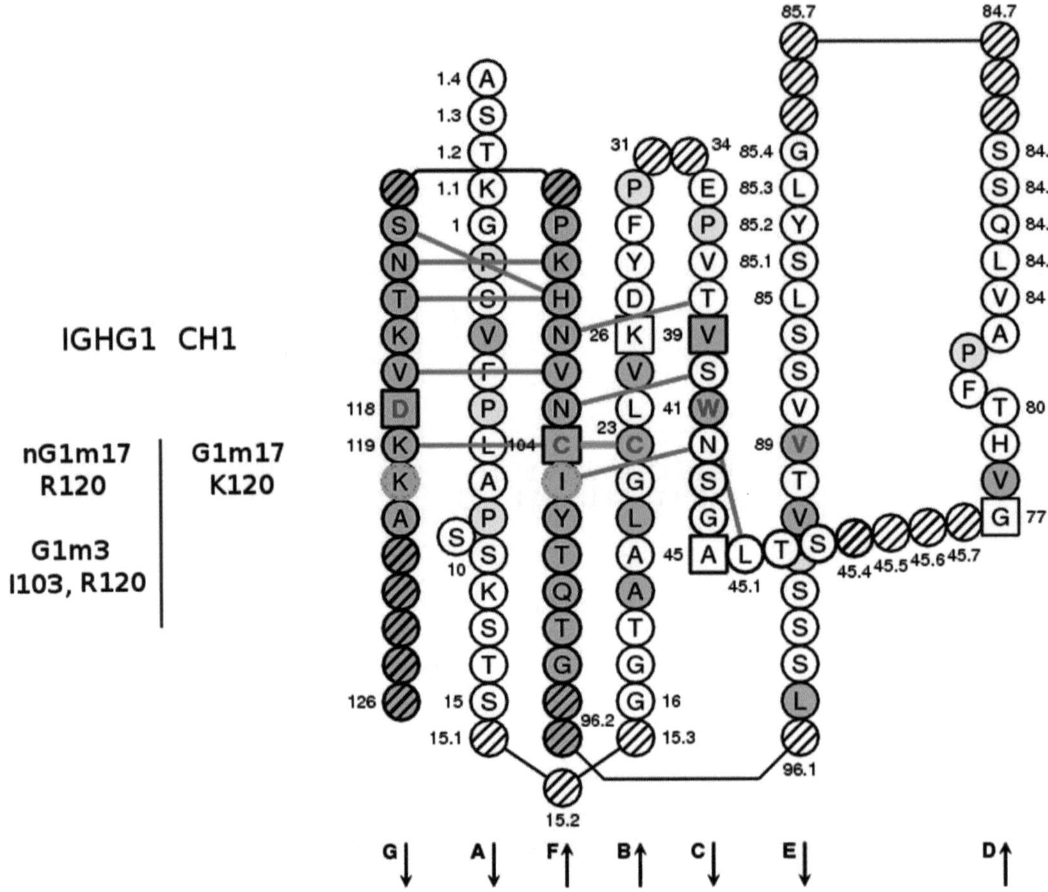


Fig. 4. IMGT Collier de Perles of the IGHG1 CH1 domain. The CH1 domain is from the b12 antibody (IMGT/3Dstructure-DB, code PDB:1hzh, http://www.imgt.org) (16, 17). The IMGT Collier de Perles is shown on two layers, with hydrogen bonds shown as *green lines* online. Hatched positions correspond to gaps according to the IMGT unique numbering (14). The lysine at position 120 (K120) corresponds to the G1m17 allotype. The isoleucine I103 is specific for the gamma1 chain isotype. If an arginine is expressed at position 120 (R120), the simultaneous presence of R120 and I103 corresponds to the expression of the G1m3 allotype.

*3.1.3. G1m3, G1m17, and nG1m17*

G1m3 was first identified by Steinberg and Wilson in 1963 (23), then further characterized by Gold et al. (24, 25). G1m3, located on the CH1 domain, corresponds to an arginine at position 120 (IGHG1 CH1 Arg R120) (132) (Figs. 4 and 5). The expression of G1m3 requires the presence of an amino acid specific for gamma1, because the CH1 Arg R120 is also present on the gamma3 and gamma4 chains (Fig. 1a). It seems likely from the analysis of 3D structures of Fab and of the b12 antibody, the only complete human IG so far crystallized (IMGT/3Dstructure-DB, code PDB:1hzh) (16, 17) (see Note 7) that the isoleucine at position 103 (IGHG1 CH1 Ile I103) is the amino acid involved in the expression of the G1m3 allotype (Figs. 4 and 5).

G1m17 (26), located in the CH1 domain, corresponds to lysine at position 120 (IGHG1 CH1 Lys K120) (132). G1m17 is

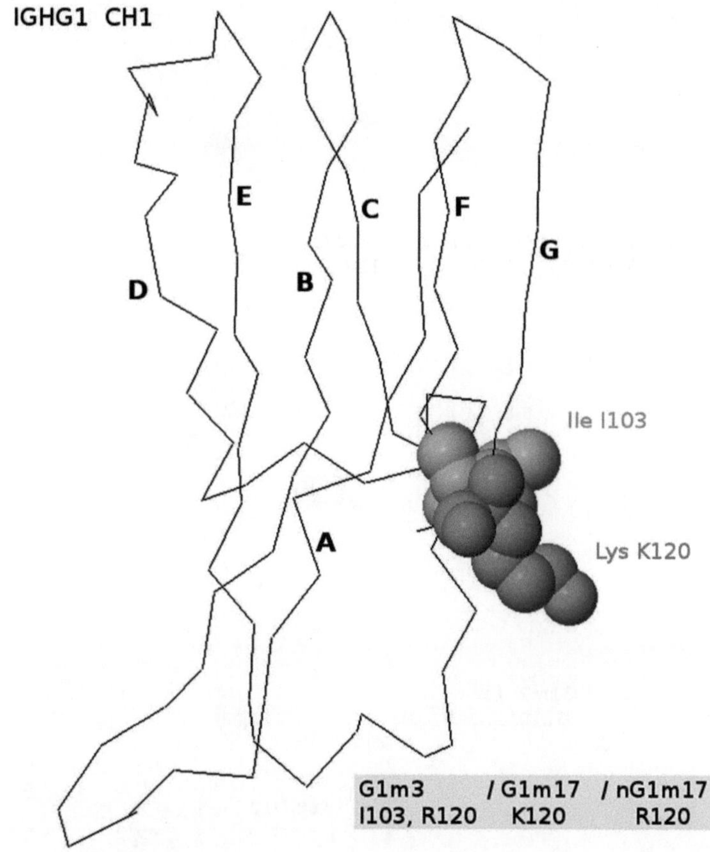


Fig. 5. Three-dimensional structure of the IGHG1 CH1 domain. The CH1 domain is from the b12 antibody (IMGT/3Dstructure-DB, code PDB:1hzh, http://www.imgt.org) (16, 17). The lysine K120 (strand G) and the isoleucine I103 (strand F) are shown. The K120 corresponds to the G1m17 allotype. The simultaneous presence of I103 (specific of the gamma1 isotype) and of arginine R120 corresponds to the G1m3 allotype. The R120 corresponds to the nG1m17 isoallotype.

mutually exclusive with ("antithetical to") G1m3 and is present on gamma1 chains which are G1m3-negative.

The isoallotype nG1m17 corresponds to arginine at position 120 in the CH1 (IGHG1 CH1 Arg R120). It is detectable on isolated gamma3 and gamma4 chains where R120 is present but without the gamma1-specific determinant CH1 Ileu I103 (threonine T103 is found instead in the other subclasses) (Fig. 1a).

#### 3.1.4. G1m27 and G1m28

G1m27 and G1m28 have only been demonstrated to be present on the gamma1 chains in Negroid populations (96); however, it is not excluded that these "surnumerary" allotypes may explain some uncommon haplotypes found in other populations (52, 53, 94, 95, 102). G1m27 most probably corresponds to IGHG1 CH3 Ileu I101 (resulting from an amino acid change V101 > I), and G1m28 to IGHG1 CH3 Arg R115, Tyr Y116 (with an amino acid change H115 > R) (see Subheading 5.1.7).

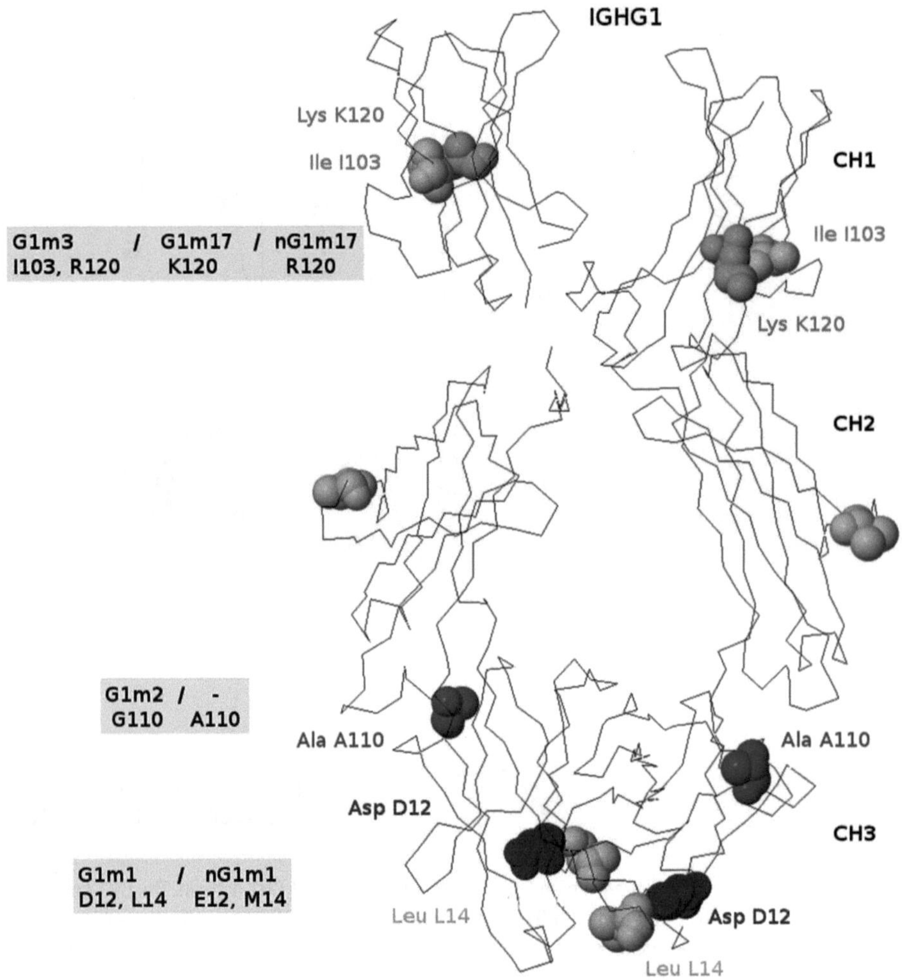


Fig. 6. G1m allotypes localizations on gamma1 chains. The CH1, CH2, and CH3 domains of the b12 gamma1 chains are shown (IMGT/3Dstructure-DB, code PDB:1hzh, http://www.imgt.org) (16, 17), with the positions involved in the G1m allotypes. The CH2 position 45.1 is not related to the G1m allotypes, but indicates the amino acid position that should be responsible for the G2m23 allotype, or of its absence (G2m..), on a gamma2 chain.

### 3.2. Correspondence Between G1m Alleles and IGHG1 Alleles

The heavy gamma1 chains of IgG1 may express four typical G1m alleles (combinations of G1m allotypes): G1m3, G1m3,1, G1m17,1, and G1m17,1,2 (and three additional G1m alleles, Gm17,1,27, Gm17,1,28, and Gm17,1,27,28, the last two identified in Negroid populations (96)). The C region of the G1m3,1, G1m17,1, and G1m17,1,2 chains differs from that of the G1m3 chains by two, three, and four amino acids, respectively. The structural correlations with amino acids are illustrated in Fig. 6. The correspondence between the G1m alleles and IGHG1 alleles is shown in Table 4. Thus, IGHG1*01 and IGHG1*02 (see Note 3) are G1m17,1, IGHG1*03 is G1m3, IGHG1*04, IGHG1*05, and IGHG1*06 are G1m17,1,27, G1m17,1,28, and G1m17,1,27,28, respectively, IGHG1*07 is G1m17,1,2, and IGHG1*08 is G1m3,1. In Table 4, amino acids corresponding to G1m allotypes are shown in bold. The nG1m1

**Table 4**
**Correspondence between the G1m alleles and IGHG1 alleles**

| | | Amino acid positions[b] | | | | |
|---|---|---|---|---|---|---|
| **G1m alleles[a]** | **IGHG1 alleles** | **Domain CH1** | | **CH3** | | |
| | | **IMGT 103**<br>Exon (82)<br>Eu *199* | **120**<br>(97)<br>*214*<br>G1m17/nG1m17[c]<br>G1m3[c] | **12**<br>(16)<br>*356*<br>G1m1/nG1m1 | **14**<br>(18)<br>*358* | **110**<br>(91)<br>*431*<br>G1m2/- |
| G1m17,1<br>G1m17,1,27<br>G1m17,1,28<br>G1m17,1,27,28 | IGHG1*01, IGHG1*02<br>IGHG1*04<br>IGHG1*05p<br>IGHG1*06p | Ile I103 atc | **Lys K120** aaa | **Asp D12** gat | **Leu L14** ctg | Ala A gct |
| G1m3<br>*nG1m1*<br>*nG1m17* | IGHG1*03 | **Ile I103** atc | **Arg R120** aga | Glu E gag | Met M atg | Ala A gct |
| G1m17,1,2 | IGHG1*07p[d] | Ile I103 atc | **Lys K120** (aaa) | **Asp D12** (gat) | **Leu L14** (ctg) | **Gly G110** (ggt) |
| G1m3,1<br>*nG1m17* | IGHG1*08p[d] | **Ile I103** atc | **Arg R120** (aga) | **Asp D2** (gat) | **Leu L14** (ctg) | Ala A (gct) |

[a]In Negroid populations, the G1m17,1 allele frequently includes G1m27 and G1m28, leading to new G1m alleles, G1m17,1,28 and G1m17,1,27,28, as demonstrated serologically (96) (see Subheading 5.1.7). They were assigned to IGHG1*05p and IGHG1*06p, respectively, following the sequencing of IGHG1*04 (164) (IMGT/GENE-DB, http://www.imgt.org). The letter "p" indicates that these alleles have not yet been sequenced at the nucleotide level, and therefore are not shown in IMGT Repertoire, Alignments of alleles: *Homo sapiens* IGHG1 (http://www.imgt.org) (5, 6). Amino acid changes and codons for G1m27 (CH3 Ileu I101) and G1m28 (most probably CH3 Arg R115, Tyr Y116) are not shown

[b]Positions in bold are according to the IMGT unique numbering for C domain (14); between parentheses, exon numbering (11), and in italics, Eu numbering (correspondence between C numberings, in IMGT Scientific chart, http://www.imgt.org) (5, 6)

[c]The presence of R120 is detected by anti-nG1m17 antibodies, whereas the simultaneous presence of I103 and R120 in the gamma1 chains is detected by anti-Gm3 antibodies

[d]IGHG1*07p and IGHG1*08p amino acids, and codons between parentheses, are expected (GL and MPL) (11). The letter "p" indicates that these alleles have not yet been sequenced at the nucleotide level, and therefore are not shown in IMGT Repertoire, Alignments of alleles: *Homo sapiens* IGHG1 (http://www.imgt.org) (5, 6)

and nG1m17 isoallotypes present on the Gm1-negative and Gm-17 negative gamma-1 chains (and on other gamma chains, Table 2) are shown in italics.

## 4. G2m

### *4.1. G2m Allotype*

G2m23 (27) is the only allotype shown on the IgG2 heavy chains, and the gamma2 chains are either G2m23 or G2m.. (two dots indicate that a specimen was tested and found to be negative for G2m23 (48, 52, 53)) (see Note 8). G2m23 is localized on the CH2 domain (detectable on the Fc of G2m23 myeloma proteins but not on isolated CH3 domains) (134). Amino acid sequence and 3D structure comparisons show that the G2m23 allotype is correlated with methionine 45.1 ('.1' for first position in the transverse CD strand (14)) in the CH2 (IGHG2 CH2 Met M45.1),

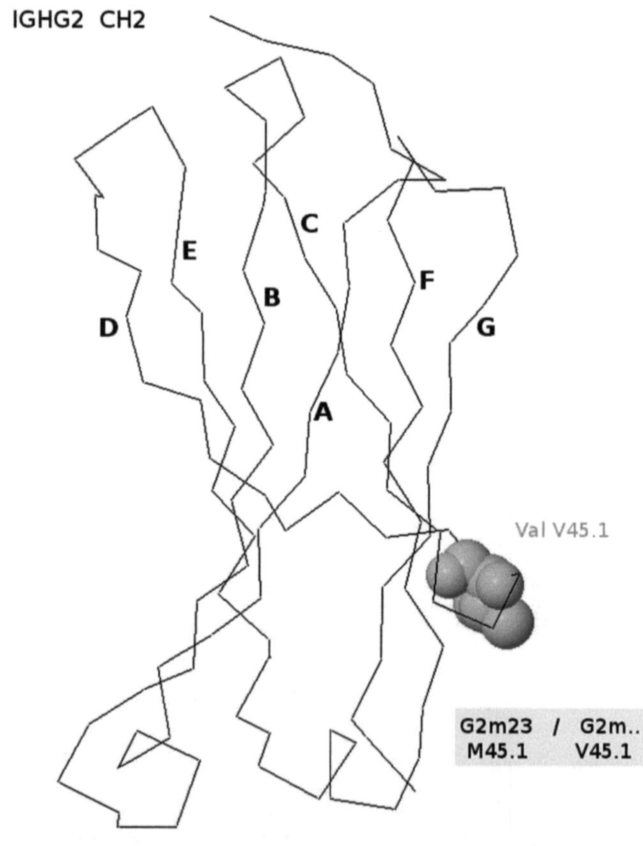


Fig. 7. Three-dimensional structure of the IGHG2 CH2 domain. CH2 position 45.1 (first position of the transversal CD strand) corresponds to the G2m23/G2m.. allotype. Valine V45.1 corresponds to G2m.., whereas a methionine corresponds to G2m23.

**Table 5**
**Correspondence between the G2m alleles and IGHG2 alleles**

| | | Amino acid position[a] | |
|---|---|---|---|
| **G2m alleles** | **IGHG2 alleles** | **Domain** | **CH2** |
| | | **IMGT**<br>Exon<br>Eu | **45.1**<br>(52)<br>*282*<br>G2m23/G2m.. |
| G2m23 | IGHG2*02 | | **Met M45.1** atg |
| G2m.. | IGHG2*01, IGHG2*03, IGHG2*04, IGHG2*05, IGHG2*06 | | Val V45.1 gtg |

[a]Positions in bold are according to the IMGT unique numbering for C domain (14); between parentheses, exon numbering (11), and in italics, Eu numbering (correspondence between C numberings, in IMGT Scientific chart, http://www.imgt.org) (5, 6)

whereas the absence of the allotype (G2m..) is correlated with valine 45.1 (IGHG2 CH2 Val V45.1) (11, 15) (Fig. 7).

The G2m23-positive gamma2 chains are also characterized by the presence of threonine 92 in the CH1 domain (IGHG2 CH1 Thr T92) (11, 15). In contrast, the G2m23-negative chains and the gamma chains of other IgG subclasses have proline 92 in the CH1 domain (IGHG2 CH1 Pro P92) (11, 15) (Fig. 1a). Being located on the CH1 domain, this amino acid change is not involved in the expression of the G2m23 allotype, but owing to the strong linkage on the same chain, the CH1 Thr T92 codon has been used for the molecular characterization of the G2m23 chains (130).

### 4.2. Correspondence Between the G2m Alleles and IGHG2 Alleles

The G2m alleles are characterized by the presence or absence of the G2m23 allotype. Only the IGHG2*02 allele is G2m23. The other alleles IGHG1*01, IGHG2*03, IGHG2*04, IGHG2*05 and IGHG2*06 are G2m23-negative (or G2m..) (Table 5) (see Note 9).

## 5. G3m

### 5.1. G3m Allotypes

#### 5.1.1. G3m Allotypes and IGHG3 Sequences

The G3m allotypes make the gamma3 chain the most polymorphic IG chains in humans. Thirteen G3m allotypes are characterized: G3m5, G3m6, G3m10, G3m11, G3m13, G3m14, G3m15, G3m16, G3m21, G3m24, G3m26, G3m27, G3m28 (Table 1). Three isoallotypes (nG3m5, nG3m11, and nG3m21) have also been characterized (Table 2).

Amino acids which could give rise to subclass-specific epitopes and to G3m allotypes were identified following the first complete nucleotide sequence of the IGHG3 gene, by Huck et al. (104). The IGHG3 gene was from a healthy Tunisian individual (EZZ, TOU II-4) homozygous for a multigene IGHC deletion (encompassing IGHG1 to IGHG4) and homozygous for the G3m5* allele (G3m5,10,11,13,14,26,27, or G3mb0,b1,b3,b4,b5,u,v) (104). The IGHG3 EZZ translation was compared with amino acid sequences of heavy chain disease (HCD) gamma3 proteins (ZUC (146), Wis (147), OMM (148)), of myeloma gamma3 chains (Goe (149) and JIR (150)), and of gamma chains of other subclasses (104). Although only G3m5*, G3m21*, and G3m16* (see Subheading 5.2) could be compared, the analysis confirmed that the number of amino acid changes was lower than the number of allotypes and suggested that the conformational structure of a combination of amino acids was required to explain several allotypes.

In 1989, Huck et al. published the sequence of a new allele from a healthy Tunisian individual (LAT) homozygous for the G3m24* allele (G3m5,6,11,24,26 or G3mb0,b1,c3,c5,u) and demonstrated that this allele results from a gene conversion event (106). In 2001, Dard et al. sequenced 51 full-length genomic IGHG3 alleles from healthy individuals from African, Siberian, West Asian, and European population samples whose sera have been typed for the Gm allotypes (113). Different levels of molecular diversity were observed for the G3m alleles. EZZ (104) and LAT (106) were included in the analysis. Analysis of 19 DNA sequences of the G3m5* allele yielded 11 different IGHG3 alleles; similar analysis of 10 DNA sequences of the G3m21* allele yielded 4 distinct IGHG3 alleles; in contrast, the 9 DNA sequences of the G3m24* allele were monomorphic (113). These data allowed the first identification of the amino acids involved in the G3m allotypes; however, detailed correlations remained to be defined. In the following paragraphs, we report, for the first time, the full elucidation of the G3m allotypes and amino acid correlations, taking into account conformational structures that may involve two or even three amino acids (Fig. 8).

#### *5.1.2. G3m6, G3m10, G3m11, nG3m11, G3m13, G3m24, G3m27*

A first mosaic of G3m allotypes on the CH3 can be defined around G3m11. G3m11 is characterized by a serine at position 44 of the CH3 (IGHG3 CH3 Ser S44), whereas nG3m11 depends on an asparagine at the same position (IGHG3 CH3 Asn N44) (113).

Haplotype analysis shows that four allotypes, G3m6, G3m10, G3m13, and G3m24, depends on the presence of G3m11 (49–53).

Extensive analysis of the sequence (104, 106, 113) and genetic data demonstrate that:

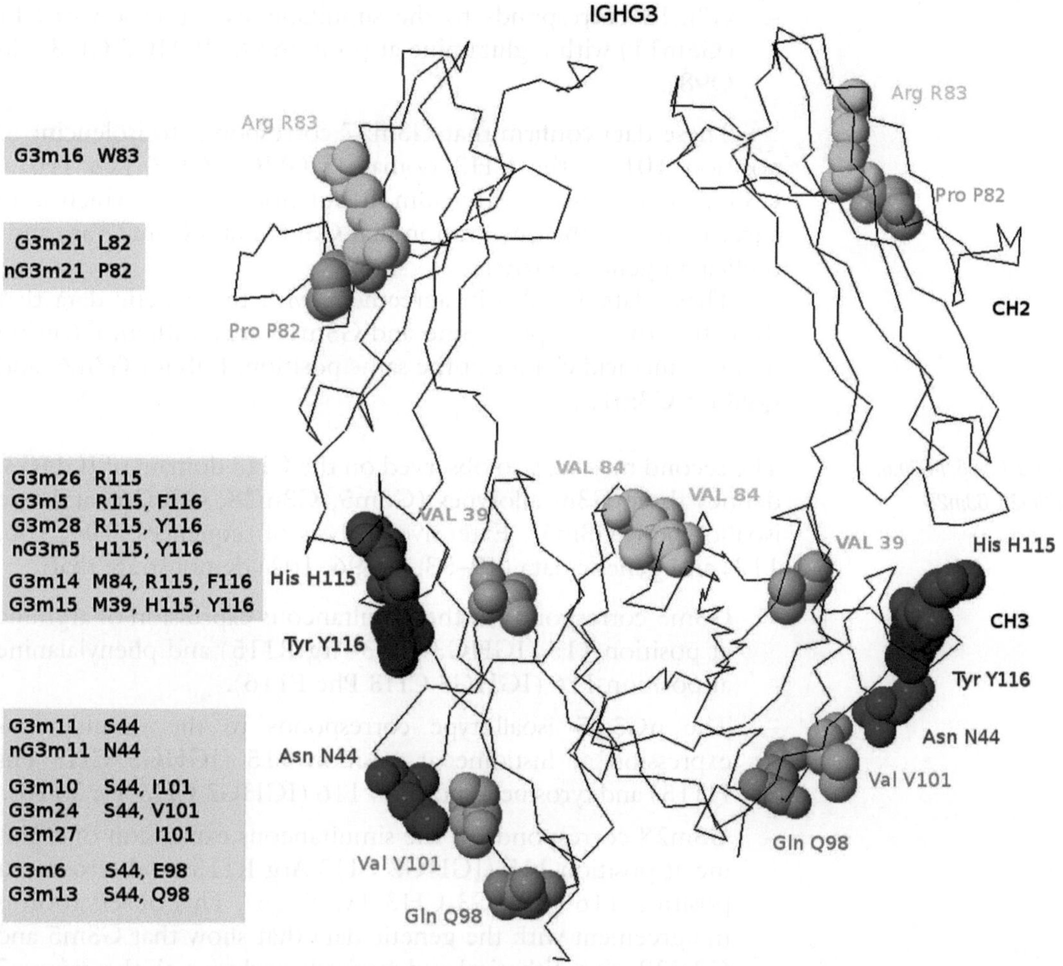


Fig. 8. G3m allotypes localizations on gamma3 chains. G3m allotypes are described in Subheading 5.1. G3m16 (tryptophan Trp W83) and G3m21 (leucine Leu L82), nG3m21 (proline Pro P82) are located on the CH2. The other G3m allotypes form two mosaics on the CH3. G3m26 (R115), G3m5 (R115, F116), G3m28 (R115, Y116), nG3m5 (H115, Y116), G3m14 (M84, R115, F116) and G3m15 (M39, H115, Y116) form a first mosaic. G3m11 (S44), nG3m11 (N44), G3m10 (S44, I101), G3m24 (S44, V101), G3m27 (I101), G3m6 (S44, E98), G3m13 (S44, Q98) form a second mosaic.

- G3m10 corresponds to the simultaneous expression of S44 (G3m11) with an isoleucine at position 101 (IGHG3 CH3 Ile I101).
- G3m24 corresponds to the simultaneous expression of S44 (G3m11) with a valine at position 101 (IGHG3 CH3 Val V101).
- G3m6 corresponds to the simultaneous expression of S44 (G3m11) with a glutamate at position 98 (IGHG3 CH3 Glu E98).

- G3m13 corresponds to the simultaneous expression of S44 (G3m11) with a glutamine at position 98 (IGHG3 CH3 Gln Q98).

These data confirm that G3m27 corresponds to isoleucine at position 101 in the CH3 domain (IGHG3 CH3 Ileu I101). G3m27 is expressed with G3m10 but not G3m24, which is in agreement with the observation that G3m24 and G3m27 are antithetical in genetic analysis.

These data are also in agreement with the genetic data that show that the allotypes G3m6 and G3m13 are antithetical (owing to an amino acid change at the same position, E98 for G3m6, and Q98 for G3m13).

*5.1.3. G3m5, nG3m5, G3m28, G3m26*

The second mosaic, also observed on the CH3 domain of IGHG3, defines three G3m allotypes (G3m5, G3m28, G3m26) and one isoallotype (nG3m5). Extensive analysis of sequences (104, 106, 113) and genetic data (49–53, 89–96, 102) demonstrate that:

- G3m5 corresponds to the simultaneous expression of arginine at position 115 (IGHG3 CH3 Arg R115) and phenylalanine at position 116 (IGHG3 CH3 Phe F116).
- The nG3m5 isoallotype corresponds to the simultaneous expression of histidine at position 115 (IGHG3 CH3 His H115) and tyrosine at position 116 (IGHG3 CH3 Tyr Y116).
- G3m28 corresponds to the simultaneous expression of arginine at position 115 (IGHG3 CH3 Arg R115) and tyrosine at position 116 (IGHG3 CH3 Tyr Y116). This observation is in agreement with the genetic data that show that G3m5 and G3m28 are antithetical and mutually exclusive on the gamma3 chains.

These data confirm that G3m26 corresponds to arginine at position 115 (IGHG3 CH3 Arg R115). This explains the high frequency of G3m26, present on all Gm5-positive (R115, F116) and G3m28-positive (R115, Y116) gamma3 chains, and its absence, the arginine being replaced by a histidine, on G3m15-positive gamma3 chains which are nG3m5 (H115,Y116).

*5.1.4. G3m14 and G3m15*

G3m14 has been the subject of discussion concerning its localization on either the CH2 or CH3 domain with contradictory serological data (discussed in (50)). Extensive analysis of previously published data of usual and uncommon haplotypes, supported by familial studies (47–53, 89–95, 102), led us to postulate that G3m14 corresponds to the simultaneous presence on CH3 of a methionine at position 84 (IGHG3 CH3 Met M84) with the G3m5 mosaic (CH3 Arg R115, Phe F116).

Gm15 was reported to be located first on the CH2 domain. In 1983, Matsumoto et al. postulated that G3m15 correlates with histidine at position Eu 435 (IGHG3 CH3 H115) and G3m16 with methione at position Eu 379 (IGHG3 CH3 M39), on JIR, a G3m15,16-positive myeloma gamma3 protein (150). In 1986, Matsumoto et al. reported that the G3m15 is located on the CH3 domain of Kam, another G3m15,16-positive myeloma gamma3 protein (151). Dard et al. (113) showed that His H115 alone cannot be responsible for G3m15, as it is found in all the nG3m5 chains, and suggested a role for Met M39. Based on these observations, and in a similar way as for Gm14, we postulate that G3m15 corresponds to the simultaneous presence on CH3 of Met M39 (IGHG3 Met M39) with the nG3m5 mosaic (CH3 His H115, Tyr Y116).

Interestingly, they are the two allotypes, G3m14 and G3m15, localization of which have been controversial for a long time, that require an amino acid at a position that interferes with the binding site but is not directly located at the epitope site. This emphasizes the importance of the conformational configuration, but at a degree that was not suspected.

*5.1.5. G3m16 and G3m21*

Two allotypes, G3m16 and G3m21, are localized on the CH2 domain. G3m16 correlates with a tryptophane at position 83 (IGHG3 CH2 Trp W83), whereas G3m16-negative chains have an arginine at that position (113). G3m21 correlates with a leucine at position 82 (IGHG3 CH2 Leu L82), whereas nG3m21 correlates with Pro P82 (113) (IMGT Repertoire, Alignments of alleles, *Homo sapiens* IGHG3, http://www.imgt.org (5, 6)).

*5.1.6. "Silent" G3m Allotypes*

Among data obtained by Dard et al. (113), one sequence was noted as unusual as it presents an asparagine (N44) (IGHG3*08 in IMGT Repertoire, Alignments of alleles, *Homo sapiens* IGHG3, http://www.imgt.org (5, 6)), whereas a serine (S44) was expected, given the G3m5* phenotype. The individual, Mand114, is heterozygous for a normal G3m5* haplotype associated to the unusual haplotype (the one that was sequenced) (113). We postulate that the unusual haplotype corresponds to G3m5,14,26, with an absence of G3m (10,11,13), as previously demonstrated in the Tunisian family 275 (95, 102). Two nucleotide substitutions in codon 44 (as a result of mutations or of a genic conversion) are the most probable explanation for these silent G3m (10, 11,13) allotypes.

*5.1.7. "Surnumerary" Gm27 and Gm28 Allotypes*

In Caucasoid and Mongoloid populations, G3m28 is frequently associated with G3m21, although exceptions have been shown (38, 52, 53, 94, 95, 102). In contrast, Negroid populations are G3m21-negative and, interestingly, for individuals who are Gm28-positive, this allotype appears as "surnumerary." It has

**Table 6**
**Correlation between G3m allotypes and isoallotypes and amino acids**

| G3m allotypes and isoallotypes | Amino acid position[a] Domain | CH2 | | CH3 | | | | | | |
|---|---|---|---|---|---|---|---|---|---|---|
| | IMGT<br>Exon<br>Eu | **82**<br>(61)<br>*291* | **83**<br>(62)<br>*292* | **39**<br>(39)<br>*379* | **44**<br>(44)<br>*384* | **84**<br>(57)<br>*397* | **98**<br>(79)<br>*419* | **101**<br>(82)<br>*422* | **115**<br>(95)<br>*435* | **116**<br>(96)<br>*436* |
| G3m5 | | | | | | | | | Arg R cgc | Phe F ttc |
| nG3m5 | | | | | | | | | His H cac | Tyr Y tac |
| G3m6 | | | | | Ser S agc | | Glu E gag | | | |
| G3m10 | | | | | Ser S agc | | | Ileu I atc | | |
| G3m11 | | | | | Ser S agc | | | | | |
| nG3m11 | | | | | Asn N aat | | | | | |
| G3m13 | | | | | Ser S agc | | Gln Q cag | | | |
| G3m14 | | | | | | Met M atg | | | Arg R cgc | Phe F ttc |
| G3m15 | | | | Met M atg | | | | | His H cac | Tyr Y tac |
| G3m16 | | | Trp W tgg | | | | | | | |
| G3m21 | | Leu L ctg | | | | | | | | |
| nG3m21 | | Pro P ccg | | | | | | | | |
| G3m24 | | | | | Ser S agc | | | Val V gtc | | |
| G3m26 | | | | | | | | | Arg R cgc | |
| G3m27 | | | | | | | | Ileu I atc | | |
| G3m28 | | | | | | | | | Arg R cgc | Tyr Y tac |

[a]Positions in bold are according to the IMGT unique numbering for C domain (14); between parentheses, exon numbering (11), and in italics, Eu numbering (correspondence between C numberings, in IMGT Scientific chart, http://www.imgt.org (5, 6))

**Table 7**
**The six most prevalent G3m alleles**

| WHO/IUIS/IMGT nomenclature | Simplified form |
|---|---|
| G3m5,10,11,13,14,26,27 | G3m5* |
| G3m5,6,10,11,14,26,27 | G3m6* |
| G3m5,6,11,24,26 | G3m24* |
| G3m10,11,13,15,27 | G3m15* |
| G3m10,11,13,15,16,27 | G3m16* |
| G3m21,26,27,28 | G3m21* |

been demonstrated in Lat-IV-5 (homozygous for G3m24*) and Sno (homozygous for G3m6*) that the surnumerary allotype Gm28 is expressed on the gamma1 chains (96). Thus, in Negroid populations, Gm28 represents a G1m28 allotype. The amino acid change on the gamma1 chain, nG3m5 (H115, Y116) to G1m28 (R115, Y116), most probably corresponds to a single nucleotide mutation (a344 > g, H115 > R) (Table 6).

The presence of surnumerary Gm27 has also been demonstrated on the gamma1 chain of Lat IV-5 and Sno representing a G1m27 allotype (96). The amino acid change on the gamma1 chain most probably corresponds to a single nucleotide mutation (g301 > a, V101 > I).

Both Gm27 and Gm28 are qualified as "alloallotype," being an allotype for two different gamma chains, gamma1 (G1m27, G1m28) and gamma3 (G3m27, G3m28), depending on the populations.

*5.1.8. IGHG3 Hinge CNV Exon Polymorphism*

For the gamma3 chains, an additional polymorphism results from differing numbers (CNV) of hinge exons. The hinge is encoded by 2–5 exons, depending on the alleles (104, 106, 112, 113). Thus, the hinge region can vary from 27 to 83 amino acids and can influence structural conformations.

### 5.2. G3m Alleles and the "IMGT G3m Allele Butterfly" Representation

The thirteen G3m allotypes are inherited in different combinations or G3m alleles. The six most prevalent G3m alleles are shown in Table 7 and illustrated in Fig. 9, as "IMGT G3m alleles butterfly" representation. For convenience, these most common G3m alleles can be written in a simplified form indicated with an asterisk (see Note 10 for correspondence between the WHO/IUIS/IMGT nomenclature and previous designation).

### 5.3. Correspondence Between the G3m Alleles and IGHG3 Alleles

The correspondence between the G3m alleles and IGHG3 alleles is shown in Table 8.

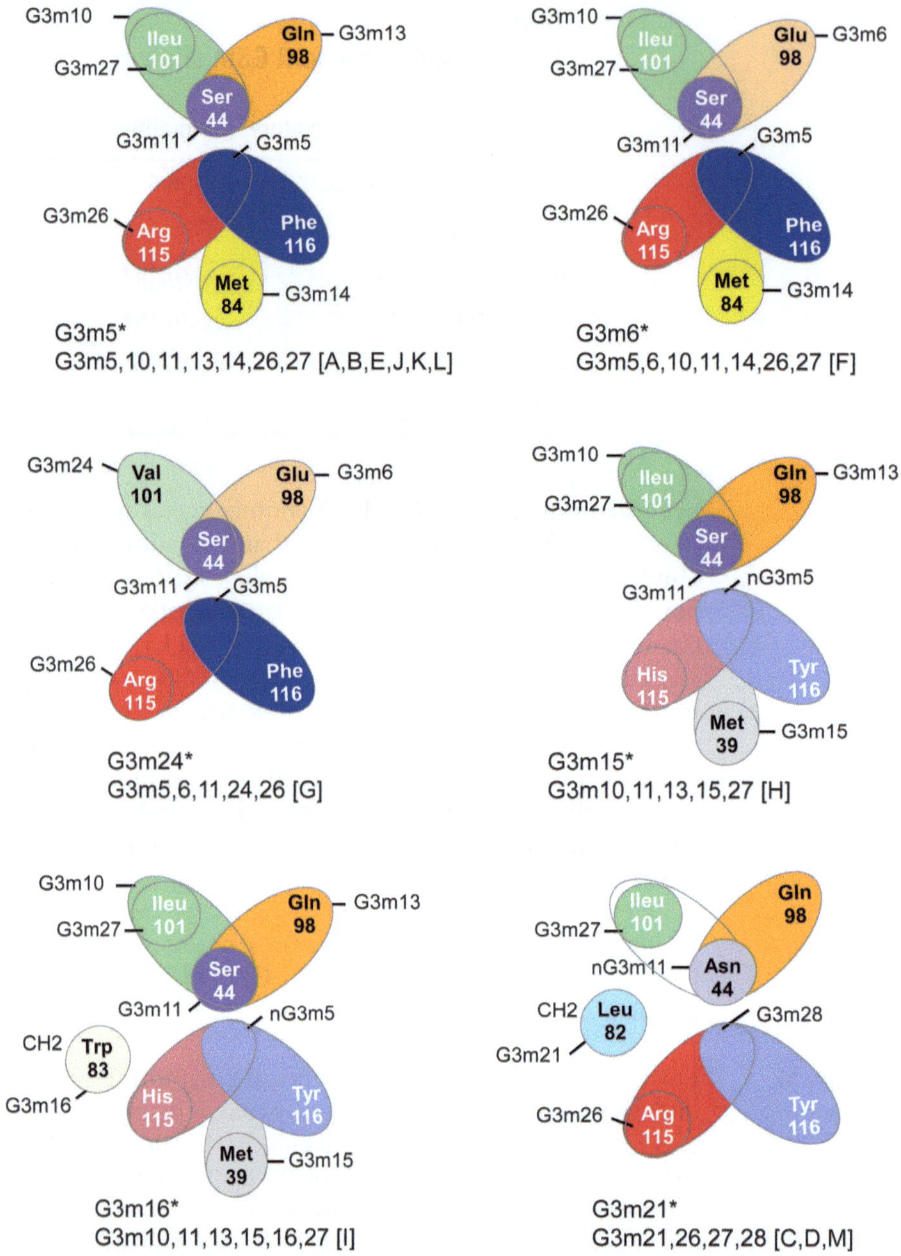


Fig. 9. "IMGT G3m allele butterfly" representation. The six most prevalent G3m alleles (Table 7) are shown. The first G3m mosaic on the CH3 domain of IGHG3 (detailed in Subheading 5.1.2) is illustrated by the top part of each butterfly representation and corresponds to G3m11/nG3m11, G3m27, and the antithetical G3m10/G3m24, and G3m13/G3m6 allotypes. The second G3m mosaic on the CH3 domain of iGHG3 (detailed in Subheading 5.1.3) is illustrated by the bottom part of each butterfly representation and corresponds to G3m26, and the antithetical G3m5/nG3m5/G3m28 allotypes. Amino acids involved in the allotype expression (Table 6) and their position according to the IMGT unique numbering for C domain (14) are indicated. Two allotypes are on the CH2 domain, G3m16 (Trp W83) and G3m21 (Leu L82). For each G3m allele butterfly, G3m alleles are indicated with the simplified form (e.g., G3m5*) and the full nomenclature (Table 7). Haplotypes to which the G3m alleles belong are indicated between *square brackets* (Table 10) (see Note 11).

## Table 8
## Correspondence between the G3m alleles and IGHG3 alleles

| G3m alleles and IGHG3 alleles | Amino acid position[a, b] Domain | CH2 | | CH3 | | | | | | |
|---|---|---|---|---|---|---|---|---|---|---|
| | IMGT<br>Exon<br>Eu | **82**<br>(61)<br>*291* | **83**<br>(62)<br>*292* | **39**<br>(39)<br>*379* | **44**<br>(44)<br>*384* | **84**<br>(57)<br>*397* | **98**<br>(79)<br>*419* | **101**<br>(82)<br>*422* | **115**<br>(95)<br>*435* | **116**<br>(96)<br>*436* |
| G3m5* (G3m5,10,11,13,14,26,27)<br>*nG3m21*<br>IGHG3*01, IGHG3*05, IGHG3*06, IGHG3*07, IGHG3*09, IGHG3*10, IGHG3*11, IGHG3*12 | | Pro P ccg | Arg R cgg | Val V gtg | **Ser S** agc | **Met M** atg | **Gln Q** cag | **Ileu I** atc | **Arg R** cgc | **Phe F** ttc |
| G3m6* (G3m5,6,10,11,14,26,27)<br>*nG3m21*<br>IGHG3*13 | | Pro P ccg | Arg R cgg | Val V gtg | **Ser S** agc | **Met M** atg | **Glu E** gag | **Ileu I** atc | **Arg R** cgc | **Phe F** ttc |
| G3m24* (G3m5,6,11,24,26)<br>*nG3m21*<br>IGHG3*03 | | Pro P ccg | Arg R cgg | Val V gtg | **Ser S** agc | Val V gtg | **Glu E** gag | **Val V** gtc | **Arg R** cgc | **Phe F** ttc |
| G3m15* (G3m10,11,13,15,27)<br>*nG3m5*, *nG3m21*<br>IGHG3*17 | | Pro P ccg | Arg R cgg | **Met M** atg | **Ser S** agc | Val V gtg | **Gln Q** cag | **Ileu I** atc | **His H** cac | **Tyr Y** tac |
| G3m16* (G3m10,11,13,15,16,27)<br>*nG3m5*, *nG3m21*<br>IGHG3*18, IGHG3*19 | | Pro P ccg | **Trp W** tgg | **Met M** atg | **Ser S** agc | Val V gtg | **Gln Q** cag | **Ileu I** atc | **His H** cac | **Tyr Y** tac |
| G3m21* (G3m21,26,27,28)<br>*nG3m11*<br>IGHG3*14, IGHG3*15, IGHG3*16 | | **Leu L** ctg | Arg R cgg | Val V gtg | Asn N aat | Met M atg | Gln Q cag | **Ileu I** atc | **Arg R** cgc | **Tyr Y** tac |

[a]Positions in bold are according to the IMGT unique numbering for C domain (14); between parentheses, exon numbering (11), and in italics, Eu numbering (correspondence between C numberings, in IMGT Scientific chart, http://www.imgt.org (5, 6))

[b]The amino acid change asparagine/lysine at position 79 in the CH3 domain (IGHG3 CH3 Asn/Lys N79/K) (exon numbering (52), Eu numbering *392*) is not reported in the table as no specific antibody (and therefore no allotype) has been characterized. It should be noted that the asparagine Asn N79, if present, belongs to a N-glycosylation site in alleles IGHG3*01 to *05, *08 to *12, *14, and *16)

## 6. nG4m Isoallotypes

### 6.1. nG4m(a) and nG4m(b)

No allotype has been defined for the gamma4 chains of the IgG4 subclass. The only serologically defined polymorphism corresponds to the isoallotypes nG4m(a) and nG4m(b), described on the CH2 domain (138). These antithetical determinants of the gamma4 chains behave as allotypes in the IgG4 subclass, but they are present on the other subclasses and therefore must be considered as isoallotypes.

It has been postulated that nG4m(a) was correlated to leucine 309 (IGHG4 CH2 Leu L92) and isoallotype nG4m(b) to a deletion at that position (152). However, comparison with the translation of IGHG4 sequences did not confirm that deletion and instead showed that it was an amino acid change of leucine into valine (IGHG4 CH2 Val V92) which explained the "disappearance" of the leucine and was responsible for the expression of nG4m(b) chains (1, 104). The nG4m(a) epitope (IGHG4 CH2 Leu L92) is expressed on the gamma1 and gamma3 chains, whereas the nG4m(b) epitope (IGHG4 CH2 Val V92) is expressed on the gamma2 chains (Table 2).

### 6.2. Correspondence Between nG4m Alleles and IGHG4 Alleles

The nG4m(a) allele corresponds to IGHG4*01, IGHG4*03, and IGHG4*04, whereas the nG4m(b) allele corresponds to IGHG4*02 (Table 9).

**Table 9**
**Correspondence between the nG4m alleles and IGHG4 alleles**

| | | Amino acid positions[a] | |
|---|---|---|---|
| G4m alleles | IGHG4 alleles | Domain | CH2 |
| | | **IMGT**<br>Exon<br>Eu<br>nG4m(a)/nG4m(b) | **92**<br>(79)<br>*309* |
| nG4m(a) | IGHG4*01, IGHG4*03, IGHG4*04 | Leu L92 <u>c</u>tg | |
| nG4m(b) | IGHG4*02 | Val V92 <u>g</u>tg | |

[a]Positions in bold are according to the IMGT unique numbering for C domain (14); between parentheses, exon numbering (11), and in italics, Eu numbering (correspondence between C numberings, in IMGT Scientific chart, http://www.imgt.org (5, 6))

## 7. Gm Haplotypes

### *7.1. Description of the Main Gm Haplotypes*

The G1m, G2m, and G3m alleles are inherited in fixed combinations or Gm haplotypes. Table 10 shows the eleven most prevalent Gm haplotypes. The nomenclature of the Gm haplotypes takes into account the IGHG gene order in the locus (97, 114, 115). The Gm allotypes are written in the linkage order of the IGHG subclass genes, i.e., IGHG3, IGHG1, and IGHG2, with semicolons separating the subclasses and comas separating the allotypes; G2m23 is the only allotype defined on gamma 2, two dots being used to indicate that a specimen was tested and found to be negative for G2m23 (47, 48, 52, 53).

**Table 10**
**Prevalent Gm haplotypes**

| Populations | Gm haplotypes (Prevalent Gm haplotypes[a]) | Simplified form[b] | Complete description |
|---|---|---|---|
| Caucasoid | A | Gm5*;3;23 | Gm5,10,11,13,14,26,27;3;23 |
| | B | Gm5*;3;.. | Gm5,10,11,13,14,26,27;3;.. |
| Caucasoid and Mongoloid | C | Gm21*;17,1;.. | Gm21,26,27,28;17,1;.. |
| | D | Gm21*;17,1,2;.. | Gm21,26,27,28;17,1,2;.. |
| Negroid | E | Gm5*;17,1;.. | Gm5,10,11,13,14,26,27;17,1;.. (+G1m28)[c] |
| | F | Gm6*;17,1;.. | Gm5,6,10,11,14,26,27;17,1;.. (+G1m28)[c] |
| | G[c] | Gm24*;17,1;.. | Gm5,6,11,24,26;17,1;.. (+G1m28)[c] |
| Khoisan[d] | H | Gm15*;17,1;.. | Gm10,11,13,15,27;17,1;.. |
| Mongoloid | I | Gm16*;17,1;.. | Gm10,11,13,15,16,27;17,1;.. |
| | J | Gm5*;3,1;23 | Gm5,10,11,13,14,26,27;3,1;23 |
| | K | Gm5*;3,1;.. | Gm5,10,11,13,14,26,27;3,1;.. |

[a]Prevalent haplotypes are characteristic of given populations. This does not mean that they are totally absent from other populations. They can be found to frequency usually <0.01 and represent rare alleles without metissage

[b]The current simplified form of the Gm haplotypes only contains one number for the G3m allele. 24* was previously designated as 6,24*, and 16* as 15,16*

[c]The presence of the G1m28 allotype (96) (see Subheading 5.1.7) is frequently observed in association with haplotypes E, F, and G. In contrast, the presence of G1m27 can only be confirmed in homozygotes for haplotype G (haplotype G is negative for G3m27, whereas haplotypes E and F are positive for G3m27) (96, 106). As the assignment to one or the other haplotype in heterozygous individuals is not possible in usual typing, G1m28 allotype is usually indicated as "+G1m28," in genotype description. In homozygous individuals, as demonstrated in (96), the haplotype is Gm24*;17,1,27,28;.. in Lat IV-5, and Gm6*;17,1,27,28;.. in Sno. The G1m28 also explains the uncommon haplotypes found in Tunisian families (94, 95, 102)

[d]The Khoisan population regroups the San (or Bushmen), native people, hunters/gatherers of southwestern Africa, and the Khoikhoi (or Hottentots), pasturalists who had lived in southern Africa since the fifth century AD

In haplotypes A and B, the G3m5* allele is inherited with the G1m3 allele, with or without G2m23, respectively. In haplotypes C and D, the G3m21* allele is inherited with G1m17,1 or G1m17,1,2, respectively (without G2m23). In haplotypes E, F, G, and H, the G3m alleles (G3m5*, G3m6*, G3m24*, and G3m15*) differentiate the four haplotypes since they are all associated with the G1m17,1 allele (without G2m23). The haplotype I corresponds to Gm16*;17,1;.. whereas the haplotypes J and K correspond to the G3m5* allele inherited with the G1m3,1 allele, with or without G2m23, respectively (Table 10). Less frequent haplotypes include, for example, haplotypes L (Gm5*;17,1,2;..) and M (Gm21*;17,1;23), identified in Lebanese and Tunisian populations (47, 52, 53) (see Note 11 for correspondence between the WHO/IUIS/IMGT nomenclature and previous designation for the Gm haplotypes).

### 7.2. Prevalent Gm Haplotypes in Different Populations

The eleven most prevalent Gm haplotypes are differently represented in the Negroid, Khoisan, Caucasoid, and Mongoloid populations (Table 10). Thus, Gm5*;3;23 [A] and Gm5*;3;.. [B] are only typical of the Caucasoid populations. Two haplotypes Gm21*;17,1;.. [C] and Gm 21*;17,1,2;.. [D] are shared by the Caucasoid and Mongoloid populations. A unique set of haplotypes characterizes the Negroid populations, Gm5*;17,1,.. [E], Gm6*;17,1;.. [F], and Gm24*;17,1,.. [G]. The haplotype Gm15*;17,1;.. [H] (with or without G3m16) is characteristic of the Khoisan population of southern Africa. Three Gm haplotypes only occur in the Mongoloid populations, Gm16*;17,1;.. [I] largely in the northern hemisphere, Gm5*;3,1;23 [J] and Gm5*;3,1;.. [K] in the southern hemisphere.

Haplotypes E, F, and G in the Negroid populations have been found with G1m27 and G1m28 on gamma1 (demonstrated on isolated chains of Lat-IV-5 (haplotype G) and Sno (haplotype F)) (96) (see Subheading 5.1.7).

### 7.3. From Gm Phenotypes to Gm Genotypes and Haplotypes

Gm phenotypes and deduced Gm genotypes and haplotypes from the Tunisian population (53) are shown as examples in Table 11. The observed diversity (26 phenotypes, and 28 deduced genotypes, contributed by 8 haplotypes) is explained by the geographical localization of Tunisia at the carrefour of many population migrations and civilizations (Table 11).

### 7.4. Gm Haplotype Frequency in Different Populations

Gm haplotype frequencies from different populations are shown, as examples, in Table 12.

**Table 11**
**Gm phenotypes observed in the Tunisian population and deduced Gm haplotypes**

| Gm phenotypes[a] | Gm genotypes[b] | Observed[c] |
|---|---|---|
| 5,10,11,13,14,26,27;3;23 | A/A ou A/B | 117 |
| 5,10,11,13,14,26,27;3;.. | B/B | 7 |
| 5,10,11,13,14,21,26,27,28;1,3,17;23 | A/C | 93 |
| 5,10,11,13,14,21,26,27,28;1,3,17;.. | B/C | 17 |
| 5,10,11,13,14,26,27;1,3,17;23 | A/E | 45 |
| 5,10,11,13,14,26,27;1,3,17;.. | B/E | 8 |
| 5,6,10,11,13,14,24,26,27;1,3,17;23 | A/G | 3 |
| 5,6,10,11,13,14,24,26,27;1,3,17;.. | B/G | 1 |
| 5,6,10,11,13,14,26,27;1,3,17;23 | A/F | 4 |
| 21,26,27,28;1,17;23 | C/M | 2 |
| 21,26,27,28;1,17;.. | C/C | 18 |
| 5,10,11,13,14,21,26,27,28;1,17;23 | E/M | 2 |
| 5,10,11,13,14,21,26,27,28;1,17;.. | C/E | 13 |
| 5,10,11,13,14,21,26,27,28;1,2,3,17;23 | A/D | 17 |
| 5,10,11,13,14,21,26,27,28;1,2,3,17;.. | B/D | 2 |
| 21,26,27,28;1,2,17;23 | D/M | 1 |
| 21,26,27,28,1,2,17;.. | D/D ou C/D | 6 |
| 5,10,11,13,14,21,26,27,28;1,2,17;.. | D/E | 3 |
| 5,10,11,13,14,26,27;1,17;.. | E/E | 1 |
| 5,6,10,11,13,14,24,26,27;1,17;.. | E/G | 1 |
| 5,6,10,11,13,14,26,27;1,17;.. | E/F | 1 |
| 5,6,11,21,24,26,27,28;1,17;.. | C/G | 1 |
| 5,6,10,11,14,21,26,27,28;1,17;..;23 | C/F | 1 |
| 10,11,13,15,16,21,26,27,28;1,17,.. | C/I | 1 |
| 5,10,11,13,14,15,16,26,27;1,3,17 | A/I | 1 |
| 5,10,11,13,14,15,16,26,27;1,3,17;.. | B/I | 1 |
| Total | | 367 |

[a]In Gm phenotypes, allotypes are given in increasing numbers, in the order G3m, G1m, G2m, and separated by semicolons between chains of different subclasses
[b]Gm haplotypes (A to M) are described in Subheading 7 (Table 10) (see Note 11)
[c]Five unusual phenotypes, each one found in one individual, were the starting point of familial studies and are not included in this table (53)

**Table 12**
**Gm haplotype frequencies among Middle Eastern, European, African, and Asian populations**

| | Gm haplotypes | | | | | | | | |
|---|---|---|---|---|---|---|---|---|---|
| | Caucasoid | Caucasoid Mongoloid | | Negroid | | Khoisan | Mongoloid | | |
| Populations[a] | A,B | C | D | E | F,G | H | I | J,K | References |
| Tunisian | 0.602–0.618 | 0.226–0.243 | 0.025–0.051 | 0.083–0.101 | 0.018–0.022 | – | 0.004–0.007 | – | (53) |
| Lebanese | 0.692–0.748 | 0.137–0.197 | 0.007–0.033 | 0.007–0.053 | 0.000–0.037 | – | 0.013–0.042 | – | (47, 49, 52) |
| Hungary, Czechoslovakia | 0.776–0.777 | 0.138–0.147 | 0.049–0.076 | 0.005–0.013 | 0.005–0.013 | – | 0.005–0.014 | – | (69, 70) |
| Austria, Germany, Italy Sardinia | 0.725–0.831 | 0.120–0.190 | 0.049–0.085 | – | – | – | – | – | (60, 66, 73) |
| Ethopia Sidamos | 0.157 | 0.236 | 0.018 | 0.400 | 0.135 | 0.027 | 0.027 | – | (65) |
| Angola | – | – | – | 0.793 | 0.207 | – | – | – | (59) |
| Mozambique | – | – | – | 0.716 | 0.260 | 0.024 | – | – | (59) |
| San | – | 0.120 | – | 0.295 | 0.030 | 0.555 | – | – | (71) |
| Khoikhoi | – | – | 0.048 | 0.429 | 0.190 | 0.333 | – | – | (71) |
| Japan | – | 0.437 | 0.151 | – | – | – | 0.261 | 0.151 | (90) |

[a]More information on these populations and other populations are available in (1) and in the original references. *See* also (47–87)

## 8. A2m Allotypes

#### *8.1. A2m1 and A2m2*

Two allotypes of the IGHA2 gene have been described, A2m1, identified by two groups, independently (39, 40), and A2m2 (41). A2m1 and A2m2 are antithetical and located on the CH1 domain. A2m1 corresponds to a proline at position 115 (IGHA2 CH1 Pro P115) and is also correlated to a proline at position 124 (IGHA2 CH1 Pro P124) (153) (Fig. 1b). A2m2 corresponds to a serine at position 115 (IGHA2 CH1 Ser S115) and is also correlated to an arginine at position 124 (IGHA2 CH1 Arg R124) (154, 155) (Fig. 10a).

#### *8.2. A2m1 and A2m2 Allotype Frequency*

The frequency of the A2m1 and A2m2 allotypes varies a lot between and within most populations (53, 77, 82, 90, 94). In Caucasoid populations, almost all individuals are homozygous for the A2m1 allotype. The A2m2 allotype, rare in Caucasoid populations, is present with a frequency of 0.40–0.75 in Mongoloid populations (78) and 0.60–0.85 in Negroid populations (79).

#### *8.3. A2m1 and A2m2 Allotype Determination by RFLP*

A2m1 and A2m2 allotypes can be determined at the DNA level by RFLP using appropriate restriction enzymes (101). The amino acid responsible for the A2m2 allotype, serine 115, is encoded by nucleotides which are part of an *Eco*RI restriction site (101) (Table 13). Due to a nucleotide substitution, this site is absent in the A2m1 allele. Thus, whereas the restriction enzyme *Pst*I yields two fragments containing the IGHA1 (1.2 kb) and IGHA2 (2 kb) genes (97, 114) when DNA samples are probed with a Cα probe, double digests *Eco*RI–*Pst*I show two different patterns: one similar to the *Pst*I one for the A2m1 allele and the other with a new 0.9 kb band for the A2m2 allele due to the existence of the *Eco*RI site (101). The determination of A2m alleles by RFLP is particularly useful when reagents are not readily available for the serological determination of the allotypes. Moreover, it is the only way to identify A2m alleles when no serum is available (for instance cell lines).

#### *8.4. Sequence Identity and Conformational Difference for A2m1 and the Alpha1 Isotypic Epitope*

The sequence of the A2m1 chain is identical to the sequence of the alpha 1 chain at positions 115 (CH1 Pro P115) and 124 (CH1 Pro P124) (109) (Fig. 1b). However, the IGHA2 A2m1 allotype and the IGHA1 isotypic epitope are recognized by different antibodies (Erna van Loghem, GL, MPL), due to a difference in the disulfide bridge. Indeed, in IgA1 (as in IgA2 A2m2), the cystein (CH1 Cys C123) is normally involved in a heavy-light (H-L) disulfide bridge. In contrast, in IgA2 A2m1, there is no H-L disulfide bridge to the cysteine (CH1 Cys C123) due to a conformational hindrance of the Pro P124, and the two light chains are directly linked to each other (102).

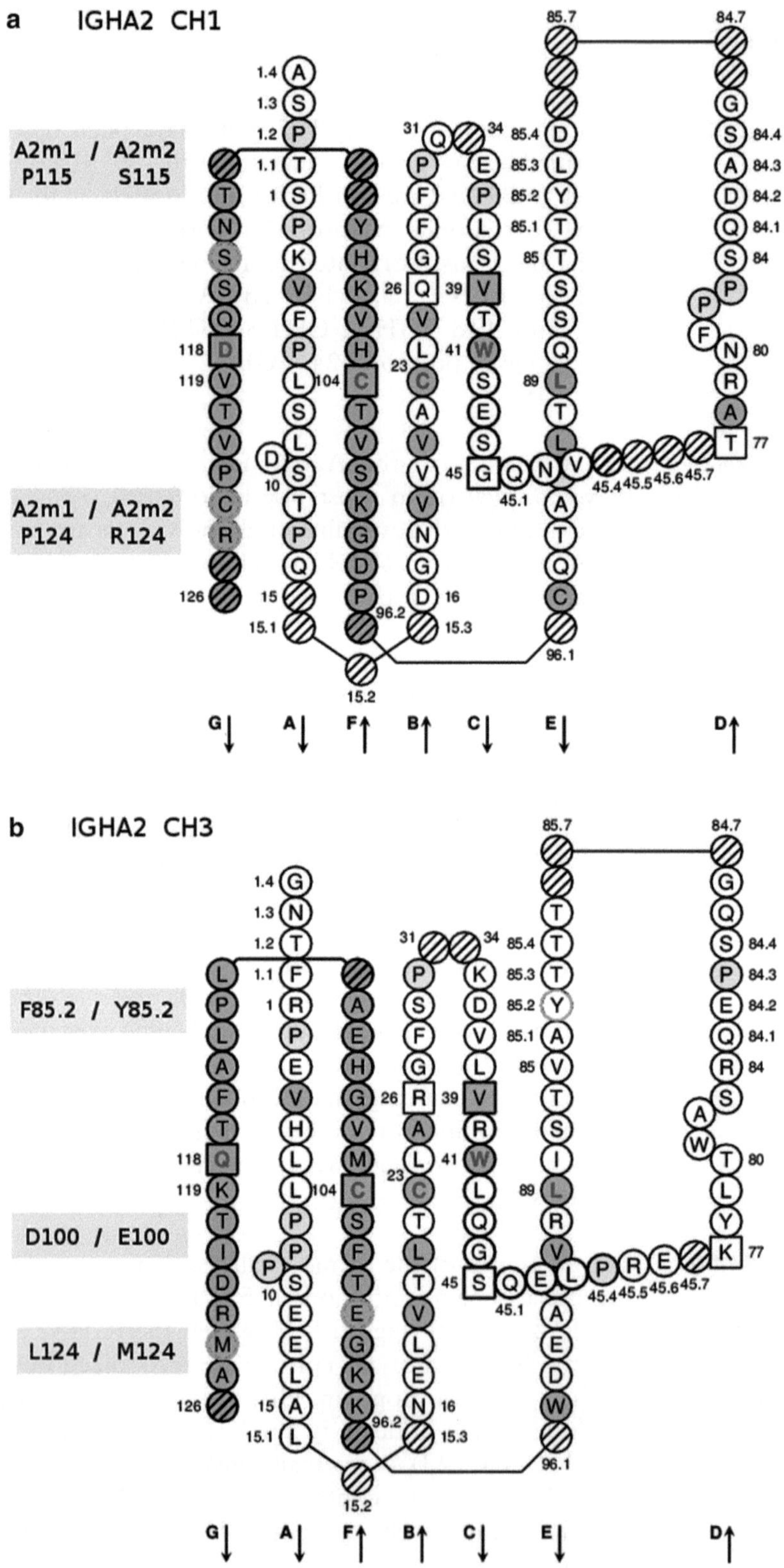
a IGHA2 CH1
A2m1 / A2m2
P115 S115
A2m1 / A2m2
P124 R124
G A F B C E D
b IGHA2 CH3
F85.2 / Y85.2
D100 / E100
L124 / M124
G A F B C E D

### 8.5. A2m3 Allotype Antithetical to nA2m3

The C-terminal region (CH3 domain and/or CHS region) of the IGHA2*02 allele (TOU II-5) (11) (Fig. 10b) was shown to be immunogenic and to correspond to a new allotype-designated A2m3, as it was antithetical to the nA2m3 isoallotype (previously called nA2m(2)) (unpublished data, Erna van Loghem, GL and MPL). One or several of the following IGHA2 amino acid changes may be involved in the A2m3 allotype/nA2m3 isoallotype expression, Tyr Y85.2/Phe F85.2, Glu E100/Asp D100, Met M124/Leu L124 (in the CH3), Ileu I134/Val V134, or Ala A143/Val V143 (in the CHS region) (IMGT Repertoire, Alignments of alleles, *Homo sapiens* IGHA2, http://www.imgt.org (5, 6)) (Fig. 1b).

### 8.6. Correspondence Between A2m Alleles and IGHA2 Alleles

The correspondence between A2m alleles and IGHA2 alleles is shown in Table 13. Three A2m alleles, A2m1, A2m2,3, and A2m2, are defined based on their allotypes. A2m1 corresponds to the IGHA2*01 allele, A2m2,3 to the IGHA2*02 (TOU II-5) allele, and A2m2 to the IGHA2*03 allele.

## 9. Km Allotypes

### 9.1. Definition

Allotypes have been identified for the human IGKC gene and are designated as Km (for "kappa marker") (previously Inv) (42, 43).

There are three kappa chain allotypes designated Km1, Km2, and Km3 that define three alleles. In 1961, Ropartz described the first IG light chain allotype Inv(a) (42), now called Km2. One year later, the Inv(l) allotype, now called Km1, was described by the same group (43). In 1962, Steinberg et al. described the third Km allotype, Inv(b) (44), now called Km3. They found that sera negative for Km1 and Km2 were always positive for Km3, and that sera negative for Km3 were always positive for Km1 and mostly also for Km2. Thus, the three Km allotypes define three alleles, Km3, Km1,2, and Km1 (detailed in Subheading 9.3)

Fig. 10. IMGT Colliers de Perles of the IGHA2*02 CH1 and CH3 domains. The CH1 and CH3 domains are from IGHA2*02 (IMGT/DomainDisplay, IMGT/GENE-DB (11, 15)) (IMGT®, http://www.imgt.org). The IMGT Colliers de Perles are shown on two layers. Hatched positions correspond to gaps according to the IMGT unique numbering (14). (**a**) CH1 domain. The serine at position 115 (S115) corresponds to A2m2, with the arginine at position 124 (R124) also correlating to that allotype (11, 101, 155). A proline at positions 115 (P115) and 124 (P124) would correspond to the A2m1 allotype (11, 101, 155). (**b**) CH3 domain. One or several of the following amino acids in the CH3 domain, tyrosine Tyr at position 85.2 (Y85.2), glutamate Glu at position 100 (E100), methionine Met at position 124 (M124), and/or in the CHS (not shown), isoleucine Ileu I134, alanine Ala A143 may be involved in the A2m3 allotype (11, 15, 155). One or several of the following amino acids, in the CH3 domain, phenylalanine Phe F85.2, aspartate Asp D100, leucine Leu L124, and/or in the CHS (not shown), valine Val V134 and valine Val V143 are involved in the antithetical nA2m3 allotype (11, 15, 155).

**Table 13**
**Correspondence between A2m alleles and IGHA2 alleles**

| A2m alleles | IGHA2 alleles | Domain | CH1 | | | CH3 | | | CHS | |
|---|---|---|---|---|---|---|---|---|---|---|
| | | Amino acid positions[a] | | | | | | | | |
| | | IMGT<br>Exon<br>Bur | **115**<br>(93)<br>*212* | **123**<br>(101)<br>*220* | **124**<br>(102)<br>*221* | **85.2**<br>(70) | **100**<br>(87) | **124**<br>(110) | **134**<br>(117) | **143**<br>(126) |
| A2m1<br>*nA2m3* | IGHA2*01 | | **Pro P** ccc | Cys C tgc | **Pro P** cca | Phe F ttc | Asp D gac | Leu L ttg | Val V gtc | Val V gtg |
| A2m2,3[b] | IGHA2*02 | | **Ser S** tcc | Cys C tgc | **Arg R** cga | Tyr Y tac | Glu E gag | Met M atg | Ile I atc | Ala A gcg |
| A2m2<br>*nA2m3* | IGHA2*03 | | **Ser S** tcc | Cys C tgc | **Arg R** cga | Phe F ttc | Asp D gac | Leu L ttg | Val V gtc | Val V gtg |

[a]Positions in bold are according to the IMGT unique numbering for C domain (14), between parentheses: exon numbering (11) and in italics: Bur numbering (164) (correspondence between C numberings, in IMGT scientific chart, *Homo sapiens* IGHA2, http://www.imgt.org (5, 6))
[b]The allotype A2m3 was identified serologically on the C-terminal region (CH3 and/or CHS) of TOU II-5 (Erna van Loghem, GL and MPL)

***9.2. Km Allotype Determination, Km Phenotypes, and Km Genotypes***

The three Km allotypes, Km1, Km2, and Km3, are determined by the hemagglutination inhibition technique (47, 50, 51, 53). Given the rarity of anti-Km2 and anti-Km3 reagent antibodies, only the Km1 allotype is tested in most of the population studies. Km genotypes and observed phenotypes depend on the number of tested allotypes. In Table 14, are shown:

- The six Km genotypes defined by their Km alleles.
- The five Km phenotypes observed when sera are tested for the three allotypes Km1, Km2, and Km3.
- The three Km phenotypes observed when sera are only tested for allotypes Km1 and Km2.
- The two Km phenotypes observed when sera are only tested for allotype Km1.

***9.3. Km Phenotypes and Km Allele Frequencies in Different Populations***

The two allotypes Km1 and Km2 mostly cooccur and are present in 10–20% of Caucasoid (47, 53, 54, 67), 40–60% of Negroid (79), and 30–60% of Mongoloid (78) populations (Table 15) (1). Km allele frequency in the different populations is given in Table 16. Details on extensive Km analysis in populations from Lebanon

**Table 14**
**Km genotypes and observed Km phenotypes depending on the tested Km allotypes**

| | Km phenotypes | | |
|---|---|---|---|
| Km genotypes | Sera tested for allotypes Km1, Km2, and Km3 | Sera only tested for allotypes Km1 and Km2 | Sera only tested for allotype Km1 |
| Km1/Km1 | Km1 | Km1,-2 | Km1 |
| Km1/Km3 | Km1,3 | | |
| Km1/Km1,2 or Km1,2/Km1,2 | Km1,2 | Km1,2 | |
| Km1,2/Km3 | Km1,2,3 | | |
| Km3/Km3 | Km3 | Km-1,-2 | Km-1 |

**Table 15**
**Km phenotype**

| | Populations | | |
|---|---|---|---|
| Km phenotype frequency | Caucasoid | Negroid | Mongoloid |
| Km3 | 80–90 | 40–60 | 40–70 |
| Km1,2 | 10–20 | 40–60 | 30–60 |

**Table 16**
**Km allele frequency**

| | Populations | | |
|---|---|---|---|
| Km allele frequency | Caucasoid | Negroid | Mongoloid |
| Km3 | 0.90–0.94 | 0.80–0.50 | 0.80–0.50 |
| Km1,2 | 0.06–0.08 | 0.20–0.50 | 0.20–0.50 |
| Km1 | 0.01 | 0.01 | 0.01 |

(6,076 alleles studied in 8 different communities) and Tunisia (756 alleles) (47, 52, 53) are available in IMGT Repertoire, Allotypes, *Homo sapiens* IGKC, http://www.imgt.org (5, 6)).

### *9.4. Correspondence Between Km Alleles and IGKC Allele Names*

Km allotypes correspond to amino acid changes in the C region of the kappa chain (C-KAPPA) at position IMGT 45.1 and 101 (156–158) (Fig. 11) (IMGT Repertoire, Alignments of alleles, *Homo sapiens* IGKC, http://www.imgt.org) (5, 6)).

Km1 correlates with valine at position 45.1 ('.1' for first position in the transverse CD strand (14)) (IGKC Val V45.1) and leucine at position 101 (IGKC Leu L101), Km1,2 correlates with alanine at position 45.1 (IGKC Ala A45.1) and leucine at position 101 (IGKC Leu L101), and Km3, the most frequent allotype, correlates with alanine at position 45.1 (IGKC Ala A45.1) and valine at position 101 (IGKC Val V101). Correspondence between Km alleles and IGKC allele names is shown in Table 17.

Km3 corresponds to four IGKC alleles, IGKC*01, *02, *03, and *05, Km1,2 to the IGKC*04 allele, and Km1 to the IGKC*06 allele.

## 10. Notes

1. An "incomplete" antibody binds to erythrocytes or bacteria but does not produce agglutination.
2. No allotypes have been found on the gamma4 and alpha1 chains of the IgG4 and IgA1 subclasses, respectively. Only one allotype, Em1, has been discovered on the epsilon chain of the IgE (159). As the concentration of IgE is very low, Em1 cannot be typed using the hemagglutination inhibition method, as the other allotypes, but instead using a radioimmunoassay with a monoclonal antibody (124). Em1 is very common in all populations and therefore not very informative. It has not been characterized at the amino acid level and currently is not determined. Allotypic markers have not been reported for IG lambda

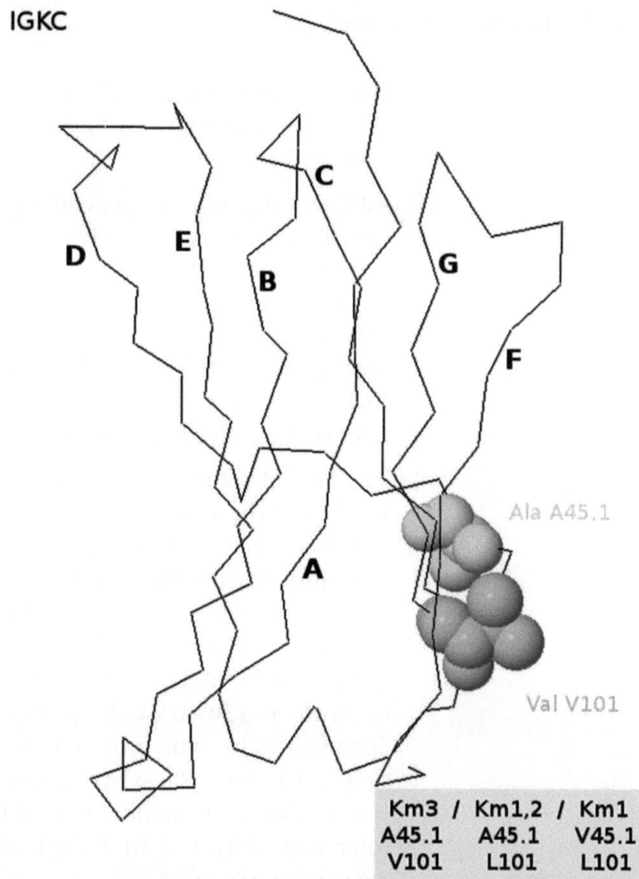


Fig. 11. Three-dimensional structure of IGKC*01. The C-KAPPA domain is from the b12 antibody (IMGT/3Dstructure-DB, code PDB:1hzh, http://www.imgt.org) (16, 17). The alanine Ala A45.1 (strand CD) and the valine Val V101 (strand F) are shown. The A45.1 and V101 correspond to the Km3 allotype. The A45.1 and L101 correspond to Km1,2, and the V45.1 and L101 to Km1.

## Table 17
## Correspondence between Km alleles and IGKC alleles

| Km alleles | IGKC alleles | Amino acid positions[a] | | |
|---|---|---|---|---|
| | | **IMGT**<br>Exon<br>Eu/Kabat | **45.1**<br>(46)<br>*153* | **101**<br>(84)<br>*191* |
| Km3 | IGKC*01, IGKC*02, IGKC*03, IGKC*05 | | Ala gcc | Val gtc |
| Km1,2 | IGKC*04 | | Ala gcc | Leu ctc |
| Km1 | IGKC*06[b] | | Val (gtc) | Leu (ctc) |

[a]Positions in bold are according to the IMGT unique numbering for C domain (14); between parentheses, IMGT exon numbering (11), and in italics, Eu/Kabat numbering (correspondence between C numberings, in IMGT Scientific chart, http://www.imgt.org) (5, 6))

[b]IGKC*06 (not sequenced at the nucleotide level) corresponds to Km1 allele and has amino changes A45.1 > V and V101 > L (compared to IGKC*01). The expected codons (shown between parentheses) are gtc (V45.1) and ctc (L101), respectively (IMGT Repertoire, http://www.imgt.org, GL and MPL, 13/05/2003)

(IGL) chains; however, there are multiple lambda chain isotypes and the number of IGLC genes vary between individuals (11, 160–163).

3. Alleles of a gene, or "gene alleles," correspond to polymorphic variants of a gene that differ by at least one nucleotide in their coding region (10, 11). Gene alleles are part of the concepts of classification of IMGT-ONTOLOGY (7, 8). They include the IMGT gene symbol with an asterisk, followed by a number starting from *01, e.g., IGHG1*01, IGHG1*02, etc. Gene alleles are available in IMGT/GENE-DB (15) and in IMGT Repertoire, Alignments of alleles, http://www.imgt.org (5, 6).

4. The WHO numeric nomenclature (45, 46) was established in 1976. For the G3m, the number is based on the chronological order of their discovery. The correspondence with the previous alphanumeric designation is the following: G3m5 or G3m(b1), G3m6 or G3m(c3), G3m10 or G3m (b5), G3m11 or G3m(b0), G3m13 or G3m(b3), G3m14 or G3m(b4), G3m15 or G3m(s), G3m16 or G3m(t), G3m21 or G3m(g1), G3m24 or G3m(c5), G3m26 or G3m(u), G3m27 or G3m(v), G3m28 or G3m(g5). Specificities for which there is no more antisera include Gm (7, 9, 18, 19, 20, 22), whereas Gm (8) is a marker of uncertain status. Correspondence with older designations is available in reference (50) and in IMGT Repertoire, Allotypes, http://www.imgt.org (5, 6).

5. As isoallotypes are present in several subclasses, typing of isoallotypes can only be done on isolated proteins. This is the case of the nG4m(a) and nG4m(b) isoallotypes (see Subheading 6).

6. Alanine is present at position 110 of CH3 in G1m2-negative gamma1 chains and in the gamma chains of the other IgG subclasses (Fig. 1a); however, CH3 Ala A110 is not an isoallotype as no antibody reagent has been characterized.

7. The presence of CH1 Ala A121 (IMGT numbering) in the 3D structure is a file error in PDB. It should be a valine (V) as in the b12 Fab (IMGT/3Dstructure-DB code PDB:1n0x_H). The sequence of the C region of the b12 heavy gamma1 chain (1hzh_H) should be IGHG1*01 100% in its entirety (IMGT/3Dstructure-DB entry card for 1hzh, http://www.imgt.org) (16, 17).

8. G2m23 (27) was detected by using an antiserum produced in a nonhuman primate. Since then no polyclonal human anti-G2m23 has been found (124).

9. A G2m23-positive serum can be from a homozygous individual G2m23/G2m23 or from a heterozygous individual G2m23/G2m... Because there is no antiserum to detect G2m.., the hemagglutination inhibition method cannot distinguish between sera from homozygotes or from heterozygotes.

10. Correspondence between the WHO/IUIS/IMGT nomenclature and the previous designation for the G3m alleles.

| WHO/IUIS/IMGT nomenclature | | Previous designation | |
|---|---|---|---|
| **Simplified form[a]** | **Complete description** | **Simplified form[b]** | **Complete description** |
| G3m5* | G3m5,10,11,13,14,26,27 | G3m(b)* | G3m b0,b1,b3,b4,b5,u,v |
| G3m6* | G3m5,6,10,11,14,26,27 | G3m(c3)* | G3m b0,b1,b4,b5,c3,u,v |
| G3m24* | G3m5,6,11,24,26 | G3m(c5)* | G3m b0,b1,c3,c5,u |
| G3m15* | G3m10,11,13,15,27 | G3m(s)* | G3m b0,b3,b5,s,v |
| G3m16* | G3m10,11,13,15,16,27 | G3m(t)* | G3m b0,b3,b5,s,t,v |
| G3m21* | G3m21,26,27,28 | G3m(g)* | G3m g1,g5,u,v |

[a]G3m24* was also designated as G3m6,24*, and G3m16* as G3m15,16*
[b]G3m(c5)* was also designated as G3m(c3,c5)*, and G3m(t)* as G3m(s,t)*

11. Correspondence between the WHO/IUIS/IMGT nomenclature and the previous designation for the Gm haplotypes. Only the simplified form is indicated. The correspondence for the detailed description of the G3m alleles is given in Note 10.

| Gm haplotypes | WHO/IUIS/IMGT nomenclature[a] | Previous designation[b] |
|---|---|---|
| A | Gm5*;3;23 | Gmb*;f;n |
| B | Gm5*;3;.. | Gmb*;f;.. |
| C | Gm21*;17,1;.. | Gmg*;z,a;.. |
| D | Gm21*;17,1,2;.. | Gmg*;z,a,x;.. |
| E | Gm5*;17,1;.. | Gmb*;z,a;.. |
| F | Gm6*;17,1;.. | Gmc3*;z,a;.. |
| G | Gm24*;17,1;.. | Gmc5*;z,a;.. |
| H | Gm15*;17,1;.. | Gms*;z,a;.. |
| I | Gm16*;17,1;.. | Gmt*;z,a;.. |
| J | Gm5*;3,1;23 | Gmb*;f,a;n |
| K | Gm5*;3,1;.. | Gmb*;f,a;.. |
| L | Gm5*;17,1,2;.. | Gmb*;z,a,x;.. |
| M | Gm21*;17,1;23 | Gmg*;z,a;n |

[a]24* was previously designated as 6,24*, and 16* as 15,16*
[b]c5* was previously designated as c3,c5*, and t* as s,t*

## Acknowledgments

We thank Géraldine Folch for the "IMGT G3m allele butterfly" representation, Chantal Ginestoux and Saida Hadi-Saljoqi for their help, and François Ehrenmann for the 3D structure figures. We are very grateful to the IMGT® team for its expertise and constant motivation. This chapter is a tribute to Erna van Loghem, Liliane Rivat and Claude Ropartz.

### References

1. Lefranc M-P, Lefranc G (1990) Molecular genetics of immunoglobulin allotype expression. In: Shakib F (ed) The human IgG subclasses: molecular analysis of structure, function and regulation (chapter 4). Pergamon, Oxford, UK, pp 43–78
2. Lefranc M-P (2011) Antibody nomenclature: from IMGT-ONTOLOGY to INN definition. MAbs 3(1):1–2
3. Jefferis R, Lefranc M-P (2009) Human immunoglobulin allotypes: possible implications for immunogenicity. MAbs 1(4):332–338
4. Magdelaine-Beuzelin C, Vermeire S, Goodall M, Baert F, Noman M, Van Assche G, Ohresser M, Degenne D, Dugoujon JM, Jefferis R, Rutgeerts P, Lefranc M-P, Watier H (2009) IgG1 heavy chain-coding gene polymorphism (G1m allotypes) and development of antibodies-to-infliximab. Pharmacogenet Genomics 19:383–387
5. Lefranc M-P (2008) IMGT®, the international ImMunoGeneTics information system® for immunoinformatics. Methods for querying IMGT® databases, tools and Web resources in the context of immunoinformatics. Mol Biotechnol 40:101–111
6. Lefranc M-P, Giudicelli V, Ginestoux C, Jabado-Michaloud J, Folch G, Bellahcene F, Wu Y, Gemrot E, Brochet X, Lane J, Regnier L, Ehrenmann F, Lefranc G, Duroux P (2009) IMGT®, the international ImMunoGeneTics information system®. Nucleic Acids Res 37:D1006–D1012
7. Giudicelli V, Lefranc M-P (1999) Ontology for immunogenetics: IMGT-ONTOLOGY. Bioinformatics 15:1047–1054
8. Duroux P, Kaas Q, Brochet X, Lane J, Ginestoux C, Lefranc M-P, Giudicelli V (2008) IMGT-Kaleidoscope, the formal IMGT-ONTOLOGY paradigm. Biochimie 90:570–583
9. Lefranc M-P, Giudicelli V, Regnier L, Duroux P (2008) IMGT®, a system and an ontology that bridge biological and computational spheres in bioinformatics. Brief Bioinform 9:263–275
10. Lefranc M-P (2000) Nomenclature of the human immunoglobulin genes. In: Coligan JE, Bierer BE, Margulies DE, Shevach EM, Strober W (eds) Current protocols in immunology. Wiley, Hoboken, NJ, pp A.1P.1–A.1P.37
11. Lefranc G, Lefranc M-P (2001) The immunoglobulin FactsBook. Academic Press, London, UK, pp 1–458
12. Lefranc M-P (2007) WHO-IUIS nomenclature subcommittee for immunoglobulins and T cell receptors report. Immunogenetics 59:899–902
13. Lefranc M-P (2008) WHO-IUIS nomenclature subcommittee for immunoglobulins and T cell receptors report August 2007, 13th International Congress of Immunology, Rio de Janeiro, Brazil. Dev Comp Immunol 32:461–463
14. Lefranc M-P, Pommié C, Kaas Q, Duprat E, Bosc N, Guiraudou D, Jean C, Ruiz M, Da Piédade I, Rouard M, Foulquier E, Thouvenin V, Lefranc G (2005) IMGT unique numbering for immunoglobulin and T cell receptor constant domains and Ig superfamily C-like domains. Dev Comp Immunol 29:185–203
15. Giudicelli V, Chaume D, Lefranc M-P (2005) IMGT/GENE-DB: a comprehensive database for human and mouse immunoglobulin and T cell receptor genes. Nucleic Acids Res 33:D256–D261
16. Kaas Q, Ruiz M, Lefranc M-P (2004) IMGT/3Dstructure-DB and IMGT/StructuralQuery, a database and a tool for immunoglobulin, T cell receptor and MHC structural data. Nucleic Acids Res 32:D208–D210
17. Ehrenmann F, Kaas Q, Lefranc M-P (2010) IMGT/3Dstructure-DB and IMGT/DomainGapAlign: a database and a tool for immunoglobulins or antibodies, T cell receptors, MHC, IgSF and MhcSF. Nucleic Acids Res 38:D301–D307

18. Kaas Q, Lefranc M-P (2007) IMGT Colliers de Perles: standardized sequence-structure representations of the IgSF and MhcSF superfamily domains. Curr Bioinform 2:21–30
19. Kaas Q, Ehrenmann F, Lefranc M-P (2007) IG, TR and IgSf, MHC and MhcSF: what do we learn from the IMGT Colliers de Perles? Brief Funct Genomic Proteomic 6:253–264
20. Grubb R (1956) Agglutination of erythrocytes coated with "incomplete" anti-Rh by certain rheumatoid arthritic sera and some other sera. The existence of human serum groups. Acta Pathol Microbiol Scand 39:195–197
21. Grubb R, Laurell AB (1956) Hereditary serological human serum groups. Acta Pathol Microbiol Scand 39:390–398
22. Harboe M, Lundevall J (1959) A new type in the Gm system. Acta Pathol Microbiol Scand 45:357–370
23. Steinberg AG, Wilson JA (1963) Studies on hereditary gamma globulin factors: evidence that Gm (b) in Whites and Negroes is not the same and that Gm-like is determined by an allele at the Gm locus. Am J Hum Genet 15:96–105
24. Gold ER, Ropartz C, Rivat L, Rousseau PY (1965) Gm(f)–a determinant of human gamma-globulin. Vox Sang 10:299–302
25. Gold ER, Mandy WJ, Fudenberg HH (1965) Relation between Gm(f) and the structure of the gamma-globulin molecule. Nature 207(5001):1099–1101
26. Litwin SD, Kunkel HG (1966) A gamma-globulin genetic factor related to Gm(a) but localized to a different portion of the same heavy chains. Nature 210:866
27. Kunkel HG, Yount WJ, Litwin SD (1966) Genetically determined antigen of the Ne subgroup of gamma-globulin: detection by precipitin analysis. Science 154(752):1041–1043
28. Harboe M (1959) A new hemagglutinating substance in the Gm system, anti-$Gm^b$. Acta Pathol Microbiol Scand 47:191–198
29. Steinberg AG, Giles BD, Stauffer R (1960) A Gm-like factor present in Negroes and rare or absent in whites: its relation to Gma and Gmx. Am J Hum Genet 12:44–51
30. Ropartz C, Rivat L, Rousseau PY (1963) Le Gm(b) et ses problèmes. Vox Sang 8:717–723
31. Steinberg AG, Goldblum R (1965) A genetic study of the antigens associated with the Gm(b) factor of human γ-globulin. Am J Hum Genet 17:133–147
32. Martensson L, van Loghem E, Matsumoto H, Nielsen J (1966) Gm(s) and Gm(t): genetic determinants of human gamma-globulin. Vox Sang 11:393–418
33. Natvig JB (1966) Gm(g)–a "new" gamma-globulin factor. Nature 211:318–319
34. van Loghem E, Martensson L (1967) Genetic (Gm) determinants of the γ2c (Vi) subclass of human IgG immunoglobulins. A study with special reference to Gm(c3) and Gm(c5), and their relationship with the Gm(b) determinants. Vox Sang 13:369–392
35. van Loghem E, Grobbelaar BG (1971) A new genetic marker of human IgG3 immunoglobulin. Evolutionary dissociation of Gm allotypes. Vox Sang 21:405
36. Schanfield MS, Fudenberg HH (1974) Gm (Ray), a new allotypic marker on human IgG3. Vox Sang 26:133–140
37. Blanc M, Dugoujon JM, Ruffié J (1976) [A new genetic marker for human IgG3 usually associated with Gm (21) factor found in the caucasian and mongolian populations]. In French. Un nouveau marqueur génétique des IgG3 humaines habituellement associé au facteur Gm(21) dans les populations caucasoides et mongoloides. C R Acad Sci Paris 283:1461–1463
38. van Loghem E, Blanc M, de Lange G (1977) Human IgG3 allotypes, with special reference to a new allotype related to G3m(g) (G3m(21)). J Immunogenet 4:371–383
39. Vyas GN, Fudenberg HH (1969) Am(1), the first genetic marker of human immunoglobulin A. Proc Natl Acad Sci USA 64:1211–1216
40. Kunkel HG, Smith WK, Joslin FG, Natvig JB, Litwin SD (1969) Genetic marker of the gamma-A2 subgroup of γA immunoglobulins. Nature 223:1247–1248
41. van Loghem E, Wang AC, Shuster J (1973) A new genetic marker of human immunoglobulins determined by an allele at the α2 locus. Vox Sang 24:481–488
42. Ropartz C, Lenoir J, Rivat L (1961) A new inheritable property of human sera: the Inv factor. Nature 189:586–587
43. Ropartz C, Rivat L, Rousseau PY (1962) Deux nouveaux facteurs dans les systèmes héréditaires de gammaglobuline: le Gm(e) et l'Inv(l). Proceedings of the 9th Society of blood Transfusion. Karger Baset, Mexico, p 455
44. Steinberg AG, Wilson JA, Lanset S (1962) A new human gamma globulin factor determined by an allele at the Inv locus. Vox Sang 7:151–156
45. WHO (1976) Review of the notation for the allotypic and related markers of human immunoglobulins. WHO meeting on human immunoglobulin allotypic markers. J Immunogenet 3:357–362

46. WHO. Review of the notation for the allotypic and related markers of human immunoglobulins (1976) WHO meeting on human immunoglobulin allotypic markers, held July 16–19, 1974, Rouen, France. Report amended June 1976. Eur J Immunol 6:599
47. Lefranc G, Loiselet J, Rivat L, Ropartz C (1976) Gm, Km and ISf allotypes in the Lebanese population. Acta Anthropogenet 1:34–45
48. Lefranc G, Rivat L, Rivat C, Loiselet J, Ropartz C (1976) Evidence for "deleted" or "silent" genes homozygous at the locus coding for the constant region of the γ3 chain. Am J Hum Genet 28:51–61
49. Lefranc G, Rivat L, Salier JP, van Loghem E, Aydenian H, Zalzal P, Chakhachiro L, Loiselet J, Ropartz C (1977) Recombination, mutation, or constitutive expression at a Gm locus and familial hypergammaglobulinemia. Am J Hum Genet 29:523–536
50. Lefranc G (1978) Allotypes et haplotypes des immunoglobulines dans les communautés libanaises: intérêt exceptionnel en immunogénétique et séro-anthropologie [in French]. PhD Thesis. Université de Rouen, France
51. Lefranc G (1978) Immunoglobulin allotypes and haplotypes in the Lebanese communities: discussion of unusual genetic events and population structure. PhD Thesis. Université de Rouen, France, pp 1–137
52. Lefranc G, Rivat L, Serre JL, Lalouel JM, Pison G, Loiselet J, Ropartz C, de Lange G, van Loghem E (1978) Common and uncommon immunoglobulin haplotypes among Lebanese communities. Hum Genet 41:197–209
53. Lefranc G, de Lange G, Rivat L, Langaney A, Lefranc M-P, Ellouze F, Sfar G, Sfar M, van Loghem E (1979) Gm, Am and Km immunoglobulin allotypes of two populations in Tunisia. Hum Genet 50:199–211
54. Ropartz C, Rivat L, Rousseau PY, Baitsch H, van Loghem J (1963) The Gm and Inv systems in Europe. Acta Genet Stat Med 13:109–123
55. Ropartz C, Rousseau PY, Rivat L (1963) Les groupes de gamma-globulines Gm et Inv : Etude génétique et anthropologique. Bull Soc Anthropol Paris 4(Xie ser.):458–469
56. Steinberg AG, Matsumoto H (1964) Studies on the Gm, Inv, Hp and Tf serum factors of Japanese populations and families. Hum Biol 36:77–85
57. Taleb N, Ruffie J (1968) Hémotypologie des populations jordaniennes. Bull Mém Soc Anthrop Paris 3(XIIe sér.):269–282
58. Ropartz C, Rivat L, Rousseau PY, Lauridsen UB, Persson I (1970) A survey of 9 Gm-factors, the Inv and the ISf systems in Danes. Hum Hered 20:275–280
59. Jenkins T, Zoutendyk A, Steinberg AG (1970) Gammaglobulin groups (Gm and Inv) of various Southern African populations. Am J Phys Anthropol 32:197–218
60. Mayr WR, Mickerts D (1970) Der menschliche Gammaglobulin-Polymorphismus. Acta Biol Med Germ 25:475–482
61. Bonné B, Godber M, Ashbel S, Mourant AE, Tills D (1971) South-Sinai Beduin. A preliminary report on their inherited blood factors. Am J Phys Anthropol 34:397–408
62. Ropartz C, Rivat L, Rousseau PY, Legueult LC (1972) Frequency of Gm, Inv and ISf phenotypes in the population of 4 Yugoslavian villages. Hum Hered 22:508–518
63. Salzano FM, Steinberg AG, Tepfenhart MA (1973) Gm and Inv allotypes of Brazilian Cayapo Indians. Am J Hum Genet 25:167–177
64. Steinberg AG (1973) Contribution of the Gm and Inv allotypes to the characterization of human populations. Israel J Med Sci 9:1249–1256
65. Steinberg AG (1973) Gm and Inv allotypes of some Sidamo Ethiopians. Am J Phys Anthropol 39:403–408
66. Wiebecke D (1973) Die frequenczen von Gm (1,2,3,5) und Inv (1) in der Bevölkerung der Bundesrepublik Deustchland. Humangenetik 18:175–180
67. Fraser GR, Volkers WS, Bernini LF, van Loghem E, Meera Khan P, Nijenhuis LE (1974) Gene frequencies in a Dutch population. Hum Hered 24:435–448
68. Daveau M, Rivat L, Langaney A, Afifi N, Bois E, Ropartz C (1975) Gm and Inv allotypes in French Guiana Indians. Hum Hered 25:88–92
69. Schanfield MS, Gergely J, Fudenberg HH (1975) Immunoglobulin allotypes of European populations. I. Gm and Km(Inv) allotypic markers in Hungarians. Hum Hered 25:370–377
70. Schanfield MS, Herzog P, Fudenberg HH (1975) Immunoglobulin allotypes of European populations. II.Gm, Am and Km(Inv) allotypic markers in Czechoslovakians. Hum Hered 25:382–392
71. Steinberg AG, Jenkins T, Nurse GT, Harpending HC (1975) Gammaglobulin groups of the Khoisan peoples of Southern Africa: evidence for polymorphism for a $Gm^{1,5,13,14,21}$ haplotype among the San. Am J Hum Genet 27:528–542
72. Lalouel JM, Loiselet J, Lefranc G, Chaiban D, Chakhachiro L, Rivat L, Ropartz C (1976) Genetic differentiation among Lebanese communities. Acta Anthropogenet 1:15–33

73. Piazza A, van Loghem E, de Lange G, Curtoni ES, Ulizzi L, Terrenato L (1976) Immunoglobulin allotypes in Sardinia. Am J Hum Genet 28:77–86
74. Gershowitz H, Neel JV (1978) The immunoglobulin allotypes (Gm and Km) of twelve Indian tribes of Central and South America. Am J Phys Anthropol 49:289–301
75. Rivat L, Rivat C, Cook CE, Steinberg AG (1978) Gm(28). Un nouvel allotype du système Gm présent sur les IgG3: Intérêt particulier de son étude dans les populations négroides. Ann Immunol Inst Pasteur 129:33–45
76. Steinberg AG, Cook CE (1981) The distribution of the human immunoglobulin allotypes. Oxford University Press, Oxford
77. Chaabani H, Helal AN, van Loghem E, Langaney A, Benammar Elgaaied A, Rivat Peran L, Lefranc G (1984) Genetic study of Tunisian Berbers. I. Gm, Am and Km immunoglobulin allotypes and ABO blood groups. J Immunogenet 11:107–113
78. de Lange G, Zhong FM, Henke J, Feng ZC, Bernhardt R, van Leeuwen F, van Eede P (1985) Immunoglobulin allotypes in a Chinese population: comparison of haplotype frequencies with other Asian groups. J Immunogenet 12:191–195
79. van Loghem E (1986) Immunoglobulin markers. In: Cavalli-Sforza LL (ed) African pygmies (chapter 14). Academic Press, Orlando, p 201
80. Helal AN, Rivat-Peran L, van Loghem E, de Lange G, Langaney A, Lefranc G (1988) Further contribution of common Gm-Am haplotypes and Km alleles in the characterization of the Tunisian population. Exp Clin Immunogenet 5:1–14
81. Helal AN, de Lange G, van Loghem E, Lefranc G (1988) Uncommon Gm haplotypes in the Tunisian population: further contribution to the genetics of the IgG immunoglobulins. Exp Clin Immunogenet 5:24–38
82. Soua Z, Ghanem N, Salem B, Lefranc G, Lefranc M-P (1989) Frequencies of the human immunoglobulin IGHA2*M1 and IGHA2*M2 alleles corresponding to the A2m(1) and A2m(2) allotypes in the French, Lebanese, Tunisian and Black African populations. Nucleic Acids Res 17:3625
83. Zhao TM, Lee TD (1989) Gm and Km allotypes in 74 Chinese populations: a hypothesis of the origin of the Chinese nation. Hum Genet 83:101–110
84. Blanc M, Sanchez-Mazas A, Van Blyenburgh NH, Sevin A, Pison G, Langaney A (1990) Interethnic genetic differentiation: Gm polymorphism in eastern Senegal. Am J Hum Genet 46:383–392
85. Sukernik RI, Osipova LP, Schanfield MS (1992) Distribution of GM allotypes and deleted IGHG1 haplotypes in the Sel'kups in comparison to the Forest Nentsi of northwestern Siberia. Exp Clin Immunogenet 9:15–23
86. Schanfield MS (1992) Immunoglobulin allotypes (GM and KM) indicate multiple founding populations of Native Americans: evidence of at least four migrations to the New World. Hum Biol 64:381–402
87. Yacoubi Loveslati B, Sanchez-Mazas A, Ennafaa H, Marrakchi R, Dugoujon J-M, Lefranc M-P, Ben Ammar Elgaaied A (2001) A study of Gm allotypes and immunoglobulin heavy gamma chain IGHG genes in Berbers, Arabs and sub-Saharan Africans from Jerba Island, Tunisia. Eur J Immunogenet 28:531–538
88. Geha RS, Malakian A, Lefranc G, Chaiban D, Serre JL (1976) Immunologic reconstitution in severe combined immunodeficiency following transplantation with parental bone marrow. Pediatrics 58:451–455
89. van Loghem E, Natvig JB (1970) Uncommon Gm gene complexes. Vox Sang 18:421–434
90. van Loghem E, Natvig JB, Matsumoto H (1970) Genetic markers of immunoglobulins in Japanese families. Inheritance of associated markers belonging to one IgA and three IgG subclasses. Ann Hum Genet 33:351–359
91. Lefranc G, Dumitresco SM, Salier JP, Rivat L, de Lange G, van Loghem E, Loiselet J (1979) Familial lack of the IgG3 subclass: gene elimination or turning off expression and neutral evolution in the immune system. J Immunogenet 6:215–221
92. Salier JP, Rivat L, Daveau M, Lefranc G, Breton P, De Menibus CH, Henocq A, Fudenberg HH (1980) Quantitative studies of Gm allotypes. V. Simultaneous presence of latent Gm allotypes and deficient Gm genes in a family with hypogammaglobulinaemic probands. J Immunogenet 7:123–135
93. van Loghem E, Sukernik RI, Osipova LP, Zegers BJM, Matsumoto H, De Lange G, Lefranc G (1980) Gene deletion and gene duplication within the cluster of human heavy chain genes. Selective absence of IgG subclasses. J Immunogenet 7:285–299
94. Lefranc M-P (1980) Les allotypes Gm, Am et Km des immunoglobulines humaines dans deux échantillons de la population Tunisienne (Mahdia et Sfax): contribution à la connaissance séro-anthropologique de cette population et à la génétique des immunoglobulines [in French] Thesis, Série 3° cycle n°16, Université Paris Sud, France, pp 1–108

95. Lefranc G, Lefranc M-P, Helal AN, Boukef K, Chaabani H, Gandoura MS, van Loghem E (1982) Unusual heavy chains of human IgG immunoglobulins: rearrangements of the CH domain exons. J Immunogenet 9:1–9
96. van Loghem E, de Lange G, van Leeuwen AM, van Eede PH, Nijenhuis LE, Lefranc M-P, Lefranc G (1982) Human IgG allotypes co-occurring in more than one IgG subclass. Vox Sang 43:301–309
97. Lefranc M-P, Lefranc G, Rabbitts TH (1982) Inherited deletion of immunoglobulin heavy chain constant region genes in normal human individuals. Nature 300:760–762
98. Lefranc M-P, Lefranc G, de Lange G, Out TA, van den Broek PJ, van Nieuwkoop J, Radl J, Helal AN, Chaabani H, van Loghem E, Rabbitts TH (1983) Instability of the human immunoglobulin heavy chain constant region locus indicated by different inherited chromosomal deletions. Mol Biol Med 1:207–217
99. Lefranc G, Chaabani H, van Loghem E, Lefranc M-P, de Lange G, Helal AN (1983) Simultaneous absence of the human IgG1, IgG2, IgG4 and IgA1 subclasses: immunological and immunogenetical considerations. Eur J Immunol 13:240–244
100. Flanagan JG, Lefranc M-P, Rabbitts TH (1984) Mechanisms of divergence and convergence of the human immunoglobulin alpha1 and alpha2 constant region gene sequences. Cell 36:681–688
101. Lefranc M-P, Rabbitts TH (1984) Human immunoglobulin heavy chain A2 gene allotype determination by restriction fragment length polymorphism. Nucleic Acids Res 12:1303–1311
102. Lefranc M-P (1984) Recombinaisons, délétions et conversions de gènes de la région constante des chaînes lourdes des immunoglobulines humaines [in French]. PhD Thesis. Université Montpellier 2, France
103. Lefranc M-P, Helal AN, de Lange G, Chaabani H, van Loghem E, Lefranc G (1986) Gene conversion in human immunoglobulin γ locus shown by unusual location of IgG allotypes. FEBS Lett 196:96–102
104. Huck S, Fort P, Crawford DH, Lefranc M-P, Lefranc G (1986) Sequence of a human immunoglobulin γ3 heavy chain constant region gene: comparison with the other human Cγ genes. Nucleic Acids Res 14:1779–1789
105. Lefranc M-P, Lefranc G (1987) Human immunoglobulin heavy-chain multigene deletions in healthy individuals. FEBS Lett 213:231–237
106. Huck S, Lefranc G, Lefranc M-P (1989) A human immunoglobulin IGHG3 allele (Gmb0, b1, c3, c5, u) with an IGHG4 converted region and three hinge exons. Immunogenetics 30:250–257
107. Keyeux G, Lefranc G, Lefranc M-P (1989) A multigene deletion in the human IGH constant region locus involves highly homologous hot spots of recombination. Genomics 5:431–441
108. Lefranc M-P, Hammarström L, Smith CI, Lefranc G (1991) Gene deletions in the human immunoglobulin heavy chain constant region locus: molecular and immunological analysis. Immunodefic Rev 2:265–281
109. Bensmana M, Chuchana P, Lefranc G, Lefranc M-P (1991) Sequence of the CH1 and hinge-CH2 exons of the human immunoglobulin IGHA2 A2m(2) allele: comparison with the nonallelic and allelic IGHA genes. Cytogenet Cell Genet 56:128
110. Lefranc M-P, Hammarström L, Smith CIE, Lefranc G (1993) Gene deletions in the human immunoglobulin heavy chain constant region locus: molecular and immunological analysis. In: Rosen FS, Seligmann M (eds) Immunodeficiencies (chapter 5). Harwood Academic Publishers, Newark, New Jersey, USA, pp 99–109
111. Wiebe V, Helal A, Lefranc M-P, Lefranc G (1994) Molecular analysis of the T17 immunoglobulin CH multigene deletion (del A1-GP-G2-G4-E). Hum Genet 93:520–528
112. Dard P, Huck S, Frippiat JP, Lefranc G, Langaney A, Lefranc M-P, Sanchez-Mazas A (1997) The IGHG3 gene shows a structural polymorphism characterized by different hinge lengths: sequence of a new 2-exon hinge gene. Hum Genet 99:138–141
113. Dard P, Lefranc M-P, Osipova L, Sanchez-Mazas A (2001) DNA sequence variability of IGHG3 alleles associated to the main G3m haplotypes in human populations. Eur J Hum Genet 9:765–772
114. Flanagan JG, Rabbitts TH (1982) Arrangement of human immunoglobulin heavy chain constant region genes implies evolutionary duplication of a segment containing γ, ε and α genes. Nature 300:709–713
115. Rabbitts TH, Flanagan JG, Lefranc M-P (1983) Flexibility and change within the human immunoglobulin gene locus. In: Chater KF et al (eds) Genetic rearrangement. Croom Helm, London, UK, pp 143–154
116. Ghanem N, Lefranc M-P, Lefranc G (1988) Definition of the RFLP alleles in the human immunoglobulin IGHG gene locus. Eur J Immunol 18:1059–1065
117. Ghanem N, Dugoujon JM, Bensmana M, Huck S, Lefranc M-P, Lefranc G (1988)

Restriction fragment haplotypes in the human immunoglobulin IGHG locus and their correlation with the Gm polymorphism. Eur J Immunol 18:1067–1072

118. Ghanem N, Dugoujon JM, Lefranc M-P, Lefranc G (1989) BstEII restriction fragment alleles and haplotypes of the human IGHG genes with reference to the BamHI/SacI RFLPs and to the Gm polymorphism. Exp Clin Immunogenet 6:39–54

119. Ghanem N, Bensmana M, Dugoujon JM, Constans J, Lefranc M-P, Lefranc G (1989) BamHI and SacI RFLPs of the human immunoglobulin IGHG genes with reference to the Gm polymorphism in African people. Evidence for a major polymorphism. Hum Genet 83:37–4418

120. Hammarström L, Ghanem N, Smith CIE, Lefranc G, Lefranc M-P (1990) RFLP of human immunoglobulin genes. Exp Clin Immunogenet 7:7–19

121. Dard P, Sanchez-Mazas A, Dugoujon JM, de Lange G, Langaney A, Lefranc M-P, Lefranc G (1996) DNA analysis of the immunoglobulin IGHG loci in a Mandenka population from eastern Senegal: correlation with Gm haplotypes and hypotheses for the evolution of the Ig CH region. Hum Genet 98:36–47

122. Osipova LP, Posukh OL, Wiebe VP, Miyazaki T, Matsumoto H, Lefranc G, Lefranc M-P (1999) BamHI-SacI RFLP and Gm analysis of the immunoglobulin IGHG genes in the Northern Selkups (west Siberia): new haplotypes with deletion, duplication and triplication. Hum Genet 105:530–541

123. Gold ER, Fudenberg HH (1967) Chromic chloride: a coupling reagent for passive hemagglutination reactions. J Immunol 99(5): 859–866

124. de Lange G (1988) Monoclonal antibodies against human immunoglobulin allotypes. PhD Thesis. London, Amsterdam, pp 1–175

125. Zelaschi D, Newby C, Parsons M, van West B, Cavalli-Sforza LL, Herzenberg LA, Herzenberg LA (1983) Human immunoglobulin allotypes: previously unrecognized determinants and alleles defined with monoclonal antibodies. Proc Natl Acad Sci USA 80:3762–3766

126. Kurth JH, Bowcock AM, Erlich HA, Nevo S, Cavalli-Sforza LL (1991) Km typing with PCR: application to population screening. Am J Hum Genet 48(3):613–620

127. Balbin M, Grubb A, Abrahamson M, Grubb R (1991) Determination of allotypes G1m (f) and G1m (z) at the genomic level by subclass-specific amplification of DNA and use of allele-specific probes. Exp Clin Immunogenet 8:88–95

128. Balbin M, Grubb A, de Lange GG, Grubb R (1994) DNA sequences specific for Caucasian G3m (b) and (g) allotypes: allotyping at the genomic level. Immunogenetics 39:187–193

129. Brusco A, de Lange GG, Boccazzi C, Carbonara AO (1995) Molecular characterization of G2m (n+) and G2m (n-)allotypes. Immunogenetics 42:414–417

130. Hougs L, Svejgaard A, Barington T (2001) The first constant-domain (CH1) exon of human IGHG2 is polymorphic and in strong linkage disequilibrium with the (CH2) exon polymorphism encoding the G2m(n+) allotype in Caucasians. Immunogenetics 52:242–248

131. Frangione B, Franklin EC, Fudenberg HH, Koshland ME (1966) Structural studies of human γG myeloma proteins of different antigenic subgroups and genetic specificities. J Exp Med 124:715–732

132. Press EM, Hogg NM (1970) The amino-acid sequences of the Fd fragments of two human γ1 heavy chains. Biochem J 117:641–660

133. Burton RM, Deutsch HF (1970) The structure of peptides of Fc-fragments from γG-globulins of known allotypic specificity. Immunochemistry 7:145–156

134. Natvig JB, Turner MW (1971) Localization of Gm markers to different molecular regions of the Fc fragment. Clin Exp Immunol 8:685–700

135. Michaelsen TE, Frangione B, Franklin EC (1977) The amino acid sequence of a human immunoglobulin G3m(g) pFc' fragment. J Immunol 119:558–563

136. Pardo AG, Rosenwasser ES, Frangione B (1978) The primary structure of a human immunoglobulin G2 (IgG2) pFc'fragment. J Immunol 121:1040–1044

137. Natvig JB, Kunkel HG, Joslin FG (1969) Delineation of two antigenic markers, "non a" and "non g" related to the genetic antigens of human gamma globulins. J Immunol 102:611–617

138. Kunkel HG, Joslin FG, Penn GM, Natvig JB (1970) Genetic variants of γG4 globulin. A unique relationship to other classes of γG globulin. J Exp Med 13:508–520

139. van Loghem E, de Lange G (1972) 'non-b', antigenic determinant of IgG. Vox Sang 22:193–199

140. Gaarder PI, Natvig JB (1972) Two new antigens of human IgG, "non $b^0$" and "non $b^1$", related to the Gm system. J Immunol 108:617–621

141. van Loghem E, de Lange G (1976) The first example of an isoallotype of human IgG located on the Fd fragment. Scand J Immunol 5:1015–1019

142. van Loghem E, de Lange G, Koistinen J (1976) The first isoallotype of human IgA proteins. An antigenic determinant occurring as allotype in the IgA2 subclass and as isotype in the IgA1 subclass. Scand J Immunol 5:161–164
143. van Loghem E (1971) Formal genetics of the immunoglobulin systems. Ann N Y Acad Sci 190:136–149
144. Wang AC, Shuster J, Fudenberg HH (1969) Evolutionary origin of the Gm"a" peptide of immunoglobulins. J Mol Biol 41:83–86
145. Cook CE, Steinberg AG (1979) An amino acid substitution in the γ1 chain of human immunoglobulin G associated with the Gm (2) allotype. Mol Immunol 16:555–558
146. Wolfenstein-Todel C, Frangione B, Prelli F, Franklin EC (1976) The amino acid sequence of "heavy chain disease" protein ZUC. Structure of the Fc fragment of immunoglobulin G3. Biochem Biophys Res Commun 71:907–914
147. Frangione B, Rosenwasser E, Prelli F, Franklin EC (1980) Primary structure of human γ3 immunoglobulin deletion mutant: γ3 heavy-chain disease protein Wis. Biochemistry 19:4304–4308
148. Alexander A, Steinmetz M, Barritault D, Frangione B, Franklin EC, Hood L, Buxbaum JN (1982) Gamma heavy chain disease in man: cDNA sequence supports partial gene deletion model. Proc Natl Acad Sci USA 79(10):3260–3264
149. Recht B, Frangione B, Franklin E, van Loghem E (1981) Structural studies of a human γ3 myeloma protein (GOE) that binds Staph protein A. J Immunol 127:917–923
150. Matsumoto H, Ito S, Miyazaki T, Ohta T (1983) Structural studies of a human γ3 myeloma protein (JIR) bearing the allotypic marker Gm(st). J Immunol 131: 1865–1870
151. Matsumoto H, Ito S, Miyazaki T, Kawai N (1986) Structural studies of another human IgG3 myeloma protein (Kam) carrying the allotypic markers Gm(s,t) and its alteration induced by chemical modification. In: Brinkmann B, Henningsen K (eds) Advances in forensic haemogenetics, Springer Verlag, Berlin-Heidelberg, Germany vol I. p 153
152. Abel CA, Despont JP (1974) An amino acid deletion associated with the IgG4b allotype of human IgG4 myeloma proteins. J Immunogenet 1:79–82
153. Tsuzukida Y, Wang CC, Putnam FW (1979) Structure of the A2m(1) allotype of human IgA. A recombinant molecule. Proc Natl Acad Sci USA 76:1104–1108
154. Toraño A, Putnam FW (1978) Complete amino acid sequence of the alpha 2 heavy chain of a human IgA2 immunoglobulin of the A2m (2) allotype. Proc Natl Acad Sci USA 75(2):966–969
155. Flanagan JG, Lefranc M-P, Rabbitts TH (1984) Mechanisms of divergence and convergence of the human immunoglobulin alpha 1 and alpha 2 constant region gene sequences. Cell 36(3):681–688
156. Baglioni C, Alescio Zonta L, Cioli D, Carbonara A (1966) Allelic antigenic factor Inv(a) of the light chains of human immunoglobulins: chemical basis. Science 152:1517–1519
157. Steinberg AG, Milstein CP, McLaughlin CL, Solomon A (1974) Structural studies of an Inv (1, -2) kappa light chain. Immunogenetics 2:1–10
158. Milstein CP, Steinberg AG, McLaughlin CL, Solomon A (1974) Amino acid sequence change associated with genetic marker Inv(2) of human immunoglobulin. Nature 248:160–161
159. van Loghem E, Aalberse RC, Matsumoto H (1984) A genetic marker of human IgE heavy chains, Em(1). Vox Sang 46:195–206
160. Ghanem N, Dariavach P, Bensmana M, Chibani J, Lefranc G, Lefranc M-P (1988) Polymorphism of immunoglobulin lambda constant region genes in populations from France, Lebanon and Tunisia. Exp Clin Immunogenet 5:186–195
161. Lefranc M-P, Lefranc G (1992) Les Immunoglobulines humaines. In: Breton-Gorius J, Reyes F, Rochant H, Rosa J, Vernant JP (eds) L'hématologie de Bernard Dreyfus (chapter 20). Médecine-Sciences Flammarion, pp 197–254
162. Lefranc M-P, Pallarès N, Frippiat J-P (1999) Allelic polymorphisms and RFLP in the human immunoglobulin lambda light chain locus. Hum Genet 104:361–369
163. Lefranc M-P, Lefranc G (2004) Immunoglobulin lambda (IGL) genes of human and mouse. In: Honjo T, Alt FW, Neuberger MS (eds) Molecular biology of B cells. Academic Press, Elsevier Science Amsterdam, The Netherlands, pp 37–59
164. Goetze AM, Zhang Z, Liu L, Jacobsen FW, Flynn GC (2011) Rapid LC-MS screening for IgG Fc modifications and allelic variants in blood. Mol Immunol 49:338–352
165. Liu YS, Low TL, Infante A, Putnam FW (1976) Complete covalent structure of a human IgA1 immunoglobulin. Science 193(4257):1017–1020

# INDEX

## A



## B



Frank T. Christiansen and Brian D. Tait (eds.), *Immunogenetics: Methods and Applications in Clinical Practice*, Methods in Molecular Biology, vol. 882, DOI 10.1007/978-1-61779-842-9, © Springer Science+Business Media New York 2012

## M



## N



## O

## P



## Q



## R

## S



## T

MIX
Papier aus verantwortungsvollen Quellen
Paper from responsible sources
FSC® C105338

If you have any concerns about our products,
you can contact us on
**ProductSafety@springernature.com**

In case Publisher is established outside the EU,
the EU authorized representative is:
**Springer Nature Customer Service Center GmbH**
**Europaplatz 3, 69115 Heidelberg, Germany**

Printed by Libri Plureos GmbH
in Hamburg, Germany